Biological Bases of Brain Function and Disease

Biological Bases of Brain Function and Disease

Edited by

Alan Frazer, Ph.D.
Chairman, Department of Pharmacology
University of Texas Health Science Center at San Antonio
San Antonio, Texas
Formerly with
Departments of Psychiatry and Pharmacology
University of Pennsylvania School of Medicine
  and Philadelphia Veterans Affairs Medical Center
Philadelphia, Pennsylvania

Perry B. Molinoff, M.D.
A. N. Richards Professor and
Chairman, Department of Pharmacology
University of Pennsylvania School of Medicine
Philadelphia, Pennsylvania

Andrew Winokur, M.D., Ph.D.
Professor, Departments of Psychiatry and Pharmacology
University of Pennsylvania School of Medicine
Philadelphia, Pennsylvania

Raven Press 🐦 New York

Raven Press, Ltd., 1185 Avenue of the Americas, New York, New York 10036

Made in the United States of America

Library of Congress Cataloging-in-Publication Data

Biological bases of brain function and disease/ editors, Alan Frazer,
  Perry B. Molinoff, Andrew Winokur.
     p. cm.
    Includes bibliographical references and index.
    ISBN 0-7817-0085-X (pbk.).—ISBN (invalid) 0078170089Z (hardcover)
    1. Neurobiology. 2. Neuropsychology. 3. Neuropsychiatry. 4. Mental
Disorders—pathophysiology. 5. Synapses—physiology. I. Frazer, Alan.
II. Molinoff, Perry B. III. Winokur, Andrew. 1944–
    [DNLM: 1. Brain—physiology. 2. Brain—pathophysiology. 3. Brain
Diseases. WL 300 B6142 1993]
  QP355.2.B56 1993
  612.8′2—dc20
  DNLM/DLC
  for Library of Congress   93-16859
                                                  CIP

9 8 7 6 5 4 3 2 1

Contents

I. Principles of Neurobiology

II. Synaptic Transmitters and Modulators

III. Complex Functions of the Brain

Contributing Authors

Thomas W. Abrams, Ph.D.
Department of Biology
University of Pennsylvania
514 Goddard Laboratories
Philadelphia, Pennsylvania 19104-6018

Steven E. Arnold, M.D.
Departments of Psychiatry and Neurology
University of Pennsylvania School of Medicine
10 Gates Building
Hospital of the University of Pennsylvania
Philadelphia, Pennsylvania 19104-4283

William A. Ball, M.D., Ph.D.
Department of Psychiatry
University of Pennsylvania School of Medicine
11 Founders Pavilion
Hospital of the University of Pennsylvania
Philadelphia, Pennsylvania 19104-4283

Mark S. Bauer, M.D., Ph.D.
Department of Psychiatry and Human Behavior
Brown University School of Medicine
Department of Veterans Affairs Medical Center
Providence, Rhode Island 02908-4799

Marc A. Dichter, M.D., Ph.D.
Departments of Neurology and Pharmacology
University of Pennsylvania School of Medicine
and Graduate Hospital
Pepper Pavilion, Suite 900
Philadelphia, Pennsylvania 19146

James H. Eberwine, Ph.D.
Departments of Pharmacology and Psychiatry
University of Pennsylvania School of Medicine
68 John Morgan Building
Philadelphia, Pennsylvania 19104-6084

William D. Essman, Ph.D.
Departments of Psychiatry and Pharmacology
University of Pennsylvania School of Medicine
320 John Morgan Building
Philadelphia, Pennsylvania 19104-6084

Steven J. Fluharty, Ph.D.
Departments of Animal Biology and
* Pharmacology*
School of Veterinary Medicine
University of Pennsylvania
Philadelphia, Pennsylvania 19104-6046

Alan Frazer, Ph.D.
Department of Pharmacology
University of Texas Health Science Center
* at San Antonio*
7703 Floyd Curl Drive
San Antonio, Texas 78284-7764

Raquel E. Gur, M.D., Ph.D.
Department of Psychiatry
University of Pennsylvania School of Medicine
10 Gates Building
Hospital of the University of Pennsylvania
Philadelphia, Pennsylvania 19104-4283

Ruben C. Gur, Ph.D.
Department of Psychiatry
University of Pennsylvania School of Medicine
10 Gates Building
Hospital of the University of Pennsylvania
Philadelphia, Pennsylvania 19104-4283

Howard I. Hurtig, M.D.
Department of Neurology
Graduate Hospital
Philadelphia, Pennsylvania 19146
* and*
Department of Neurology
University of Pennsylvania School of Medicine
3400 Spruce Street
Philadelphia, Pennsylvania 19104

Jeffrey N. Joyce, Ph.D.
Departments of Psychiatry and Pharmacology
University of Pennsylvania School of Medicine
127 Clinical Research Building
Philadelphia, Pennsylvania 19104-6141

Karen M. Kumor, M.D.
Department of Clinical Pharmacology
Miles, Inc.
400 Morgan Lane
West Haven, Connecticut 06516

Irwin Lucki, Ph.D.
Departments of Psychiatry and Pharmacology
University of Pennsylvania School of Medicine
3600 Market Street, Room 808
Philadelphia, Pennsylvania 19104-2649

Perry B. Molinoff, M.D.
Department of Pharmacology
University of Pennsylvania School of Medicine
154 John Morgan Building
Philadelphia, Pennsylvania 19104-6084

Adrian R. Morrison, D.V.M., Ph.D.
Department of Animal Biology
School of Veterinary Medicine
University of Pennsylvania
3800 Spruce Street
Philadelphia, Pennsylvania 19104-6045

Charles P. O'Brien, M.D., Ph.D.
Department of Psychiatry
University of Pennsylvania School of Medicine
and
Philadelphia Veterans Affairs Medical Center
3900 Chestnut Street
Philadelphia, Pennsylvania 19104-6178

Gary E. Pickard, Ph.D.
Departments of Psychiatry and Neuroscience
University of Pennsylvania School of Medicine
50A Clinical Research Building
Philadelphia, Pennsylvania 19104-6141

R. Arlen Price, Ph.D.
Departments of Psychiatry and Genetics
University of Pennsylvania School of Medicine
145B Clinical Research Building
Philadelphia, Pennsylvania 19104-6141

Terry D. Reisine, Ph.D.
Departments of Pharmacology and Psychiatry
University of Pennsylvania School of Medicine
103 John Morgan Building
Philadelphia, Pennsylvania 19104-6084

Michael B. Robinson, Ph.D.
Departments of Pediatrics and Pharmacology
University of Pennsylvania School of Medicine
and
Children's Seashore House
Children's Hospital of Philadelphia
34th Street and Civic Center Boulevard
Philadelphia, Pennsylvania 19104-4399

Richard J. Ross, M.D., Ph.D.
Department of Psychiatry
University of Pennsylvania School of Medicine
Philadelphia Veterans Affairs Medical Center
University and Woodland Avenues
Philadelphia, Pennsylvania 19104

Patricia J. Sollars, Ph.D.
Center for Sleep and Respiratory Neurobiology
University of Pennsylvania School of Medicine
991 Maloney Building
Hospital of the University of Pennsylvania
Philadelphia, Pennsylvania 19104-4283

Daryth D. Stallone, Ph.D., M.P.H.
Johns Hopkins University
School of Hygiene and Public Health
615 N. Wolfe Street
Baltimore, Maryland 21205

Albert J. Stunkard, M.D.
Department of Psychiatry
University of Pennsylvania School of Medicine
133 South 36th Street
Philadelphia, Pennsylvania 19104-3246

Michael M. White, Ph.D.
Department of Physiology
Medical College of Pennsylvania
2900 Queen Lane
Philadelphia, Pennsylvania 19129

Peter C. Whybrow, M.D.
Department of Psychiatry
University of Pennsylvania School of Medicine
305 Blockley Hall
Philadelphia, Pennsylvania 19104-6021

Andrew Winokur, M.D., Ph.D.
Departments of Psychiatry and Pharmacology
University of Pennsylvania School of Medicine
11 Gates Building
Hospital of the University of Pennsylvania
Philadelphia, Pennsylvania 19104-4283

List of Abbreviations

ACh	acetylcholine	DBH	dopamine-β-hydroxylase
ACTH	adrenocorticotropic hormone	DIMS	disorders of initiating and maintaining sleep
AD	Alzheimer's disease	DMI	desmethylimipramine or
AHP	afterhyperpolarization		desipramine
AMPA	α-amino-3-hydroxy-5-methyl-4-isoxazolepro-pionic acid	DNA	deoxyribonucleic acid
		DOES	disorders of excessive somnolence
BCCE	β-carboline-3-carboxylate ethyl ester	DRL	differential reinforcement of low rates
BEAM	brain electric activity mapping	DS	depolarizing shift
		DTA	discriminated taste aversion
BED	binge eating disorder	DZ	dizygotic (fraternal)
BMI	body mass index	EAA	excitatory amino acid
cAMP	cyclic AMP	EEG	electroencephalography,
CBF	cerebral blood flow		electroencephalogram
CCK	cholecystokinin	EMG	electromyogram
cDNA	complementary DNA	EOG	electrooculogram
CDP	chlordiazepoxide	EP	evoked potentials
CNQX	6-cyano-7-nitroquinoxaline-2,3-dione	EPSP	excitatory postsynaptic potential
CNS	central nervous system	FDA	Food and Drug Adminis-
COMT	catechol-O-methyltrans-ferase		tration
		FDG	^{18}F-fluorodeoxyglucose
CPP	3-(($\pm$)-2-carboxypiperazin-4yl)propyl-1-phosphonate	FR	fixed ratio
		FRF	follicle-stimulating
CPS	complex partial seizure		hormone-
CRE	cAMP-responsive element		releasing factor
CREB	cAMP-responsive element-binding protein	FSH	follicle-stimulating hormone
CRF	corticotropin-releasing factor	G6PD	glucose-6-phosphate dehydrogenase
cRNA	complementary ribonucleic acid	GABA	γ-aminobutyric acid
		GABA-T	GABA-α-oxoglutarate transaminase
CS	conditioned stimulus		
CSF	cerebrospinal fluid	GAD	glutamate decarboxylase
CT	computed tomography	GIF	growth hormone
CVA	cerebrovascular accident		release-inhibiting factor
D-AP5	D-2-amino-5-phosphono-pentanoate	GnRH	gonadotropin-releasing hormone
D-AP7	D-2-amino-5-phosphono-heptanoate	GRE	glucocorticoid-responsive element
DA	dopamine	GTP	guanosine triphosphate

5-HT	5-hydroxytryptamine, serotonin
HD	Huntington's disease
HnRNA	heteronuclear RNA
HP	hyperpolarization
HPA	hypothalamic-pituitary-adrenal
HRP	horseradish peroxidase
IAP	islet-activating protein
ICSH	interstitial cell-stimulating hormone
IL-1	interleukin-1
IPSP	inhibitory postsynaptic potential
ISI	interstimulus interval
L-AAD	L-aromatic amino acid decarboxylase
LGN	lateral geniculate nucleus
LH	luteinizing hormone
LHRH	luteinizing hormone-releasing hormone
LPL	lipoprotein lipase
LTP	long-term potentiation
m-CPP	*meta*-chlorophenylpiperazine
MAO	monoamine oxidase
MAOI	monoamine oxidase inhibitor
MHC	major histocompatibility complex
MK-801	(+)-5-methyl-10,11-dihydro-5*H*-dibenzocyclohepten-5,10-imine maleate
MPP^+	1-methyl-4-phenyl-pyridinium
MPTP	1-methyl-4-phenyl-1,2,3,6-tetrahydropyridine
MRI	magnetic resonance imaging
mRNA	messenger RNA
MSR	membrane-spanning regions
MZ	monozygotic (identical)
NE	norepinephrine
NFTs	neurofibrillary tangles
NHANES	National Health and Nutrition Examination Survey
NMDA	*N*-methyl-D-aspartate
NO	nitric oxide
NPY	neuropeptide Y
NREMS	non-REM sleep
NTS	nucleus of the tractus solitarius
6-OHDA	6-hydroxydopamine
8-OH-DPAT	8-hydroxy-2-(di-n-propylamino)tetralin
OCD	obsessive-compulsive disorder
PCP	phencyclidine
PCR	polymerase chain reaction
PD	Parkinson's disease
PET	positron emission tomography
PFH	perifornical region of the lateral hypothalamus
PGO	ponto-geniculo-occipital
PIF	prolactin release-inhibiting factor
PMS	premenstrual syndrome
PNMT	phenylethanolamine-*N*-methyltransferase
PRC	phase-response curve
PRF	prolactin-releasing factor
PTSD	post-traumatic stress disorder
PVN	paraventricular nucleus
PYY	peptide YY
QUIS	quisqualatae
rCBF	regional cerebral blood flow
RDC	Research Diagnostic Criteria
REM	rapid eye movement
REMS	rapid eye movement sleep
RFLP	restriction fragment length polymorphism
RHT	retinohypothalamic tract
RNA	ribonucleic acid
SAD	seasonal affective disorder
SCG	superior cervical ganglion
SCN	suprachiasmatic nucleus
SIDS	sudden infant death syndrome
SKF 10047	*N*-allylnormetazocine
SPECT	single photon emission computed tomography
SPS	simple partial seizure
STH	somatotropic hormone
T_3	triiodothyronine
T_4	thyroxine
TCA	tricyclic antidepressant

TFMPP	trifluoromethylphenylpiperazine	**TSH**	thyroid-stimulating hormone
TH$_4$	tetrahydrobiopterin	**UR, UCR**	unconditioned response
THC	Δ-9-tetrahydrocannabinol	**US, UCS**	unconditioned stimulus
TRF	thyrotropin-releasing factor	**VMH**	ventromedial hypothalamus
TRH	thyrotropin-releasing hormone	**VPA**	valproic acid
		VR	variable ratio

Foreword

This impressive volume is the successor to a textbook, *Biological Bases of Psychiatric Disorders,* edited by Alan Frazer and Andrew Winokur in the late 1970s; together, the two texts bracket the most remarkably productive era to date in the history of brain science. That the earlier text retained its useful shelf life for nearly 15 years is a tribute to the scientific foresight of the editors; that the current work likely will be dated in half that time should be seen as a tribute as well, one which must be shared with all the contributors to this volume who clearly have accepted their responsibilities as teachers and mentors, especially to the next generation of brain researchers.

The future vigor of the many professions and disciplines dedicated to the understanding, treatment, and prevention of brain and behavior disorders is linked inextricably to the soundness of our scientific foundations. And at a moment in time when the *achievability* of goals set for a presidentially proclaimed "Decade of the Brain" is discussed routinely in public forums and the popular media, it is a pleasure to introduce a volume that testifies so persuasively to the growth and substance of those foundations. Comparing the content of the earlier textbook with that of the current work reveals not only a considerable expansion of the knowledge base but, even more important, an increasingly well-honed appreciation of the questions that must be asked. The expansion is even more pronounced when one considers that this review of the biology of normal and abnormal brain function reflects just part of the growth of the field, referring only in passing to equally impressive progress in studies of the psychological and environmental elements of brain–behavior relationships. Thus, despite its emphasis, the frequency of references to psychosocial factors and considerations will reassure those who fear reductionistic explanations of the brain and all that it encompasses.

When introducing a state-of-the-science volume in one's own field, it is tempting to be provocative, to predict how the contents will have evolved by the time the next edition is published. But in the field of brain research, the pace of progress and the array of unresolved issues are such that reflection is more appropriate. It is difficult, today, to recall that only a few decades ago, the biology and function of the brain in behavior were commonly viewed as being more the province of Isaac Asimov than of the academic research community. Yet by the late 1970s, the reverberations of the then decade-long psychopharmacology revolution had been felt throughout neuroscience, creating whole new disciplines in the process, from molecular neurogenetics to "receptorology." It was this intellectual fecundity which gave rise a decade back to the observation, only partly facetious, that if the rate of growth continued stably, the membership of the Society for Neuroscience would exceed the U.S. population by the end of the century. For a time, it seemed the only factor limiting growth would be the availability of research support. Unfortunately, other more insidious threats have arisen, including, for example, creeping scientific illiteracy in the population-at-large. While funding remains a challenge throughout the biomedical and behavioral sciences, it is satisfying to be able to say that the brain sciences have competed aggressively and successfully. Even more encouraging is the fact that the advent of effective drugs for the treatment of mental disorders actually set off several "revolutions," each of which is critical in its own way to the continued vigor of brain research.

One revolution has been ideological. Unambiguous if inexplicable evidence of the therapeutic efficacy of medications on mental disorders was decisive in legitimizing these conditions and, conversely, in repudiating the standing conventional wisdom that mental illness reflected character flaws or was exclusively a product of environmental disadvantage. For better and worse, such beliefs had been the underpinnings of psychiatric science in the U.S. for much of this century. In the absence of a handle on the biology of neurobiological disorders, the "can-do" optimism of American researchers and clinicians had steered them toward psychosocial explanations of effective treatments. Indisputably productive in selected areas, this approach also proved to be damaging, with effects ranging from misplaced blame for the origin of mental disorders to the construction of elaborate but misleading diagnostic formulations based on presumed etiologies. Inevitably, this path dead-ended: in a thicket of controversy involving new philosophies concerning service delivery, new financing systems, and well-intentioned concern for the rights of patients labeled but not helped by diagnoses, therapeutic optimism dissipated and the impetus for the scientific study of functional brain disorders began to wane. Thus, the demonstrable efficacy of psychotherapeutic drugs gave impetus to the study of a biological basis to functional brain disorders that was striking, enlightening, and invigorating.

A second revolution was methodologic. The use of psychotropic medications as research tools was soon recognized to be as important as their use for therapeutic purposes. Proper use of the tools, however, demanded unprecedented rigor in clinical diagnoses, sophisticated models for clinical and genetic epidemiological research, and ever more elegant approaches to research design and data analysis. While early advances in the basic mechanisms of brain function invigorated neuroscience across the board, the subtlety of questions inherent in studies of brain-behavior relationships further increased demand for sophistication and precision in research targeted to mental illness *and health.* As is implicit in the content of this volume, the more we learn about normal brain mechanisms and functions, the better we will understand dysfunctional mechanisms and, in turn, position ourselves to design means of treating and ameliorating neuropsychiatric disease with specificity and precision.

For the mental health sciences, the road back was not easy. Even as the National Institute of Mental Health (NIMH), by far the principal source of support for mental disorder-related research, continued to build a solid foundation for growth in neuroscience, uncertainty about the mission of the NIMH during the early '70s prompted many investigators to seek support from other sources. Yet, as the earlier textbook attests, the core of our field was able to construct a scientific framework which ensured that psychiatry and the mental health disciplines would be contributors to as well as beneficiaries of the explosion in brain science.

Indeed, the introduction of effective psychopharmacological treatments sparked more than a demand for methodologic rigor alone; rather, its third revolutionary impact was to serve as a major stimulus for neuroscience itself. Clinical observations begat questions and, in turn, answers in the form of new basic disciplines (molecular neurobiology), new technologies (brain imaging), and new clinical applications and emphases ("tailoring" of treatments, both pharmacological and psychological). Our field will not coast on the momentum of psychopharmacological innovations, but is equipped to assume a leading role into the next century through such ambitious initiatives as NIMH's Human Brain Project, designed to facilitate a world-wide system of neuroscience information management and exchange through linked computer databases.

Together, these various "revolutions" and the progress achieved through each have yielded yet another potent effect: the wherewithal for a frontal assault on the ignorance and stigma that have so long impeded broad public support for the study of brain and behavior and applications of new knowledge to the treatment of mental disorders. Only in retrospect can we appreciate fully what a dramatically salutary effect these new perspectives had on the stirrings and coalescence of an authentic, passionate, and committed network of advocates for nurturing and promoting brain and behavioral research. Inspired by experience and catalyzed by evidence of renewed scientific optimism, organizations such as the National Alliance for the Mentally Ill and the National Depressive and Manic Depressive Association emerged to support and further the work of groups such as the National Mental Health Association. Driven by conviction and a sense of urgency, these advocates have exerted decisive influence on the budgetary fortunes of the NIMH and, more recently, on our symbolically significant reunion with the National Institutes of Health. Still to be fully tested is the role which these and other advocacy organizations can play in educating policy makers and the public about the formidable menace to future brain-behavior research that is embodied in such anti-intellectual agendas as that of the animal rights movement.

The willingness of our advocates to engage this issue with the same fervor that has been so successful in the funding arena will be contingent largely on how they perceive the response of the scientific community to the threat. And here, I am particularly pleased to see the forthrightness with which the editors and contributors to this volume acknowledge the indispensable role of appropriate animal models in brain research. This field, and most notably, research being conducted nearer the applied end of the basic-clinical spectrum, has been specifically targeted by the animal rights movement, presumably under the assumption that while the public may view animal models as needed for the development of new artificial heart valves, many individuals may be less certain as to the relevance of animal research in studying the human brain. To combat misperceptions, those who conduct brain research must be unflinchingly honest and articulate about the need for and achievements realized through animal studies.

This book reports on an extraordinary, unfinished scientific odyssey, but one which will be seen through only if those who embark upon it remain alert to the larger social, political, and human contexts in which science works.

Frederick K. Goodwin, M.D.
Director
National Institute of Mental Health

Preface

Biological Bases of Brain Function and Disease developed out of a course that the editors and many of the contributing authors have taught annually to undergraduates at the University of Pennsylvania since 1976. The course, "Biological Bases of Psychiatric Disorders," has attracted a diverse cross-section of students who share a common interest in learning both basic information about brain function and the practical implications of this body of knowledge for neuropsychiatric illnesses and their treatment. Thus, it goes beyond an introduction to biological mechanisms regulating behavior to address processes that might contribute to behavioral pathology. It also includes information on clinical phenomenological characteristics of specific illnesses and criteria used to make particular diagnoses. To understand the biology and treatment of major depressive disorder, for example, students are encouraged to understand the difference between a common mood state characterized as feeling "down-in-the-dumps" and the complex array of mood, cognitive, behavioral, and physiological symptoms that accompany significant clinical depression.

Since no one book covered such a breadth of information for undergraduate students, we developed a text entitled *Biological Bases of Psychiatric Disorders* which was published in 1977. The textbook not only included chapters on neuroanatomy, neurophysiology, neuropharmacology, and neuropsychology, but also described normal and abnormal behavior including those characteristic of specific psychiatric illnesses. Since 1977, however, a striking amount of information has become available in both the preclinical and clinical arenas. The brain is now known to contain numerous substances that regulate behavior (e.g., G proteins, multiple subtypes of receptors, second messengers, peptides). These substances were mentioned briefly, if at all, in the original text. Moreover, application of the tools of molecular biology has revolutionized our understanding of neuroscience and is now being applied to genetic studies of neuropsychiatric illnesses. These techniques hardly existed in the mid-1970s. Although considerable additional progress is needed to attain a comprehensive understanding of the pathobiology of neuropsychiatric illnesses, numerous advances have occurred over the past 15 years in the diagnosis, treatment, and management of these diseases and in the availability of techniques to study the brain in health and disease.

This new textbook addresses many contemporary issues of modern neuroscience and psychopharmacology. The text intentionally covers a broad expanse of material so that the student may specifically appreciate a progression of disciplines from basic neuroscience (neuroanatomy, neurophysiology, neurochemistry, neuropharmacology, and molecular biology) to analysis of complex physiology and behavior (sleep, circadian function, neuroendocrinology, learning, and memory), to research strategies available to investigate neural mechanisms involved in the control of complex behaviors (genetics, behavioral pharmacology, neuropsychology, and neuroimaging techniques). The book concludes with chapters that deal explicitly with a number of behavioral, neurological, and psychiatric disorders. The illnesses that are included are described in terms of clinical description, pathophysiological basis, and accessibility to treatment.

We hope the content and organization of the book will help students appreciate the dynamic energy permeating the field of neuroscience. Our goal is to encourage insight into the crucial interplay between intensive laboratory investigation and the application of new discoveries to the treatment of neuropsychiatric disease. It is our firm belief that the development of more effective and safer therapeutic options for the treatment of neurological and psychiatric disorders depends on an understanding of this interplay. Finally, this text may help to increase awareness of diverse, challenging, and gratifying career paths that are available to students as laboratory scientists, clinical investigators, or primary health care providers working in the areas of basic and behavioral neuroscience.

The editors would like to thank all the authors for their efforts in making their respective chapters understandable to an undergraduate audience. We also thank Theresa Filtz, Virginia Boundy, and Catherine Buettner for producing a number of the figures in the book. Dr. Graham Lees of Raven Press kindly offered sage advice throughout the planning and implementation of this text. Finally, we would like to express particular gratitude to Lotte Gottschlich for her extraordinary organizational skill, editing acumen, and unflagging persistence throughout this entire project.

Alan Frazer
Perry B. Molinoff
Andrew Winokur

Neuroanatomy

Steven E. Arnold

Now I can kind of understand the mechanical work of the brain—stimulating breathing, moving blood, directing protein traffic. It's all chemistry and electricity. A motor. I know about motors.

But this three-pound raw-meat motor also contains all the limericks I know, a recipe for how to cook a turkey, the remembered smell of my junior-high locker room, all my sorrows, the ability to double-clutch a pickup truck, the face of my wife when she was young, formulas like $E = MC^2$, and $A^2 + B^2 = C^2$, the Prologue to Chaucer's Canterbury Tales, *the sound of the first cry of my firstborn son, the cure for hiccups, the words to the fight song of St. Olaf's College, fifty years' worth of dreams, how to tie my shoes, the taste of cod-liver oil, an image of Van Gogh's "Sunflowers," and a working understanding of the Dewey Decimal System. It's all there in the MEAT.*

Robert Fulghum,
It Was on Fire When I Lay Down on It
(New York: Ivy Books, 1988, p. 39)

▶ Key Concepts ──────────────────

- The nerve cell, or neuron, is the basic building block of the brain.

- The brain sits within the bony cranium, surrounded and protected by membrane layers called meninges.

- The cerebrum is the largest portion of the brain and lies above the brain stem and cerebellum.

- The cerebral cortex is the part of the brain that supports mental activity and distinguishes us as cognizant beings.

- The basal ganglia, cell groups of the basal forebrain and amygdala, are gray matter nuclei deep within the cerebral hemispheres.

- The diencephalon, lying at the center of the cerebral hemispheres, includes the thalamus and hypothalamus.

- The mesencephalon and rhombencephalon together composed the brain stem and cerebellum.

- The brain's connectional organization allows multiple excitatory and inhibitory inputs to be integrated into a single mental experience.

- Each of the sensory modalities has specific pathways for processing sensory information that ultimately converge with other modalities in multimodal association areas.

- The limbic system consists of a group of interconnected cortical and subcortical regions at the center of the brain.

- Because of its extraordinarily extensive connections and turnaround position in the hierarchical streams of sensory processing, the hippocampal system is situated to coordinate and integrate multiple aspects of our sensory experience—in actual perception and recognition and in imagination and memory.

- Subcortical regions play a major role in such general cognitive functions as attention and motivation.

- The primary motor cortex directly controls all voluntary movement.

This chapter surveys the basic anatomic areas of the brain—brain stem, diencephalon, basal ganglia, and cerebral cortex—that together define and control our lives as sentient beings. The subdivisions of these brain parts are reviewed and the connections of some of these different regions described to furnish an understanding of how information regarding sensory experience and the body's internal milieu are processed in the brain, stored and manipulated, and then expressed in activity.

The last quarter of this century has witnessed extraordinary advances in our knowledge of the neuroanatomic, neurophysiological, and neurochemical mechanisms underlying mental processes. Equally important have been developments in cognitive psychology and artificial intelligence. There has been a move away from strict behaviorist models of psychology, which viewed the mind and brain as an impenetrable black box and made the relationship between stimulus and response the only tenable object of investigation. Instead, there is now acceptance of the mind and its physical organ, the brain, as a legitimate focus of study. In this scheme, behavior is an observable activity that allows one to make inferences about the individual's mind or cognition. Behavioral neuroscience now holds that mental, emotional, and behavioral processes arise from neuronal activity. Multiple distinct and overlapping networks of neurons support this neuronal activity and thus the many aspects of our mental and behavioral life, such as perception, memory, emotion, judgment, and the control of muscle activity.

The modern era of the study of the relationship between brain and behavior began in the mid-1800s with the French neurologist, surgeon, and anthropologist Paul Broca. In autopsy studies of brains of stroke victims who had lost the ability to speak, Broca found

Biological Bases of Brain Function and Disease, edited by Alan Frazer, Perry B. Molinoff, and Andrew Winokur. Raven Press, Ltd., New York © 1994.

that a lesion in the "third frontal convolution on the left leads to loss of the language faculty" (see Chapter 15). There was much enthusiasm for this idea at the time, perhaps fueled by competition with the popular phrenologists, which led neurologists to postulate brain "centers" that could be independently responsible for particular mental abilities (such as language, memory, and music). But other physicians, including Sigmund Freud in his early years as a neurologist, astutely observed that lesions in a variety of brain regions could disturb language. In the first half of this century, evidence accumulated that made the notion of independent brain centers untenable. This backlash against localization reached its peak in the 1950s, when it was believed that there was little intrinsic organization to the brain and that areas of the brain were equipotential and interchangeable in terms of the cognitive functions they could subserve.

The pendulum began to swing back again in the 1960s. The development of methods for tracing neural pathways enabled neuroscientists to study the intricate connections among different areas of the brain in animals. Equally important were the clinical observations being made by behaviorally oriented neurologists such as Norman Geschwind in Boston. From his clinical observations of patients with language problems after strokes in different areas of the brain, Geschwind postulated that lesions in particular parts of the brain can give rise to specific neuropsychological deficits because the lesion disconnects interactive parts of the brain. A brain lesion that was correlated with a behavioral disturbance had been previously interpreted as identifying the "center" responsible for that behavior. Now a lesion was recognized only as a probe into the hypothetical network of anatomic regions designed to cooperatively perform a specified function. Both experimental and clinical studies have led to our current concept of the brain as comprising multiple, highly complex, but very specific neural networks that interact and modulate one another to support the richness of our mental life and interactions with the world.

ANATOMIC CONSIDERATIONS

When the brain is cut in cross section, one immediately sees regions of dull-appearing *gray matter* and regions of glistening *white matter* (Fig. 1). Nerve cell bodies make up the gray matter, which is found in the outer surface, or *cortex,* of the brain and in groupings, or *nuclei,* deep within the brain. White matter is composed of bundles of nerve fibers that travel between different regions of gray matter and into the spinal cord.

The Neuron

The nerve cell, or neuron, *is the basic building block of the brain.* The human brain contains more than 50 billion neurons along with a variety of glial cells that help support and maintain the physical and physiological integrity of neurons. Each neuron is a highly asymmetrical, three-dimensional structure that is specialized to receive and transmit nerve impulses. Extending from the neuronal cell body are multiple branching *dendrites,* which are short, tapering processes that receive incoming nerve impulses. Each neuron gives rise to a single *axon,* which carries impulses away from the cell body to other parts of the brain or spinal cord. Impulses are then conveyed from the axon terminal to dendrites of other neurons in an appropriate tar-

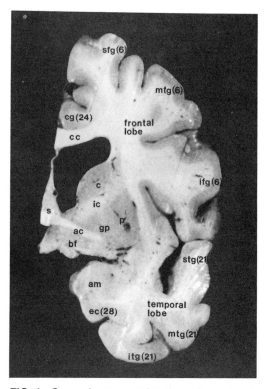

FIG. 1. Coronal cross section through one hemisphere of the human brain at the level of the hypothalamus and basal ganglia. The cortical gyri with their corresponding numbered cytoarchitectural areas (see Fig. 3) at this level are labeled sfg, mfg, and ifg, which refer to the superior, middle, and inferior frontal gyri; stg, mtg, and itg refer to the superior, middle, and inferior temporal gyri; ec is the entorhinal cortex; and cg is the cingulate gyrus. The corpus callosum (cc) and anterior commissure (ac) are important white matter tracts that connect the two hemispheres. The internal capsule (ic) conveys impulses between the cortex and brain stem and spinal cord. Caudate (c), putamen (p), and globus pallidus (gp) are subcortical nuclei comprising the basal ganglia. Amygdala (am), septal (s), and basal forebrain (bf) nuclei have widespread connections to cortical and limbic areas.

get area of the brain (see Chapter 3, Fig. 1). The point at which one neuron's axon terminal meets another neuron's dendrite is called a *synapse.* A chemical called a *neurotransmitter* is released by the axon terminal to electri-

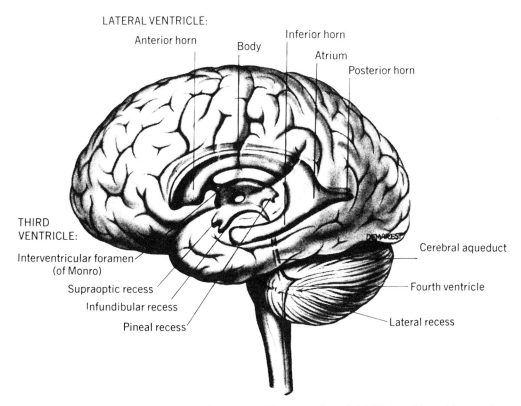

LATERAL VENTRICLE:

Anterior horn

Body

Inferior horn

Atrium

Posterior horn

THIRD VENTRICLE:

Interventricular foramen (of Monro)

Supraoptic recess

Infundibular recess

Pineal recess

Cerebral aqueduct

Fourth ventricle

Lateral recess

FIG. 2. Lateral view of the ventricles of the brain. There are four fluid-filled cavities within the brain that communicate with each other and the subarachnoid space through small apertures. Clear, colorless cerebrospinal fluid circulates through this system to bathe and cushion the brain. Cerebrospinal fluid is produced by highly vascularized tufts of tissue, called the choroid plexus, extending into each of the ventricles. From Noback CR, Demarest R. *The human nervous system.* New York: McGraw-Hill, 1981:21, with permission from McGraw-Hill.

cally excite or inhibit the target dendrite, thus causing the target neuron either to "fire" or to be inhibited in its ability to fire. Axons can be long (sometimes several feet in length, e.g., for motor neurons projecting from the spinal cord to muscles in the foot) and they may be sheathed in a lipoprotein insulation called *myelin.* Myelinated axons carry nerve impulses very quickly. Thin, nonmyelinated or poorly myelinated axons are generally shorter and slower in their conduction velocity (see Chapter 3).

Meninges and Ventricles

The brain sits within the bony cranium, surrounded and protected by three membrane layers called meninges. The outermost layer, the *dura mater,* is a tough, leathery covering that is partly attached to the inside of the skull. The innermost layer, the *pia mater,* is a thin, delicate, vascularized coating that is intimately attached to the surface of the brain. Between the pia mater and the middle layer, the *arachnoid,* is a layer of cerebrospinal fluid (CSF) that bathes the brain and provides a soft fluid protective cushion. The CSF is produced in and flows from the internal fluid cavities of the brain, the *ventricles* (Fig. 2). There are four ventricles—two lateral ventricles, one in each cerebral hemisphere; the third ventricle, found as a midline slitlike cavity in the diencephalon; and the fourth ventricle, found farther down in the brain stem.

Cerebrum

The cerebrum *is the largest portion of the brain and lies above the brain stem and cerebellum.* It is composed of the cerebral cortex, the basal ganglia, and the diencephalon, all of which are more or less symmetrically divided into two cerebral hemispheres. *The* cerebral cortex *is the part of the brain that supports mental activity and distinguishes us as cognizant beings.* The largest portion of the brain is the telencephalon, which comprises the two cerebral hemispheres. The *cerebral cortex* is a thin expanse of gray matter that covers the entire outer surface of each cerebral hemisphere. Neurons are arranged in six variably patterned layers throughout the cerebral cortex. Based on the types, quantities, and arrangement of neurons within an area, the cerebral cortex has been divided into *cytoarchitectural* regions (Fig. 3). One of the striking features of the human brain is the elaborate pattern of convolutions, or folds (also known as *sulci* and *gyri*) (Fig. 4). Folding allows a tremendous increase in the amount of surface area that can fit into a small space and reflects the evolutionary advance of the human brain relative to other species. It is the cerebral cortex that mediates all of our conscious sensation, perception, memory, thinking, and action.

There are four lobes in each cerebral hemisphere. The *occipital lobe* is the hindmost portion and contains regions of cortex that are important in visual perception and processing (Brodmann areas 17, 18, and 19; see Fig. 3). The *parietal lobe* constitutes the upper, lateral part of each hemisphere and mediates somatic sensation processing and the integration of somatic and visual information (Brodmann areas 3, 1, 2, 5, 7, 39, 40). The *temporal lobe* contains areas of cortex involved in auditory and visual processing (Brodmann areas 20, 21, 28, 35–38, 41, 42), as well as the entorhinal cortex, *hippocampus,* and *amygdala,* which are crucial structures for learning, memory, higher integration, and emotion. The *frontal lobe* constitutes almost 50% of the volume of each cerebral hemisphere in humans (Brodmann

areas 4, 6, 8–12, 25, 44–47). While its function was mysterious for many years, it is now recognized that in addition to its role in motor activity and language, it is important for higher integrative functions, personality traits, emotionality, and executive control (the translation of thought into action).

The basal ganglia, *consisting of the* caudate, putamen, globus pallidus, *and* claustrum, *the cell groups of the* basal forebrain, *and the amygdala are gray matter nuclei deep within the cerebral hemispheres.* The basal ganglia are most strongly connected to motor areas (cortical areas 4 and 6, motor nuclei of the *thalamus* and the *substantia nigra* in the midbrain) and are especially important in modulating the initiation, smoothness, and precision of motor activity. The basal forebrain and amygdala, along with the hippocampus (a phylogenetically old and intricate part of the cerebral cortex in the temporal lobe), are key components of the limbic system and are important for memory and emotion. The two cerebral hemispheres are connected by the *corpus callosum,* a massive white matter bridge composed of axons that transduce impulses from side to side.

At the center of the cerebral hemispheres lies the diencephalon, *which includes the thalamus and the* hypothalamus. The thalamus is a complex grouping of individual nuclei that are important components of a variety of sensory, motor, cognitive, and emotional functional systems. Thalamic nuclei serve as relay stations, or gateways, for both sensory input and motor output. The hypothalamus also comprises several nuclei that maintain the organism's internal milieu via autonomic, endocrine, chronobiological, and appetitive mechanisms.

Brain Stem and Cerebellum

The mesencephalon *and* rhombencephalon *together compose the brain stem and cerebellum.* The mesencephalon, or *midbrain,* is a short area at the top of the brain stem that contains nuclei controlling eye and pupil activity and the important dopaminergic nuclei

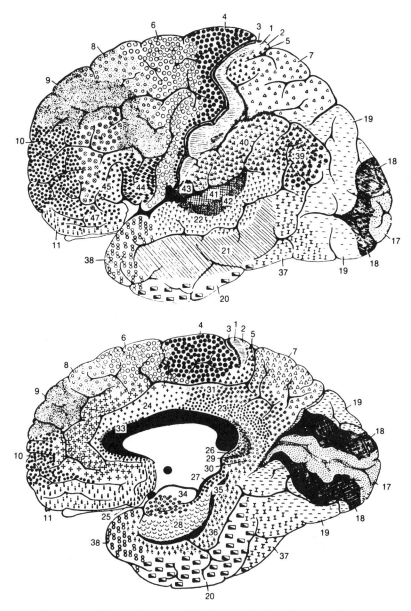

FIG. 3. Brodmann's cytoarchitectural map of the human brain. The top figure shows the lateral surface of the brain hemisphere and the lower figure shows the medial surface. Numbered areas represent regions with different microscopic appearance, many of which have been found to correlate with functional specialization. From Brodal A. *Neurological anatomy in relation to clinical medicine.* 3rd Ed. New York: Oxford University Press; 1981, with permission.

of the substantia nigra and *ventral tegmentum* (see Chapter 6). The cell bodies of neurons that contain the chemical neurotransmitter dopamine are in the midbrain. Derangement of the dopamine system has been invoked as a cause of a variety of neuro-

logical and psychiatric disorders, such as Parkinson's disease (see Chapter 23) and schizophrenia (see Chapter 18). The rhombencephalon consists of the *pons, medulla,* and *cerebellum* (or hindbrain). The pons is the midportion of the brain stem and con-

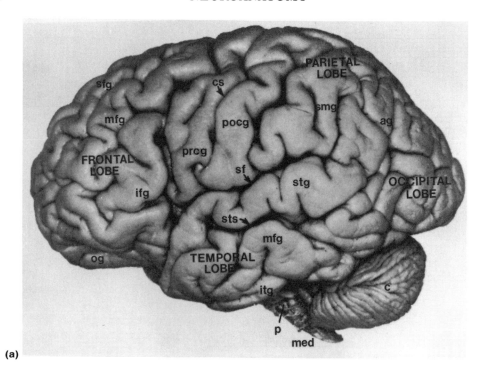

(a)

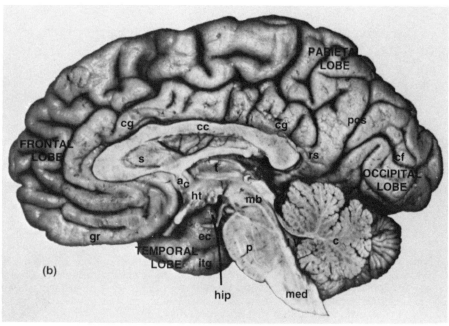

(b)

tains nuclei that control face, eye, and jaw movement and sensation as well as the *locus coeruleus* and portions of the *reticular activating system*. The locus coeruleus is a nucleus that contains cells that are the main source of the neurotransmitter norepinephrine (see Chapter 6). Abnormal norepinephrine activity may be related to depression (see Chapter 17) and anxiety states (see Chapter 19). The reticular activating system is a complex and loosely arranged collection of cells in the brain stem that maintains our level of arousal and attention.

The medulla is the lowermost portion of the brain stem adjoining the top of the spinal cord. It contains nuclei involved in hearing, balance, swallowing, head and neck movements, and various autonomic functions such as heart rate, blood pressure, and respiration.

The cerebellum is a large structure situated above the pons and medulla and beneath the occipital lobes of the cerebrum. It has two hemispheres connected by a central portion, the *vermis*. The cerebellum has an elaborate intrinsic anatomy of cortex and nuclei. Functionally, it is important in coordination of movement, posture, and balance.

Throughout the length of the brain stem are many different white matter tracts containing axons that connect the brain with the rest of the body. Because of the many highly compacted nuclei and dense axonal traffic flowing through the brain stem, damage to this area by stroke or tumor has wide-ranging, devastating effects on the individual.

ORGANIZATION OF THE CONNECTIONS OF THE BRAIN

The brain's connectional organization allows multiple excitations and inhibitory inputs to be integrated into a single mental experience. When you experience an object in the environment—say, your father cooking —even the briefest experience is incredibly complex. There is his visual image with its color, shape, spatial juxtaposition to the stove, and characteristic way he moves; the auditory image of the sounds of his voice, the food sizzling, spatula clanging, and the words he's speaking with all the various tones, pitches, and changing volume; the complex smells of the food and perhaps his aftershave; the feel of the heat on your skin and smoke in your eyes; the feel of your stomach growling and salivation starting. Not only are there these immediate perceptions, but also the wealth of remembrances and associations that this current image stimulates. Somehow, you integrate the multiple inputs into a

FIG. 4. Lateral (a) and medial (b) views of brain delineating anatomic structures, lobes, and names of the major gyri and sulci.

ac = anterior commissure	mtg = middle temporal gyrus
ag = angular gyrus	og = orbital gyrus
c = cerebellum	p = pons
cc = corpus callosum	pocg = post-central gyrus
cf = calcarine fissure	pos = parieto-occipital sulcus
cg = cingulate gyrus	prcg = precentral gyrus
cs = central sulcus	rs = retrosplenial region
ec = entorhinal cortex	s = septum
gr = gyrus rectus	sf = sylvian fissure
ht = hypothalamus	sfg = superior frontal gyrus
ifg = inferior frontal gyrus	smg = supramarginal gyrus
itg = inferior temporal gyrus	stg = superior temporal gyrus
mb = midbrain	sts = superior temporal sulcus
med = medulla	t = thalamus
mfg = middle frontal gyrus	IV = fourth ventricle

Adapted with permission from DeArmond SJ, Fusco MM, Dewey MM. *Structure of the human brain, a photographic atlas.* 3rd Ed. New York: Oxford University Press, 1989.

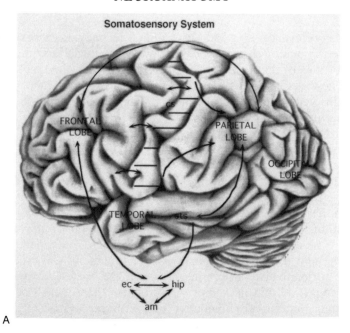

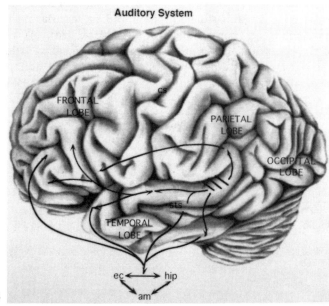

FIG. 5. Highly simplified maps of the lateral surface of the brain showing cortical steps of sensory processing for (a) somatosensory, (b) auditory, and (c) visual systems. The hatching indicates the primary sensory area for each modality (i.e., where the sensory information first reaches the cortex). (For the visual system, most of the primary cortex is not represented, as it lies in the calcarine fissure on the medial surface of the brain.) Projections from the primary areas to successive association areas are indicated with arrows. Almost all communication between different areas of the brain is bidirectional. In comparing the figures from each modality, one sees that the prefrontal cortex, inferior parietal cortex, and superior temporal sulcus receive input from all three sensory modalities. These are multimodal association areas. Connections from these areas as well as from modality-specific higher order association areas all converge into the hippocampal region, part of the limbic system in the ventromedial temporal lobe. The hippocampus as well as the entorhinal cortex and some nuclei of the amygdala are closely connected with each other and other limbic regions and are critical structures for memory.

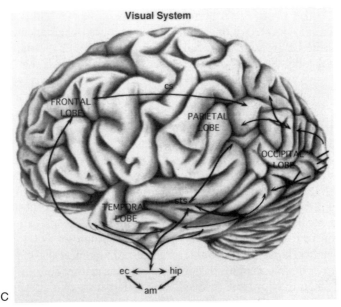

C

FIG. 5. *Continued.*

meaningful experience and you move, right foot first, left second, toward the plate coming to the table. Each aspect of the environment excites distinct populations of neurons in geographically distinct areas of the brain, and the brain organizes these into a unified mental experience and controls the execution of appropriate action. To understand how the integration comes about, one has to have an appreciation of the neuroanatomic pathways through which information is processed.

A variety of tract tracing methods have been used in experimental animals to delineate the course of projections connecting neurons in one brain region to another. An *anterograde* transport technique can be used to determine the area to which neurons in a particular brain region project. Radioactively labeled amino acids injected into the brain will be taken up by neurons at the injection site and over the course of a few days the amino acids will be anterogradely (moving forward) transported within axons all the way to the terminals. The course and termination sites can then be visualized by autoradiography. If the interest is in the sources of innervation of a particular region, *retrograde* techniques are used. Horseradish peroxidase or one of

many fluorescent dyes is taken up at an injection site and retrogradely (moving back) transported back to the neuron bodies, which are identified by light or fluorescence microscopy.

Primary Sensory Cortices and Unimodal and Multimodal Association Areas

Each of the sensory modalities has specific pathways for processing sensory information that ultimately converge with other modalities in multimodal association areas. The environment impinges on us through our eyes, ears, nose, mouth, and skin. Information regarding sensory experience is conveyed by distinct nerve pathways to specialized areas of the brain stem, thalamus, and cortex. Of all the sensory modalities, the anatomy and physiology of the visual system are perhaps the best studied. In visual processing, light impinges on the retina and nerve impulses are created. These are conveyed via the optic nerves and tracts to the lateral geniculate nucleus of the thalamus and to nuclei in the upper brain stem (to mediate pupillary reflexes). After synapsing in the lateral geniculate, impulses are conveyed to the primary visual cortex (area 17) located along the banks of the calcarine fissure on the medial side of the occipital lobe. Neurons in these areas then send axons to the immediately surrounding primary visual *association areas* (areas 18 and 19) in the occipital lobe (Fig. 5c). There are connections of the upper occipital lobe with "higher order" cortical association areas in the parietal lobe (areas 7 and 39) and from there to the lateral prefrontal cortical association areas (areas 8, 9, and 46). This pathway is specialized for the processing of visually perceived motion and spatial relationships. A person who has a brain injury that damages this network may have trouble seeing the whole array of objects in his or her visual field. The person may only be able to focus on one object, or one part of an object, for a moment before it disappears and he or she focuses on another. This phenomenon is called *simultanagnosia;* in practice, it is relatively rare.

The inferior visual pathway is composed of a series of connections from the lower occipital cortices forward along the inferior and lateral aspects of the occipital and temporal lobes toward the tip of the temporal lobe and in toward the hippocampal region. In the earlier visual association cortices (areas 18 and 19), basic color, shape, depth, and texture are appreciated. As impulses excite other higher order association areas farther along the connectional pathways into the temporal lobe toward the hippocampal region (areas 37, 20, and 21), meaning becomes attributed to the visual perception. This attribution arises because the neurons in the association areas are themselves connected to multiple other parts of the brain, and are thus in a position to integrate or converge multiple neural inputs. Lesions in the occipitotemporal region may cause a visual agnosia in which the individual can see an object but not recognize it (see Chapter 15). For instance, one may not be able to visually distinguish a pig from a dog, or often be able to visually recognize the specific identity of one's own face in a mirror.

Each sensory modality has a primary cortical area and system of connections for sensory processing. The connections within each modality are schematically represented in Fig. 5. In general, the nerve impulses from sensory portals reach their primary sensory cortical areas as follows: vision in the calcarine cortex of the occipital lobe, audition in Heschel's gyrus, areas 41 and 42, in the temporal lobe (Fig. 5b), somatic sensation in areas 3, 1, and 2 of the postcentral gyrus of the parietal lobe (Fig. 5a), smell in the prepyriform/periamygdaloid cortex of the medial temporal lobe, and taste in the parietal operculum, area 43, of the postcentral gyrus. An important feature of primary visual, auditory, and somatosensory cortices is their topographical organization. In the somatosensory system, the primary cortex is somatotopically organized such that specific portions of the cortex receive input from particular parts of the body (Fig. 6), while the visual calcarine cortex is retinotopically organized, and the auditory cortex in Heschel's gyrus is tonotopically organized.

Each primary sensory region has connections to modality-specific association areas, where convergence or integration of the different attributes of the sensory experience takes place. At further points, axons from different sensory modality-specific association areas begin to converge in what are referred to as *multimodal association areas* and from there project into limbic cortical areas. In these areas, it has been found that neurons that fire in response to visual stimulation, for example, are intermingled with neurons that respond to auditory stimulation, and that some neurons actually respond to any of multiple sensory stimulations. Some may respond in coordination with changes in motor output in addition to sensory input. There are two major nonlimbic multimodal association areas. The temporoparietal area includes the inferior parietal lobule and the banks of the superior temporal sulcus. The prefrontal area includes the vast expanses of cortex anterior to the motor cortices in the frontal lobe. Projections from the unimodal and multimodal association areas then converge at even higher order multimodal association areas that are part of the limbic system.

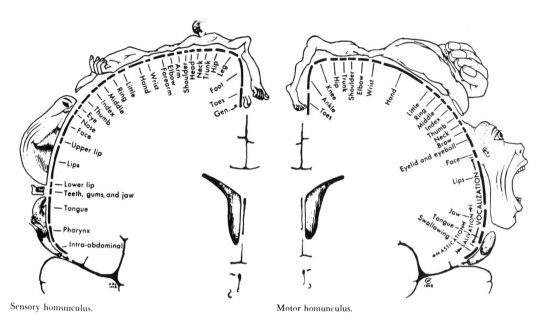

Sensory homunculus.   Motor homunculus.

FIG. 6. Motor and sensory homunculi. Each homunculus depicts the location and extent of body representation in the primary motor and sensory cortices. Note the relatively large amount of cortex devoted to motor innervation of the hand and face, and sensory innervation of the lips, tongue, and pharynx. Reprinted with the permission of Macmillan Publishing Company from *The cerebral cortex of man* by Wilder Penfield and Theodore Rasmussen. Copyright 1950 Macmillan Publishing Company; copyright renewed (c) 1978 Theodore Rasmussen.

Limbic System

The limbic system consists of a group of interconnected cortical and subcortical regions at the center of the brain. The concept of the limbic system was first set forth in 1937 by James Papez, who proposed that the "hypothalamus, the anterior thalamic nucleus, the cingulate gyrus, the hippocampus, and their interconnections constitute a harmonious mechanism which may elaborate the functions of central emotion as well as participate in emotional expressions." Over time, the limbic system has been expanded to include the cortices of the cingulate gyrus; the parahippocampal gyrus; the hippocampus; the orbitofrontal, medial frontal, and retrosplenial regions; and subcortical structures including the hypothalamus, anterior and medial nuclei of the thalamus, amygdala, septal nuclei, basal forebrain nuclei, habenula, and portions of the mesencephalon (Fig. 7). The different parts of the limbic system are inter-connected to varying degrees with each other and also have widespread connections with areas throughout the brain. In addition to their interconnections, the limbic structures also have their own connections with nonlimbic regions that distinguish them from one another both anatomically and functionally.

In terms of cognitive processing, the most important limbic regions are in the ventro-medial temporal lobe—the hippocampus, amygdala, and immediately surrounding areas of cortex (areas 28 and 35–38). A host of connections from sensory-specific and multimodal association areas in all four lobes converge onto the hippocampal region. After a series of intrinsic connections, neurons in the hippocampal region send powerful feedback projections to the association areas as well as to other subcortical limbic structures where emotive forces are activated. The hypothalamus, for example, controls the autonomic nervous system that regulates car-

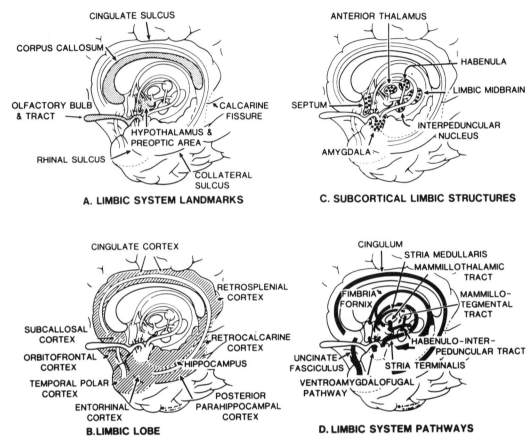

FIG. 7. Limbic system. Reproduced from Damasio AR, Van Hoesen GW. Emotional disturbances associated with focal lesions in the frontal lobe. From Heilman KM, Satz P, *Neuropsychology of human emotion.* New York: Guilford Publications; 1983 with permission.

diovascular, smooth muscle, and glandular activity. Indeed, almost all corticocortical connections are reciprocal, with feedback pathways returning projections to their sources of feedforward innervation as well as to other cortical points.

Because of its extraordinarily extensive connections and its turnaround position in the hierarchical streams of sensory processing, the hippocampal system is situated to coordinate and integrate multiple aspects of our sensory experience—in actual perception and recognition, and in imagination and memory. Individuals who have had extensive damage to the hippocampal regions bilaterally have dense amnesia with an inability to learn any new material or to appropriately

and fully recall past experiences (see Chapter 15). The human, conscious experiences of our environment require more than the integration of bits of color, shape, sound, and smell, which, as we have seen, are mediated by many anatomically distinct brain regions. They also require placement of those perceptions in the context of past experience. A particular memory does not exist whole as a piece of RNA in a single cell in the hippocampus, for instance. Rather, just like a raw perceptual experience (with the separate attributes of color, shape, tone, etc.) being processed in separate but coordinated networks, the bits and pieces that constitute our memories are also stored in assemblies of neurons, in lower order, sensory-specific association areas. A remembered event is reexperienced in our imagination because of the simultaneous coactivation of multiple, geographically separated ensembles of neurons in different brain regions. The vividness, complexity, and specificity of a remembered experience depend on the extent of the coordinated activation of multiple sensory-specific association areas by multiple, higher order association areas. Recognizing a shirt generically as an article of clothing might only require the activation of lower order visual association areas by some midlevel association areas. But the most elaborate and complex experiences, such as recognizing a specific shirt in a drawer as the one you received on your 23rd birthday as a gift from your parents who had just returned from their second trip to Hawaii, would require the most widespread activation and must be mediated by neurons in an association area with widespread connections, such as the hippocampus (Fig. 8).

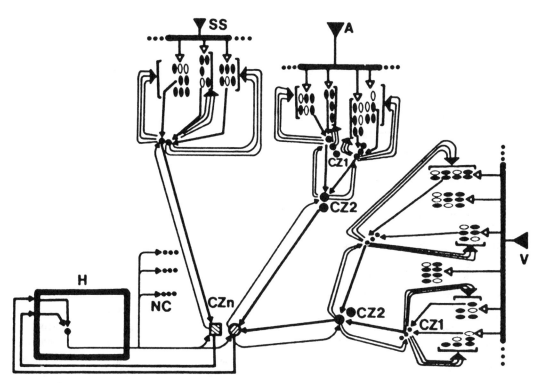

FIG. 8. Simplified schematic diagram of some aspects of a model for the neural architecture subserving cognition. V, SS, and A depict early and intermediate sensory cortices in visual, somatosensory, and auditory modalities. In each of those sensory sectors, separate functional regions are represented by open and filled dots. Note feedforward projections (thick lines) from those regions toward several orders of convergence zones (association areas) (CZ1, CZ2, CZn), and note also feedback projections from each CZ level toward originating regions (thin lines). H depicts the hippocampal system, one of the structures where signals related to a large number of activity sites can converge. Note outputs of H toward the last station of feedforward convergence zones (CZn) and noncortical neural neurotransmitter nuclei. Feedforward and feedback pathways should not be seen as rigid channels. They are conceived as facilitated lines that become active when concurrent firing in early cortices of CZs takes place. Furthermore, those pathways terminate over neuron ensembles, in distributed fashion, rather than on specific single neurons. Reproduced from Damasio AR. *Neural Comput* 1989;1:123–132, with permission from MIT Press.

Subcortical Nuclei

Subcortical regions play a major role in such general cognitive functions as attention and motivation. While the specific aspects of conscious experience are mediated by cortical networks, innervation from subcortical regions can have a strong, more generalized influence on the cortical neural activity. For instance, cholinergic neurons in the *nucleus basalis of Meynert* situated in the basal forebrain project widely to the cerebral cortex, and their activity releases the neurotransmitter acetylcholine in the cortex. Acetylcholine (see Chapter 6) may be considered a neuromodulator that makes neurons more receptive to other inputs. Thus, the level of activity of cholinergic neurons in the basal forebrain can affect the overall information-processing capacity of the cerebral cortex. Other subcortical regions that project widely to cerebral cortex include the neurons of the pontomesencephalic reticular formation (acetylcholine), brain stem *raphe nuclei* (serotonin), nucleus locus coeruleus (norepinephrine), substantia nigra and ventral tegmentum (dopamine), intralaminar nuclei of the thalamus, and neurons in the medial and lateral hypothalamus. Because each of these regions contains a relatively small group of neurons with very widespread projections, they are in a position to rapidly modulate the processing capacity of the entire cerebral cortex. Alterations in these systems can enhance or diminish such general functions as arousal and attention, mood, motivation, and level of anxiety.

Motor Output

The primary motor cortex directly controls all voluntary movement. Motor activity allows us to manipulate our environment. Cortical areas that are important in motor activity occupy a large portion of the lateral and medial surfaces of the frontal lobes. Primary motor cortex (area 4), premotor and supplementary motor areas (areas 6 and 8), and motor speech area (Broca's area, areas 44 and 45) have connections with primary somatosensory cortex and with limbic, multimodal, and unimodal association areas throughout the brain. The premotor and supplementary motor areas are tightly interconnected and function in the complex planning, preparation, and initiation of motor activity. The basal ganglia, motor nuclei of the thalamus and brain stem, and cerebellum are also strongly connected to motor cortices and have an important role in motor integration. They are essential for the precise timing, speed, accuracy, and smoothness of movements. The primary motor cortex lies in the precentral gyrus and directly controls voluntary movement. Like the somatosensory cortex, the primary motor strip is somatotopically organized, with specific regions controlling activity of specific muscle groups in the limbs and trunk (Fig. 6). Axons from neurons of the primary motor cortex gather to form the corticospinal tract, which descends through the cerebrum and brain stem to synapse directly with motor neurons in the spinal cord. Motor neurons then innervate specific individual muscles.

SUMMARY

Neural activity in the brain occurs in cortical and subcortical nuclei that are interconnected in highly complex networks. Sensory organs translate physical and chemical stimuli into neural impulses that are conducted along specific pathways, relayed at synapses of subcortical nuclei, and then directed to primary sensory cortices. These neural impulses undergo a type of distributed parallel processing in which the multiple attributes of an object or event are integrated, compared with past experience, and manipulated. This occurs largely by way of precisely coordinated feedforward and feedback interactions among sensory-specific, multimodal, and limbic association cortices. Neurotransmission throughout the brain is influenced by the activity of various subcortical neurotransmitter systems. There is a constant interplay among sensory cortices, motor cortices, and motor-related subcortical structures (especially basal ganglia, motor nuclei of the thalamus, and cerebellum), allowing sensory experience to drive and influence motor output and thus manipulate the environment.

BIBLIOGRAPHY

Original Articles

Damasio AR. The brain binds entities and events by multiregional activation from convergence zones. *Neural Comput* 1989;1:123–132.

Damasio AR. Time-locked multiregional retroactivation: a systems-level proposal for the neural substrates of recall and recognition. *Cognition* 1989;33(1–2): 25–62.

Geschwind N. Disconnexion syndromes in animals and man. *Brain* 1965;88:237–294, 585–644.

Jones EG, Powell TPS. An anatomical study of converging sensory pathways within the cerebral cortex of the monkey. *Brain* 1970;93:793–820.

Kawamura K, Naito J. Corticocortical projections to the prefrontal cortex in the rhesus monkey investigated with horseradish peroxidase techniques. *Neurosci Res* 1989;1:89–103.

Mesulam M-M, Van Hoesen GW, Pandya DK, Geschwind N. Limbic and sensory connections of the inferior parietal lobule (area PG) in the rhesus monkey: a study with a new method for horseradish peroxidase histochemistry. *Brain Res* 1977;136:393–414.

Papez JW. A proposed mechanism of emotion. *Arch Neurol Psychiatry* 1937;38:725–743.

Van Hoesen GW. The parahippocampal gyrus. New observations regarding its cortical connections in the monkey. *Trends Neurosci* 1982;(5):345–350.

Books and Reviews

Brodal A. *Neurological anatomy in relation to clinical medicine.* 3rd Ed. New York: Oxford University Press; 1981.

Carpenter M. *Core text of neuroanatomy.* Baltimore: Williams & Wilkins; 1978.

Damasio H, Damasio AR. *Lesion analysis in neuropsychology.* New York: Oxford University Press; 1989.

Heimer L. *The human brain and spinal cord.* New York: Springer-Verlag; 1983.

Mesulam, M. *Principles of behavioral neurology.* Philadelphia: FA Davis; 1985.

Raine CS. Neuroanatomy. In: Siegel GJ, Agranoff BW, Albers RW, Molinoff PB, eds. *Basic neurochemistry,* 5th ed. New York: Raven Press; 1994 (in press).

2

Excitability and Conduction

Michael M. White

Briefly, the hypothesis is that the action potential depends on a rapid sequence of changes in the permeability to the sodium and potassium ions. It makes use of the observation that potassium is concentrated inside most excitable cells, whereas sodium and chloride are relatively dilute. The resting potential is explained by supposing that the cell membrane is moderately permeable to the potassium and chloride ions, but is relatively impermeable to sodium and to the internal anions. Any sodium which leaks into the cell is assumed to be pumped out by a secretory process which must ultimately depend on metabolism. A large but transient increase in the permeability to sodium occurs when the fibre is depolarized by an electrical stimulus or by flow of current from an adjacent region of active nerve. Sodium ions therefore enter the fibre at a high rate, and reverse the potential difference across the cell membrane. They also provide the current for depolarizing adjacent regions of resting nerve. The increase in the permeability to sodium is followed by a similar rise in the permeability to potassium. This accelerates the rate at which these ions leave the fibre and helps to restore the membrane potential to its resting value. The interchange of sodium and potassium provides the immediate source of energy for the propagation of nervous impulses, but it must be reversed by a metabolic process during the period of recovery which follows a burst of electrical activity. Since nervous activity is usually intermittent, it must be supposed that nerve fibres spend a large part of their lives paying off the debt which they have incurred during the passage of electrical impulses.

A. L. Hodgkin,
The ionic basis of electrical activity in nerve and muscle
Biol. Rev. 1951;26:340

▶ Key Concepts

- Membrane potentials are generated by the combination of unequal ion distribution across the membrane and selective ion permeabilities.

- Alterations in membrane permeability properties lead to changes in the membrane potential.

- The voltage clamp allows the direct measurement of permeability changes.

- Membrane permeability is little affected by hyperpolarization, but it changes dramatically in response to depolarization.

- Permeability is dependent on the presence of specific proteins in the cell membrane called ion channels.

- The nerve impulse propagates along the axon.

- A local depolarization at a synapse initiates an impulse.

■ Chapter Overview ─────────────

This chapter describes the physiochemical processes that give rise to membrane potentials. This is followed by a description of results and conclusions coming from a series of experiments carried out using the squid giant axon. These experiments led to a refinement of Bernstein's membrane theory and form the basis of our understanding of the generation and propagation of the nerve impulse.

Although the ancient Egyptians recognized the brain and nerves as discrete structures, they considered them to be of little functional consequence. In particular, they considered the brain to be of so little importance that they discarded it during the mummification process, while retaining a number of other organs. Hippocrates (400 B.C.) was the first to suggest that the brain was an important structure and postulated that it was the sole source of emotions. One of the earliest descriptions of the nervous system was by Galen (200 A.D.), who considered the nervous system to be a system of pneumatic tubes conducting *animal spirits* to various parts of the body from the cerebral ventricles. Where did these animal spirits come from? Digested food was transferred from the gut to the liver, where it was used to make *natural spirits.* The natural spirits were passed to the right side of the heart for conversion to *vital spirits,* which were pumped with the arterial blood to the ventricles of the brain, where they were converted to *animal spirits.*

As naive as this formulation seems to us today, it was accepted as fact for the next 1,500 years. One could explain a number of phenomena in terms of this scheme. For example, the cessation of nerve function when one blocked blood flow to the brain was due to the blockade of the transport of vital spirits to the brain.

All of this changed in the eighteenth and nineteenth centuries. Luigi Galvani found

that electrical shocks could cause a muscle to twitch. He suggested that the "nerve power" was electricity. However, at that time there was no way to measure electrical signals, and this remained mere speculation. The invention of the galvanometer made it possible to measure small current flows due to differences in potential (voltage) between the two terminals of the device; however, investigators failed to detect any current flow in biological tissues. Finally, in 1840, DuBois-Reymond improved the sensitivity of the galvanometer so that it could measure the miniscule currents that flowed in nerves. He measured the so-called *injury current* that is observed when one of the leads of the current-measuring device is placed at a site where the nerve is damaged and the other is placed at a position where the tissue is normal. A small, steady-state current that flows from the undamaged to the damaged part of the nerve was observed. When the nerve was stimulated with an electrical shock, the sign and magnitude of the current changed transiently, a phenomenon that DuBois-Reymond termed *negative variation* (Fig. 1A). When the experiment was repeated using an undamaged nerve, no steady-state current could be detected; however, when the fiber was stimulated, the galvanometer once again measured a small, transient change in current (Fig. 1B) due to a change in the local extracellular potentials.

In 1902 Julius Bernstein formulated the "membrane theory" to explain the basic mechanisms behind electrical activity seen in both nerve and muscle. At rest, an excitable cell had a potential, the *resting potential,* that

Biological Bases of Brain Function and Disease, edited by Alan Frazer, Perry B. Molinoff, and Andrew Winokur. Raven Press, Ltd., New York © 1994.

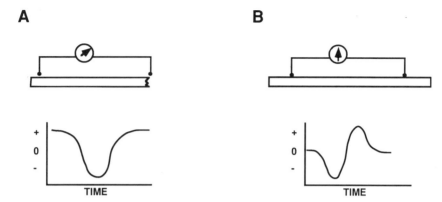

FIG. 1. Extracellular currents recorded in response to nerve stimulation using a galvanometer. **(A)** A damaged nerve is used, with one lead of the galvanometer placed at the site of damage and the other some distance away. A constant current flowing from the undamaged to the damaged portion (the injury current) is detected. Upon stimulation, this current transiently changes from a positive to a negative value, the so-called negative variation. **(B)** When an undamaged nerve is used, no steady-state current is observed. However, upon stimulation, the current first becomes negative, then positive, before returning to a zero current condition.

appeared as a voltage between the inside and outside of the cell. This potential came from the unequal distribution of cations between the inside and outside of the cell (high [K$^+$] and low [Na$^+$] inside, high [Na$^+$] and low [K$^+$] outside), coupled with a high membrane permeability for K$^+$ but not for Na$^+$. A nerve impulse was generated by a transient loss of this ionic selectivity and the resting potential disappeared, a phenomenon he termed *membrane breakdown*. The basic features of this theory are correct, even though at the time it was impossible to actually measure these membrane potentials, since nerve and muscle cells were too small for the apparatus available at the time. In 1936, J. Z. Young "rediscovered" the squid giant axon, whose diameter (0.5 to 1 mm) is approximately 100 times larger than that of other nerves (in fact, these axons are so large that they were mistaken for blood vessels by earlier anatomists). Armed with this new preparation and theories to explain how nerves generated electrical activity, two groups—Hodgkin, Huxley, and Katz in England, and Curtis and Cole in the United States—began a program of experiments in the late 1930s and 1940s that

led to our understanding of the basic processes involved in the generation and propagation of electrical impulses in the nervous system.

PHYSIOCHEMICAL PROCESSES

Membrane potentials are generated by the combination of unequal ion distribution across the membrane and selective ion permeabilities. Bernstein's membrane theory proposed that a voltage exists between the inside and the outside of nerve cells. The basic theory that governs the generation of such potentials was first laid out by Nernst in 1888. Consider the following situation: two compartments containing a salt KA with concentrations C_1 and C_2 separated by a "semipermeable" membrane such that only K$^+$ can cross the membrane (Fig. 2). If the K$^+$ concentrations are unequal, then K$^+$ ions will diffuse from the chamber of higher concentration to the chamber of lower concentration until the concentrations are equal. Note that if the membrane were permeable to both K$^+$ and A$^-$, both would diffuse to the

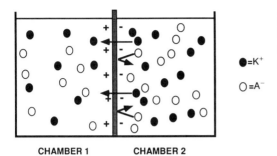

CHAMBER 1   CHAMBER 2

●=K$^+$

○=A$^-$

FIG. 2. A K$^+$-selective membrane separating two chambers containing a solution of the salt KA, with the concentration of KA in chamber 2 being twice that of chamber 1. This concentration difference promotes the movement of K$^+$ from chamber 2 to chamber 1, but since A$^-$ cannot cross the membrane, the charge imbalance sets up a diffusion potential such that the voltage in chamber 2 is negative with respect to that in chamber 1.

chamber of lower concentration; however, the semipermeable nature of the membrane prevents A$^-$ from crossing. The driving force for the diffusion process can be described as a chemical potential, ΔG_{chem}:

$$\Delta G_{chem} = RT \ln \frac{C_2}{C_1}$$

where R is the gas constant and T is the absolute temperature (Kelvin). The sign of the potential indicates the direction that is favored. If $C_1 = C_2$, then there is no tendency for K$^+$ to move from one compartment to the other, and $\Delta G_{chem} = 0$. If $C_2 > C_1$, K$^+$ would move from compartment 2 to compartment 1, and ΔG_{chem} is positive; if $C_1 > C_2$, ΔG_{chem} is negative. This relationship will hold for any diffusible component regardless of its charge. However, since in this particular example only a positively charged particle can cross the membrane, a charge imbalance will occur if K$^+$ diffuses across the membrane. If this happens, the separation of charge produces an electrical potential, sometimes called a *diffusion potential,* which will in turn affect the movement of the charged particle across the membrane. The difference in electrical

potential between the two chambers, ΔG_{elec}, can be defined as the amount of work required to move a charged particle through an electric field:

$$\Delta G_{elec} = zF(V_2 - V_1)$$

where z is the valence of the ion ($z = 1$ for K$^+$ and $z = -1$ for A$^-$), F is the Faraday constant, and V_1 and V_2 are the voltages in chambers 1 and 2, respectively. At equilibrium, the electrical and diffusive forces will balance each other and the sum of the two potentials will equal 0:

$$\Delta G_{chem} + \Delta G_{elec} = 0$$

$$RT \ln \frac{C_2}{C_1} + zF(V_2 - V_1) = 0$$

$$V_2 - V_1 = -\frac{RT}{zF} \ln \frac{C_2}{C_1}$$

$$V_2 - V_1 = -\frac{59.2}{z} \log \frac{C_2}{C_1}$$

In this equation the temperature is 25°C (298° K) and the voltage is in millivolts. Equilibrium potentials will vary with temperature and the ratio of the concentration of the permeable ion in compartment 2 to that in compartment 1. For example, if there is a tenfold K$^+$ concentration gradient between chambers 2 and 1 ($C_2/C_1 = 10$), then a membrane potential of -59 mV will be set up. If the diffusing particle is uncharged, or if no concentration gradient is present, then no potential will be set up. An equilibrium diffusion potential set up by only one type of ion is denoted as E_X, where X is the ion involved. If one were able to apply a voltage across the semipermeable membrane by connecting a battery across the membrane so that ($V_2 - V_1$) no longer equaled E_X, the system would no longer be at equilibrium and ions would begin to move across the membrane. The direction in which an ion moves depends on its charge and the new value of $V_2 - V_1$. If $V_2 - V_1 > E_X$, then cations would move from chamber 2 to chamber 1, while if $V_2 < V_1$, cations would move from chamber 1 to chamber 2.

Diffusion potentials are the basis of pH measurements by pH meters. A pH electrode contains a special type of glass that is selectively permeable to protons. A solution of known [H^+] is inside the electrode, and the diffusion potential generated after placing the electrode in a solution of unknown [H^+] allows one to determine the magnitude of the concentration gradient in H^+ ions. Since the proton concentration inside the electrode is known, this makes the determination of the [H^+] concentration in the solution outside the electrode a simple matter, and the pH meter does the conversion from mV to pH.

For a more complicated system, which may have several different ionic species, the equilibrium potential for each ion present can still be written. An example would be the ion concentrations for the squid giant axon (Table 1).

Bernstein proposed that this type of diffusion potential existed in nerve cells. In this case, chamber 1 is the extracellular solution and chamber 2 is the inside of the cell. If the cell membrane can be considered to be selectively permeable only to K^+, as Bernstein hypothesized, then a membrane potential that is negative inside the cell relative to the outside (remember, cells have [K^+] inside that is higher than that of the extracellular solution) should exist. This membrane potential should be sensitive only to the K^+ concentration gradient and insensitive to changes in the concentration of other ions (i.e., the membrane potential should be the same as the K^+ equilibrium potential):

$$V_m = V_{in} - V_{out} = E_K = -59 \log \left(\frac{[K]_{in}}{[K]_{out}} \right)$$

The introduction of the squid giant axon as an experimental preparation made it possible to test this hypothesis, since it was actually possible to insert a small electrode inside the axon and directly measure the potential under defined ionic conditions. Curtis and Cole in the United States and Hodgkin and

TABLE 1. *Ionic concentrations and equilibrium potentials for the squid giant axon*

Ion	[X]$_{in}$ (mM)	[X]$_{ext}$ (mM)	E_X (mV)
Na^+	72	455	+48
K^+	345	10	−90
Cl^-	61	540	−55
Ca^{++}	$<10^{-7}$	10	>+64

Katz in England measured the value of the resting potential of the squid giant axon as a function of extracellular [K^+] (which could be varied experimentally), and found that at high [K^+]$_{ext}$, the membrane potential followed E_K, but that it was more positive than E_K at low values of [K^+]$_{ext}$. The deviation from E_K at low [K^+]$_{ext}$ was interpreted to mean that the axon membrane is primarily K^+-selective at rest but is also slightly permeable to other ions. For a system such as a nerve cell, which contains a membrane permeable to several ionic species, an equation called the Goldman–Hodgkin–Katz equation can be derived:

$$V_m = \left(\frac{RT}{F} \right)$$

$$\times \ln \frac{P_K[K]_{ext} + P_{Na}[Na]_{ext} + P_{Cl}[Cl]_{in}}{P_K[K]_{in} + P_{Na}[Na]_{in} + P_{Cl}[Cl]_{ext}}$$

where P_X is called the *permeability coefficient* and is a measure of how permeable the membrane is to a given ion X. The actual value of the resting potential is set, then, by the concentrations of each ion and its respective permeability coefficient. For a membrane that is permeable only to K^+, $P_{Na} = P_{Cl} = 0$, and the membrane potential is set by E_K and is thus approximately −90 mV. Similarly, if the membrane were permeable only to Na^+, the membrane potential would be approximately +50 mV, the value of E_{Na}. For a system that has a finite permeability to several different ions, such as biological membranes, an intermediate situation exists, with the product of the permeability coefficient and the ion concentration determining the potential. In the case of the squid giant axon at rest,

$P_K/P_{Na}/P_{Cl}$ is 1:0.04:0.45. Since $[K]_{in}$ is high, $P_K[K]_{in}$ is the dominant term in the denominator. At high values of $[K]_{ext}$, $P_K[K]_{ext}$ is also the dominant term in the numerator, and $V_m = E_K$. At low values of $[K]_{ext}$, including physiological levels, the $P_K[K]_{ext}$ term becomes small enough that the other terms in the numerator become nonnegligible, and V_m deviates from E_K. In the case of the squid giant axon, the resting potential is on the order of -50 mV.

Although the above discussion deals with the squid giant axon, similar behavior is found for essentially all biological membranes. In general, biological membranes are more permeable at rest to K^+ than to Na^+ and thus have a resting potential that is negative inside. In addition, while the actual values of the permeability coefficients for individual ions as well as their ratios may vary among cell types, the Goldman–Hodgkin–Katz equation has been found to be an adequate description of the resting potential.

Alterations in membrane permeability properties lead to changes in the membrane potential. The Goldman–Hodgkin–Katz equation shows that membrane potential can be changed by altering either the concentration or the permeability of one or more ions. Since the time course of the change of the membrane potential during an action potential is rapid, occurring in as little as 1 msec, we can safely assume that the first possibility is implausible and that the changes in membrane potential during an action potential are due to changes in the permeability properties of the cell membrane. According to Bernstein's hypothesis, the action potential is generated by a transient total breakdown in the ionic selectivity of the membrane. At rest, the cell membrane is permeable to K^+, and thus a diffusion potential equal to E_K is set up. During an action potential, however, the membrane becomes completely nonselective, and the membrane potential is 0 mV. After the action potential, the membrane returns to its K^+-selective state, and once again a K^+ diffusion potential is set up. While the work of

Hodgkin and Katz showed that the generation of the resting potential involved more than just permeability to K^+ ions, K^+ permeability could still be considered the major determinant of the resting potential.

Once accurate recordings of the action potential in squid giant axon were carried out using intracellular electrodes, Hodgkin and Katz and Curtis and Cole found that the membrane potential during an action potential did not go to 0 mV as predicted by Bernstein's hypothesis, but instead reached values of $+30$ to $+50$ mV (Fig. 3). In addition, the membrane potential went below the resting level immediately after the action potential and then returned to the resting potential. This undershoot is called an *afterhyperpolarization* (AHP). In a series of elegant experiments in which the effects of alterations in the ionic composition of the extracellular solution on the action potential were measured, Hodgkin and Katz found that while the resting potential was relatively insensitive to the extracellular Na^+ concentration, the amplitude of the action potential was very sensitive to $[Na]_{ext}$. For example, replacing two-thirds of the NaCl in the extracellular solution with dextrose (to preserve the tonicity of the solution) made the resting potential only 2 mV more negative (to -52 mV) but reduced the amplitude of the action potential by 44 mV, so that the value of the membrane potential during the peak of the action potential just barely reached 0 mV, instead of $+45$ mV. They also observed that the rate of rise (i.e., the speed of the depolarization of the membrane) of the action potential was decreased when $[Na]_{ext}$ was decreased. If a smaller fraction of the external Na^+ was removed, the reduction in the amplitude of the action potential and the rate of rise of the action potential were smaller. All of these effects were reversible, and the action potential returned to normal on changing the external solution back to one containing a normal concentration of Na^+. Essentially no effect on the peak of the action potential was observed when the external K^+ concentration was varied, al-

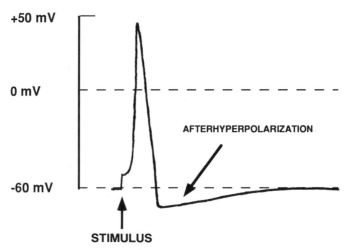

FIG. 3. An action potential recorded from a squid giant axon. The arrow marks the point at which a brief depolarizing current was applied to the axon to elicit an action potential. Note that the peak of the action potential is much more positive than 0 mV and that the afterhyperpolarization brings the membrane potential to a value more negative than the resting potential. The entire record covers a period of 25 msec, and the width of the action potential is approximately 3 msec.

though the AHP was increased when the K^+ concentration was decreased.

Careful analysis of the dependence of the effects of extracellular Na^+ and K^+ on the resting potential, the amplitude of the action potential, and the amplitude of the AHP allowed determination of the relative ionic permeabilities of the membrane during the action potential using the Goldman–Hodgkin–Katz equation (Table 2). From these experiments, Hodgkin and Katz proposed what they termed the "sodium hypothesis," in which the membrane does not go from K^+-selective to nonselective during an action potential (as Bernstein proposed), but rather goes from K^+-selective to Na^+-selective. When the membrane becomes Na^+-selective, Na^+ ions start to cross the membrane from the outside (high $[Na^+]$) to the inside (low $[Na^+]$). It is this entry of Na^+

that causes the membrane potential to approach E_{Na}. The amount of Na^+ that must cross the membrane to cause this large (>100 mV) change in membrane potential can be calculated to be approximately 10^{-12} mol Na^+/cm^2 of membrane. For a squid giant axon with a diameter of 1 mm, entry of this much Na^+ would increase the intracellular Na^+ concentration by less than 10^{-7} M, an inconsequential amount that would have no effect on E_{Na}. Similarly, repolarization of the membrane due to K^+ exit once the membrane is again K^+-selective would involve movement of the same amount of K^+.

VOLTAGE CLAMP

The voltage clamp allows the direct measurement of permeability changes. Experiments that measure the effects of changes in external solution on the action potential established many of the basic concepts of the ionic basis of the action potential. In these types of experiments, current is delivered to the axon, and the resulting changes in membrane potential are monitored. Results of early work had shown that a stimulus had to be of the proper sign and magnitude to elicit

TABLE 2. *Relative permeability coefficients for the squid giant axon*

Condition	P_K	P_{Na}	P_{Cl}
Rest	1.0	0.04	0.45
AP peak	1.0	20.0	0.45
AHP	1.8	0	0.45

an action potential. The stimulus had to cause the membrane to depolarize (i.e., the membrane potential became less negative); stimuli that hyperpolarized the membrane did not elicit an action potential. In addition, the action potential was shown to be *all or none:* once a threshold value of the stimulus was reached, the size and shape of an elicited action potential was independent of the amplitude of the stimulating current, and stimuli less than the threshold level did not elicit an action potential. However, these types of measurements do not allow easy study of the mechanisms that underlie the permeability changes. To study the excitation process in detail, a different type of experimental approach is required, the *voltage clamp.* In a voltage clamp experiment, a constant voltage is applied to the cell membrane, and the current that flows across the cell membrane is measured as a function of time. This current is a measure of the permeability of the membrane to ions under whatever conditions the experiment is carried out. Detailed analysis of the properties of currents can thus be used to obtain information about the permeability changes themselves.

An idealized voltage clamp consists of three components (Fig. 4): (1) a circuit for measuring the transmembrane potential, (2) a command amplifier that compares the measured value of V_m to whatever value the experimenter wishes (V_{comm}) and then injects a current proportional to this difference into the cell, and (3) a circuit for measuring the current that flows across the cell membrane. A voltage clamp is an example of a negative feedback device, which means that the output of the command amplifier is proportional to the difference in the inputs, which in this case are V_m and V_{comm}. The command amplifier will inject current into the cell until $V_m = V_{comm}$; it therefore "clamps" the transmembrane potential at V_{comm}. Any current that flows across the membrane would cause the membrane potential to change. If a cell is voltage-clamped, the command amplifier will inject a current equal and opposite to that flowing across the membrane to compensate for that flow to maintain the desired voltage.

This type of negative feedback device can be compared with a more familiar one: a home heating and cooling system. A desired room temperature is set at the thermostat. If the actual room temperature is lower than the desired temperature, the furnace delivers heat to the house until the desired temperature is reached; likewise, if room temperature is higher than the desired temperature, the air conditioning system cools the house by removing heat until the setpoint is reached. The amount of heat that must be delivered or removed will depend on the properties of the

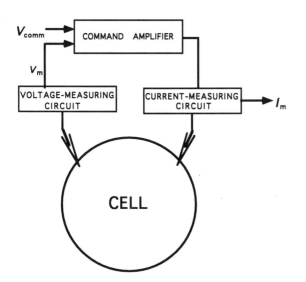

FIG. 4. Basic components of a voltage clamp. Two separate electrodes are placed in a cell to measure the voltage and to inject current into the cell, respectively. Command amplifier compares the measured membrane potential (V_m) to the desired potential (V_{comm}), and then injects a current into the cell that is proportional to the difference between the two potentials. An additional circuit measures the amount of current that is injected (I_m). Under ideal conditions, this injected current is equal and opposite to the current flowing across the cell membrane at any given time.

house, such as how well it is insulated; a poorly insulated house will require much more heat to be delivered per unit time to maintain a certain temperature than a well-insulated one. If the steady-state condition is disturbed by, say, the opening of a window in winter, the furnace must deliver more heat to maintain the desired temperature while the window is open.

Membrane permeability is little affected by hyperpolarization, but it changes dramatically in response to depolarization. In a classic series of papers, Hodgkin and Huxley reported the results of an elegant set of experiments using this technique to study the permeability changes in the squid giant axon during excitation. They clamped the axon membrane potential at a holding potential near the resting potential of the axon (−65 mV) and measured the current that flowed across the cell membrane in response to rapidly changing the voltage to a new value for a brief period (5–25 msec) after which they returned it to the original holding potential. When the membrane potential was changed from −65 mV to −130 mV (a 65-mV hyperpolarization), only a small change in the steady-state current was seen. If, on the other hand, the potential was jumped to 0 mV (a 65-mV depolarization), a large transient inward current followed by a maintained outward current was seen (Fig. 5) (the direction of the current refers to the way that a cation would move, so an inward current is one in which cations would move into the cell). Since the current flow is a measure of the permeability of the membrane, this means that while the membrane permeability changes little in response to hyperpolarization, it changes dramatically in response to depolarization.

This type of experiment was repeated for a series of different depolarizing voltage steps. An early transient current could be detected in response to depolarizations more positive than −40 mV. It reached its largest peak amplitude at approximately −10 mV, and it then became smaller as the voltage was made more positive, until it reversed its polarity at

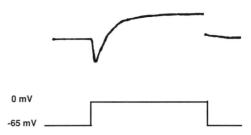

FIG. 5. Current elicited from a voltage-clamped squid giant axon in response to a 15-msec-long voltage step from −65 mV to 0 mV. Note the transient inward current (shown as a downward-going current in the trace) followed by an outward current that lasts as long as the voltage is held at 0 mV. The inward current is carried by Na^+ ions and would not be detected if extracellular Na^+ were replaced by an impermeant ion like choline, while the maintained outward current is carried by K^+ ions.

around +50 mV (close to E_{Na}) to become a transient outward current. The late maintained outward current became evident at voltages more positive than −20 mV and increased in amplitude as the voltage became more depolarized. Based on this behavior, Hodgkin and Huxley postulated that the transient current (inward for $V_m < E_{Na}$, outward for $V_m > E_{Na}$) was carried by Na^+ ions, while the maintained outward current was carried by K^+. The identification of the transient current as being carried by Na^+ was further borne out by examining the effect of alterations in the extracellular Na^+ concentration. Replacement of Na^+ with choline eliminated the transient inward current with no effect on the maintained outward current; if the Na^+ was only partially replaced by choline, the transient current was reduced but not eliminated. Experiments carried out later using a perfused axon preparation, in which the composition of the internal solution could be controlled, demonstrated that the maintained outward current was indeed carried by K^+ ions.

Detailed analysis of the properties of the transient inward current led Hodgkin and Huxley to postulate that two parallel processes were involved in the generation of this current. After the cell membrane was depolarized, a process they termed *activation* led to the opening of the Na^+ permeability pathway, and an inward current was generated. At the same time a slower process termed *inactivation* was initiated and this eventually led to the closing of the Na^+ permeability pathway. The net result was a transient inward current. Both processes are voltage-dependent with respect to both the extent and the speed of occurrence. Once inactivated, the Na^+ permeability pathway could not be reactivated until the membrane potential had returned to its resting value for a brief period.

Analysis of the properties of the outward K^+ current showed that the K^+ permeability pathway showed a similar type of voltage-dependent activation, although it was a slower process than that for the Na^+ permeability pathway. However, there was no inactivation process, which meant that as long as the voltage was maintained at an appropriate depolarized potential, a steady outward current carried by K^+ ions would flow across the membrane.

While Hodgkin and Huxley's analysis of the changes in the permeability properties of the squid giant axon did not deal with the actual nature of the elements of the cell membrane that were responsible for these permeability changes, further studies over the years have shown that these permeability pathways are specific proteins in the cell membrane called ion channels. The proteins responsible for the changes in Na^+ permeability are called *Na^+ channels,* while those responsible for the changes in K^+ permeability are called *K^+ channels.* These proteins can respond to changes in the membrane potential to produce pores in the membrane that allow either Na^+ or K^+ to pass through them. Detailed models as to how these proteins can respond to changes in the transmembrane potential, as well as the structure of the pore within the channel, have been proposed. Determination of the structural features of the channel proteins that underlie the various aspects of ion channel function is the focus of intense scientific investigation at this time.

Hodgkin and Huxley's models for the properties of both the Na^+ and K^+ permeability pathways allowed them to adequately describe the time and voltage dependence of the currents measured under voltage clamp conditions. Since both activation and inactivation of the Na^+ pathway are faster than the activation process for K^+ permeability, one initially observes a transient inward current in response to depolarization. As the Na^+ current starts to decay due to the inactivation process, the more slowly developing outward K^+ current appears, and by the end of a long (i.e., 25 msec) depolarization, all of the Na^+ channels have inactivated and only the outward K^+ current remains. As the membrane voltage returns to its resting value, the voltage-dependent K^+ permeability pathway is inactivated.

The *tour de force* of Hodgkin and Huxley's analysis of the electrical properties of the squid giant axon was to use the information on the time and voltage dependence of the Na^+ and K^+ currents studied under voltage clamp conditions to reconstruct the action potential. The model they derived to describe the properties of the voltage clamp currents also could predict action potentials virtually indistinguishable from those recorded from the squid giant axon. Once the axon membrane potential passes a certain threshold value, Na^+ channels start to open and Na^+ ions flow inward. This inward current causes a further depolarization, which opens more Na^+ channels, which causes more depolarization, and so on until the membrane becomes predominantly Na^+-selective and the membrane potential approaches E_{Na}. This entire process takes only a few milliseconds. Meanwhile, the more slowly occurring Na^+ channel inactivation process starts to take place, decreasing the Na^+ permeability of the axon, and the membrane potential starts to move away from E_{Na} back toward the resting level. Finally, the even slower process of K^+ channel activation starts to occur, which further increases the rate of return to the resting level. As the membrane potential becomes more negative, K^+ channels start to close, but since the closing rate is slow with respect to the rate of repolarization, enough K^+ channels are open when the membrane potential reaches the original resting potential that the K^+ permeability is higher than before the action potential took place, and the membrane potential becomes more negative than V_{rest}, which causes the afterhyperpolarization. As the K^+ channels close, the membrane potential goes back to V_{rest}. It takes a brief time at the resting potential (approximately 20 msec) for the Na^+ channels to recover from the inactivated state; during this period of time, called the *refractory period,* another action potential cannot be elicited.

Alan Hodgkin and Andrew Huxley received the 1963 Nobel Prize for Physiology and Medicine for their pioneering work. While more detailed studies of the properties of the Na^+ and K^+ channels of nerves from a number of preparations have shown that some of the fine details of the Hodgkin–Huxley formulation are open to question, the basic picture is correct. In addition, examination of action potentials from a number of excitable tissues has shown that the Hodgkin–Huxley formulation (developed from the squid giant axon experiments) can be applied to essentially all types of excitable cells, since axons have essentially only one function: to rapidly conduct an all-or-none impulse in response to an appropriate stimulus. In addition to this uniformity of mechanism as applied to nerve cells, variations of this conceptual framework can be applied to other excitable tissues such as muscle. For example, the action potentials from cardiac ventricular muscle have a very long plateau phase that can last for 50 to 100 msec before the potential starts to return to rest. This is due to the presence of a third type of channel, a slowly inactivating Ca^{++} channel, which maintains the membrane in a depolarized state during the plateau phase. Nonetheless, the action potential can still be described by a modification of the Hodgkin–Huxley scheme with the addition of this third type of channel.

ACTION POTENTIAL

The nerve impulse propagates along the axon. The Hodgkin–Huxley experiments were carried out using preparations in which a thin wire ran inside the axon along its entire length. This was done to make the axon *isopotential* (i.e., the transmembrane potential was the same along the entire length of the axon) and was required to accurately voltage-clamp the axon. Such an axon will fire an action potential in response to the proper stimulus; however, since the axon is isopotential, the membrane potential rises and falls at the same time at all points along the axon. This behavior is in contrast to an axon under normal conditions, in which a stimulus applied at one point elicits an action potential at the stimulus point which then propagates along the axon at a finite speed governed by the properties of the individual axon. This propagation can be easily understood if we consider the axon to consist of a number of identical segments next to each other, with each segment being capable of producing an action potential if that segment is depolarized beyond threshold. Stimulation of the axon at one end evokes an action potential in that segment. The current flowing through that section of the axon during the action potential depolarizes the adjacent section, which then fires an action potential, which depolarizes the next section, etc. Each section fires an action potential slightly after the preceding section, which gives the impression that the evoked action potential "travels" down the axon from the stimulus site. The inactivation process of the Na^+ channels, which prevents a given section from producing an action potential during the refractory period, imposes a unidirectionality on this conduction such that the wave of excitation travels away from the site of stimulus.

For axons to serve as an effective signaling system, the propagation of the impulse must be rapid with respect to the distance the signal must travel. Two different strategies have evolved to achieve a rapid rate of conduction. In the case of invertebrates, which have relatively few (compared to vertebrates) axons and much shorter pathlengths for the impulse to travel, fast signaling is achieved by having large-diameter axons, such as the 1-mm-diameter squid giant axon. In the case of vertebrates, this strategy would be impractical, since it would be difficult to accommodate the number of large-diameter axons needed to carry out all of the electrical signaling that takes place throughout the body. Vertebrate axons have an entirely different mechanism for ensuring rapid signaling. They are surrounded by myelin, which is formed by Schwann cells wrapped tightly around the axon. This myelin sheath provides an insulating layer not unlike the plastic insulation found on electrical wire. This insulation is broken every 0.2 to 1 mm for a length of about 5 μm at regions called *nodes of Ranvier.* It is at the nodal region that Na^+ channels are concentrated, and it is in this region that an action potential can be elicited. The insulation provided by the Schwann cell layer allows the change in membrane potential caused by the action potential in one node to extend to the next node to elicit an action potential in that node, and so on. In this type of situation, termed *saltatory conduction,* the action potential seems to "hop" from one node to the other. The rapid signaling achieved by saltatory conduction means that myelinated axons no longer need large diameters to obtain rapid signaling, and typical vertebrate axons (including the Schwann cell sheath) have diameters on the order of only 1 to 20 μm.

A local depolarization at the synapse initiates an impulse. For the above events to take place, the membrane must be depolarized beyond threshold to initiate an action potential. While in a laboratory situation this is done by injecting a depolarizing current into the axon, some other mechanism obviously underlies this initiating depolarization in the body. The process of impulse initiation involves synaptic transmission and is discussed in detail in Chapter 3. Briefly, excitatory neurotransmitters such as acetylcholine and glutamic acid bind to specific receptors on the postsynaptic side of the synapse and induce a conformational change in the receptor molecule. This conformational change causes the opening of a cation-selective channel that results in an increased permeability to both Na^+ and K^+ ions, which leads to a depolarization of the postsynaptic cell at the synapse. It is this depolarization, called an *excitatory postsynaptic potential* (EPSP), which provides the initial depolarization needed to initiate an action potential at this part of the cell.

Inhibitory neurotransmitters such as glycine and γ-aminobutyric acid (GABA), have the opposite effect. In vertebrates, these transmitters lead to an increase in the Cl^- permeability of the postsynaptic membrane called an *inhibitory postsynaptic potential* (IPSP). Since E_{Cl} is usually more negative than the resting potential, this would result in a hyperpolarization, which does not elicit an action potential. At first glance it is not obvious why such a process would be at all useful, but when one realizes that many neurons can receive multiple synaptic inputs, the existence of both excitatory and inhibitory inputs allows for a sophisticated degree of integration of neuronal inputs at individual synapses.

SUMMARY

Signaling throughout the nervous system involves brief alterations in the transmembrane potential. This transmembrane potential, in which the inside of the cell is negative with respect to the outside of the cell, is produced by a combination of ionic gradients due to unequal distribution of ions between the inside and the outside of the cell, and the selective permeability of the cell membrane at rest to K^+ ions. Action potentials, which are transient reversals in the polarity of the membrane potential, are brought about by a brief alteration in the ionic selectivity of the cell membrane, such that Na^+ is the most permeant ion during this period.

A detailed characterization of the ion permeability of the squid giant axon by Hodgkin and Huxley using the technique of voltage clamping showed that the entire cycle of permeability changes could be understood in terms of the properties of two independent permeability pathways, one for Na^+ and the other for K^+. They were able to completely reconstruct the events that take place during this cycle of permeability changes. A similar analysis of the excitation process of nerves in a number of other species (including humans) has shown that the basic processes described by Hodgkin and Huxley for the squid giant axon apply to other systems as well.

BIBLIOGRAPHY

Original Articles

Hodgkin AL, Huxley AF. Currents carried by sodium and potassium ions through the membrane of the giant axon of *Loligo. J Physiol (London)* 1952; 116:449–472.

Hodgkin AL, Huxley AF. The components of membrane conductance in the giant axon of *Loligo. J Physiol (London)* 1952;116:473–496.

Hodgkin AL, Huxley AF. The dual effect of membrane potential on sodium conductance in the giant axon of *Loligo. J Physiol (London)* 1952;116:497–506.

Hodgkin AL, Huxley AF. A quantitative description of membrane current and its application to conduction and excitation in nerve. *J Physiol (London)* 1952; 117:500–544.

Books and Reviews

Catterall WA. Structure and function of voltage-sensitive ion channels. *Science* 1988;242:50–61.

Hille B. *Ionic channels of excitable membranes.* Sunderland, MA: Sinauer Associates; 1984.

Hille B, Catterall WA. Electrical excitability and ion channels. In: Siegel GJ, Agranoff BW, Albers RW, Molinoff PB, eds. *Basic neurochemistry* 5th ed. New York: Raven Press; 1994 (in press).

Katz B. *Nerve, muscle and synapse.* New York: McGraw-Hill; 1966.

3

Synaptic Transmission
General Considerations

Steven J. Fluharty

The night before Easter Sunday of that year (1920) I awoke, turned on the light, and jotted down a few notes on a tiny slip of thin paper. Then I fell asleep again. It occurred to me at six o'clock in the morning that during the night I had written down something most important, but I was unable to decipher the scrawl. The next night, at three o'clock, the idea returned. It was the design of an experiment to determine whether or not the hypothesis of chemical transmission that I had uttered seventeen years ago was correct. I got up immediately, went to the laboratory, and performed a simple experiment on a frog heart according to the nocturnal design. . . . These results unequivocally proved that the nerves do not influence the heart directly but liberate from their terminals specific chemical substances which, in their turn, cause the well-known modifications of the function of the heart characteristic of the stimulation of its nerves.

O. Loewi,
An Autobiographic Sketch: Perspectives in Biology and Medicine
(London: Pergamon Press, 1960, p. 3)

- The nerve cell, or neuron, is the fundamental unit of the nervous system.

- Despite apparent diversity, all nerve cells function in much the same way.

- The concept of chemical mediation of synaptic transmission, which is now axiomatic in modern biology, was not always readily accepted.

- Definitive demonstration of the chemical mediation of synaptic transmission was provided by Loewi.

- It was confirmed that nerve stimulation leads to the release of acetylcholine.

- It is now possible to state the modern view of synaptic transmission.

- There are five criteria that must be met for a chemical to be designated a neurotransmitter.

- In the last decade, the number of candidate neurotransmitters has more than tripled.

- All known neurotransmitters fall into the same three categories.

This chapter begins with a review of some of the most important experiments that have contributed to the modern view of synaptic transmission. The contemporary view of the chemical events underlying neurotransmission are then used to develop a set of criteria that must be met for a chemical substance in the brain to be considered a neurotransmitter. Some of the special properties of neurotransmitters that permit these compounds to mediate cell-to-cell communication in the nervous system are also reviewed. Finally, the general classes of chemicals that fulfill these criteria and appear to function as neurotransmitters in the mammalian nervous system are identified. The unique properties of particular types of neurotransmitters will be discussed in greater detail in subsequent chapters (see Chapters 6–8).

The experimental findings that were generated as a consequence of the German pharmacologist Otto Loewi's predawn imagination (see epigraph) are generally credited with demonstrating the chemical mediation of synaptic transmission. However, the scientific community was only prepared to accept this idea as a result of experiments conducted almost 100 years before Loewi's landmark studies.

THE GENERALIZED NEURON

The nerve cell, or neuron, *is the fundamental unit of the nervous system.* Before beginning a historical overview, it will be useful to briefly review the general properties of nerve cells. There are several different types of neurons, each of which has specialized properties related to its particular function (Fig. 1). For instance, sensory neurons transmit information into the central nervous system (*afferents*) from specialized sensory transducers such as the retina, olfactory epithelium, and hair cells of the cochlea. There are also motor neurons that transmit information out of the central nervous system (*efferent*) to smooth or skeletal muscle and endocrine glands. In

Biological Bases of Brain Function and Disease, edited by Alan Frazer, Perry B. Molinoff, and Andrew Winokur. Raven Press, Ltd., New York © 1994.

between sensory afferent and motor efferent neurons are *interneurons.* Together, these three types of cells provide all of the machinery necessary for simple reflexes such as the "knee jerk." Finally, a fourth type of nerve cell is called a neuroendocrine cell because it is able to release chemical substances into the general circulation rather than into the extracellular fluid of synapses. As such, these neurons, which are found in the hypothalamus, have a wide sphere of influence.

Despite apparent diversity, all nerve cells function in much the same way. It is possible to divide a generalized neuron into three anatomic and functional zones (see Fig. 1). The first of these zones is referred to as the *chemoreceptive zone* and consists of the *soma,* or cell body, and the *dendritic processes* of the neuron. These regions of the nerve cell contain high densities of neurotransmitter receptors and ion channels (see Chapter 4). The chemoreceptive zone is the part of the neuron that receives and integrates inputs from other parts of the nervous system. The receptors are, in effect, extracellularly facing proteins that bind neurotransmitters released from other nerve cells with high affinity and specificity (see Chapter 4). Ion channels are pores in the membrane that allow the regulated influx and efflux of ions (see Chapter 2). In many instances, when a neurotransmitter occupies a receptor, it influences the probabil-

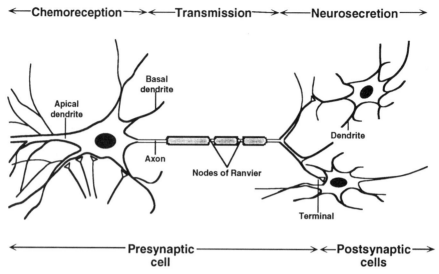

←——Chemoreception——→ ←——Transmission——→ ←——Neurosecretion——→

Basal dendrite

Apical dendrite

Dendrite

Axon

Nodes of Ranvier

Terminal

←——————————— Presynaptic —————————→ ←—Postsynaptic—→
cell   cells

FIG. 1. Schematic diagram of a generalized neuron indicating the three functional zones responsible for the functional properties of the cell.

ity that ion channels will open or close, thus altering the excitability of the neuron (see Chapter 2). These modulatory influences can be exerted directly, as in the case of ligand-gated ion channels, or indirectly, through the receptor-mediated generation of *intracellular second-messenger molecules.*

All of the inputs from other regions of the nervous system that impact on this chemoreceptive zone are summed algebraically according to the principle of *temporal and spatial summation.* The ionic changes that result from the actions of one neurotransmitter influencing membrane permeability can summate with those resulting from other neurotransmitters within a certain time frame and within neighboring regions of the dendritic tree. The net effect of the ionic fluxes induced by several neurotransmitters acting at more or less the same time may be to induce an *all-or-none action potential* in the second functional zone of the neuron.

The second region is referred to anatomically as the *axon* and functionally as the *transmission zone.* This is the largest portion of the neuron and it can extend over a distance as long as 10 m, which is the distance traveled by the motor neurons in the nervous system of the blue whale that mediate the sweeping movements of its tail. The transition from soma to axon begins with an *initial segment* or *axon hillock;* this is the region of the neuron in which an action potential can arise. More precisely, if the temporal and spatial summation of ionic conductance changes occurring in the chemoreceptive zone are sufficient to exceed the threshold for depolarization of the axon hillock, then an all-or-none action potential will be initiated that will be propagated down the entire length of the axon without diminution (see Chapter 2). Thus, the axon exhibits two functional properties that differ from those of dendrites. First, its informational unit, the action potential, is not graded the way synaptic potentials are in the chemoreceptive zone. Second, once initiated, the action potential is propagated without loss of electrochemical potential. This occurs because the axon contains a continuous gradient of voltage-sensitive sodium channels and each responds to the oncoming wave of depolarization by opening and allowing the entry of sodium, thus perpetuating a depolarization down the entire length of the axon. The presence of myelin on some neurons facilitates this conductive process (see Chapter 2).

Eventually, a propagated wave of depolarization invades the terminal region of the axon, the third and final zone of a generalized neuron. This region consists of specialized nerve terminals and is the *neurosecretory zone* of the neuron. The nerve terminal actually emerges from the end of the axon as an elaborate outgrowth that possesses its own unique attributes necessary for neurotransmitter release. Some neurotransmitters are synthesized in cell bodies and are transported to the nerve terminal region along *microtubules.* Once in the nerve terminal, most neurotransmitters are stored in specialized subcellular particles called *vesicles.* Vesicular storage has many important advantages. For instance, in some neurotransmitter systems such as neurons containing biogenic amines (see Chapter 6), the vesicle is an important site for the continued manufacture of the neurotransmitter because synthetic enzymes are contained within these structures. Vesicular storage is also important in the maintenance of neurotransmitter levels insofar as it prevents their degradation by intraneuronal enzymes. Finally, vesicles provide a releasable pool of neurotransmitter because they both prevent leakage of neurotransmitter in the absence of nerve stimulation and are involved in a release process called *exocytosis.*

Exocytotic release of biologically active molecules was first described for a number of hormone-secreting cells, but it now appears equally applicable to neurons (Fig. 2). When an action potential propagates down to the neurosecretory zone, *voltage-sensitive calcium channels* open, allowing entry of calcium. By activating the microtubular apparatus and neurofilament proteins in the nerve cell, this ion promotes the migration of neurotransmitter-containing vesicles to regions of the nerve terminal membrane called *active zones.* The vesicles then fuse with the membrane and eventually rupture, dispensing their contents—the neurotransmitter and related proteins—into the synaptic cleft. The

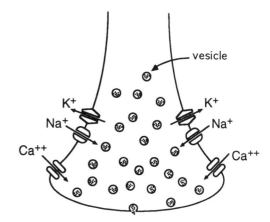

FIG. 2. Schematic diagram depicting the arrival of a depolarizing stimulus in the nerve terminal, the subsequent influx of ions, and the exocytotic release of neurotransmitter from vesicular stores. From Kandel ER, Schwartz JH. *Principles of neural science 2nd ed.* New York: Elsevier; 1985.

newly released neurotransmitter can then interact with receptors on adjacent nerve cells. Thus, vesicles provide neurons with packages of neurotransmitter whose release is regulated by changes in ionic currents, assuring that neurons only convey information when stimulated. While exocytosis is likely to be the most common mechanism of neurotransmitter release, it is important to point out that the release of some neurotransmitters, such as amino acids and acetylcholine, may also take place from cytoplasmic stores, and other alternative mechanisms of regulated release may be possible under certain circumstances.

In summary, the synapse consists of three important elements: a presynaptic nerve terminal that releases a neurotransmitter when invaded by a wave of depolarization propagated down the axon; a physical space of approximately 200 Å across which the released neurotransmitter must diffuse; and a postsynaptic membrane that contains the relevant proteins including receptors, ion channels, and other components of effector mechanisms (see Chapter 4). These components allow the cell to respond to a neurotransmitter and thus ensure that information

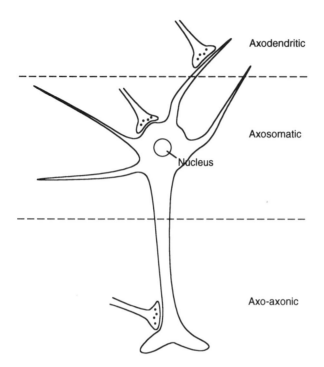

FIG. 3. Various types of synaptic contacts observed in the nervous system.

flows from one cell to the next. As mentioned above, synapses usually exist between nerve terminals and dendrites, although this need not be the case. For instance, there are dendo-dendritic, axo-axonic, and axo-somatic synapses (Fig. 3), as well as recurrent collaterals in which the same neuron sends a portion of its axon back to synapse on its own cell body, thus providing a self-regulatory control within neural circuits. Nonetheless, despite the diversity of these cytoarchitectural arrangements, the rules governing the chemical mediation of nerve impulse flow are largely the same.

HISTORICAL VIEW OF SYNAPTIC TRANSMISSION

The concept of chemical mediation of synaptic transmission, which is now axiomatic in modern biology, was not always readily accepted. Some of the earliest experiments that first suggested the involvement of chemical processes in neuronal communication were performed in the mid-1800s by the German physiologist H. von Helmholtz. von Helm-

holtz was studying the velocity of neural conduction using a simple preparation—the isolated sciatic nerve–gastrocnemius muscle of the frog. In one series of experiments, von Helmholtz applied electrical stimulation to one portion of the nerve and recorded the time that elapsed before the muscle contracted. He then moved the electrode to a more distal site on the nerve and once again recorded the temporal delay between stimulation and muscle contraction. In this fashion, von Helmholtz was able to calculate the approximate speed at which the stimulation traveled along the axon—20 m/sec. The suggestion that chemical processes were involved was provided when von Helmholtz repeated this simple experiment at a lower ambient temperature and noted that the conduction velocity decreased significantly. On the basis of these findings von Helmholtz concluded that some aspect of the nerve–muscle communication was likely to be chemical in nature because chemical reactions are more influenced by temperature than are electrical events.

The famous French physiologist Claude Bernard also investigated neural transmission using the frog sciatic nerve–gastrocnemius muscle preparation. Bernard was studying the action of curare, the poison widely used by several South American tribes to kill their prey. These tribes extracted the alkaloid from its indigenous plant sources and dipped arrowheads in the poison to render their weapons lethal. Bernard knew that curare produced muscular paralysis, and his experiments were designed to determine what aspect of nerve–muscle interaction was affected. He modified the isolated nerve-muscle preparation in such a way as to bathe portions of the nerve or muscle in curare. He then stimulated the nerve and recorded the muscle contraction. He observed that if the axon was bathed in curare, the muscle would still contract in response to stimulation. Similarly, when the muscle itself was placed in the curare, stimulation still elicited a contraction. Only when the junction between the nerve and the muscle was placed in the curare-containing solution was the stimulation-induced contraction prevented. This demonstration of the chemical vulnerability of the neuromuscular junction provided one of the first indications that the events occurring within synapses differed from those in nerve and muscle.

The early work of von Helmholtz, Bernard, and others was suggestive, but definitive demonstration of the chemical mediation of synaptic transmission was provided by Loewi. The innovative experiments of Otto Loewi (see epigraph) also involved an isolated nerve-muscle preparation from the frog, but he used the tenth cranial nerve, the vagus nerve, and the muscle was the heart. The unique variation of Loewi's experiments was that each study used two of these nerve–muscle preparations—one heart was designated the "donor" heart, while the other heart was referred to as the "recipient." Loewi arranged his perfusion bath so that the extracellular fluid for the donor heart superfused the recipient organ (Fig. 4). He then stimulated the vagus nerve of the donor heart, but not that of the recipient heart, and recorded the characteristic slowing of heart rate that we know results from the release of acetylcholine from vagal nerve terminals. The more significant effect, however, is what Loewi observed in the recipient heart, namely, that its heart rate also declined in the

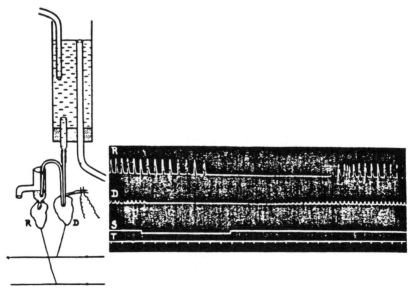

FIG. 4. Illustration of Loewi's original experiments investigating the neurohumoral control of cardiac function. Adapted from Bain A. *Quart J Med Exp Physiol Med Sci* 1932;22:269–274.

absence of any direct nerve stimulation. On the basis of this simple yet elegant experiment, Loewi concluded that nerve stimulation triggered the release of a chemical substance, which he called *Vagusstoff,* now known as acetylcholine, that was responsible for eliciting the change in heart rate; thence, the modern view of the chemical mediation of synaptic transmission was born. An interesting historical note is that Loewi's observations were not immediately accepted because of difficulties in replicating these observations in mammals. It was later learned that these problems were due to the much greater activity of cholinesterases in mammals than in frogs, which resulted in degradation of the released acetylcholine before it was delivered to the superfused recipient heart in mammalian preparations. Once this fact was appreciated, Loewi's observations were easily replicated by the addition of cholinesterase inhibitors to prolong the life of the liberated acetylcholine.

MODERN VIEW OF SYNAPTIC TRANSMISSION

It was confirmed that nerve stimulation leads to the release of acetylcholine. After the completion of Loewi's studies only a few additional details needed to be discovered for the modern view of synaptic transmission to emerge. Much of this research was performed in Great Britain just before World War II. The first of these studies was performed by Sir Walter Dale and his colleagues in the 1930s. By this time Loewi's *Vagusstoff* had been identified as acetylcholine (Loewi was instrumental in this discovery as well) and had been shown to be involved in synaptic transmission at the neuromuscular junction. Indeed, the earlier work of Bernard led to the realization that curare blocked the actions of acetylcholine by acting as an antagonist at nicotinic receptors. By using a very sensitive bioassay, Dale was able to demonstrate that nerve stimulation did in fact lead to the release of acetylcholine from nerve terminals,

thus confirming Loewi's original hypothesis. Dale went on to demonstrate that the release of acetylcholine was dependent on extracellular calcium, although the physiological significance of that fact was not fully appreciated for several more years.

Dale also performed one final study that is now the standard bearer for any chemical substance thought to function as a neurotransmitter (see section on Criteria). In this study Dale first demonstrated that nerve stimulation produced the expected muscle contraction. Subsequently, he discovered that the application of exogenous acetylcholine to the muscle elicited the same contraction as did nerve stimulation even in the absence of any stimulation. This property of neurotransmitters is referred to as *synaptic mimicry* and is the most important criteria to be satisfied by any substance that is a putative transmitter.

The final series of studies that set the stage for the widespread acceptance of Loewi's original hypothesis were performed by Bernard Katz and his colleagues beginning in the 1950s. Katz was already well known for helping to delineate the mechanisms mediating axonal conductance (see Chapter 2). By this time significant technical advances had occurred, permitting the development of micropipettes for the precise delivery of acetylcholine (ACh) to selected regions within the neuromuscular junction. Using this technique, Katz was able to demonstrate that the synapse was *unidirectional.* More specifically, when Katz applied ACh to the presynaptic nerve terminal or to more distal sites on the muscle itself, no contraction was elicited. On the other hand, when he applied the ACh directly onto the neuromuscular junction, the muscle contracted just as if the nerve had been stimulated. The positional sensitivity of the synapse to the actions of ACh paralleled the known sensitivity of this preparation to the poison curare that had been demonstrated years before by Claude Bernard. Katz hypothesized that this specificity resulted from the presence of ACh receptors located on the muscle fibers immediately across from the nerve terminal and not elsewhere within the synapse.

It is now possible to state the modern view of synaptic transmission. To summarize the modern view of synaptic transmission: A wave of depolarization is propagated down the axon and invades the nerve terminal. The change in membrane potential causes the opening of voltage-sensitive calcium channels, allowing an influx of calcium down its concentration gradient. The resulting increase in intracellular calcium levels promotes the recruitment of neurotransmitter-containing vesicles to the active release zones of the nerve terminal. The vesicles fuse with nerve terminal membranes and eventually rupture, probably due to the force generated by contracting neurofilaments. Once the vesicles rupture, the soluble contents of the vesicle including the neurotransmitter are released into the synapse such that they can diffuse across the cleft and the transmitter interacts with receptors located on postsynaptic membranes. The binding of the neurotransmitter to these receptors causes changes in ionic conductances and activates intracellular processes in the receptive cell to effect responses. Finally, the action of the neurotransmitter is terminated by diffusion and inactivation processes that include degradatory enzymes and/or removal of the neurotransmitter from the synapse by uptake into neurons or surrounding cells.

CRITERIA FOR NEUROTRANSMITTERS

There are five criteria that must be met for a chemical to be designated a neurotransmitter. On the basis of our understanding of the events underlying synaptic transmission, these criteria are as follows: The first criterion is that *the putative transmitter must be present within presynaptic nerve terminals* and, in most instances, be contained within vesicles. As a corollary, it is presumed that the neurotransmitter is actually synthesized within the nerve. This can usually be demonstrated following the development of antibodies that react with enzymes involved in the synthetic process.

The second criterion follows from the first, namely, that *the putative neurotransmitter must be released from the nerves during stimulation.* Since this is likely to occur via exocytosis, it is further assumed that such release will be calcium-dependent. Although not an explicitly stated criterion, most neurotransmitter systems exhibit another important property related to release and referred to as *synthesis–secretion coupling.* For neurons to continue to release transmitter when the frequency of stimulation is increased, synthetic processes must increase as well, and such adaptations must occur rapidly lest the neuron be depleted of the transmitter. In the short term this is usually achieved by increasing the activity of the rate-limiting step in the synthesis of the neurotransmitter; this step may be an enzyme such as tyrosine hydroxylase for the catecholamines or the neuronal uptake of an essential precursor such as choline for acetylcholine (see Chapter 6). Long-term mechanisms that respond to chronic changes in neuronal firing also exist. These mechanisms usually involve increased gene transcription for essential enzymes or other proteins involved in the synthetic process.

Since neurotransmitters must interact with receptors to elicit a biological response, the third criterion requires that *high-affinity receptors be present on the surface of cells responsive to the putative neurotransmitter.* The presence of such receptors is usually verified by the use of radioligand binding and quantitative autoradiography together with techniques that assess changes in membrane conductances or biochemical second-messenger systems (see Chapter 4). In a few instances, the detection of binding sites or receptors has preceded the discovery of an endogenous neurotransmitter that interacts with these sites. The best example of such an occurrence was a consequence of the report that the mammalian brain apparently contained receptors for the opiate-derived drug morphine (see Chapter 20). On the basis of this observation it was suggested that the brain might produce its own morphine-like compounds that were the endogenous ligands for this receptor. Such speculation was correct, and it was not long after the discovery of the morphine receptor that the endogenous opiates—the endorphins, dynorphins, and enkephalins—were isolated and confirmed as neurotransmitters.

For neurotransmitters to retain their information-carrying capacity in the nervous system, it is necessary both that their release occur only during nerve stimulation and that their duration of action be terminated soon after release has ceased. This latter quality forms the basis of the fourth criterion, namely, that there be *mechanisms for the inactivation of neurotransmitters in or around the vicinity of the synapse.* Inactivation of neurotransmitter action usually results from degradation by enzymes or from the removal of the neurotransmitter from the synapse by diffusion or by specific uptake mechanisms; such uptake may occur into both neuronal and nonneuronal cells. Moreover, in some neurotransmitter systems, degradatory enzymes and uptake mechanisms act in a cooperative fashion. For example, when catecholamines are released into the synapse, they are recaptured by neurons via high-affinity uptake systems. Once inside the neuron, the catecholamine can be repackaged into vesicles for later release or, alternatively, be deaminated by the intraneuronal enzyme monoamine oxidase. Hence, reuptake of neurotransmitter can help to conserve the transmitter for later use, thus ensuring biological economy.

The fifth and final criterion is the most important of all and was referred to earlier as *synaptic mimicry.* To fulfill this criterion it is necessary to demonstrate that the neurotransmitter has a functional effect that mimics effects induced by stimulation of the nerve that contains the putative transmitter. These experiments usually involve stimulation of the nerve and recording of postsynaptic potentials. The putative transmitter is then applied to responsive cells in the absence of stimulation and responses are once again recorded. If the neurotransmitter mediates the response, its functional effects should be indistinguishable from those induced by stimulation. Moreover, synaptic responses should be obtained with exogenous application of transmitter at levels that approximate those resulting from endogenous release. This experimental strategy should sound familiar because it is the same approach employed by Dale and colleagues when they demonstrated that ACh was involved in synaptic transmission at the neuromuscular junction.

GENERAL CLASSES OF NEUROTRANSMITTERS

In the last decade, the number of candidate neurotransmitters has more than tripled. The establishment of a set of criteria for determining when a given chemical substance in the nervous system actually functions as a neurotransmitter has greatly facilitated the search for new transmitters. Fortunately, while the number of identified transmitters is increasing, these newly described compounds have joined the ranks of previously established neurotransmitters so that all known transmitters can be conveniently classified into three main categories. Each of these categories is based on the common structural and functional properties of its members. This chapter will conclude with a brief review of these three types of transmitters to prepare the reader for a more complete discussion in subsequent chapters.

All known neurotransmitters fall into the same three categories. The simplest category is that of the amino acid neurotransmitters (see Chapter 7). Amino acid neurotransmitters are the most prevalent type of transmitter and may be present in as many as 80% of the synapses in the mammalian nervous system. Amino acids are actually present in all cells as a consequence of ongoing metabolic processes. However, in neurons that utilize amino acids as neurotransmitters, there appears to be a mechanism that permits these cells to shunt some portion of the amino acids away from the metabolic cascades to a functional pool—a process that is likely to involve sequestration of the amino acid into synaptic vesicles for stimulation-induced release. In still other instances, however, slight modifications of amino acids may occur in neurons, resulting in another transmitter compound that remains classified as an amino acid. The best-understood example of this scenario is the decarboxylation of glutamate that results in the intraneuronal production of γ-aminobutyric acid (GABA). Thus, in some neurons, an otherwise excitatory amino acid neurotransmitter, glutamate, is modified by the enzyme glutamic acid decarboxylase to produce one of the major inhibitory amino acid neurotransmitters—GABA (see Chapter 7).

In other neurons, amino acids are concentrated within the cell and used as substrates for the production of neurotransmitters. These amino acids are not themselves neurotransmitters. Instead, they are modified by a series of intraneuronal enzymes to produce the *monoamines.* As a class, the monoamines include the catecholamines, dopamine, norepinephrine, and epinephrine, as well as the major indoleamine, serotonin. This class includes some of the most-studied neurotransmitters that figure prominently in neurological and psychiatric diseases (see Chapters 17–19, 22, and 23), despite the fact that only a small percentage of central synapses actually employs a monoamine as a neurotransmitter. Acetylcholine synthesized from choline is a biogenic amine (see Chapter 6).

The final class of neurotransmitters is the collection of amino acids that compose the *peptides.* This is the most numerous class of neurotransmitters and exhibits tremendous structural diversity, with members containing as few as three amino acids and as many as 50 or more. Regardless of their eventual size, the production of peptide neurotransmitters is different from that of other classic transmitters because it begins with a large precursor molecule, called a *preproprotein,*

that is an initial gene product (see Chapter 8). This large protein is then cleaved into smaller fragments that individually can function as neurotransmitters. Some of this enzymatic cleavage can actually take place intravesicularly. Thus, many neurons possess the capacity to generate families of functionally and structurally related peptide neurotransmitters. Peptides also appear to be present in a relatively small proportion of synapses in the central nervous system compared to the widespread distribution of the amino acids. In addition, peptides have been colocalized within nerve cells that also contain a more classic neurotransmitter such as a biogenic amine. Moreover, the two transmitter substances are localized in different types of vesicles that release their respective contents in response to different frequencies of nerve stimulation. Thus, one or both types of neurotransmitter may be released under different physiological conditions, further increasing the communicative capacity of these unique synapses.

SUMMARY

The fundamental unit of the nervous system is the nerve cell or neuron. All neurons possess unique anatomical and biochemical properties that permit these cells to (1) receive and integrate electrochemical signals from other neurons or sensory cells in the periphery, (2) transmit these electrochemical signals over long distances, and (3) release chemicals referred to as neurotransmitters that activate or inhibit other neurons or effector cells located across the synapse. The chemical mediation of such synaptic transmission is now well accepted. Briefly, synaptic transmission begins with the entry of calcium into the nerve terminal triggered by depolarization. Calcium facilitates the fusion of neurotransmitter-containing vesicles with the terminal membrane such that the vesicle ruptures and releases the transmitter into the synaptic cleft. The liberated transmitter can then interact with receptors located on adjacent cells. Based on this understanding of the cellular events underlying synaptic transmission, it has been possible to establish a set of five criteria to aid in the unequivocal verification of putative transmitters in the nervous system, as well as to facilitate the continued identification of neurotransmitters yet to be discovered.

BIBLIOGRAPHY

Original Articles

Dale HH, Feldberg W, Vogt M. Release of acetylcholine at voluntary motor nerve endings. *J Physiol.* London: 1936;86:353–380.

Katz B, Miledi R. The development of acetylcholine sensitivity in nerve-free segments of skeletal muscle. *J Physiol.* London: 1964;170:389–396.

Katz B, Miledi R. The release of acetylcholine from nerve endings by graded electric pulses. *Proc Roy Soc London* 1967;B167:23–38.

Katz B, Miledi R. The timing of calcium action during neuromuscular transmission. *J Physiol.* London: 1967;189:535–544.

Loewi O. On the humoral propagation of cardiac nerve action. *Pflugers Arch* 1921;189:239–242.

Loewi O, Navratil E. On the humoral propagation of cardiac nerve action: the fate of the vagus substance. *Pflugers Arch* 1926;214:678–688.

Books and Reviews

Bernard C. (Trans. HC Greene). *An introduction to the study of experimental medicine.* New York: Dover; 1957.

Dale HH. *Adventures in physiology, with excursions into autopharmacology, a selection from the scientific publications of Sir Henry Hallett Dale.* London: Pergamon Press; 1953.

Erulkar SD. Chemically mediated synaptic transmission: an overview. In: Siegel GJ, Agranoff BW, Albers RW, Molinoff PB, eds. *Basic neurochemistry,* 5th ed. New York: Raven Press; 1994 (in press).

Kandel ER, Schwartz JH. *Principles of neural science.* 2nd Ed. New York: Elsevier; 1985.

Katz B. *Nerve, muscle and synapse.* New York: McGraw-Hill; 1966.

Katz B. *The release of neural transmitter substances.* Liverpool: Liverpool University Press; 1969.

Loewi O. *An autobiographic sketch: perspectives in biology and medicine.* London: Pergamon Press; 1960.

von Helmholtz H. *Popular scientific lectures.* London: Longmans; 1889.

Receptors and Effector Mechanisms

Perry B. Molinoff

I need not recount in full the theory I have put forward to account for these facts. But two points in it must be mentioned. First that two special substances at least (receptive substances) are present in the neural region of the muscle, and that nerve impulses can only cause contraction by acting on a receptive substance. Secondly that the receptive substances form more or less easily dissociable compounds.

J. N. Langley,
On the contraction of muscle, chiefly in relation to the presence of "receptive" substances: Part IV., The effect of curare and of some other substances on the nicotine response of the sartorious and gastrocnemius muscles of the frog.
J. Physiol. 1909;39:236

- At least three major classes of neurotransmitters exist.

- Although there are many receptors for each of the conventional transmitters, the number of subtypes is limited.

- The distribution of receptors can be assessed by quantitative autoradiography.

- Direct binding assays are assays in which tissue homogenates are incubated with a radioligand that has a high affinity for the receptor.

- Indirect binding assays are used to study the interactions of competing nonradiolabeled drugs with receptors.

- Receptor subtypes exist in a wide variety of neurotransmitter receptor systems.

- One superfamily involves receptors that cause changes in membrane permeability.

- Another superfamily is characterized by a specific role of guanine nucleotides in mediating the physiological effects associated with these receptors.

- Many hormones and neurotransmitters act through changes in levels of cAMP and other second messengers.

- Increases in the turnover of membrane phospholipids generate biologically active second messengers.

In this chapter, receptors are identified as belonging to one of a limited number of families. In most cases, receptors act to change membrane permeability or to activate one of several second-messenger systems. In addition to identifying classes of transmitters and second-messenger systems, this chapter describes various approaches for the quantitative study of receptors and their subtypes.

A receptor is defined as the membrane constituent that has the ability to recognize a specific neurotransmitter or hormone. We know that receptors for neurotransmitters, hormones, and drugs exist on the surface membrane of a variety of classes of excitable cells and that occupancy of a receptor by an appropriate agonist results in an identifiable physiological response. Operationally, receptors are defined in terms of the physiological response with which they are associated. Radiolabeled compounds (*ligands*) are now available that permit the direct demonstration of particular classes of receptors in biochemical assays. This approach makes it possible to study the direct interaction between a drug and the receptor in question, whereas with the use of a physiological response to identify and/or characterize a receptor, there are a number of intervening steps between binding of the ligand and elicitation of the response. These intervening steps can markedly affect the presumed properties of the receptor. On the other hand, the interaction of a radioactively labeled substance with a constituent present in a preparation only documents the existence of a binding site, and such data, in the absence of an observed physiological response, cannot be taken as evidence for the existence of a particular type of receptor.

It is well recognized that receptive substances exist on the cell surface. Although at the beginning of this century, the process of chemical neurotransmission had not yet been described, the British physiologists John Langley and Sir Henry Dale and their colleagues suggested that receptive substances must exist on the surface of excitable cells. These and other investigators recognized that many drugs had the ability to excite nerves or muscles, and they hypothesized that there must be an element on the cell that is able to recognize the drug. In 1923, the German physiologist Otto Loewi demonstrated the release of chemical substances from a perfused frog heart (see Chapter 3). In mammals, including humans, acetylcholine and norepinephrine are the inhibitory and excitatory neurotransmitters acting on the heart.

Transmitters or drugs that interact with a given type of receptor and elicit a particular class of response are usually called *agonists.* In contrast, substances that interact with the same or an overlapping site on the receptor and block the effects of an agonist without inducing responses of their own are called *antagonists.* There are now many examples of agents that interact at the same site to cause a partial stimulation of response, and such substances are termed *partial agonists.* They are usually characterized in terms of the level of response observed relative to that of the most efficacious agonist. In most but not all cases the maximal response is observed with the naturally occurring endogenous agonist.

CLASSES OF NEUROTRANSMITTERS

At least three major classes of neurotransmitters exist. The three major classes of neurotransmitters are described as follows (Table

Biological Bases of Brain Function and Disease, edited by Alan Frazer, Perry B. Molinoff, and Andrew Winokur. Raven Press, Ltd., New York © 1994.

1) (see Chapter 3): The so-called *biogenic amines* include acetylcholine (ACh) and the catecholamines dopamine, norepinephrine, and epinephrine. Epinephrine (see Chapter 6) is a hormone released from the adrenal medulla, and it may also be a transmitter in the central nervous system (CNS). Dopamine, in addition to being a precursor for the synthesis of norepinephrine and epinephrine, is a naturally occurring transmitter that has significant physiological effects in the CNS (see Chapters 6 and 23). Other biogenic amines include ACh, which is the predominant neurotransmitter at ganglionic sympathetic and parasympathetic synapses and at synapses on skeletal muscles, and serotonin (5-hydroxytryptamine; 5-HT), which also appears to be a neurotransmitter, particularly in the CNS (see Chapter 6). A variety of *amino acids* (see Chapter 7) serve as neurotransmitters, particularly in the CNS. Glutamate (and aspartate) are major excitatory neurotransmitters, while γ-aminobutyric acid (GABA) and glycine are major inhibitory transmitters. A large number of *peptides* (see Chapter 8) have now been shown to be transmitters in both the CNS and the gastrointestinal tract. The complexity resulting from the large number of transmitters is exacerbated by the existence of multiple classes of receptors responding to each of the known transmitters. Subtypes of receptors for biogenic amines are discussed in Chapter 6, of receptors for amino acids in Chapter 7, and of peptides in Chapter 8 (Table 1).

TABLE 1. *Classes of neurotransmitters*

Biogenic amines
    Dopamine, norepinephrine, epinephrine
    Acetylcholine
    Serotonin
Amino acids
    GABA
    Glutamate
    Glycine
Peptides
    Substance P
    Endorphin
    Somatostatin

GABA, γ-aminobutyric acid.

Although there are many receptors for each of the conventional transmitters, the number of subtypes is limited. Identification of receptor subtypes was initially based on the differing physiological effects observed in studies, for example, of naturally occurring agonists such as epinephrine and norepinephrine. This approach was used by Ahlquist in 1948. In his experiments, differing responses to a series of naturally occurring and endogenously prepared agents led to the conclusion that there are two principal subtypes of receptor for catecholamines, named α- and β-adrenergic receptors. Similar studies led Lands and his colleagues to identify responses mediated by β-adrenergic receptors as being due to activation of β_1 or β_2 receptors. Responses mediated by β_1 receptors include the positive effects of catecholamines acting on the heart while responses mediated by β_2 receptors include relaxation of smooth and bronchiolar smooth muscle. A different approach was taken by Langer and his colleagues. They showed that the α-adrenergic receptor responsible for contraction of smooth muscle had different properties from an α-adrenergic receptor on the presynaptic nerve terminal which modulated the release of norepinephrine. The former receptor was called an α_1-adrenergic receptor while the presynaptic autoreceptor was termed an α_2-adrenergic receptor. More recently, pharmacological studies have been carried out using agonists and antagonists that show different degrees of selectivity for various types of receptor. Studies of the binding of radioligands and of receptor-linked second-messenger systems have made it possible to quantitatively describe the properties of receptors. Kebabian and Calne noted that in some systems dopamine activated adenylyl cyclase while in other systems it had no effect. The receptor linked to stimulation of adenylyl cyclase was called a D_1 receptor, while that which in initial studies had no effect on adenylyl cyclase was called a D_2 receptor. It is now known that there are multiple subtypes of dopamine receptor, some of which are linked to stimulation of adenylyl cyclase activity and some to inhibition, while others act through second-messenger systems that have yet to be identified. Ultimately, the tools of the molecular biologist have made it possible to clone and sequence receptors and the DNA encoding specific types of receptors. It is now clear that receptors are highly conserved across species. The molecular biological approach has confirmed the existence of receptor subtypes as suggested by the results of studies of the pharmacological and biochemical properties of receptors. On the other hand, cloning of receptor genes has revealed the existence of new subtypes of receptors and has identified potential therapeutic targets for the treatment of neuropsychiatric disease (see Chapter 23).

APPROACHES FOR THE STUDY OF RECEPTORS

The distribution of receptors can be assessed by quantitative autoradiography. To utilize the technique of quantitative autoradiography, sections of tissue are incubated with a radioactively labeled compound in either the presence or absence of a competing drug. After binding of the radioligand has reached equilibrium, the sections are washed and then apposed to x-ray film. After an appropriate exposure, the x-ray film is developed, and the specific regions within the tissue that contain binding sites for the radioligand are identified.

Binding assays carried out with homogenates of a particular tissue or brain region provide a means of assessing the biochemical and pharmacological properties of a receptor. For this technique, a radioligand with appropriate specificity labeled to a high specific activity must be available. The most useful isotopes for these types of experiments are ^{125}I and ^{3}H. ^{14}C is not useful for studies of receptor biochemistry because its specific activity is far too low. In practice, membranes are incubated with an appropriate radioligand either in the absence or presence of a competing ligand. Binding observed in the absence of a competing ligand is called *total binding,* that observed in the presence of a competing

ligand is called *nonspecific binding,* and the difference between total and nonspecific binding represents *specific binding* to the receptor. Nonspecific binding can be due to ionic or hydrophobic interactions or can be due to other specifiable constituents of the cell including biosynthetic or degradative enzymes or proteins included in the storage or release of the transmitter. In some cases, biochemical responses can be linked directly to activation of specific receptors. Examples of such responses include activation or inhibition of the enzyme adenylyl cyclase, activation of phospholipase C resulting in increased intracellular levels of inositol polyphosphates and inorganic calcium, and changes in the conductance of the membrane for specific ions. In some cases, physiological responses mediated by particular receptors can be assessed, and it is sometimes possible to define behavioral responses (see Chapter 14) associated with activation of particular receptors or receptor subtypes.

Direct binding assays are assays in which tissue homogenates are incubated with a radioligand that has a high affinity for the receptor. In a direct binding assay, the amount of radioligand bound is graphed as a function of drug concentration (Fig. 1). Nonspecific binding, defined by carrying out duplicate assays in the presence of a saturating concentration of a competing drug, is in most cases linear (nonsaturating). The two parameters of particular interest are the B_{max}, which is the *density of binding sites* or the *amount of radioligand bound at an infinite concentration of a radioligand,* and the K_d value, which is the *concentration of radioligand that occupies half of the receptors.* In practice, it is difficult to determine the B_{max} directly because nonspecific binding increases (see Fig. 1) as the concentration of ligand is increased. Thus, at the high concentrations of radioligand necessary to define the B_{max}, the data become relatively less reliable. An alternative approach is to transform the data by the method of Scatchard. In this approach, the ratio of the amount of radioligand bound to the free concentration of ligand is plotted as a function of the amount of radioligand

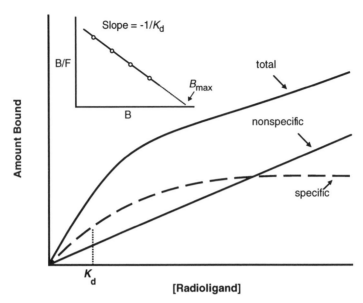

FIG. 1. Bound radioligand plotted as a function of radioligand concentration. Nonspecific binding is defined in the presence of a high concentration of a competing drug. Transformation of specific binding (----) by the method of Scatchard (*inset*) makes it possible to determine the K_d and B_{max}.

bound. In the simplest case, the data will fit a single straight line, the slope of which is $-1/K_d$; the intercept of the abscissa provides a measure of the B_{max}. Intuitively, the ratio of bound to free will become zero as free becomes exceedingly large, and it is exactly under this condition that the amount bound will approach B_{max} (Fig. 1).

Indirect binding assays are used to study the interactions of competing nonradiolabeled drugs with receptors. The direct approach described above is feasible if a radioligand is available with high specific activity and the appropriate affinity and specificity to label the site in question. In many cases, an investigator will be interested in studying the interactions of a number of competing drugs with the receptor in question despite the fact that the competing drugs have not been radiolabeled. An *indirect binding assay* is used in this case. To carry out an experiment of this type, tissue is incubated with a constant amount of radioligand in the presence of increasing amounts of a competing drug (inhibitor). The IC_{50} value, defined as the concentration of the inhibiting drug that blocks

one-half of the specific binding of the radioligand, is determined (Fig. 2). It should be noted that the IC_{50} will increase if the concentration of the radioligand is increased. To eliminate the ambiguity that would result from comparison of IC_{50} values obtained in different laboratories using different drugs as radioligands or using different concentrations of the same radioligand, IC_{50} values are converted to K_i values by dividing the IC_{50} value by the factor $(1 + L/K_d)$. In this equation, L is the concentration of radioligand and K_d is a measure of the affinity of the receptor for the radioligand determined independently by saturation/Scatchard analysis (see above).

The overall reaction being utilized in studies of the binding of a radioligand is

$$D + R \underset{k_{-1}}{\overset{k_1}{\rightleftarrows}} DR$$

In this equation, D refers to the concentration of a drug or radioligand, R is the concentration of receptors, and DR represents the concentration of the drug–receptor complex.

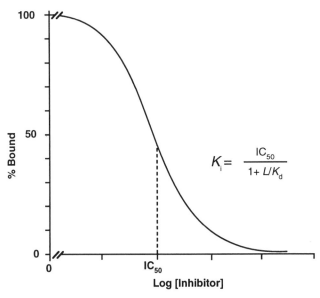

FIG. 2. Analysis of competition data. The IC_{50} is determined by inhibiting the binding of a fixed concentration of a radioligand (L) by increasing concentrations of an inhibitor. Since the IC_{50} is a function of the concentration of the radioligand, it is converted to a K_i value using the equation $K_i = IC_{50}/(1 + L/K_d)$ as described by Cheng and Prusoff. In this equation the K_d of the receptor for the radioligand is determined as described in Figure 1.

As previously noted, K_d is the concentration of drug (or radioligand) that occupies one-half of the total available receptors. Thus, when the concentration of D is equal to K_d, the concentration of free receptor (R) is equal to the concentration of drug–receptor complex $[DR]$. Alternative descriptions of K_d are as follows: (1) K_d is equal to $[DR]/([R] + [D])$. (2) The kinetics of the interaction are such that K_d is equal to the ratio of the rate constant for dissociation to the rate constant for association, $(k_{-1})/(k_{+1})$. (3) Finally, a general equation can be written that relates the amount of drug bound to B_{max}, K_d, and D. This equation is

$$\text{Bound} = \frac{B_{max} \times D}{K_d + D}$$

The inclusion of a competitive inhibitor as in an indirect binding assay results in a change in the apparent K_d value. Specifically, the observed apparent K_d value is increased by a factor of $(1 + i/K_i)$, where i is the concentration of competitor and K_i is a measure of the affinity of the receptor for the competing drug. The basic equation becomes

$$\text{Bound} = \frac{B_{max} + D}{D + K_d(1 + i/K_i)}$$

Receptor subtypes exist in a wide variety of neurotransmitter receptor systems. Receptor subtypes have been identified pharmacologically, biochemically, and, more recently, in studies using the tools of molecular biology. As noted above, a finite number of receptor subtypes exist for a given neurotransmitter. For example, there are now three subtypes of β-adrenergic receptor and five known subtypes of muscarinic cholinergic receptor and dopamine receptor. It is virtually certain that additional subtypes will be identified. Among the generalizations that can be made are that the properties of receptors are highly conserved across species and that multiple classes of receptor for the same transmitter may coexist in the same tissue. Receptor subtypes may mediate the same or different physiological responses, and they may act through the same or different biochemical second-messenger systems. Studies of the effects of lesions and of chronic and acute drug administration have revealed that in some cases receptor subtypes are independently regulated in regions of the mammalian CNS. Pharmacological and biochemical approaches involving, for example, studies of the binding of radioligands are probably sufficient to resolve systems in which there are two subtypes of receptor for a particular transmitter. These techniques are unlikely to be sufficient in situations where there are multiple subtypes such as the five existing subtypes of muscarinic cholinergic receptor. A different approach involves expressing the gene for a particular subtype of receptor in a cell that does not normally express that receptor. It is then possible to carry out pharmacological and biochemical studies to define the properties of the receptor in question. Such studies can also permit, for example, experiments designed to identify the class(es) of G protein and/or G-protein subunit that are normally associated with a particular transmitter receptor subtype.

Biochemical approaches for the study of receptors and biochemical receptor-linked effector systems have been described above. Reference has also been made to the existence of receptor subtypes. The basic equation relating the amount of a drug or radioligand bound to a receptor as a function of the concentration of drug, the density of receptors (B_{max}), and the affinity of the receptor for the drug (K_d) is given above. This system can be generalized to account for situations in which there are multiple classes of receptors:

$$\text{Bound} = \frac{B_{max_1} \cdot D}{K_{d_1} + D} + \frac{B_{max_2} \cdot D}{K_{d_2} + D} \cdots$$

Mathematical analyses of studies of radioligand binding in systems containing multiple receptor subtypes are similar to those described above for the simple system in which there is only a single class of receptor. For example, experiments can be carried out in which the amount of ligand bound is plotted as a function of the concentration of radioligand (Fig. 3). If the radioligand has a markedly higher affinity (lower K_d value) for one subtype than the other and if both subtypes coexist, the saturation isotherm will approach equilibrium less rapidly than in the simple system in which there is only a single class of binding site. More obvious effects are observed if the data are transformed by the method of Scatchard. In the presence of more than one receptor subtype, a markedly curvilinear Scatchard plot will result (Fig. 3, inset). If an experiment is carried out analogous to the indirect binding assay described above in which a fixed concentration of a nonselective radioligand is incubated with increasing concentrations of a selective competing ligand, then one may observe a marked decrease in the slope of the competition curve (Fig. 4). Experiments of either type can be analyzed

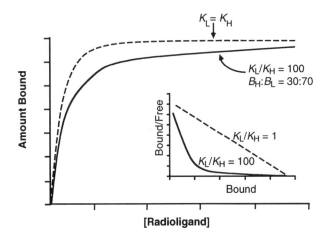

FIG. 3. Bound radioligand plotted as a function of radioligand concentration. Data are plotted for a single class of sites (----) and for two classes of sites (——). K_L/K_H is the ratio of dissociation constants such that the K_d value of the sites with a low affinity for the radioligand (K_L, 70% of the total) is 100 times that of the sites with a high affinity for the radioligand (K_H, 30% of the total). B_H and B_L define the relative densities of sites with high and low affinity for the radioligand. **Inset:** The same data are plotted by the method of Scatchard.

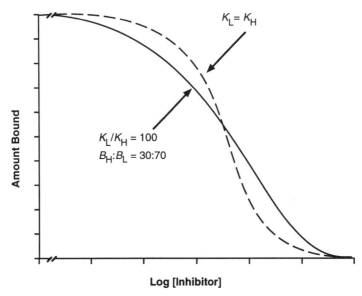

FIG. 4. Analysis of untransformed competition data. The proportion of receptor subtypes can be estimated by inhibiting the binding of a fixed concentration of a nonselective radioligand by increasing concentrations of a selective inhibitor. K_L, K_H, B_H, and B_L are defined as in Fig. 3 except that in this case H and L refer to the affinity of the sites for a selective inhibitor of the binding of the nonselective radioligand. Data are plotted when $K_L = K_H$ (one site, ---) and when $K_L/K_H = 100$ (two sites, ——).

mathematically using the technique of nonlinear least-squares regression analysis of untransformed data or the data can be transformed (e.g., by the method of Scatchard), and then linear least-squares analysis can be applied.

RECEPTOR SUPERFAMILIES

Results of physiological, pharmacological, and biochemical studies of receptors led to the conclusion that not only are there multiple classes of receptors relating to specific transmitters, but multiple subtypes of receptors are activated by each of the known transmitters. The seemingly endless complexity engendered by this multiplication of receptors and receptor subtypes has been increased by the results of molecular biological studies of a variety of classes of neurotransmitter receptors. On the other hand, it appears that receptors for neurotransmitters belong to one of two superfamilies that can be distinguished in terms of their basic mode of action.

One superfamily involves receptors that cause changes in membrane permeability. The first superfamily, exemplified by the nicotinic cholinergic receptor (Fig. 5), includes receptors that when activated result in changes in the permeability of the membrane to one or more ions. These receptors are themselves ionophores (ion channels) so that the interaction of an agonist with a nicotinic receptor results in a change in the conformation of the receptor such that ions can flow down their concentration gradients. It is now known that the nicotinic cholinergic receptor (Fig. 5) is a pentamer made up of five subunits. Two of these, the so-called α subunits, are identical, and they are relatively homologous in sequence to the β, γ, and δ subunits. The nicotinic cholinergic receptor is thus a pentameric protein with the structure $\alpha_2\beta\gamma\delta$ (Fig. 5). It is generally thought that the four hydrophobic sequences characteristic of each subunit represent transmembrance sequences. Knowledge of the sequence of the individual subunits and consideration of the results of site-specific mutagenesis in which

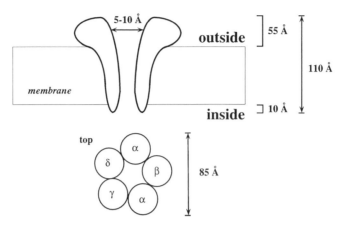

FIG. 5. Acetylcholine receptor geometry. The nicotinic acetylcholine receptor is composed of five subunits arranged in the shape of a doughnut. The relative stoichiometry of the subunits is $\alpha_2\beta\gamma\delta$.

carefully selected changes in amino acid sequences are engineered have made it possible to begin to identify specific regions of the receptor that contain the recognition site responsible for the binding of acetylcholine (ACh) and to investigate potential models for the change in the conformation of the receptor that results in increased permeability to cations. Another receptor, the so-called GABA$_A$ receptor, is clearly a member of the same family. The GABA$_A$ receptor is composed of three classes of subunit called α, β, and γ. The stoichiometry of the GABA$_A$ receptor appears to be $\alpha_2\beta\gamma$. It is interesting to note with regard to the GABA$_A$ receptor that multiple isoforms of all three subunits have been identified. These isoforms are independently distributed in regions of the CNS, raising the possibility of the existence of an enormous multiplicity of GABA$_A$ receptors. Other receptors directly linked to ion channels, such as glycine receptors and some of the receptors for excitatory amino acids, are also members of this receptor superfamily.

Another superfamily is characterized by a specific role of guanine nucleotides in mediating the physiological effects associated with these receptors. Initially, an obligatory role of guanosine triphosphate (GTP) was identified in mediating the effects of receptors acting through stimulation of adenylyl cyclase.

More recently, it was demonstrated that GTP also plays a critical role in the effects of receptors that act to inhibit adenylyl cyclase or to activate phospholipase C and thus phosphoinositide turnover. In addition, changes in membrane permeability have in some cases been shown to require the interaction of GTP with particular G proteins. In the case of the nicotinic cholinergic receptor, the receptor contains inherent within its structure the apparatus necessary for mediation of a biochemical response. In the case of effects mediated by G-protein–linked receptors, the receptor does not have biological activity in its own right. Rather, occupancy of the receptor by an appropriate agonist results in the binding of GTP to a G protein, and it is the GTP-liganded G protein that induces a physiological or biochemical response. The effect of light on rhodopsin is mediated by a G protein called transducin. At least 30 other members of the G-protein–linked receptor superfamily have been cloned and sequenced. Members of this superfamily appear to share a highly conserved general structure (Fig. 6) and have been shown to contain seven hydrophobic sequences of amino acids, usually 22 to 25 in number, consistent with the protein crossing the membrane seven times. Comparison of the sequences of the multiple members of this G-

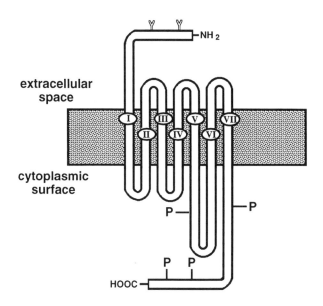

FIG. 6. Proposed structure of G-protein–linked receptors. The G-protein–linked receptors share a common structure with seven membrane-crossing helices (I–VII). Consensus sites for glycosylation (Y) are found on the extracellular amino terminus, and sites at which phosphorylation may occur (P) are located on the carboxy tail and/or on the third intracellular loop.

protein–linked receptor family reveals a high degree of homology within the seven transmembrane regions. The two portions of the molecule that show the least homology are the large third intracellular loop connecting transmembrane regions 5 and 6 and the cytoplasmic carboxy terminus. Other structural features that are seen with most if not all of the members of this family are sites for N-linked glycosylation on the N-terminal portion of the molecule thought to be in the extracellular space and sites for protein phosphorylation mediated by a variety of protein kinases on the carboxy terminus and the third intracellular loop. It has been difficult to link specific amino acid residues or specific portions of the molecule with the biological functions of these proteins. However, results of experiments using antireceptor antibodies, proteolytic enzymes, ligands with a photoactivatable group, and site-directed mutagenesis have suggested that in several cases the binding site for the ligand is within the plane of the membrane and includes parts of several of the transmembrane α helices. Portions of the third intracellular loop and the carboxyl tail appear to be involved in the interaction between the receptor and a guanine nucleotide-binding protein.

SECOND-MESSENGER SYSTEMS

Despite the ever increasing number of receptors and receptor subtypes, only a relatively limited number of receptor-mediated effector systems appear to have evolved (Table 2). These include increases and decreases in adenylyl cyclase activity, increases in

TABLE 2. *Receptor-mediated effector systems*

1. Increase in cyclic AMP formation
   a. D_1 receptors (also D_5)
   b. β-Adrenergic receptors
2. Decrease in cyclic AMP formation
   a. α_2-Adrenergic receptors
   b. D_2 receptors
   c. Muscarinic cholinergic receptors
3. Increase in phosphatidylinositol turnover
   a. α_1-Adrenergic receptors and muscarinic cholinergic receptors
   b. Phosphatidylinositol is converted into a polyphosphoinositide which is broken down into diacylglycerol and inositol trisphosphate
   c. Diacylglycerol activates protein kinase C
   d. Inositol trisphosphate releases Ca^{++} from internal stores
4. Changes in membrane permeability
   a. Increased permeability to Na^+ causes depolarization
   b. Increased permeability to Cl^- causes hyperpolarization
   c. G-protein–mediated changes in permeability to K^+ and to Ca^{++}

phosphatidylinositol turnover with liberation of inositol trisphosphate and diacylglycerol, and changes in membrane permeability. In this chapter, changes in cyclic AMP (cAMP) formation and in membrane phospholipid turnover are discussed, whereas changes in membrane permeability were discussed in Chapters 2 and 3.

Role of GTP–Binding Proteins

Many hormones and neurotransmitters act through changes in cAMP levels. The reactions involved in stimulation and inhibition of adenylyl cyclase activity are highly homologous. In several instances the same transmitter can interact with multiple receptor subtypes linked to changes in adenylyl cyclase activity. For example, dopamine (Fig. 7) can stimulate adenylyl cyclase activity through interaction with D_1 or D_5 receptors and inhibit it through interaction with D_2 receptors. D_3 and D_4 receptors are similar in sequence to D_2 receptors but have no effect on cAMP levels. Stimulation of enzyme activity results when an appropriate hormone interacts with the receptor, inducing formation of a ternary complex of agonist, receptor, and G protein. The G protein involved in stimulation of adenylyl cyclase is called G_s; it is a heterotrimeric protein containing α, β, and γ subunits. The α subunit contains a binding site for GTP, and the β and γ subunits are tightly coupled and are usually copurified. Interactions occurring within the ternary complex result in binding of GTP to the α subunit,

displacing guanosine diphosphate. The α subunit containing GTP is then able to interact with the catalytic moiety of adenylyl cyclase, activating the enzyme. Inactivation involves the hydrolysis of GTP by GTPase activity inherent in the α subunit. Nonhydrolyzable analogs of GTP, such as Gpp(NH)p, result in the persistent activation of adenylyl cyclase. Regardless of the mechanism through which adenylyl cyclase activity is increased, the net result is an increase in intracellular levels of cAMP which affect a variety of biological systems. Many of these effects are due to the ability of cAMP to bind to the regulatory subunit of an enzyme called protein kinase A. The catalytic subunit dissociates from the regulatory subunit and phosphorylates a variety of protein substrates. The phosphorylated proteins have biochemical properties different from those of nonphosphorylated homologs. Protein kinase A is one of a number of enzymes which, when activated by an appropriate stimulus, induce phosphorylation and a change in the properties of one or more substrate proteins (see below).

Similar mechanisms appear to account for the ability of hormones or transmitters to inhibit adenylyl cyclase activity. In particular, the interaction of an inhibitory hormone with the receptor induces formation of a ternary complex and the binding of GTP. The α subunit of G_i differs from the α subunit of G_s while the β/γ subunits appear to be identical. The specific mechanisms responsible for the inhibition of adenylyl cyclase have not yet been fully defined. It appears that $G_i \cdot GTP$ may interact specifically with the catalytic

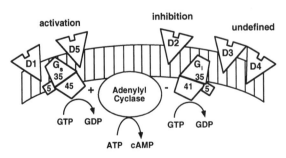

FIG. 7. Effect of dopamine on adenylyl cyclase activity. Stimulation and inhibition of adenylyl cyclase activity require binding of GTP to the α subunit of G_s and G_i, respectively.

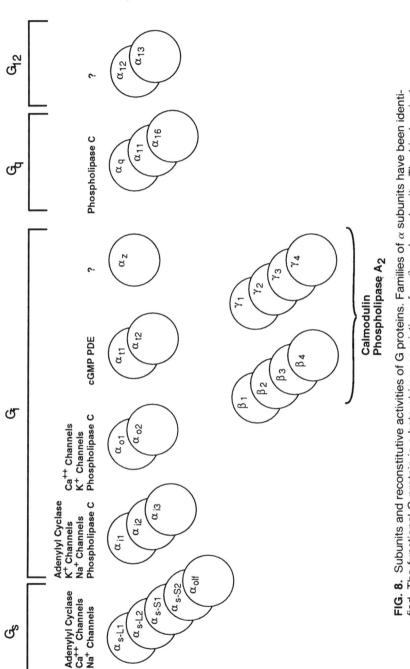

FIG. 8. Subunits and reconstitutive activities of G proteins. Families of α subunits have been identified. The functional G protein is a heterotrimer consisting of α, β, and γ subunits. The biochemical specificity of a G protein is largely a consequence of the presence of a particular α subunit. The $\beta\gamma$ heterodimer has been shown, however, to bind to Ca^{++}/calmodulin and to activate phospholipase A_2. Reproduced with permission of David R. Manning.

subunit of adenylyl cyclase, and, in addition, the β/γ subunits of G_i can by mass action interact with the α subunit of G_s, preventing activation of adenylyl cyclase. It should be stressed that there are multiple forms of each of the major subunits of G protein. At the present time there are nearly 20 known forms of G_α. There are also multiple forms of the β and γ subunits of G protein (Fig. 8). It has been possible to associate physiological or biochemical functions with some of the subunits of the various classes of G protein. It has not yet been possible to ascribe specific functions to specific complexes of particular α, β, and γ subunits. Indeed, it is not at all clear that specific trimeric complexes are found in particular classes of cells linked with particular receptors or particular biochemical responses. A useful biochemical tool involves a substance called islet-activating protein (IAP), isolated from the toxin of the bacteria *Bordetella pertussis.* IAP catalyzes the ADP ribosylation of $G_{i\alpha}$, $G_{o\alpha}$, and, to a lesser extent, $G_{t\alpha}$. Unlike choleratoxin, which results in the persistent activation of G_s, IAP results in persistent inhibition of the effects mediated by the specific G proteins that are ribosylated.

Increases in the turnover of membrane phospholipids generate biologically active second messengers. A second major biochemical second-messenger system that is receptor-controlled and involves a guanine nucleotide-binding protein is represented by receptors that activate the hydrolysis of membrane phosphoinositides. The principal reaction involves the enzyme phospholipase C, which catalyzes the cleavage of phosphatidylinositol bisphosphate (Fig. 9), yielding diacylglycerol and inositol trisphosphate. Both of the cleavage products of phosphatidylinositol bisphosphate are biologically active. Inositol trisphosphate causes mobilization of calcium from the endoplasmic reticulum, resulting in marked increases in intracellular levels of calcium. Among other effects of changing intracellular calcium is activation of a family of calcium-dependent protein kinases. The other product of the reaction, diacylglycerol, is thought to remain dissolved in the plane of the membrane where it activates a protein kinase called protein kinase C. Phosphorylation of a variety of substrates of calcium-dependent protein kinases or protein kinase C results in marked changes in the properties of the cell. In many cases it has been shown that the activation of phospholipase C and cleavage of phosphatidylinositol bisphosphate requires GTP. In some, though not all, cases, this reaction is blocked by pretreatment of cells or tissues with IAP, again suggesting a role for G proteins. In other cases, effects of GTP on responses have been seen but IAP is without effect. These responses appear to be mediated by members of the G_q class.

It is tempting to distinguish the ion channel receptors from the G-protein–linked receptors on the basis of their ability to trans-

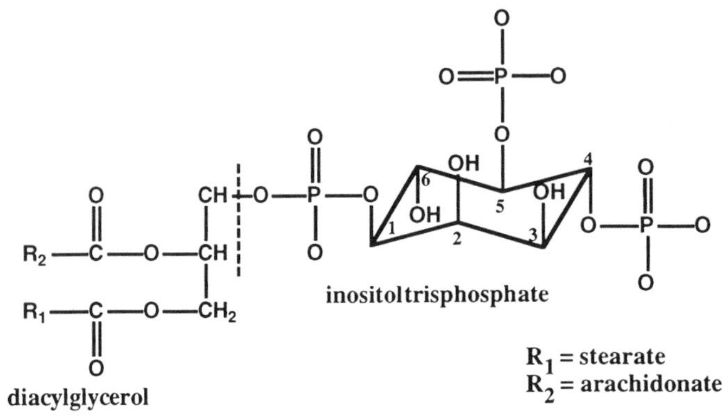

FIG. 9. Phosphatidylinositol bisphosphate. Receptor-mediated hydrolysis of phosphatidylinositol bisphosphate results in the liberation of diacylglycerol and inositol trisphosphate.

duce rapidly occurring changes in membrane permeability or conductance as compared to less rapid changes in the activity of an enzyme, whether it be adenylyl cyclase or phospholipase C. It is already clear, however, that this distinction represents a significant oversimplification. For example, there is now abundant evidence that a variety of transmitters can activate G proteins, resulting in changes in permeability to sodium, potassium, or calcium. These effects have been clearly shown to involve G proteins but they do not require activation of either adenylyl cyclase or phospholipase C, nor are they associated with changes in intracellular levels of cAMP, phosphatidylinositol bisphosphate, or diacylglycerol.

Additional effects of transmitters on membrane phospholipid pools result from the fact that enzymes such as phospholipase A_2 are regulated by cyclic nucleotides and calcium and cause release of arachidonic acid from membrane phospholipids. In addition, multiple enzymatic steps occur that result in the presence of multiple species of phosphatidylinositides. These molecules contain between one and four phosphates per molecule and express a variety of biological activities.

SUMMARY

The first studies involving in vitro binding assays with radioligands were carried out in the early 1970s. Since that time there has been an explosive growth in our understanding of receptors and receptor-linked effector mechanisms. We now know that there are a large number of transmitters, most of which have the ability to activate multiple subtypes of receptor. These receptors appear to fall into one of a limited number of superfamilies. In one of these superfamilies the receptor is itself an ion channel, while in the other the receptor is without inherent biological activity but functions through activation of a G protein which then initiates a biological response. A variety of second-messenger systems have been identified involving activation or inhibition of the enzyme adenylyl cyclase, activation of phospholipase C or

phospholipase A2, or changes in membrane conductance. The interplay between the multiple subtypes of receptor and the multiple classes of GTP-binding protein undoubtedly contributes to the complexity of the mammalian CNS.

BIBLIOGRAPHY

Original Articles

Hill AV. The possible effects of the aggregation of the molecules of haemoglobin on its dissociation curves. *J Physiol (London)* 1910;40:iv–vii.

Hokin LE, Hokin MR. Effects of acetylcholine on the turnover of phosphoryl units in individual phospholipids of pancreas slices and brain cortex slices. *Biochim Biophys Acta* 1955;18:102–110.

Books and Reviews

Agranoff BW, Fisher SK. Phosphoinositides. In: Siegel GJ, Agranoff BW, Albers RW, Molinoff PB, eds. *Basic neurochemistry,* 5th ed. New York: Raven Press; 1994 (in press).

Berridge MJ. Inositol trisphosphate and diacylglycerol: two interacting second messengers. *Annu Rev Biochem* 1987;56:159–193.

Guy HR, Hucho F. The ion channel of the nicotinic acetylcholine-receptor. *Trends Neurosci* 1987;10: 318–321.

Hepler JR, Gilman AG. G proteins. *Trends Biochem Sci* 1992;17:383–387.

Kobilka B. Adrenergic receptors as models for G protein-coupled receptors. *Annu Rev Neurosci* 1992;15: 87–114.

Limbird LE. *Cell surface receptors: a short course on theory and methods.* Boston: Martinus Nijhoff; 1985:51–96.

McGonigle P, Molinoff PB. Receptors and signal transduction: classification and quantitation. In: Siegel GJ, Agranoff BW, Albers RW, Molinoff PB, eds. *Basic neurochemistry,* 5th ed. New York: Raven Press; 1994 (in press).

Molinoff PB, Wolfe BB, Weiland GA. Quantitative analysis of drug–receptor interactions. II. Determination of the properties of receptor subtypes. *Life Sci* 1981;29:427–443.

Nestler EJ, Duman RS. G proteins and cyclic nucleotides in the nervous system. In: Siegel GJ, Agranoff BW, Albers RW, Molinoff PB, eds. *Basic neurochemistry,* 5th ed. New York: Raven Press; 1994 (in press).

Snyder SH. Drug and neurotransmitter receptors in the brain. *Science* 1984;224:22–31.

Weiland GA, Molinoff PB. Quantitative analysis of drug–receptor interactions. I. Determination of kinetic and equilibrium properties. *Life Sci* 1981; 29:313–330.

5

Molecular Biological Techniques Applied to the Study of the Central Nervous System

James H. Eberwine

The little girl gave a cry of amazement and looked about her, her eyes growing bigger and bigger at the wonderful sights she saw. . . .

L. Frank Baum,
The Wizard of Oz, 1899
(Dorothy upon emerging from her home when she landed in Oz)

▶ Key Concepts ─────────────────────────────

- All methods involved in the isolation of a specific cDNA clone require the availability of cDNA libraries.

- A cDNA library is a mixture of cloned cDNAs, made from mRNAs that were originally present within a tissue.

- Molecular biological techniques have been utilized to analyze the function of the nicotinic acetylcholine receptor.

- Molecular biological techniques have been utilized to analyze the function of the kainate receptor.

- The polymerase chain reaction technique (PCR) obviates the need for a cDNA library.

- G-protein–coupled receptors are cell surface receptors that transduce agonist binding into cellular responsiveness by causing guanylyl nucleotide-binding proteins to bind GTP.

- Protein levels in the CNS are regulated by neuromodulators.

- The standard method for measuring mRNA levels is Northern blotting.

- The RNAse protection assay improves on the sensitivity of the Northern blotting procedure.

- Cellular resolution can be provided by the technique of in situ hybridization.

- Transgenic analysis is one of the newest methods to aid our understanding of gene functioning.

This chapter describes the use of molecular biological techniques for the determination of protein sequence from cloned DNA and to study the regulation of gene expression. Experimental methods and procedures for RNA and DNA quantitation, creation of DNA libraries, cloning, and bacterial screening are discussed. Future prospects for the application of molecular biological techniques are considered.

Our understanding of the molecular basis of brain functioning has been hampered by both the genetic and the structural complexity of the brain. These complexities include a large number of phenotypically distinct cell types, genes that appear to be expressed solely in the central nervous system (CNS), and the vast number of synaptic connections that can be made by most neurons. This complexity means that issues of general importance in cellular functioning, such as how signal transduction occurs, become more complicated when applied to neurons. The appropriate question then becomes, how does input from hundreds of different synapses get transduced, integrated, and modified in single neurons, resulting in the production or control of some aspect of behavior? In the past decade, great advances have been made in studying the inner workings of the brain. New technical approaches continue to provide avenues to previously inaccessible areas of brain function. The newest approaches being applied to the study of the CNS are in the area of molecular biology.

Molecular biology is the field of science that examines or utilizes a specific set of subcellular molecules, namely, the *nucleic acids.* Nucleic acids fall into two classes: *deoxyribonucleic acid* (DNA) and *ribonucleic acid* (RNA). DNA, which is found in the nucleus and in mitochondria of cells, is the repository of all hereditary information. The central

dogma of molecular biology postulates that parts of the DNA called genes are made (transcribed) into RNA. Of the several classes of RNA known to exist, it is the messenger RNA (mRNA) that gives rise, via translation, to the proteins made within the cell. These proteins include receptors, neurotransmitter-synthesizing enzymes, reuptake transporters, cell adhesion molecules, and other cellular components that, acting in concert, enable cells to function.

The techniques of molecular biology have found wide application in the study of the CNS because of their exquisite sensitivity, permitting the study of small numbers of molecules in discrete cell populations. The sensitivity comes from the capacity of these techniques to distinguish similar DNA sequences from one another using simple hybridization paradigms (i.e., annealing of a probe with a target RNA or DNA sequence).

DETERMINATION OF PROTEIN SEQUENCE FROM CLONED DNA

All methods involved in the isolation of a specific cDNA clone require the availability of cDNA libraries. Perhaps the widest use of molecular biological techniques is in the determination of the amino acid sequences of proteins. In the absence of molecular biological methods, it is often difficult to determine the protein sequence because not enough of a rare protein can be purified to permit sequencing by conventional means. This is particularly true for proteins that are either represented in low copy number (very few

Biological Bases of Brain Function and Disease, edited by Alan Frazer, Perry B. Molinoff, and Andrew Winokur. Raven Press, Ltd., New York © 1994.

molecules) or are very hydrophobic. If a cDNA (complementary DNA) clone is available for a given protein, then it is a relatively trivial task to sequence the DNA and translate this sequence into a protein sequence. The task for most molecular neurobiologists has become not one of characterization of protein structure but rather determination of the cDNA sequence (the DNA sequence that is a copy of the mRNA that encodes the protein). Individual clones can be obtained from cDNA or genomic libraries. Therefore, the first step to be considered is the construction of a cDNA library.

Construction of a cDNA Library

A cDNA library is a mixture of cloned cDNAs, made from mRNAs that were originally present within a tissue. One assesses the quality of a cDNA library by how well a population of cDNAs parallels the original mRNA population (i.e., what percentage of individual mRNA molecules from the tissue are represented by cDNA clones). Making a cDNA library is not a trivial task even in this day of molecular biology cloning kits. Several procedures have been utilized successfully to prepare libraries; however, we will only consider one of these approaches in this chapter.

If a cDNA library is to be constructed to clone a specific protein, it is essential to know that the molecule of interest is present in the tissue from which the RNA was originally isolated. Indeed, it is usually desirable to prepare the library from a tissue that is enriched for that specific molecule. This consideration has often led investigators who are interested in cloning CNS proteins to initially clone their sequences from cDNA libraries prepared from the pituitary and the gastrointestinal tract and from various cell lines, in which a specific mRNA may be present in higher abundance and hence be more easily isolated.

Once the appropriate tissue is selected, the next phase of library construction involves the isolation of RNA (Fig. 1, step 1). Since RNA cannot be cloned as RNA and because it is easily degraded by endogenous RNA-degrading enzymes, it is necessary to convert the RNA into cDNA (Fig. 1, steps 2 and 3). The viral enzyme reverse transcriptase catalyzes the synthesis of DNA from either RNA or DNA (Fig. 1, step 3). For DNA synthesis to occur, a small DNA molecule that is complementary (i.e., will anneal) to the RNA is used as a primer. The most convenient primer for this procedure is composed of thymidine residues and is referred to as an oligo-dT primer. It hybridizes to the string of adenosine residues present at the 3' end of most mRNA molecules that encode proteins (Fig. 1, step 2). At the completion of DNA synthesis, a DNA-RNA hybrid molecule has been generated. The next step of the process replaces the RNA of the DNA-RNA hybrid with DNA (Fig. 1, steps 4 and 5). This reaction also requires the use of a primer and is catalyzed by DNA polymerase, which will synthesize a complementary DNA to the existing DNA template. This enzyme can use either RNA or DNA as a primer for cDNA synthesis. The RNA of the RNA-DNA hybrid is randomly cut with an enzyme called RNAse H to provide multiple sites at which DNA polymerase can bind and initiate cDNA synthesis (Fig. 1, step 4). The completion of this reaction results in a double-stranded DNA molecule (Fig. 1, step 5).

To construct a cDNA library it is necessary to clone the double-stranded DNA. Cloning is the amplification of DNA sequences, usually in bacteria, and is accomplished by inserting the cDNA into another DNA molecule, called a *vector*. The vector contains the information necessary to direct the propagation and amplification of the DNA when put into bacteria. As bacteria grow rapidly to a high density, it is then a simple matter to obtain a large amount of DNA. Two types of bacterial vectors are commonly used in molecular biology. One is a plasmid that replicates in individual bacteria, and the other is a bacterial virus that can infect bacteria, called a *phage.* Regardless of the type of vector chosen for construction of the cDNA library, the

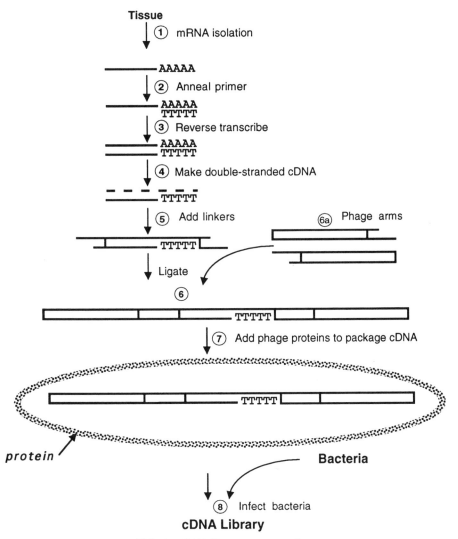

FIG. 1. cDNA library construction.

double-stranded cDNA must be placed in the vector so that when the vector is propagated, so too is the cDNA. Combining the cDNA with the vector involves a ligation reaction. To facilitate this joining, often as an intermediate step, specific, single-stranded DNA sequences are added to the double-stranded cDNA by ligation (Fig. 1, step 5). This allows the cDNA and vector to hybridize to one another. After this initial ligation, the cDNA and vector can be mixed and ligated to one another, forming a single molecule (Fig. 1, step 6).

For plasmid vectors, the ligated plasmid cDNAs are transformed into bacteria. As shown in Fig. 1, when a phage vector is used (Fig. 1, step 6a), the ligated molecules are encapsulated in phage proteins, which facilitate the uptake of the encapsulated cDNA by infection. Phage are put into a bacterial host, such that a single bacterium takes in only a single DNA molecule. It is this event that makes cloning possible. The collection of individual bacteria containing individual cDNA clones is the library. The larger the number of recombinant bacteria generated from a given amount of starting mRNA, the better is the library. Usually libraries that contain over 10^6 clones per microgram of starting mRNA are considered to be good libraries. Individual bacteria that contain the desired cDNA can be isolated from the bacteria containing other cDNAs using various screening procedures. Some of these screening procedures will be described in the next few sections of this chapter.

Cloning of the Nicotinic Acetylcholine Receptor Using Partial Amino Acid Sequence

Molecular biological techniques have been utilized to analyze the function of the nicotinic acetylcholine receptor. The nicotinic acetylcholine receptor is an aggregate of four distinct subunits in a molar ratio of 2:1:1:1

that combine to form a cation channel. The initial step in cloning this receptor was to purify the receptor to homogeneity from the electric organ of the eel, a tissue that is enriched in this receptor. The receptor subunits were separated and cleaved with proteolytic enzymes, and the amino acid sequences of several of the fragments were then determined. The resultant sequences were used to design short DNA sequences that were synthesized and radiolabeled and were then used to probe a cDNA library made from the eel electric organ. cDNA clones were isolated and the DNA sequenced. The deduced amino acid sequences that were originally generated from the purified receptor were present in the cloned sequence. This screening strategy is depicted in Fig. 2.

Knowledge of the DNA sequence and the implied amino acid sequence allowed structural models of the receptor to be generated.

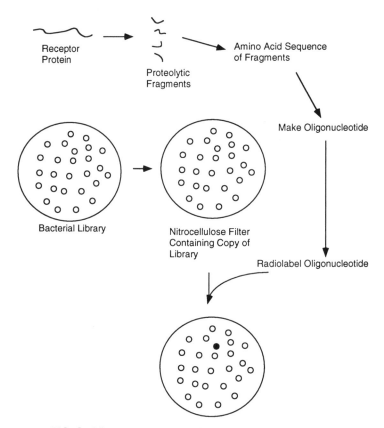

FIG. 2. Library screening with oligonucleotide probe.

The nucleotide sequences of the cloned subunits predicted protein subunit molecular weights of approximately 50,000. In each of these sequences four hydrophobic stretches of amino acids were hypothesized to be membrane-spanning regions (MSR).

Initially, the model that was proposed on the basis of this structure suggested that the hydrophobic stretches positioned the subunits to surround a central ion channel, with the amphipathic (charged) transmembrane regions forming a pore through which ions could move. Since this initial model was described, there has been intense controversy regarding the number of membrane-spanning regions of the individual subunits.

An alternative approach to this model incorporates data from electron microscopic localization of monoclonal antibodies directed to distinct regions of the receptor. A receptor subunit structure has been predicted with different, less hydrophobic regions of the receptor forming the MSR. It should be remembered that while the nucleotide and protein sequence information is predictive of structure, it is not definitive.

Molecular biological techniques have been exploited to analyze the function of the nicotinic acetylcholine (ACh) receptor by converting (expressing) the receptor mRNA sequence into functional ACh receptors in cells that normally do not express the protein.

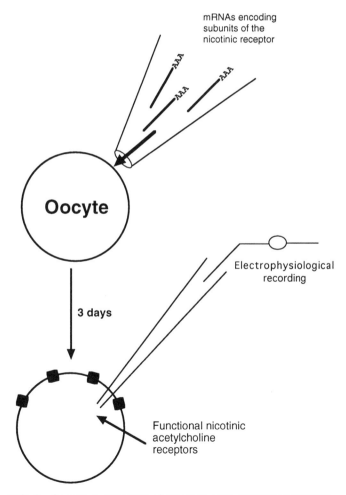

FIG. 3. Oocyte expression of nicotinic acetylcholine receptors.

These experiments initially involve the *in vitro* synthesis of RNA from cloned DNA sequences. The RNA is then injected into *Xenopus laevis* oocytes where the cellular machinery for protein synthesis translates the mRNA into protein (Fig. 3).

When the RNA from the four subunits of the nicotinic ACh receptor were mixed and injected into oocytes, the existence of functional receptors could be demonstrated using electrophysiological techniques. In attempts to distinguish the role of each of the subunits in receptor functioning, several variations on the original oocyte expression experiments were tried, including (1) use of subunits from different species (which have different properties) to form hybrid receptors and (2) use of different amounts of each subunit. In the latter set of experiments, it was found that if either the γ or the δ subunits were left out of the mRNA mixture, functional ACh receptors could still be formed. It has been hypothesized that this occurs because the γ and δ subunits are so similar in their protein sequence that one can substitute for the other. Studies such as these have been extended using site-directed mutagenesis to demonstrate that specific amino acids are involved in distinct aspects of receptor functioning.

The cloning strategy for the nicotinic ACh receptor relied on the availability of synthetic oligonucleotide sequences that could be used in the screening of a library. Each amino acid (the building blocks of proteins) is coded for by a string of three ribonucleotides, called a *codon*. These triplets, arranged in a specific order, compose the RNA sequence that gives rise to the functional protein. Each amino acid has one or more codons. Some amino acids, such as serine, have as many as six codons. The existence of more than one codon for an amino acid is referred to as *degeneracy*. It is this degeneracy that creates one of the more serious problems in this "reverse genetics" approach to isolating a desired clone. Since it is not apparent from the amino acid sequence which codon is used for a particular amino acid, it is necessary in making the oligonucleotide to use all possible codon choices or to make a guess as to the identity of the codon (Fig. 4).

If one were to use all of the choices for an amino acid sequence in an oligonucleotide, then multiple oligonucleotide sequences would have to be synthesized, each differing in the position of the degeneracy. This approach is limited in its applicability because the existence of degeneracy often dictates the synthesis of over 1,000 oligonucleotide sequences in order to take into account the total degeneracy. While the synthesis of so many oligonucleotides may appear difficult, with current technology it is often possible to synthesize all of them at the same time. The problem resides in the fact that of the thousands of sequences synthesized, only one will

Amino Acid Sequence	Phe	-	Tyr	-	Met	-	Ser	-	Gly	-	Pro	-	Ala	-	Ile
Number of Codons	2		2		1		6		4		4		4		3
Oligonucleotide Sequence	UUU C	-	UAU C	-	AUG	-	UCU C A G AGU C	-	GGU C A G	-	CCU C A G	-	GCU C A G	-	AUU C A G

Total Degeneracy $(2 \times 2 \times 1 \times 6 \times 4 \times 4 \times 4 \times 3 = 4608)$

FIG. 4. Design of oligonucleotide probe.

exactly hybridize to the appropriate cDNA sequence. This means that the specific probe is only a small fraction of the total probe used in the screening procedure, and the sensitivity of the procedure may not be sufficient to allow detection of the desired sequence. To limit the degeneracy, "guesses" are made as to which codons are likely to be used. These guesses can be based on codon usage tables that are compilations of the frequency with which specific codons are used to encode a particular amino acid. Since guesses are likely to introduce errors into the oligonucleotide sequence so that it will not exactly match the RNA molecule, such probes are generally synthesized to a longer length so that any mismatches are compensated for by the increased stability of a longer stretch of hybridization.

Cloning of a Kainate Receptor Using Oocyte Expression

Molecular biological techniques have also been utilized to analyze the function of the kainate receptor. The kainate receptor is a ligand-gated cation channel that is involved in eliciting much of the inhibitory input into the CNS. It was cloned using functional expression techniques. This strategy relies on the ability of an expression system, in this case oocytes, to effectively translate and express RNAs that are microinjected into the oocytes. An appropriate assay system to detect expression (Fig. 5) is also required for this selection scheme to work. Specifically, a rat brain cDNA library that should contain clones for the kainate receptor was divided into 18 different sublibraries, each containing cDNA from about 10,000 individual clones. As previously described for the nicotinic receptor, RNA can be made directly from cDNA clones. RNA was made from each sublibrary, and this RNA was injected into oocytes.

Several days postinjection, voltage recordings demonstrated depolarization with kainate receptor agonists in some of the sublibraries, suggesting that these sublibraries contained cDNA clones that encoded a functional kainate receptor. When depolarization was detected, the sublibrary responsible for the signal was further subdivided, RNA was synthesized, and oocyte injections followed by voltage recordings of oocytes were performed. This procedure was repeated until a single clone that produced kainate-induced depolarization was isolated. The same strategy was previously utilized to isolate cDNAs for substance K and 5-HT$_{1c}$ serotonin receptors. Such a cloning strategy can be successful in cloning receptors if the following conditions are met:

1. The functional receptor must be a single subunit.
2. The oocyte must contain the proteins necessary to permit detectable receptor functioning.
3. The cDNA library must contain cDNAs that encode the complete protein sequence.

Cloning of Proteins Using the Polymerase Chain Reaction

The polymerase chain reaction technique (PCR) obviates the need for a cDNA library. If a partial amino acid sequence is available for a protein that is to be cloned, it is possible to use another cloning strategy that does not rely on the existence of a cDNA library. This strategy utilizes the polymerase chain reaction to amplify regions of DNA between two priming sites. The methodology requires the synthesis of oligonucleotide primers that will prime DNA synthesis in both a sense and an antisense direction. The sense direction is defined as the direction in which translation occurs; hence a sense primer would be the same sequence as the mRNA sequence (Fig. 6).

The use of PCR to clone a sequence from a population of mRNAs isolated from a tissue in which the protein is made requires the conversion of the mRNA to cDNA with an antisense primer. This cDNA is subsequently copied into double-stranded DNA

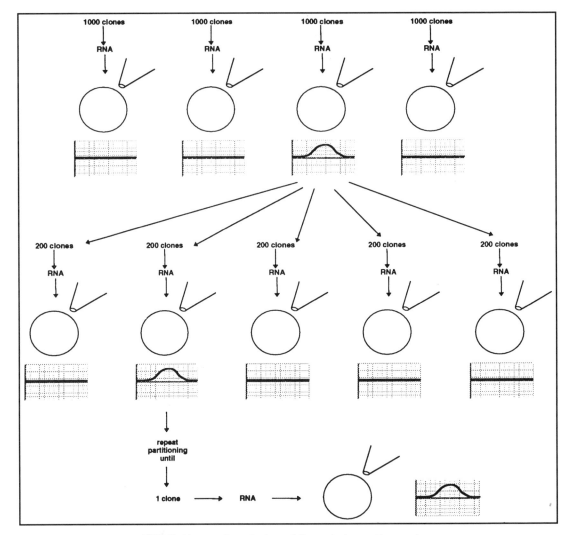

FIG. 5. Expression cloning of the substance K receptor.

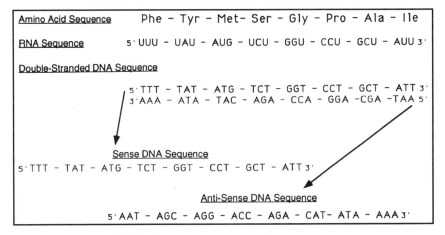

FIG. 6. Sense vs. antisense DNA probes.

using a sense primer. After the DNA is made into double-stranded molecules it is heat-denatured, and the sense and antisense primers are used to again initiate DNA synthesis. With continued repetition of these steps the sequence between the primers is amplified exponentially (Fig. 7).

PCR can also be used to amplify DNA from genomic DNA or DNA isolated from cDNA libraries. The amplified DNA can subsequently be cloned. cDNA clones isolated using PCR should be sequenced in an effort to confirm their identity. This is particularly important in this cloning strategy because of the need to detect errors induced by PCR. These errors occur as a result of the enzymatic activity of TAQ DNA polymerase, the enzyme used in performing PCR.

A PCR product can also be used to screen a cDNA or genomic library to isolate full-length clones that do not contain PCR-generated sequence errors. This eliminates the need to clone the PCR product. The substance P receptor sequence was cloned in exactly this manner. Using the sequence of the substance K receptor (as well as the sequences of other members of this family of receptors), degenerate oligonucleotide primers separated by approximately 200 bases were used to amplify sequences that would be similar to, yet distinct from, the substance K receptor. The rationale for using the substance K receptor sequence to generate oligonucleotide primers was that the sequence, pharmacology, and physiology of the kinins were similar, and hence it was presumed that this functional similarity would manifest itself as similarities in their receptor sequences.

The ease with which PCR can be performed has facilitated the cloning of members of several large gene families. Examples of this cloning strategy are illustrated by the cloning of members of the G-protein-coupled receptor family as described below.

G-Protein–Coupled Receptors

G-protein–coupled receptors are cell surface receptors that transduce agonist binding into cellular responsiveness by causing guanylyl nucleotide-binding proteins to bind GTP. The G-protein–coupled receptors encompass a gene family composed of several hundred proteins. Members of this receptor family include the adrenergic receptors, dopamine receptors, and several peptide receptors, including receptors for substance P and substance K. Muscarinic cholinergic receptors and most subtypes of serotonin receptors are also members of this family. All of these receptors share a similar predicted topology, each containing seven MSR with the N-terminal region being extracellular while the C-terminal domain is intracellular. These receptors are most similar in sequence in the MSR. Using degenerate oligonucleotide primers to various MSR, many additional members of this family were isolated. The sequences of only a few members of this family are known from biochemical purification of the receptor protein followed by library screening. However, using molecular biological approaches such as PCR (using conserved regions of the receptors as primers), the sequences of over 50 members of this receptor family have been determined. The structure of this class of receptors is presented in Chapter 4, Fig. 6.

Knowledge of receptor structure has allowed investigators to examine the role of specific regions involved in receptor function. Some of the receptors are coupled to the stimulatory guanylyl nucleotide-binding protein (G_s) while others interact with other G proteins (G_i, G_o, and G_t). Since the receptors are similar in sequence, the question of how individual receptors can specifically interact with individual G proteins is of interest. To address this issue, several types of experiment have been performed including (1) overexpression of the receptor, (2) exon shuffling, and (3) site-directed mutagenesis.

Overexpression Studies

It has been possible to insert clones for muscarinic receptors into various cell lines and to regulate the level of expression or titrate the

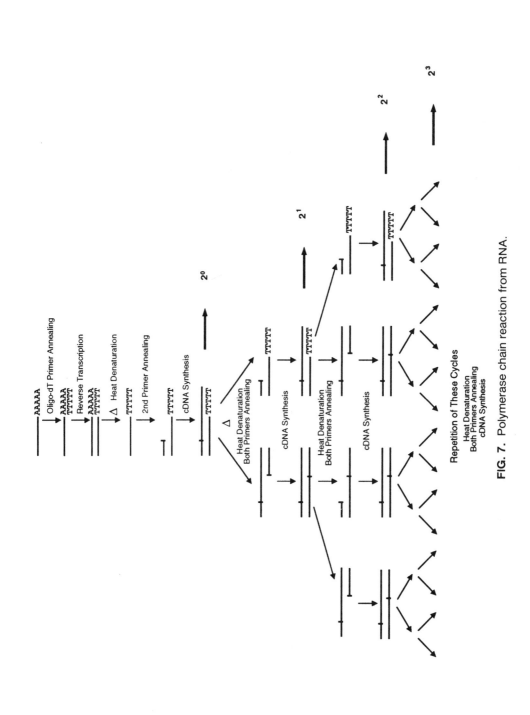

FIG. 7. Polymerase chain reaction from RNA.

amount of muscarinic receptor expressed in a given cell line. These experiments have provided insight into the specificity of signal transduction pathways. The muscarinic receptor normally couples preferentially to G_i. In these overexpression experiments, so much of the muscarinic receptor was expressed (over a million molecules per cell) that all of the G_i was in a complex with the muscarinic receptor (Fig. 8). The "leftover" muscarinic receptor was then shown to be able to interact with G_s. This experiment showed that specific receptors can interact with different G proteins.

Exon Shuffling

The conservation of the seven-MSR structure of this class of receptors suggests that spe-

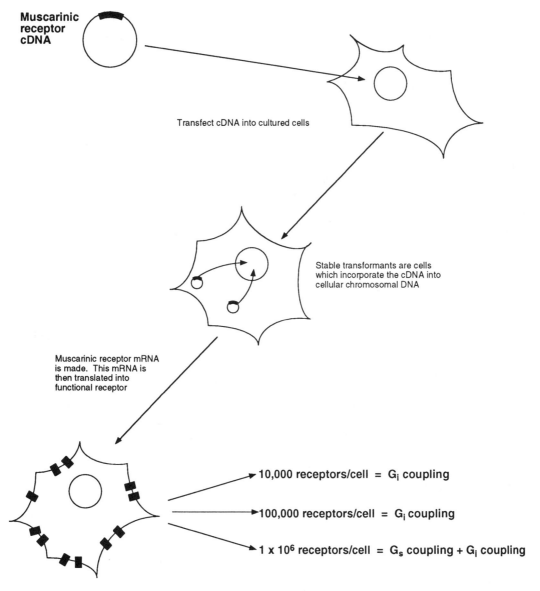

Muscarinic receptor cDNA

Transfect cDNA into cultured cells

Stable transformants are cells which incorporate the cDNA into cellular chromosomal DNA

Muscarinic receptor mRNA is made. This mRNA is then translated into functional receptor

10,000 receptors/cell = G_i coupling

100,000 receptors/cell = G_i coupling

1 x 10^6 receptors/cell = G_s coupling + G_i coupling

FIG. 8. Pharmacological consequences of overexpression of muscarinic receptors.

cific regions of these receptors may be involved in specific functions including ligand binding or coupling to the G proteins. Several investigators have approached this question by creating chimeric receptors from sequence-shuffling experiments. In these experiments, different MSR are removed from their native clone and MSR from other receptors are inserted as replacement sequences. The exchange is performed using essentially the same ligation techniques previously described in construction of a cDNA library. One such set of chimeric receptor studies has defined the region of the β-adrenergic receptor that is responsible for interacting with G_s. In these experiments, the regions between and including the second and sixth MSR were removed from the α_2-adrenergic receptor and replaced with the analogous region from the β-adrenergic receptor (Fig. 9). The chimeric receptor-bound α_2-adrenergic receptor agonists appropriately but cAMP production, rather than being inhibited, was stimulated. This experiment showed that a particular region of the β-adrenergic receptor was primarily responsible for its interaction with G_s.

Site-Directed Mutagenesis

To know precisely which amino acids are responsible for these interactions as well as those sites responsible for the binding of β-adrenergic ligands, it is useful to perform site-directed mutagenesis to change the identity of individual amino acids. The results of a number of recent studies in which the nucleotides encoding the aspartic acid at position 113 were changed to encode either an asparagine or glutamic acid suggest that the aspartic acid at amino acid number 113 is important for agonist and antagonist binding.

The genetically engineered receptors were expressed in cell lines, and the binding affinities as well as the amount of agonist needed to maximally stimulate adenylyl cyclase for a set of agonists and antagonists were determined. Such site-directed mutagenesis studies have been performed for many amino acid residues in the β-adrenergic receptor. These results suggest that a particular membrane-spanning sequence is not required for G-protein coupling but rather the presence of amphiphilic α helices of specific charge distribution is likely to dictate the type of receptor–G-protein coupling.

The power of molecular biological techniques is again illustrated in the investigation of dopamine receptors. While there has been biochemical and pharmacological evidence for the existence of two dopamine receptors, recently molecular biology confirmed the existence of at least five different genes encoding dopamine receptors. The first receptor cloned was the D_2 dopamine receptor, which was isolated by screening a rat brain cDNA library with probes made from the rat β-adrenergic receptor. This screening strategy presumed that there was sufficient sequence similarity between the two receptors that under the appropriate conditions one clone would hybridize with the other. Isolation was accomplished by low-stringency hybridization such that mismatches between similar sequences did not destabilize the hybrid between the two sequences. Indeed, other members of this receptor family have been isolated using this low-stringency hybridization strategy.

In studies of the regional distribution of the D_2 dopamine receptor with a PCR technique specific for the third cytoplasmic loop of this receptor, it became apparent that there was an additional, previously unknown form of the receptor that was extended by 87 nucleotides (29 amino acids). The significance of the extended form of the D_2 receptor is unclear, but preliminary data suggest that it is regulated independently of the short form. Since there is only one gene for the D_2 dopamine receptor, the existence of two forms of the receptor suggests that there is alternative splicing of the parent RNA, also called the heteronuclear RNA (HnRNA) (Fig. 10).

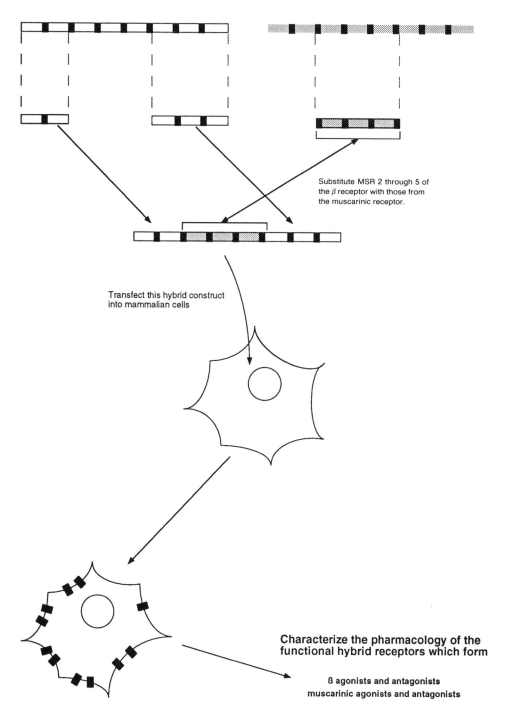

Substitute MSR 2 through 5 of the β receptor with those from the muscarinic receptor.

Transfect this hybrid construct into mammalian cells

Characterize the pharmacology of the functional hybrid receptors which form

ß agonists and antagonists
muscarinic agonists and antagonists

FIG. 9. Domain switching of G-protein–coupled receptor.

Such alternative splicing events have been shown to exist for a number of genes that are expressed in the CNS, including the *Shaker* potassium channel in the fruit fly and calcitonin gene–related peptide. These alternatively spliced mRNAs can give rise to multiple molecules with different functions. From these examples it is readily apparent that alternative splicing of brain RNAs increases the functional complexity of the CNS.

REGULATION OF GENE EXPRESSION IN THE CNS

Protein levels in the CNS are regulated by neuromodulators. In many cases the level of protein in a cell is thought to be a reflection of function. For example, if a cell has a high level of dopamine-β-hydroxylase (DBH) protein, that cell is likely to be able to make more norepinephrine (the product of DBH enzymatic activity) than a cell that contains less DBH protein. It is often difficult to measure the amount of protein in CNS structures because of the low level of expression in certain structures. The level of protein is also thought to be reflected in the abundance of its corresponding mRNA, which is indicative of gene transcription or mRNA stability changes. The amount of mRNA present within a given

CNS structure is easier to measure than the amount of protein and can be assessed using several different methods, each with its own level of sensitivity as well as its own inherent set of problems. Presentation of the techniques that facilitate mRNA quantitation as well as a discussion of the mechanism of gene regulation follow.

Northern Blotting

The standard method for measuring mRNA levels is Northern blotting. The Northern technique requires that the tissue be dispersed in a strong denaturant and the RNA separated from other cellular components. The RNA is then electrophoresed through a gel matrix to separate the RNA by size. Usually the RNA is transferred from the gel to a solid support such as nitrocellulose and is then hybridized to a radiolabeled probe that can be detected by autoradiography (Fig. 11).

When probe is present in excess and hybridization is continued for a long time, the intensity of the hybridization of the probe is a direct measure of the amount of the corresponding RNA on the blot. It is a highly sensitive procedure, detecting as little as 50 pg of mRNA. Northern blot analysis also provides

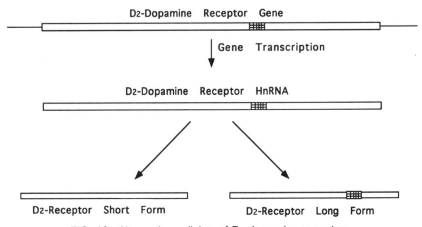

FIG. 10. Alternative splicing of D_2 dopamine receptor.

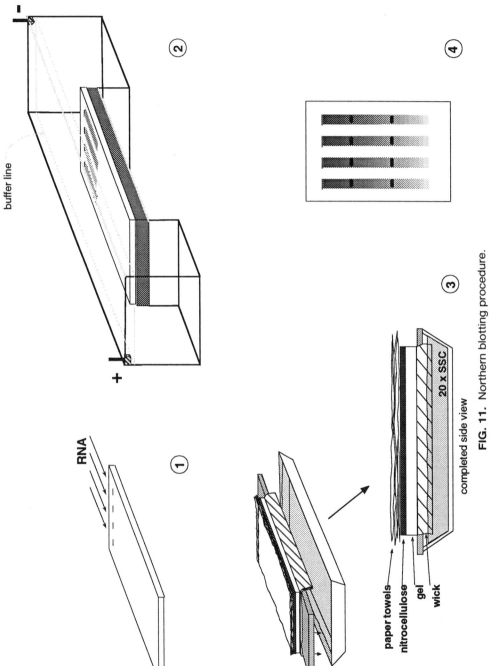

FIG. 11. Northern blotting procedure.

a direct measure of the size of the mRNA being examined. A drawback to this procedure is loss of cellular resolution, and purification of mRNA is usually required.

RNAse Protection

The RNAse protection assay improves on the sensitivity of the Northern blotting procedure. In the RNAse protection assay, a radiolabeled antisense RNA probe specific for a given mRNA is hybridized to the population of RNAs isolated from the tissue. The material that remains single-stranded, which includes cellular RNA and excess probe, is removed by digestion with RNAse so that only double-stranded RNA remains. The double-stranded RNA is analyzed by gel electrophoresis. The amount of material in hybrid form is quantitated by determining the amount of radiolabeled RNA present in the hybrid (Fig. 12).

RNAse protection assays are more sensitive than Northern blotting by at least four-fold, so that as little as 12 pg of RNA can be detected. Since the sensitivity is greater, less tissue is needed for this analysis than is needed for Northern blots. The drawbacks to using the RNAse protection assay are that it is a difficult procedure to set up, it does not provide a measure of RNA size, and, as with

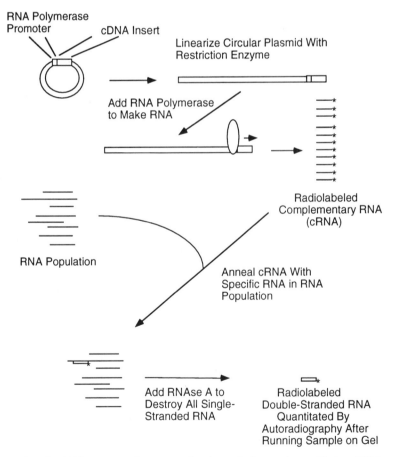

FIG. 12. RNAse protection assay to characterize and quantitate mRNA.

Northern blots, it does not provide cellular resolution. In most instances purification of mRNA is not required.

In Situ Hybridization

Cellular resolution can be provided by the technique of in situ *hybridization. In situ* hybridization is essentially a Northern analysis with the RNA still in the tissue (Fig. 13). In most procedures, the brain is sectioned through the region of interest, fixed with paraformaldehyde, and stored at $-80°C$. Fixation is necessary to prevent the RNA from diffusing out of the tissue section. Sections are prehybridized with reagents (e.g., bovine serum albumin, tRNA, etc.) that will bind to and block nonspecific sites of probe interaction. This is followed by hybridization of the section with the probe of interest.

Any type of probe that can be used for Northern blotting procedures can also be used for *in situ* hybridization. The most commonly used probes are cRNA and oligonucle-

otides. Because there is little scatter of the decay particles, ^3H and ^{35}S are preferred radiolabels for determination of the cellular localization of mRNA. In attempts to minimize the use of radioactive materials because of safety and waste disposal issues, labeling methods have been developed that incorporate chemicals such as biotin or digoxigenin to serve as molecular tags for the presence of mRNA. These methods, which are still in their infancy, are not as sensitive as those with radiolabeled probes. They have an added utility in facilitating the combined use of *in situ* hybridization with immunocytochemistry or receptor autoradiography. This decreases the amount of tissue needed for many analyses and permits detection of multiple regulatory points in the expression of any given gene.

The importance of *in situ* hybridization resides in its ability to localize mRNA within identifiable brain nuclei and even in single identifiable cells. Knowledge of cellular identity often provides insight into potential functions of the corresponding protein.

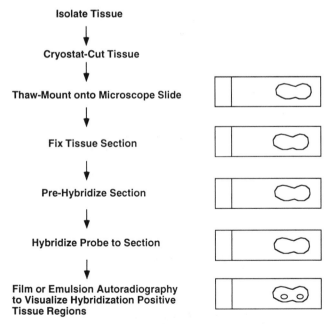

FIG. 13. Procedure for *in situ* hybridization.

Transcription Factors

Transgenic analysis is one of the newest methods to aid our understanding of gene functioning. The amount of mRNA expressed by cells is determined by regulatory regions in the gene encoding the mRNA. These regulatory regions, called *cis*-acting elements, are DNA sequences that usually reside immediately 5' to the transcription initiation site. The importance of these regions in regulating transcription became apparent when several different genes were transfected into cell lines, and it was discovered that the genes retained their original regulatory characteristics. This was in contrast to transfection with cDNAs in which native regulatory control is lost. The difference can be accounted for by the additional DNA sequence in the regulatory region of the gene. The importance of the 5' end of a gene for controlling gene regulation has been studied by removing the coding region of particular genes and replacing them with a reporter gene such as β-galactosidase. When these constructs were transfected into cells, the reporter gene was regulated in the same manner as the native gene, demonstrating that the 5' end dictated transcriptional responsiveness (Fig. 14).

Several short DNA *cis*-acting elements have been characterized at the nucleotide level using deletion analysis followed by transfection. These sequences are 8 to 20 bases long and include sequences that dictate glucocorticoid responsiveness and cAMP responsiveness. The existence of these sequences suggested that specific proteins called *trans-activating* factors exist and bind to these regions to either activate or inhibit transcription. Indeed, this hypothesis sug-

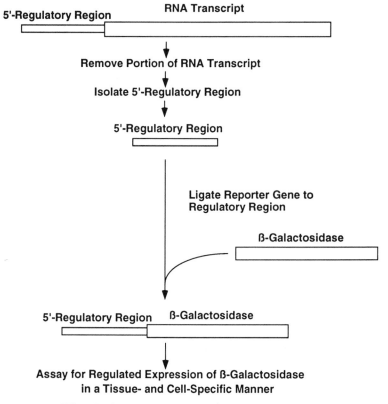

FIG. 14. Characterization of 5'-promoter regions.

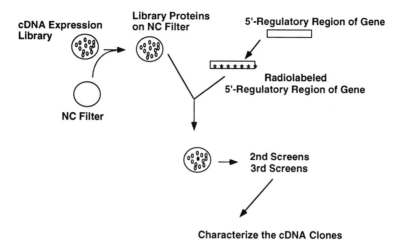

FIG. 15. Southwestern screening procedure for isolation of transcription factors.

gested a means for isolating these binding proteins.

One of the proteins that responds to an increase in cAMP accumulation by binding to the cAMP-responsive elements (CREs) of responsive genes is called CREB (cAMP-responsive element-binding protein). CREB was cloned using a partial amino acid sequence from purified protein to synthesize oligonucleotides (as discussed for the nicotinic ACh receptor) and by screening a bacterial expression cDNA library prepared from GH$_3$ cells with a radiolabeled oligonucleotide encoding the CRE. This latter technique, also called the "Southwestern blot," requires bacterial expression of functional eukaryotic proteins (Fig. 15). CREB could be isolated with this technique because the protein strongly and specifically interacted with the CRE oligonucleotide.

Analysis of the protein sequence for CREB suggested that CREB contained several potential phosphorylation sites. These sites are candidates for rapid modification by protein kinases and hence may be involved in regulating the ability of CREB to bind to endogenous CREs in the genome. In experiments utilizing site-directed mutagenesis and transfection paradigms, phosphorylation of serine 133 was shown to be necessary for CREB

protein activity. The role of phosphorylation in regulating CREB activity in vivo has been examined in an elegant series of experiments in which a cDNA corresponding to a nonphosphorylatable CREB was used to create transgenic mice. Mutated CREB cDNA was microinjected into the pronucleus of fertilized mouse eggs under control of the growth hormone promoter, which is the 5'-regulatory region of the growth hormone gene. Its presence at the 5' end of the CREB molecule restricts the expression of CREB to those cells in which the growth hormone promoter can function, namely, the somatotrophs (growth hormone–producing cells) in the anterior pituitary (Fig. 16).

Overexpression of the mutated CREB allowed it to compete for endogenous CREB binding, effectively inactivating the endogenous CREB and rendering the cells insensitive to CRE. The biological response of the transgenic animals to mutated CREB was phenotypical dwarfism resulting from atrophied pituitary glands deficient in somatotrophs. These experiments showed that activation of the CREB was necessary for normal somatotroph development. The use of transgenic analysis illustrates one of the newest ways in which molecular biological techniques have had an impact on our under-

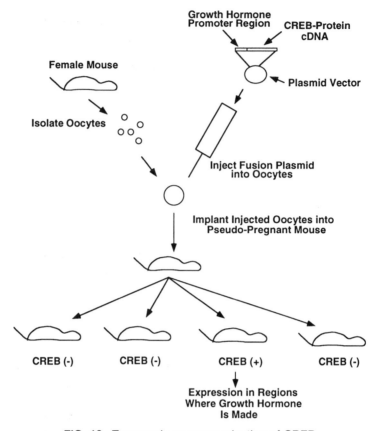

FIG. 16. Transgenic mouse production of CREB.

standing of gene functioning in a normal cellular context.

FUTURE PROSPECTS

The widespread application of molecular biological techniques to the study of the CNS will continue to provide valuable insights into the molecular mechanisms of normal and abnormal brain function. Arguably, the most important new direction for development is the joining of molecular biological techniques with cellular physiology. This combination promises to provide information about single-cell functioning in context with other cells. It is conceivable that the application of single-cell molecular biology with electrophysiological recording techniques in cells in the "live-slice" tissue prepa-

ration will provide information not only about cell physiology but also about behavior. This is intriguing because it is possible to record from cells in which at least some of the normal neuronal connectivity and glial interactions remain intact. Indeed, an understanding of the complex interaction of cells within the CNS, or the "hard wiring" of the CNS, may be experimentally approachable with these strategies.

While it is relatively easy to clone cDNAs encoding most proteins, it is often difficult to assign a physiological function to the protein. Transgenic animal production, which is currently very tedious and difficult to perform, holds promise for facilitating the discovery of protein function. This technology should permit the elimination of genes (knock-out experiments) or regulated overproduction (add-back experiments) so that the influence of alterations in the abundance of specific proteins on physiological properties can be assessed. These add-back experiments will require the isolation and characterization of cell-selective transcriptional promoters whose developmental expression is known. Of course there are caveats to this type of experiment, but important biological information should be obtainable. Indeed, such experiments are likely to lead to the development of specific gene therapy paradigms for the treatment of CNS disorders.

SUMMARY

Genes give rise to mRNA, and mRNA is the immediate precursor of proteins. Of importance to the CNS are proteins such as receptors, channels, second-messenger system enzymes, peptide neurotransmitters, growth factors, and structural proteins that give rise to the structure and functioning of the nervous system. The reductionist would argue that these molecules are the building blocks from which CNS functioning eventually results. The use of molecular biological techniques to determine the sequence of mRNA molecules facilitates the elucidation of protein sequence. These techniques also permit the cellular localization of mRNA molecules and provide methods for analysis of the abundance of mRNAs, which is often reflective of the amount of functional protein. While it is extremely difficult to determine the physiological function or functional significance of proteins, genetic engineering techniques make it possible to modify or disrupt the functioning of cloned proteins, permitting an analysis of the resultant physiological effects. Indeed, the most important contribution of molecular biology to the study of the CNS may be that it provides a methodology for examining, and eventually understanding, the molecular underpinnings of normal and abnormal brain functioning.

The techniques of molecular biology, because of their sensitivity and specificity, will continue to be important tools for examining the complexities of the CNS.

BIBLIOGRAPHY

Original Articles

Benzer S. Genetic dissection of behavior. *Sci Am* 1973;229(6):24–37.

Betz H. Ligand-gated ion channels in the brain: the amino acid receptor superfamily. *Neuron* 1990;5:383–392.

Hoeffler JP, Meyer TE, Yun Y, Jameson JL, Habener JF. Cyclic AMP responsive DNA-binding protein: structure based on a cloned placental cDNA. *Science* 1988;242:1430–1433.

Miller C. Genetic manipulation of ion channels: a new approach to structure and mechanism. *Neuron* 1989;2:1195–1205.

Stround RM, Finer-Moore J. Acetylcholine receptor structure, function, and evolution. *Annu Rev Cell Biol* 1985;1:317–351.

Sutcliffe JG. mRNA in the mammalian central nervous system. *Annu Rev Neurosci* 1988;11:157–198.

Unwin N. The structure of ion channels in membranes of excitable cells. *Neuron* 1989;3:665–676.

Books and Reviews

Berger S, Kimmel AR. *Guide to molecular cloning techniques.* Methods in Enzymology, Vol. 152. New York: Academic Press; 1987.

Molecular neurobiology. Cold Spring Harbor Symposia on Quantitative Biology, Vol. 48. Cold Spring Harbor, NY: Cold Spring Harbor Laboratory Press; 1983.

Goodman RH. Molecular probes for gene expression. In: Siegel GL, Agranoff BW, Albers RW, Molinoff PB, eds. *Basic neurochemistry,* 5th ed. New York: Raven Press, 1994 (in press).

Sambrook J, Fritsch EF, Maniatis T. *Molecular cloning: a laboratory manual.* 2nd ed. Cold Spring Harbor, NY: Cold Spring Harbor Laboratory Press; 1989.

Tobin AJ. Gene expression in the mammalian nervous system. In: Siegel GL, Agranoff BW, Albers RW, Molinoff PB, eds. *Basic neurochemistry,* 5th ed. New York: Raven Press, 1994 (in press).

Valentino KL, Eberwine JH, Barchas JD, eds. *In situ hybridization: applications to neurobiology.* New York: Oxford University Press; 1987.

Watson J, Gilman M, Witkowski J, Zoller M. *Recombinant DNA.* 2nd Ed. New York: WH Freeman (Scientific American Books); 1992.

Synaptic Transmission
Biogenic Amines

Perry B. Molinoff

Since adrenalin does not evoke any reaction from muscle that has at no time of its life been innervated by the sympathetic, the point at which the stimulus of the chemical excitant is received, and transformed into what may cause the change of tension of the muscle fibre, is perhaps a mechanism developed out of the muscle cell in response to its union with the synapsing sympathetic fibre, the function of which is to receive and transform the nervous impulse. Adrenalin might then be the chemical stimulant liberated on each occasion when the impulse arrives at the periphery.

T. R. Elliott,
On the action of adrenalin
J. Physiol. 1904;31:XX–XXI

▶ Key Concepts

- The synthesis of acetylcholine is catalyzed by the enzyme choline acetyltransferase.

- Like other neurotransmitters and neuromodulators, acetylcholine interacts with multiple subtypes of receptors.

- The synthesis of catecholamines involves four separate enzymatic reactions.

- The enzymatic metabolism of catecholamines is considerably more complex than that of acetylcholine.

- Release of catecholamines results from nerve stimulation or stimulation of the adrenal gland by cholinomimetic drugs.

- In addition to being a precursor in the synthesis of norepinephrine and epinephrine, dopamine is a transmitter in its own right.

- Histamine is formed from the amino acid L-histidine.

- The pharmacological effects of histamine, including profound hypotension and marked bronchoconstriction, are similar to responses observed during anaphylactic reactions.

- Serotonin is found in high concentrations in platelets from which it is released on aggregation.

- Our understanding of the regulation of 5-HT$_2$ receptors is less advanced than that of the regulation of the catecholamine or cholinergic receptors.

■ Chapter Overview

This chapter describes the synthesis, distribution, metabolism, and effects of the biogenic amine neurotransmitters. Drugs that affect aminergic neurotransmission are widely used for the treatment and prevention of neuropsychiatric disorders. Specific discussions of the role of biogenic amines in disease and the mechanisms of action of psychotherapeutic drugs are a major component of Chapters 17 to 23.

The *biogenic amines* (Fig. 1) include compounds that function as neurotransmitters, neurohormones, or neuromodulators in the central and/or peripheral nervous systems. The family of biogenic amines includes norepinephrine and acetylcholine, which are the transmitters at postganglionic terminals of the autonomic nervous system. Dopamine, the precursor of norepinephrine, is an important neurotransmitter in several CNS pathways, while epinephrine is a neurohormone released from the adrenal medulla. Epinephrine is also found in several nuclei in the brain stem. Increases in epinephrine levels in brain stem nuclei have been seen in experimentally induced hypertension. Histamine is a so-called *autacoid* found in high concentrations in mast cells. It also appears to function as a neurotransmitter in several CNS pathways. Serotonin (5-hydroxytryptamine; 5-HT) is an indoleamine found in high concentrations in platelets and in many CNS pathways. Drugs that affect 5-HT uptake or receptors are now coming into use for the treatment of disorders including anxiety, depression, and migraine headaches.

ACETYLCHOLINE

The synthesis of acetylcholine is catalyzed by the enzyme choline acetyltransferase. The synthesis of acetylcholine (ACh) occurs in a single step and involves two precursors, choline and acetyl coenzyme A (Fig. 2). The rate of synthesis of ACh does not, however, appear to be limited by the activity of choline acetyltransferase. Rather, the uptake of choline by a high-affinity, sodium-dependent uptake pump appears to be the rate-limiting step. Since neurons cannot synthesize choline, it must be supplied either from plasma or by hydrolysis of other choline-containing compounds. The compound hemicholinium-3 is a potent inhibitor of the high-affinity choline uptake system, and treatment with this drug leads to a marked reduction in ACh synthesis and nerve-stimulated release of ACh.

The effects of neuronally released ACh are terminated as a consequence of hydrolysis of acetylcholine by widely distributed enzymes called cholinesterases. These enzymes have been subdivided on the basis of substrate specificity into an enzyme called acetylcholinesterase and the butyryl or serum or pseudo-cholinesterases. Hydrolysis of ACh occurs after formation of an acyl enzyme which is deacetylated, resulting in reformation of the parent enzyme. Inhibitors of acetylcholinesterases are widely used therapeutically and as insecticides. Others have been developed for use in chemical warfare. In particular, the so-called alkylfluorophosphates, such as diisopropylfluorophosphate, form stable bonds with the enzyme that are essentially irreversible. This is the mechanism of action of the irreversible antagonists of acetylcholinesterase used or developed for use as nerve gases. Death following exposure to nerve gas results

Biological Bases of Brain Function and Disease, edited by Alan Frazer, Perry B. Molinoff, and Andrew Winokur. Raven Press, Ltd., New York © 1994.

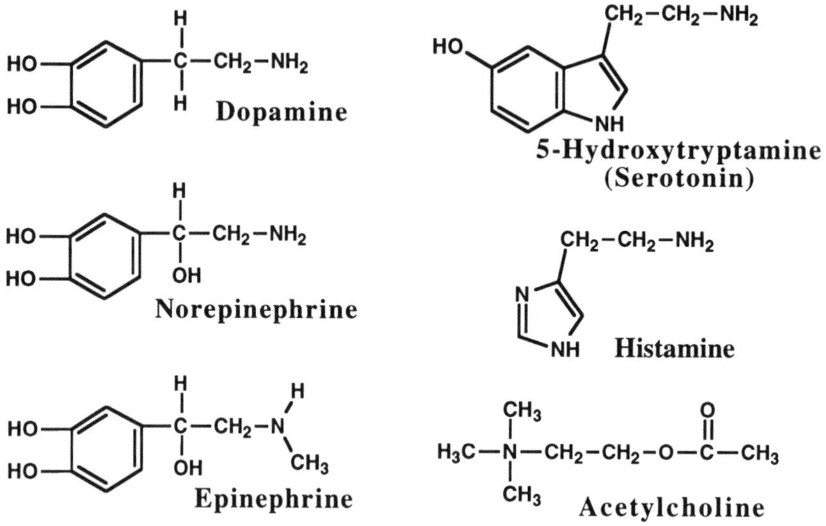

FIG. 1. Structures of biogenic amines.

from paralysis of respiratory muscles due to overstimulation by excess ACh. Other effects include excess salivary secretion and CNS stimulation leading to seizures.

ACh is widely distributed in both the central and peripheral nervous systems. In the periphery, it is the transmitter at both sympathetic and parasympathetic ganglia and is released by the splanchnic nerve to cause release of catecholamines from the adrenal medulla. ACh is also the transmitter at parasympathetic postganglionic synapses and at the neuromuscular junction. In the CNS it was shown to be the transmitter used by recurrent collaterals of motor neurons innervating Renshaw cells in the spinal cord. The use of histochemical, autoradiographic, and immunohistochemical techniques has now revealed cholinergic cells functioning as interneurons such as the intrinsic neurons in the striatum. Two major cholinergic tracts have also been identified. These include cells in the basal forebrain projecting to the nonstriatal telencephalon and cells in the pons projecting to the thalamus and other diencephalic loci.

Like other neurotransmitters and neuromodulators, acetylcholine interacts with multiple subtypes of receptors. In the case of ACh, subtypes of receptor were initially distinguished on the basis of sensitivity to muscarine or nicotine. This led to the identification of receptors as being *muscarinic cholinergic* or *nicotinic cholinergic* (Table 1). It was then observed that the nicotinic receptors in muscle had different pharmacological properties from those in ganglia. Specifically, the receptor in muscle was sensitive to curare and to

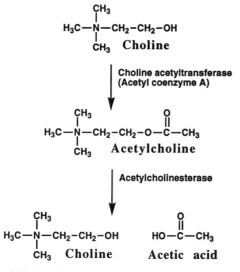

FIG. 2. Synthesis and breakdown of ACh.

TABLE 1. *Acetylcholine receptor terminology*

Receptor (antagonist)	Subtype	Second messenger
Muscarinic (atropine)	M_1 (pirenzepine) M_2 m_1, m_2, m_3, m_4, m_5	$\downarrow$cAMP/$\uparrow$PI/$\uparrow$K$^+$
Nicotinic (curare)	Muscle (decamethonium) Ganglion (hexamethonium)	Ion channels

decamethonium, while the nicotinic receptor in ganglia was less sensitive to curare and was sensitive to hexamethonium. Some muscarinic responses, defined as being blocked by atropine, were antagonized by pirenzepine while others were not. The suggestion that this reflected the existence of subtypes of muscarinic receptors was finally confirmed when results of molecular biological studies revealed at least five distinct muscarinic receptors that can be expressed in cell lines resulting in model systems with which to define their pharmacological properties.

The nicotinic cholinergic receptor was the first transmitter receptor to be purified to homogeneity. This was a consequence of the availability of snake venom toxins such as α-bungarotoxin, which has a remarkably high affinity for the receptor, along with the availability of tissue sources with high densities of these receptors, such as the electroplax of *Torpedo marmorata* and *Electrophorus electricus.* The nicotonic receptor is a pentamer containing two copies of an α subunit and one of each of three other subunits called β, γ, and δ (see Chapter 4). This results in a pentomeric receptor $(\alpha_2\beta\gamma\delta)$ with a molecular mass of approximately 280 kDa. The subunits are arranged in the form of a doughnut with a substantial portion of the protein on the extracellular surface of the membrane. The central hole of the doughnut is thought to represent the ion channel, which is impermeable to cations in its resting state. Activation results in a change in conformation and an opening of the channel. The open channel shows selectivity for cations largely on the basis of the size of the open channel. The two α subunits contain the binding sites for ACh as well as for snake venom toxins like α-bun-

garotoxin. A variety of studies utilizing both electrophysiological and biochemical techniques have shown that cooperative occupancy of both α subunits is necessary for full receptor activation.

Continued exposure of cells containing nicotinic cholinergic receptors to ACh leads to a rapid decrease in the size of the response despite the continued presence of the agonist. This diminished response is part of a process called *desensitization.* It is now believed that there are multiple states of the nicotinic receptor. These include the normal closed state, an open state capable of conducting cations, and a desensitized state. The channel can isomerize rapidly between the open and closed states and is slowly converted to a desensitized state in the continued presence of an agonist. Chronic changes in neuronal activity also have profound effects on nicotinic receptors. Thus, receptors are diffusely distributed across the surface of muscle cells in embryonic or fetal muscle. As the fibers become innervated, the distribution of receptors changes so that receptors are restricted to the region of the muscle at which the nerve muscle junction occurs, the so-called motor end-plate region. On denervation, the distribution of receptors returns to that seen in fetal muscle such that the muscle becomes uniformly sensitive to ACh.

The nicotinic receptor is structurally similar to other ligand-gated ion channels such as the GABA$_A$ receptor (see Chapter 7). The muscarinic receptor, on the other hand, has a structure similar to that of other members of the G-protein–linked superfamily of receptors (see Chapter 4). Cellular responses to stimulation of muscarinic receptors are, however, diverse. They include inhibition of adenylyl cyclase activity, stimulation of phospholipase C activity with consequent increases in phosphoinositide hydrolysis and intracellular levels of calcium, and activation of potassium channels. All of these responses involve GTP-binding proteins. The effects on adenylyl cyclase activity are almost certainly mediated through activation of G_i, while the effects on phospholipase C activity and on activation of potassium channels are mediated through G proteins that have not yet been specifically identified.

A variety of radioligands have been used to characterize nicotinic and muscarinic receptors. The most widely used ligand for the study of nicotinic receptors of the subtype found on skeletal muscle is ^{125}I-labeled α-bungarotoxin. Antagonists including quinuclidinylbenzilate and N-methylscopolamine have been used to study muscarinic receptors. Studies with pirenzepine have been critical for identification of subtypes of muscarinic receptors. Muscarinic receptors in several brain regions including cortex and hippocampus have a high affinity for pirenzepine whereas the receptors in peripheral tissues such as heart and smooth muscle as well as those in the cerebellum show a 30- to 50-fold lower affinity. The receptors in the CNS have been called M_1 receptors whereas those in the periphery are called M_2 receptors. A molecular biological approach has documented the presence of at least five subtypes of muscarinic receptor, denoted m1 through m5 (Table 1). These subtypes appear to be coupled to the various effector mechanisms that are activated by muscarinic receptors. The receptors, and the G proteins to which they are coupled, are, however, somewhat promiscuous in that multiple effects of muscarinic receptors can sometimes be elicited in cell lines expressing only a single subtype of receptor.

CATECHOLAMINES

A great deal of effort has gone into the development and application of neuroana-
tomic methods for the visualization of catecholamine-containing neurons. One of the principal methods takes advantage of the fact that catecholamines cyclize to form fluorescent products in the presence of formaldehyde. Thus, catecholamine-containing neurons can be visualized in thin sections of tissue exposed to formaldehyde vapor. An alternative approach uses antibodies elicited against the enzymes necessary for catecholamine biosynthesis. Antibodies to tyrosine hydroxylase will identify cells capable of synthesizing catecholamines. Antibodies against dopamine-β-hydroxylase (DBH) will distinguish dopamine-containing fibers that do not contain DBH from noradrenergic fibers that contain DBH. Similarly, neurons containing phenylethanolamine-N-methyltransferase, the epinephrine-forming enzyme, are presumed to be synthesizing epinephrine. The genes that encode the various biosynthetic enzymes involved in the synthesis of catecholamines have been cloned. The technique of *in situ* hybridization can therefore be used to localize mRNA for neurotransmitter-specific enzymes within particular classes of neurons (see Chapter 5).

Noradrenergic neurons arise from cell bodies clustered in the medulla oblongata, pons, and midbrain. Norepinephrine-containing fibers are divided into dorsal and ventral pathways (Fig. 3). The locus coeruleus contains the cell bodies of the neurons in the dorsal bundle. These neurons terminate in the spinal cord and cerebellum and run anteriorly through the medial forebrain bundle to innervate the cerebral cortex. Neurons from the locus coeruleus also project to the brain stem and hypothalamus.

Dopamine-containing neurons arise from cell bodies located in the midbrain and in the hypothalamus. Dopaminergic neurons are found in three major pathways called the nigrostriatal, mesolimbic, and tuberoinfundibular pathways (Fig. 4). What may be the most important dopamine-containing tract in the brain originates from cell bodies in the pars compacta of the substantia nigra. These cells terminate in a dense dopaminergic innerva-

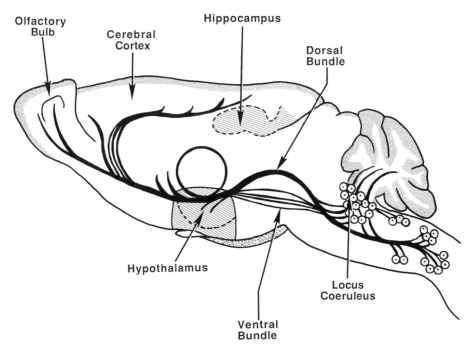

FIG. 3. Norepinephrine pathways. Adapted from Lader M. *Introduction to psychopharmacology*. A Scope publication, 1983, p. 37. The Upjohn Company © 1983.

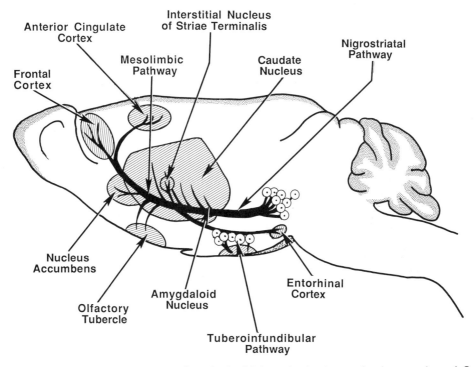

FIG. 4. Dopamine pathways. Adapted from Lader M. *Introduction to psychopharmacology*. A Scope publication, 1983, p. 34. The Upjohn Company © 1983.

tion in the striatum. Over 75% of the dopamine in the brain is found in the striatum, and it is the nigrostriatal path that degenerates in Parkinson's disease. Other dopamine-containing cell bodies result in diffuse innervation of the forebrain, septum, nucleus accumbens, and olfactory tubercle. It has been suggested that the antipsychotic neuroleptic drugs (see Chapter 18) act through blockade of the effects of dopamine on this mesocortical system. Finally, dopamine-containing cell bodies within the arcuate and periventricular nuclei of the hypothalamus innervate the pituitary and the median eminence (tuberoinfundibular pathway). These neurons are involved in regulating the release of pituitary hormones and, indeed, dopamine inhibits the release of prolactin and is what was once called prolactin inhibitory factor.

The synthesis of catecholamines involves four separate enzymatic reactions. The first reaction in catecholamine synthesis, catalyzed by tyrosine hydroxylase, is thought to be rate limiting (Fig. 5). The initial precursor of catecholamine synthesis is tyrosine, which is converted by tyrosine hydroxylase in the presence of tetrahydrobiopterin (TH_4), an external source of electrons, to L-dopa. The enzyme tyrosine hydroxylase is a mixed-function oxidase that also requires molecular oxygen from air. This enzyme has a relatively restricted distribution, being found only in catecholamine-containing neurons and chromaffin cells including those in the adrenal medulla. The enzyme is also subject to multiple regulatory influences. Short-term changes in neuronal firing induce rapid compensatory changes in the activity of the enzyme. These changes appear to reflect changes in the affinity of the enzyme for TH_4. The enzyme is also inhibited by the end products of the pathway including dopamine, norepinephrine, and epinephrine. On a longer time scale, depletion of catecholamines after chronic administration of a drug like reserpine results in a compensatory increase in the amount of tyrosine hydroxylase in sympathetic nerve endings.

The second step in the biosynthesis of catecholamines is catalyzed by the enzyme L-aromatic amino acid decarboxylase (L-AAD). This enzyme is widely distributed throughout the periphery and the CNS, and it plays a role in the biosynthesis of serotonin as well as that of norepinephrine. L-AAD utilizes pyridoxyl phosphate as a cofactor and, like tyrosine hydroxylase, it is a cytoplasmic enzyme. The usefulness of L-dopa for the treatment of Parkinson's disease is markedly increased by coadministration of carbidopa, which is an inhibitor of L-AAD that does not cross the blood–brain barrier. In the absence of carbidopa, much of an administered dose of L-dopa is destroyed by L-AAD in the liver and kidneys. The presence of tyrosine hydroxylase and L-AAD in the cytoplasm may be contrasted to the subcellular distribution of the enzyme DBH, which catalyzes the third step in the biosynthesis of catecholamines. DBH is a copper-containing enzyme that is associated with and contained within catecholamine storage vesicles. It catalyzes the conversion of dopamine to norepinephrine. DBH is a mixed-function oxidase that requires molecular oxygen from air and uses ascorbic acid as an external source of electrons.

The final step in the synthesis of catecholamines is catalyzed by the enzyme phenylethanolamine-*N*-methyltransferase (PNMT). This enzyme utilizes *S*-adenosylmethionine as a methyl donor. It is found in high concentrations in the adrenal medulla, which is bathed in high concentrations of corticosteroids released from the adrenal cortex. The resulting high concentrations of corticosteroids are necessary for the maintenance of PNMT activity. Thus, in the absence of steroids, PNMT activity virtually disappears. PNMT is found primarily in the cytoplasm. This means that dopamine must be transported across the membrane of the chromaffin granule to be β-hydroxylated. N-methylation, on the other hand, takes place in the cytoplasm while storage of the hormone epinephrine is in chromaffin granules.

The enzymatic metabolism of catechol-

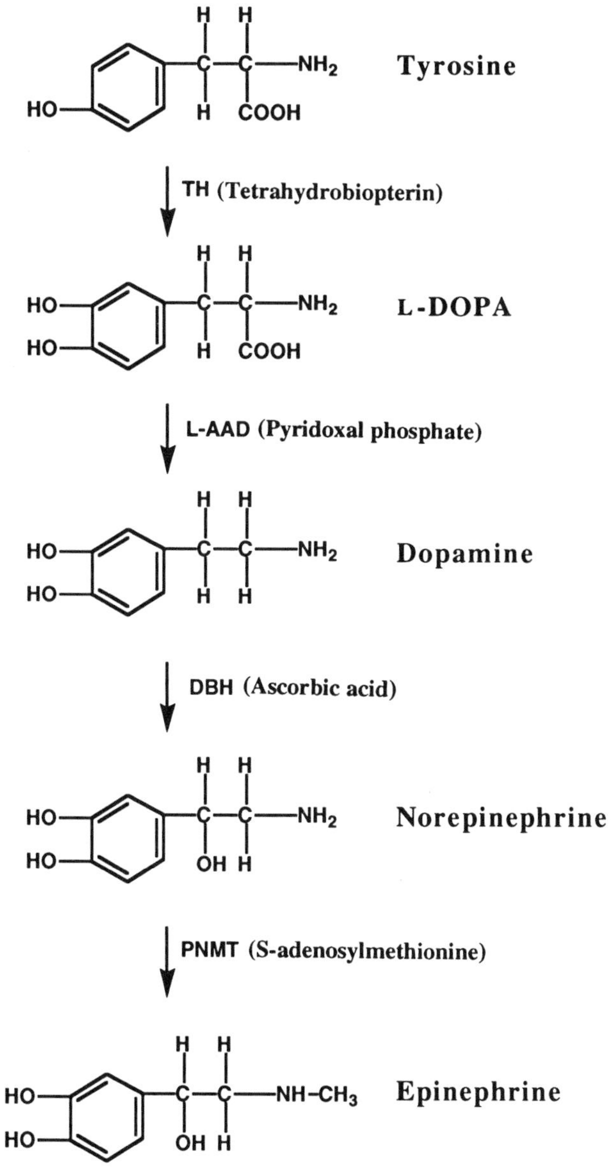

FIG. 5. Synthesis of catecholamines.

amines is considerably more complex than that of acetylcholine. Four enzymes are involved in catecholamine metabolism. The two principal enzymes are the mitochondrial enzyme monoamine oxidase (MAO) and the soluble enzyme catechol-*O*-methyltransferase (COMT) (Fig. 6). COMT catalyzes the methylation of the metahydroxyl group of epinephrine or norepinephrine to form metanephrine or normetanephrine. *S*-Adenosylmethionine is the methyl donor for this reaction. MAO catalyzes formation of an aldehyde that is relatively unstable. This aldehyde is therefore rapidly acted on by either aldehyde reductase to form a glycol or aldehyde dehydrogenase to form an acid. The product resulting from the action of either MAO or COMT can act as a substrate for the other enzyme. MAO is a mitochondrial enzyme and there are large numbers of mitochondria in adrenergic

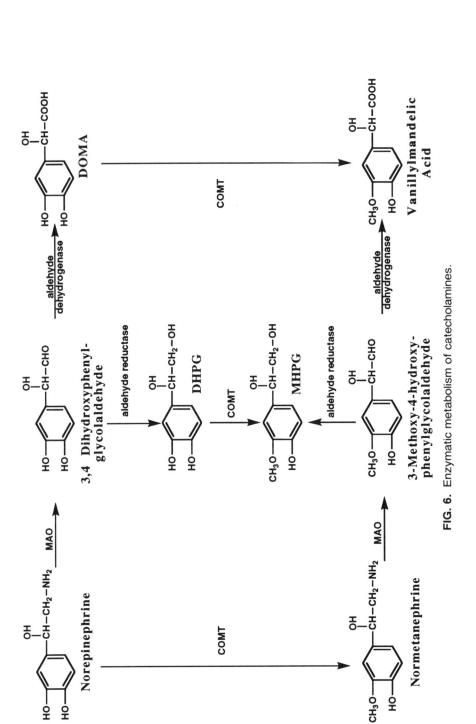

FIG. 6. Enzymatic metabolism of catecholamines.

nerve terminals. MAO thus appears to be involved in the metabolism of interneuronal catecholamines. Catecholamines that are not protected by being in storage vesicles may be oxidatively deaminated by MAO. This includes amine that has leaked out of vesicles as well as amine that has been released and then taken back up across neuronal membranes. Vanillylmandelic acid is the principal product of metabolism of norepinephrine. This compound is formed by metabolism of either norepinephrine or epinephrine since the difference between these two compounds is restricted to an *N*-methyl group that is removed by MAO. Homovanillic acid is the corresponding metabolite of dopamine. The first inhibitor of MAO to be discovered was iproniazid. It came out of an attempt to develop analogs of isoniazid for the treatment of tuberculosis. Iproniazid and other inhibitors of MAO are used for the treatment of hypertension and depression. Increased levels of catecholamine in the CNS and resulting increases in stimulation of receptors appear to account for the ability of MAO inhibitors to lower blood pressure and elevate mood.

In contrast to the effects of inhibitors of acetylcholinesterase, which markedly potentiate both endogenously released and exogenously administered ACh, inhibitors of MAO and/or COMT have relatively little influence on the magnitude or duration of the effects of catecholamines. In fact, the principal mechanism for termination of the physiological effects of catecholamines involves reuptake of catecholamine by a sodium-dependent uptake pump called uptake 1. This uptake pump has been shown to represent an important site of action of drugs used for the treatment of affective disorders (see Chapter 17). Uptake 2 is a high-capacity, low-affinity uptake system that may be involved in terminating the effects of an exogenously administered drug but is unlikely to play an important role in terminating the action of neuronally released norepinephrine (Fig. 7).

Release of catecholamines results from nerve stimulation or stimulation of the adrenal gland by cholinomimetic drugs. Catecholamine release is quantal in nature and is dependent on the presence of external calcium. ATP, DBH, and soluble proteins called chromogranins are released along with the catecholamines. Although much of the DBH is bound to the membranes of adrenergic storage vesicles or chromaffin granules, some is contained in the soluble contents of these vesi-

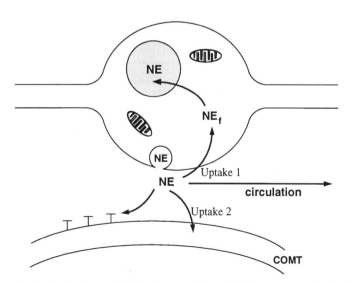

FIG. 7. Uptake of catecholamines. Uptake 1: reuptake of NE into nerve terminals—high-affinity, low-capacity system; uptake 2: extraneuronal uptake—low-affinity, high-capacity system.

cles and granules. It is the soluble enzyme that is released along with catecholamines. Storage of catecholamines in chromaffin granules in the adrenal medulla appears to be in the form of a tetracatecholamine-ATP complex, thus accounting for the release of large amounts of ATP. The release of labile molecules like ATP and large proteins including DBH and the chromogranins suggests that the mechanism of release reflects the exocytotic release of the contents of the storage vesicle (see Chapter 3).

Soon after the demonstration that norepinephrine is the predominant postganglionic sympathetic neurotransmitter, it was recognized that not all of the effects of catecholamines could be explained by interaction with a single class of receptor. Responses mediated by β-adrenergic receptors included increases in cardiac contractility and bronchodilation. These responses were also seen following administration of the exogenous catecholamine isoproterenol. In contrast, responses mediated by α-adrenergic receptors, which included contraction of the spleen and vascular smooth muscle, were not seen following administration of isoproterenol. It was subsequently realized that responses mediated by β-adrenergic receptors could be associated with two principal subtypes of receptors called β_1- and β_2-adrenergic receptors on the basis of differing sensitivities to the endogenous catecholamines epinephrine and norepinephrine. Thus, β_1-adrenergic receptors are sensitive to both norepinephrine and epinephrine, while β_2-adrenergic receptors are relatively insensitive to norepinephrine and may be thought of as hormone receptors responding to the adrenal hormone epinephrine. Subtypes of α-adrenergic receptors were first distinguished on the basis of their cellular location. The α_1-adrenergic receptor was shown to be a postsynaptic receptor mediating the excitatory effects of catecholamines on tissues such as vascular smooth muscle. In contrast, α_2-adrenergic receptors were initially described as being located on presynaptic nerve terminals, where they functioned as inhibitory autoreceptors.

Comparison of the sequences of adrenergic receptors as revealed in studies of cDNA sequences indicate that there are three subfamilies of adrenergic receptor. Subtypes of α_1-, α_2-, and β-adrenergic receptors are known to exist in various mammalian tissues (Table 2). It is likely that additional subtypes remain to be identified. Similarities in amino acid sequence, pharmacological properties, and linkage to second-messenger systems are used to distinguish between members of the three families of adrenergic receptors. The receptors differ in terms of the number of glycosylation sites, the number of phosphorylation sites, and the sizes of the third intracellular loop and the amino terminus (see Chapter 4). Nonetheless, the overall structures are remarkably similar, with the highest degree of homology being seen in the seven transmembrane α helices. Selective antagonists for α_1 and α_2 receptors like prazosin and yohimbine have been identified. The subtypes of α-adrenergic receptor have also been shown to differ in terms of the second-messenger system to which they are coupled. Thus, stimulation of α_1 receptors results in increases in phosphoinositide metabolism while stimulation of α_2 receptors results in inhibition of adenylyl cyclase activity. In contrast, stimulation of β-adrenergic receptors uniformly results in an increase in intracellular levels of cyclic AMP. The α_2 receptors are also coupled to K^+ channels, while β receptors are coupled to Ca^{2+} channels.

In addition to being a precursor in the synthesis of norepinephrine and epinephrine, dopamine is a transmitter in its own right. Several CNS pathways use dopamine as a neurotransmitter, including the nigrostriatal pathway, which degenerates in Parkinson's disease. Abnormalities of dopaminergic pathways are widely believed to be involved in the pathobiology of schizophrenia. Dopamine receptors are also found in the kidney, although their specific cellular location and function remain to be defined. Multiple subtypes of dopamine receptor have been described (Table 3). They can be distinguished by their effects on cAMP levels with D_1 and

TABLE 2. *Classification of adrenergic receptors*

Type	Agonist (antagonist)	Characteristics	No. amino acids	Second messenger
α_1-Adrenergic	NE $\geq$ EPI $\gg$ ISO			IP$_3$/DAG
α_{1A}	Phenylephrine (WB-4101)	Vasoconstriction	560-C5 (rat)	
α_{1B}	(chloroethylclonidine)	Vasoconstriction	515-C5 (rat)	
α_{1C}	Oxymetazoline (chloroethylclonidine)		466-C8 (bovine)	
α_2-Adrenergic	NE $\geq$ EPI $\gg$ ISO			
α_{2A}	Oxymetazoline	Inhibits NE and renin release, lowers blood pressure by central action	450-C10 (human)	↓cAMP K$^+$channel
α_{2B}	(prazosin) (ARC-239)		450-C2 (human)	
α_{2C}	Norepinephrine (idazoxan)		461-C4 (human)	
β-Adrenergic	ISO > EPI $\geq$ NE	Vasodilation, inhibition of uterine contraction, myocardial stimulation		↑cAMP Ca^{++} channel
β_1	ISO > EPI = NE (practolol) (ICI 89,406)	Fatty acid mobilization, cardiac stimulation	477-C10 (human)	
β_2	ISO > EPI > NE (butoxamine) (ICI 118,551)	Bronchodilation, vasodepression, inhibition of uterine contraction	413-C5 (human)	
β_3	ISO > EPI BRL-37344 (pindolol)	Lipolysis	402-C? (human)	

D_5 receptors being coupled to stimulation of cAMP synthesis while D_2 receptors are coupled to inhibition of cyclic AMP synthesis. The second messenger involved in the action of D_3 and D_4 receptors has not been identified. The D_1 and D_5 receptors appear to be members of a subfamily as do the D_2, D_3, and D_4 receptors. A variety of specific antagonists have been identified, including SCH 23390, which is a specific antagonist of D_1-

TABLE 3. *Dopamine receptor subtypes*

	D_1-like receptors	D_2-like receptors
Adenylyl cyclase	D_1, D_5—stimulate	D_{2S}, D_{2L}—inhibit D_3, D_4—no effect
Affinity for DA	$D_5 > D_1$	$D_3 > D_4 > D_2$
mRNA	D_1—diffuse D_5—hippocampus, hypothalamus	D_2—striatum D_3—olfactory tubercle, n. accumbens D_4—amygdala, f. cortex
Antagonists	SCH-23390—nonselective	Spiperone—nonselective D_3—AJ76 and UH232 D_4—clozapine
Structure	i$_3$ loop—44–56 aa C terminus 77–108 aa	i$_3$ loop—101–165 aa C terminus 16–17 aa

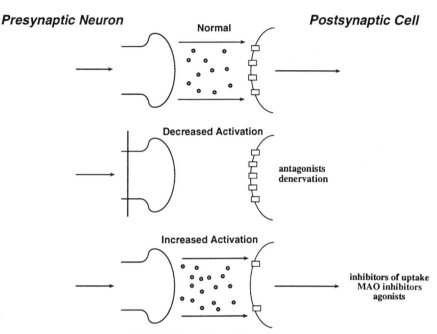

FIG. 8. Regulation of receptors.

like receptors, and the butyrophenone spiroperidol, which is a specific antagonist of D_2-like receptors.

As previously described, changes in the distribution and number of nicotinic cholinergic receptors occur as a consequence of denervation of a skeletal muscle. Changes in the number of receptors for catecholamines have also been observed following denervation. In the mammalian CNS, denervation results in an increase in the density of β_1-adrenergic receptors, as well as α_1, α_2, and D_2 dopamine receptors. No change in the density of β_2-adrenergic receptors resulted from denervation. This is probably a consequence of there being only small amounts of epinephrine in the CNS. Since norepinephrine has a relatively low affinity for β_2-adrenergic receptors, removal of sympathetic tone in the CNS does not result in a significant decrease in stimulation of β_2-adrenergic receptors. Studies carried out in a number of systems have led to the development of a model that relates changes in the density of receptors to changes in synaptic levels of transmitter (Fig. 8). Decreased receptor activation results from chronic administration of an antagonist or from surgical or chemical denervation that causes destruction of presynaptic terminals. In either experimental paradigm, there is a compensatory increase in the density of receptors without a change in their kinetic or equilibrium properties. Increased receptor activation results from a variety of pharmacological interventions including the chronic administration of agonists and, in the case of catecholamine receptors, administration of a variety of antidepressants. These include tricyclic antidepressants such as desmethylimipramine (DMI), which blocks the reuptake of catecholamines and serotonin into presynaptic nerve terminals (see Chapter 17). MAO inhibitors like pargyline block the interneuronal degradation of catecholamines, resulting in increased interneuronal levels and presumably increased release. These treatments all result in a time-dependent decrease in the density of receptors.

HISTAMINE

Histamine is formed from the amino acid L-histidine. The conversion of L-histidine to histamine (Fig. 9) is catalyzed by a specific

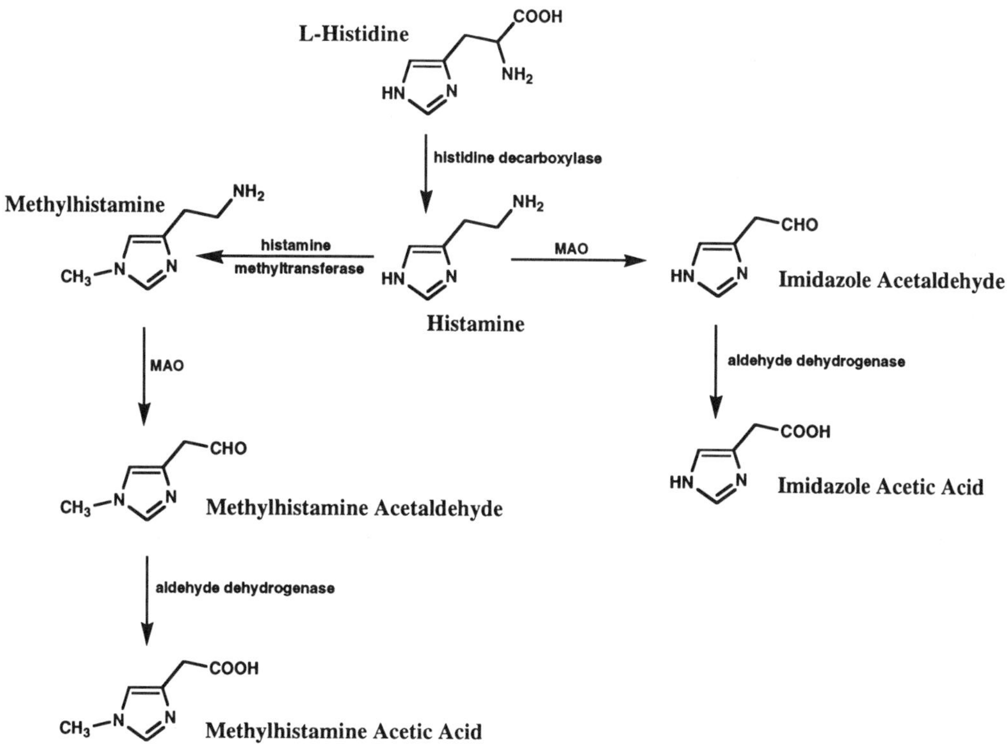

FIG. 9. Synthesis and metabolism of histamine.

histidine decarboxylase as well as by L-AAD, the enzyme that decarboxylates L-dopa. Histidine decarboxylase has been purified from rat liver and shown to have a molecular weight of 110,000. Histidine decarboxylase, like L-AAD, requires pyridoxal phosphate as a cofactor, and histidine decarboxylase is inhibited by α-fluoromethylhistidine. Cell bodies in the posterior hypothalamus project ipsilaterally to a wide distribution of areas of the brain and spinal cord. Histidine decarboxylase–containing endochromaffin-like cells are also present in the stomach, and histamine released from these cells may stimulate acid secretion, accounting for the ability of H_2 receptor antagonists to reduce acid secretion; this is the presumed mechanism by which H_2 antagonists such as cimetidine and ranitidine exert their beneficial effects on peptic ulcers. A high-affinity uptake system for histamine has not been reported. As with catecholamines, metabolism of histamine is by methylation and oxidative deamination. Methylation is carried out by a specific histamine methyltransferase, an enzyme that has been purified from both guinea pig brain and rat kidney. Oxidative deamination of histamine is catalyzed by MAO.

The pharmacological effects of histamine, including profound hypotension and marked bronchoconstriction, are similar to responses observed during anaphylactic reactions. More recently, histamine has also been shown to function as a neurotransmitter or neuromodulator in the CNS. Effects of histamine appear to be mediated through two principal subtypes of receptors; H_1 receptors are found on CNS neurons, whereas H_2 receptors play a prominent role in the control of acid secretion from the stomach. Blockade of H_2 receptors in the stomach is now the mainstay of the treatment of peptic ulcers. A variety of second-messenger systems have been implicated in the actions of histamine.

These actions include increases in cAMP levels, increases in phosphoinositide turnover, and decreases in calcium-dependent potassium conductance.

Studies of H_1 receptors in the brain have been based on studies of the binding of the antagonist pyrilamine. Results of quantitative autoradiographic studies show that the hippocampus, particularly the CA3 region, has a high density of H_1 receptors in the rat although a relatively low density is observed in guinea pig hippocampus. Attempts to investigate second-messenger systems linked to H_1 receptors have yielded conflicting results. In particular, stimulation of H_1 receptors has been associated with increases in the formation of cAMP and cyclic GMP and increased phosphoinositide turnover with associated increases in cytosolic calcium. It has not been determined whether the multiple second-messenger systems activated by H_1 receptors reflect direct effects of histamine or sequential effects of the various phosphoinositides produced on activation of phospholipase C and perhaps phospholipase A_2.

Attempts to demonstrate the presence of H_2 receptors in the CNS have been based largely on studies of histamine-stimulated increases in cAMP levels. Specific labeling of H_2 receptors has not been observed. Electrophysiological studies of effects of histamine reveal that in most cases histamine inhibits neuronal firing, causing hyperpolarization and decreased excitatory postsynaptic potentials. Studies of cultured neurons or brain slices have revealed a histamine-induced reduction in a calcium-dependent potassium conductance.

SEROTONIN

Serotonin is found in high concentrations in platelets from which it is released on aggregation. Serotonin has a wide distribution in many mammalian species and is found in neural structures of vertebrates and invertebrates. It is formed by sequential hydroxylation followed by decarboxylation of the amino acid tryptophan (Fig. 10). Tryptophan hydroxylase is a mixed-function oxidase requiring molecular oxygen from air and TH_4 as a source of electrons. Decarboxylation of 5-hydroxytryptophan is catalyzed by L-AAD in a reaction that is again dependent on pyridoxal phosphate.

Cell bodies of serotonin-containing neurons are found in the raphe nuclei of the brain stem (Fig. 11). They project widely to almost all levels of the CNS. In particular, neurons in the hippocampus and the septum (limbic structures) are innervated by neurons in the median raphe. While neurons in the dorsal raphe innervate basal ganglia structures, including the striatum and the substantia nigra, the neocortex is innervated by both the dorsal and the median raphe. Depolarization of cell bodies in the raphe results in release of serotonin, and the effects of serotonin are terminated by reuptake into presynaptic terminals. The uptake system, similar to that for other biogenic amines, is a low-capacity, high-affinity system that is both sodium- and temperature-dependent. Specific inhibitors of serotonin uptake, including drugs like sertraline and fluoxetine, have recently been identified and are used clinically as antidepressants (see Chapter 17). Obsessive-compulsive disorders, panic disorders, and migraine headaches are other diseases that are treated by drugs that affect serotonergic neurons.

Metabolism of serotonin, catalyzed by MAO, yields 5-hydroxyindoleacetaldehyde (Fig. 10). The primary metabolic pathway for serotonin then involves conversion of the aldehyde to hydroxyindoleacetic acid, a reaction catalyzed by aldehyde dehydrogenase.

An interesting additional pathway involving serotonin occurs in the pineal gland. In this tissue, the enzyme *N*-acetylserotonin-transferase converts serotonin in the presence of acetyl coenzyme A to *N*-acetylserotonin, which is *O*-methylated by hydroxyindole-*O*-methyltransferase in the presence of *S*-adenosylmethionine to form melatonin (Fig.

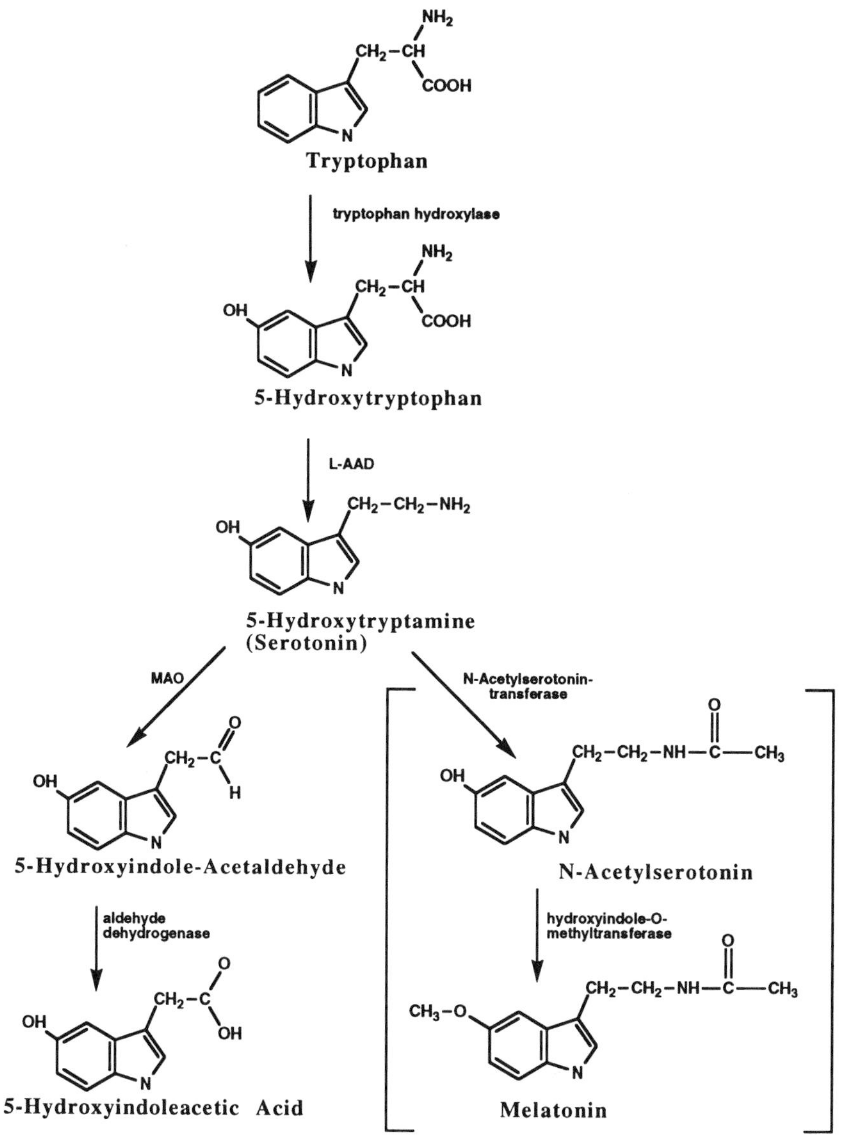

FIG. 10. Synthesis and degradation of serotonin. The conversion of serotonin to melatonin takes place in the pineal.

10). Melatonin has significant effects on skin color in frogs and has marked effects on gonadal maturation in mammals.

It is not surprising that there are multiple classes of receptors for serotonin. The nomenclature used at the present time is to identify 5-HT$_1$ receptors as those receptors with a high affinity for the endogenous agonist 5-HT. There are four distinct classes of 5-HT$_1$ receptors called 5-HT$_{1A}$, 5-HT$_{1B}$, 5-HT$_{1C}$, and 5-HT$_{1D}$ (Table 4). They have been linked to a variety of physiological and biochemical effects including increases and decreases in cAMP levels. The 5-HT$_2$ receptor has been specifically shown to increase phosphoinositide metabolism. It is identified by its high affinity for drugs like ketanserin and spiroperidol. Molecular biological studies

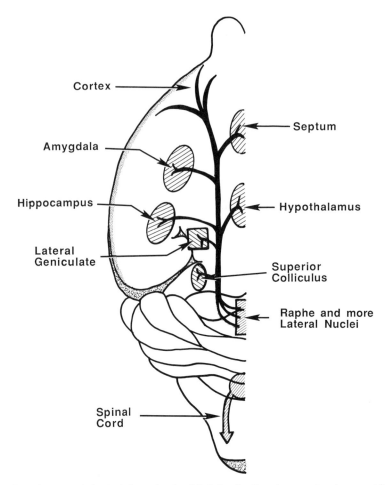

FIG. 11. 5-HT pathways. Adapted from Lader M. *Introduction to psychopharmacology.* A Scope publication, 1983, p. 39. The Upjohn Company © 1983.

have revealed that the 5-HT$_2$ receptor has a high degree of homology with the 5-HT$_{1C}$ receptor that is found in high concentrations in the choroid plexus. In addition to marked degrees of sequence similarity, both of these receptors are linked to changes in phosphoinositide metabolism and, indeed, it appears that the 5-HT$_{1C}$ receptor is more similar to the 5-HT$_2$ receptor than to the other members of the 5-HT$_1$ receptor family. The 5-HT$_3$ receptor is inhibited by ICS 205-930 and is linked to a calcium channel. The 5-HT$_4$ receptor has only recently been identified. It appears to act through increases in intracellular levels of cAMP (Table 4).

Our understanding of the regulation of 5-HT$_2$ receptors is less advanced than that of the regulation of the catecholamine or cholinergic receptors. The response of 5-HT$_2$ receptors to various experimental manipulations appears to differ from that of other biogenic amine receptors. For example, denervation of serotonergic neurons does not result in up-regulation of 5-HT$_{1A}$ or 5-HT$_2$ receptors. Similarly, administration of selective blockers of 5-HT uptake does not cause down-regulation of receptors. One could interpret both of these results as suggesting that the receptors are not under a significant endogenous tone. The lack of tone would mean that denervation would not have a marked effect on receptor stimulation and, simi-

TABLE 4. *Properties of subtypes of 5-HT receptors*

	Ligand	Effector mechanism	Tissue	Clone
5-HT$_1$	^{3}H-5-HT			
1A	^{3}H-8-OH-DPAT	cAMP↑↓	Hippocampus	+
1B	^{125}I-ICYP	cAMP↓	Rat substantia nigra; OK cells	+
1C	^{3}H-Mesulergine	PI hydrolysis	Choroid plexus	+
1D	^{3}H-5-HT	cAMP↓	Cow substantia nigra	+
5-HT$_2$	^{3}H-SPD/^{125}I-LSD/ ^{3}H-ketanserin	PI hydrolysis	Frontal cortex A$_7$R$_5$/WRK 1/C6	+
5-HT$_3$	^{3}H-ICS 205-930	Ligand-gated ion channels (Ca^{++})	N1E-115	+
5-HT$_4$		cAMP↑	Guinea pig hippocampus	−

larly, if there is a low density of serotonin-containing presynaptic neurons, blockade of 5-HT uptake might not cause significant down-regulation. More difficult to explain is the observation that the administration of 5-HT$_2$ receptor antagonists causes a rapid and persistent down-regulation of 5-HT$_2$ receptors. An understanding of the structural basis for the unexpected results obtained in studies of these effects of drugs on 5-HT receptors is likely to come from studies involving site-directed mutagenesis and the production of hybrid (chimeric) receptors. It is also possible that advances in understanding will follow the development of drugs with higher affinity and/or selectivity for particular subtypes of 5-HT receptors.

BIBLIOGRAPHY

Original Articles

Birks RI, MacIntosh FC. Acetylcholine metabolism of a sympathetic ganglion. *Can J Biochem Physiol* 1961;39:787–827.

Dale HH. The action of certain esters and ethers of choline and their relation to muscarine. *J Pharmacol* 1914;6:147–190.

Shiman R, Akino M, Kaufman S. Solubilization and partial purification of tyrosine hydroxylase from bovine adrenal medulla. *J Biol Chem* 1971;246:1330–1340.

Unwin N. The structure of ion channels in membranes of excitable cells. *Neuron* 1989;3:665–676.

Books and Reviews

Axelrod J. Noradrenaline: fate and control of its biosynthesis. *Science* 1971;173:598–606.

Bylund DB. Subtypes of α_1- and α_2-adrenergic receptors. *FASEB J* 1992;6:832–839.

Frazer A, Hensler JG. Serotonin. In: Siegel GJ, Agranoff BW, Albers RW, Molinoff PB, eds. *Basic neurochemistry*, 5th ed. New York: Raven Press; 1994 (in press).

Frazer A, Maayani S, Wolfe BB. Subtypes of receptors for serotonin. *Annu Rev Pharmacol Toxicol* 1990;30:307–348.

Gilman AG. G proteins: transducers of receptor-generated signals. *Annu Rev Biochem* 1987;56:615–649.

Green JP. Histamine. In: Siegel GF, Agranoff BW, Albers RW, Molinoff PB, eds. *Basic neurochemistry*, 5th ed. New York: Raven Press; 1994 (in press).

Hartig PR. Molecular biology of 5-HT receptors. *Trends Pharmacol Sci* 1989;10:64–69.

Hulme EC, Birdsall NJM, Buckley NJ. Muscarinic receptor subtypes. *Annu Rev Pharmacol Toxicol* 1991;30:633–673.

Kebabian JW, Calne DB. Multiple receptors for dopamine. *Nature* 1979;277:93–96.

Kobilka B. Adrenergic receptors as models for G protein-coupled receptors. *Annu Rev Neurosci* 1992;15:87–114.

Massoulié J, Bon S. The molecular forms of cholinesterase and acetylcholinesterase in vertebrates. *Annu Rev Neurosci* 1982;5:57–106.

Molinoff PB, Axelrod J. Biochemistry of catecholamines. *Annu Rev Biochem* 1971;40:465–500.

Page IH. The discovery of serotonin. *Persp Biol Med* 1976;20:1–8.

Prell GD, Green JP. Histamine as a neuroregulator. *Annu Rev Neurosci* 1986;9:209–254.

Sibley DR, Monsma FJ Jr. Molecular biology of dopamine receptors. *Trends Pharmacol Sci* 1992;13:61–69.

Taylor P, Brown JH. Acetylcholine. In: Siegel GJ, Agranoff BW, Albers RW, Molinoff PB, eds. *Basic neurochemistry*, 5th ed. New York: Raven Press; 1994 (in press).

Weiner N, Molinoff PB. Catecholamines. In: Siegel GJ, Agranoff BW, Albers RW, Molinoff PB, eds. *Basic neurochemistry*, 5th ed. New York: Raven Press; 1994 (in press).

7

Synaptic Transmission
Amino Acids

Michael B. Robinson

The improver of natural knowledge absolutely refuses to acknowledge authority, as such. For him, skepticism is the highest of duties, blind faith the one unpardonable sin.

Thomas H. Huxley,
On the Advisableness of Improving Natural Knowledge, 1866

- Over the last four decades, the excitatory amino acids (EAAs) glutamate and aspartate have gained acceptance as the predominant excitatory neurotransmitters in the mammalian CNS.

- Glutamate and aspartate, which are present in the CNS at very high levels, are essential for brain intermediary metabolism, precluding identification of a unique precursor for transmitter pools of these amino acids.

- Glutamate and aspartate are released upon depolarization and are inactivated at the synapse by uptake.

- Glutamate and aspartate depolarize neurons by interacting with at least three broad classes of receptors.

- AMPA receptors, kainate receptors, and NMDA receptors are major subtypes of EAA receptors coupled to ion channels.

- Since 1989, a number of cDNA clones have been isolated that can be used to express functional EAA receptors coupled to ion channels.

- Receptors for EAAs are also coupled to second-messenger systems and are called metabotropic receptors.

- Most of the rapid depolarizing responses in the CNS are mediated by EAAs.

- The amino acids GABA and glycine are the predominant inhibitory neurotransmitters in the mammalian CNS.

- GABA and glycine are present in the CNS at very high levels.

- GABA and glycine are released upon depolarization and are inactivated by uptake mechanisms.

- GABA and glycine hyperpolarize neurons by interacting with different receptors.

- There are two types of GABA receptors, $GABA_A$ and $GABA_B$, with the former coupled to ion channels that are permeable to chloride and the latter coupled to second-messenger systems.

- While GABA is generally thought to hyperpolarize neurons throughout the CNS, the actions of glycine tend to be restricted to caudal areas of the CNS.

- The amino acid transmitter systems have been implicated in a wide range of neurodegenerative and psychiatric disorders.

- Seizure activity can generally be thought of as the result of an imbalance between the excitatory and inhibitory amino acid systems.

- Many anxiolytics (compounds that reduce anxiety) act directly on the $GABA_A$ receptor.

This chapter describes our current understanding of the neurochemistry and physiology of synaptic transmission mediated by amino acids. The discussion begins with an elucidation of the structures of the excitatory and inhibitory amino acid neurotransmitters. This is followed by descriptions of localization and synthesis, activation/inactivation, and receptor interactions of the neurotransmitters. The final sections draw the connection between the amino acid neurotransmitters and a wide range of neurological and psychiatric disorders.

Of the several dozen established or putative *neurotransmitters,* only a few mediate rapid synaptic responses that last from 2 to 10 msec. In general, catecholamines, indoleamines, and neuropeptides generate slower signals lasting from 20 msec to 10 sec or more. Acetylcholine (ACh) and amino acids mediate most of the rapid synaptic responses in the nervous system.

ACh is the best characterized of the rapidly acting neurotransmitters (see Chapter 6). At the neuromuscular junction, muscle fibers are depolarized as a consequence of the interaction of ACh with nicotinic receptors that are coupled to cation-selective channels. Within 1 to 2 msec, the flow of sodium through this channel results in depolarization of the muscle with subsequent muscle contraction. In the mammalian central nervous system (CNS), the acidic amino acids glutamate and aspartate mediate most of the rapid depolarizing responses. Like ACh, these amino acids interact with receptors that are coupled to ion-selective channels that when activated, result in an influx of cations and depolarization. These neurotransmitters, which increase the probability of action potential initiation, are called *excitatory neurotransmitters.* The rapid depolarizing responses are balanced by rapid hyperpolarizing responses, many of which are mediated by the amino acids glycine and γ-aminobutyric acid (GABA). The receptors for glycine and GABA are coupled to ion channels that are selectively permeable to anions. Since these neurotransmitters tend to decrease the initiation of action potentials, they are called *inhibitory neurotransmitters.* Together these amino acid transmitter systems mediate most of the synaptic responses in the CNS.

Over the last two decades, our understanding of the role of these amino acids in the biology of normal and abnormal brain function has increased dramatically. The synthesis or isolation of drugs that selectively interact with the receptors for the amino acids has led to the identification, purification, and cloning of many of these receptors. In fact, cloning techniques led to the identification of subtypes of receptors that could not be identified with pharmacological approaches. Pharmacological agents that both increase and decrease the efficacy of these transmitters have been used as tools to investigate the role of amino acid neurotransmitters in mood disorders, seizure activity, and neuronal degeneration. Their use has also led to evidence of a role for amino acid neurotransmitters in memory.

STRUCTURES OF THE AMINO ACID NEUROTRANSMITTERS

Biological Bases of Brain Function and Disease, edited by Alan Frazer, Perry B. Molinoff, and Andrew Winokur. Raven Press, Ltd., New York © 1994.

The amino acids are structurally among the simplest of the neurotransmitters (Fig. 1).

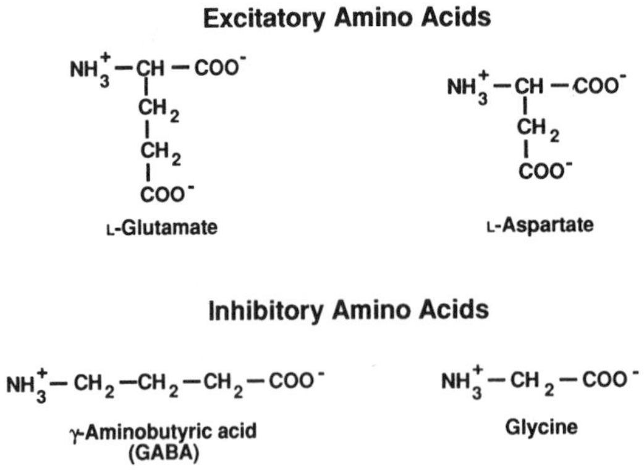

Excitatory Amino Acids

L-Glutamate   L-Aspartate

Inhibitory Amino Acids

γ-Aminobutyric acid   Glycine
(GABA)

FIG. 1. Structures of important amino acid neurotransmitters.

The excitatory amino acids (EAAs), glutamate and aspartate, have two carboxyl groups that are separated by three or two methylene groups, respectively. They also have an amino group at the α position to one of the carboxyl groups. The pK_a values of the carboxyl groups are approximately 3.5 to 4.5, and the pK_a values of the amino groups are approximately 8. Therefore, at a physiological pH of about 7.0 to 7.4, the amino and carboxyl groups are charged, but with opposite signs, and the EAAs carry a net negative charge. The inhibitory neurotransmitters, glycine and GABA, have one amino group and one carboxyl group that are separated by one or three methylene carbons, respectively. The pK_a values of the amino and carboxyl groups are similar to those for glutamate and aspartate. At physiological pH, both are charged, but with opposite signs, and the net charge of these compounds is zero.

EXCITATORY AMINO ACIDS

Over the last four decades, the excitatory amino acids (EAAs) glutamate and aspartate have gained acceptance as the predominant excitatory neurotransmitters in the mammalian CNS. The acceptance of neurotransmitter status for glutamate and aspartate in the mammalian CNS has been very slow. In 1952, Hayashi and his colleagues, in an attempt to understand epilepsy, demonstrated

that application of glutamate to the cortex resulted in excitation. It was not until the 1960s that Curtis, Watkins, and their colleagues systematically examined the structure–activity relationships of depolarizing substances related to glutamate. Active compounds had two acidic groups optimally separated by a two- or three-carbon chain with an amino group at the α position to one of the acidic groups. These are the structural features of glutamate and aspartate (Fig. 1), both of which are present in very high concentrations in brain tissue. During the last two decades, attempts to demonstrate that these amino acids meet all of the criteria for neurotransmitter status have met with varying success. In the 1970s and 1980s, calcium-dependent release of glutamate and aspartate was demonstrated, and an active uptake system to regulate extracellular concentrations of these amino acids was identified. The synthesis and/or isolation of EAA analogs has led to the identification of at least four broad subtypes of EAA receptors. The results of physiological, pharmacological, and biochemical studies suggest that glutamate and aspartate are the predominant excitatory neurotransmitters in the mammalian CNS. Potent and selective antagonists for some of the subtypes of EAA receptors are still lacking, but as selective agents become available, the role of these systems in neuronal function will be further clarified.

Localization and Synthesis

Glutamate and aspartate, which are present in the CNS at very high levels, are essential for brain intermediary metabolism, precluding identification of a unique precursor for transmitter pools of these amino acids. The high levels and ubiquitous distribution of glutamate and aspartate in brain tissue defy the traditional concept of a neurotransmitter. Most neurotransmitters are heterogeneously distributed in brain tissue. It is presumed that areas containing large amounts of a particular compound use that compound as a neurotransmitter. Levels of glutamate (approaching 10 mmol/kg of tissue) and aspartate (1 to 2 mmol/kg of tissue) in brain are at least 1,000-fold higher than the levels of other established neurotransmitters, including dopamine, ACh, and serotonin. While the levels of dopamine, ACh, and serotonin measured in various brain regions can vary as much as 20-fold, the levels of glutamate and aspartate generally vary by less than 3-fold.

A presynaptic localization of these amino acids is supported by results from biochemical and immunohistochemical investigations. Glutamate is enriched in synaptic vesicles, the subcellular organelles that are associated with the storage and release of neurotransmitter. Antibodies generated against glutamate and aspartate have been used for immunohistochemical localization. It is possible to localize glutamate- and aspartate-like immunoreactivity to axons and presynaptic terminals. However, since the antibodies can recognize other molecules with similar structural characteristics, this approach can result in false positives. This makes the unequivocal interpretation of the specificity of the staining impossible. In spite of these potential false positives, there is generally a close correlation between the distribution of glutamate- and aspartate-like immunoreactivity in neurons and other markers for EAA transmission. Extensive mapping of glutamate- and aspartate-like immunoreactivity in the hippocampal formation has been carried out. In this structure, glutamate-like immunoreactivity is enriched in projection neurons and aspartate-like immunoreactivity is enriched in interneurons.

Most neurotransmitters are synthesized through a single pathway. Generally, one of the enzymes in the pathway can be regulated to control the level of neurotransmitter. Furthermore, most neurotransmitters do not have major roles in intermediary metabolism. Both glutamate and aspartate serve as neurotransmitters and as intermediates in CNS metabolism. They are precursors for α-ketoglutarate and oxaloacetate, intermediates in the Krebs cycle, and like the other amino acids are incorporated into proteins as building blocks. Glutamate is also the immediate precursor for the inhibitory neurotransmitter GABA.

To date, no single pathway has been shown to control the synthesis of neurotransmitter pools of these EAAs. Glutamate and aspartate, nonessential amino acids that do not cross the blood–brain barrier, are synthesized from precursors that pass from blood to brain (Fig. 2). Glutamate can be directly synthesized from α-ketoglutarate by reductive amination or by transamination. It can also be directly synthesized from glutamine. Glutamate can be indirectly synthesized from proline and ornithine via Δ^1-pyrroline-5-carboxylic acid and glutamate γ-semialdehyde. By following the rates of metabolism for these various metabolites, it is possible to show that there are multiple metabolic pools of glutamate and aspartate that turn over at markedly different rates. Evidence is available suggesting that glutamine serves as the predominant precursor for glutamate acting as a transmitter. Aspartate can also be synthesized from several precursors, including oxaloacetate, glutamate, glutamine, and asparagine. It is not clear which compound serves as a precursor for aspartate acting as a neurotransmitter.

Release and Inactivation

Glutamate and aspartate are released upon depolarization and are inactivated at the synapse by uptake. After preincubation of brain slices or isolated nerve terminals with radiolabeled glutamate or the metabolically inert analog of glutamate, D-aspartate, Ca^{++}-dependent release of radioactivity can be evoked by depolarization. Alternatively, release of endogenous glutamate and aspartate can be detected by collecting perfusates and analyzing the amino acids released using high-pressure liquid chromatographic techniques that have high sensitivity. It is also possible to measure release in vivo by placing the

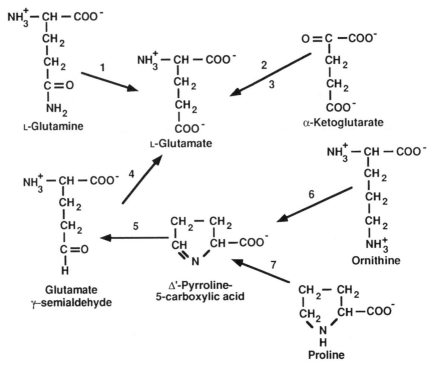

FIG. 2. Metabolic routes for the synthesis of glutamate. The enzymes for the different metabolic steps are: 1, glutaminase; 2, glutamate dehydrogenase; 3, aspartate transaminase; 4, glutamate γ-semialdehyde oxidase; 5, Δ'-pyrroline-5-carboxylic acid dehydrogenase; 6, ornithine transaminase; 7, proline oxidase.

tip of a small dialysis probe into the brain region of interest. With this technique, known as in vivo microdialysis, it is possible to electrically stimulate the projections to an area or to directly infuse a depolarizing agent and collect material that is released. In most areas of the brain, Ca^{++}-dependent release of glutamate and/or aspartate is observed. In some cases release can be reduced by prior lesioning of a defined neuronal pathway, suggesting that the lesioned pathway is the source of the release.

A high signal-to-noise ratio at the synapse is ensured by preventing accumulation of the neurotransmitter in the extracellular environment. Most of the available evidence suggests that glutamic and aspartic acids are present in the extracellular space at concentrations below 1 μM, which concentrations are at least 1,000-fold lower than the levels in total brain tissue (see above). Low extracellular

concentrations of most neurotransmitters are maintained either by extracellular enzymes, which convert the neurotransmitter to inactive metabolites, or by an uptake process, which removes the transmitter from the extracellular space. The predominant route of inactivation of neuronally released amino acids is via uptake into presynaptic terminals and into glial cells. Since the concentrations of glutamate and aspartate are higher inside than outside the cell, the uptake has to be coupled to an energy source. As is observed for other neurotransmitters, this uptake is coupled to the transmembrane sodium gradient. Sodium travels down its concentration and membrane potential gradients. The energy derived from this transport of sodium provides the energy for the movement of the amino acid against its concentration gradient. Current evidence suggests that both glutamate and aspartate are removed from the synapse by the same high-affinity transporters.

Recent results have led to the conclusion that there are multiple subtypes of sodium-dependent EAA transport systems. Results of pharmacological studies have been confirmed by the recent cloning of three different cDNAs that express sodium-dependent high-affinity L-[³H]glutamate transport. Based on the hydrophobicity of the amino acid sequence for one of these molecules, the protein is predicted to span the plasma membrane eight times such that both the amino and carboxy termini of the protein are on the intracellular side of the plasma membrane (Fig. 3). The amino acid sequences of these transporters are not similar to the sequences of the sodium-dependent transporters for norepinephrine, serotonin, dopamine, and GABA. Currently, it is not clear why multiple subtypes of EAA transporters exist, but the cloning of these transporters should facilitate their characterization.

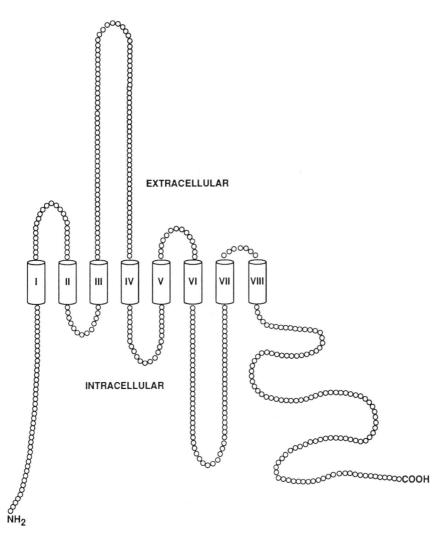

FIG. 3. Schematic model of the sodium-dependent glutamate transporter. The protein is predicted to span the membrane eight times based on hydrophobicity analysis with both the amino and carboxy termini on the intracellular side of the membrane.

Receptors for Glutamate and Aspartate

Glutamate and aspartate depolarize neurons by interacting with at least three broad classes of receptors, although it is not clear whether they preferentially activate any one of the receptor subtypes in vivo. In synaptic pathways thought to use glutamate or aspartate as neurotransmitters, depolarization of postsynaptic neurons occurs within 1 to 2 msec of stimulation of the presynaptic fiber. The depolarization lasts for 5 to 10 msec. Although some of the other established neurotransmitters depolarize neurons, the time course of depolarization is not sufficiently rapid to account for very rapid responses. Like the nicotinic ACh receptor, the receptors for glutamate and aspartate are coupled to ion channels that are selectively permeable to cations including sodium.

A number of agents that interact with EAA receptors have either been isolated from natural sources or been synthesized. These agents have been used to differentiate three major subtypes of EAA receptors that are coupled to ion channels. The receptors are named for agonists that are not endogenous to the brain and that were originally thought to activate specific subtypes of receptors. They include the *N*-methyl-D-aspartate (NMDA), kainate, and α-amino-3-hydroxy-5-methyl-4-isoxazole propionic acid (AMPA) receptors. With the use of antagonists, the receptors activated by these agonists have been differentiated. Prior to 1990, the third receptor (AMPA) was called the quisqualate receptor. Because quisqualate also activates EAA receptors that are coupled to second-messenger systems, AMPA is becoming the more widely used name for the receptor subtype specifically coupled to ion channels. The pharmacology, ion selectivity, and distribution of these subtypes of receptors are distinct. There are also EAA receptors that are coupled to inhibition of adenylyl cyclase activity or to stimulation of the turnover of phosphatidylinositol. The properties of the known EAA receptors are summarized in Table 1 and discussed below.

The pharmacological and physiological properties of the receptor subtypes will be examined, and the recent advances in the isolation of genes that code for specific subtypes of these receptors will be discussed.

AMPA Receptor

AMPA, a synthetic analog of glutamate, is a potent and selective agonist at one of the subclasses of EAA receptors. The receptor activated by AMPA is not blocked by antagonists of the NMDA receptor, including D-2-amino-5-phosphonopentanoate (D-AP5), 3-((±)-2-carboxypiperazin-4yl)propyl-1-phosphonate (CPP), and D-2-amino-5-phosphonoheptanoate (D-AP7). This differentiates the receptor activated by AMPA from the receptor activated by NMDA. Responses evoked by AMPA are not blocked by γ-D-glutamylglycine, a compound that blocks receptors activated by kainate, but are blocked by compounds that are somewhat selective antagonists at the AMPA receptor, including glutamate diethylester and 6-cyano-7-nitroquinoxaline-2,3-dione (CNQX). The ion channel associated with the AMPA receptor is selectively permeable to monovalent cations.

Three observations suggest that the AMPA receptor mediates most of the rapid excitatory synaptic responses in the mammalian CNS:

1. The kinetics of channel opening and closing are consistent with the time course for the rapid excitatory synaptic responses in the CNS. After binding of the agonist, the channel opens rapidly and closes within 3 to 8 msec.
2. The autoradiographic distribution of [³H]-AMPA binding suggests that these receptors are widely distributed throughout the CNS.
3. CNQX blocks rapid synaptic transmission in many pathways in the CNS.

TABLE 1. *Properties of the subtypes of EAA receptors*

Receptor subtypes	Agonists	Antagonists	Transduction mechanism	Role
AMPA	Quisqualate, AMPA	GDEE, CNQX	Ion channel	Synaptic transmission?
Kainate	Kainate, domoate	γ-D-Glu-Gly, CNQX	Ion channel	Synaptic transmission (?); presynaptic receptors (?); toxicity, epilepsy
NMDA	NMDA, quinolinate, ibotenate	Competitive D-AP5 D-AP7 CPP γ-D-Glu-Gly Noncompetitive PCP Tyletamine Ketamine MK-801 SKF 10047	Ion channel	Generally not involved in synaptic transmission; implicated in long-term potentiation, neurotoxicity
mGluR1α mGluR1β mGluR5	*trans*-ACPD, ibotenate, quisqualate	Noncompetitive? AP3 L-AβHA	Inositol phosphate production	?
mGluR2	?			
mGluR3	?		Negatively coupled to adenylyl cylase	?
mGluR4	L-AP4			mGluR4 may be a
mGluR6	?			presynaptic receptor

Abbreviations: AP3, 1-amino-3-phosphonopropionate; L-AβHA, L-aspartate-β-hydroxamate; *trans*-ACPD, ($\pm$)-1-aminocyclopentane-*trans*-1,3-dicarboxylic acid (Note: *trans*-ACPD is also called *cis*-($\pm$)-1-aminocyclopentane-1,3-dicarboxylic acid by IUPAC nomenclature); γ-D-Glu-Gly, γ-D-glutamylglycine; L-AP4, L-2-amino-4-phosphonobutanoate. *trans*-ACPD, ibotenate, and quisqualate all stimulate the production of inositol phosphates; this stimulation can be blocked by AP3 and L-AβHA. It is not known whether these compounds are selective for mGluR1$_\alpha$, mGluR1$_\beta$, or mGluR5.

Kainate Receptor

Kainic acid is a glutamate analog that was originally isolated from the seaweed of *Diginea simplex* and is one of the most potent EAA receptor agonists. The receptor activated by kainate is insensitive to inhibition by compounds that block the NMDA receptor, including D-AP5, CPP, and D-AP7. It is differentiated from quisqualate receptors by its insensitivity to glutamate diethylester and its sensitivity to γ-D-glutamylglycine. Although the kainate receptor can be differentiated from the AMPA and NMDA receptors, selective antagonists for the kainate receptor have not been identified. The channel associated with this receptor complex is similar to that of the AMPA receptor; it is selectively permeable to monovalent cations and is generally thought to have negligible permeability for divalent cations. Although this receptor has been localized to a limited number of specific brain regions, without specific antagonists it has not been possible to demonstrate that this receptor mediates synaptic responses in these pathways.

NMDA Receptor

The NMDA receptor contains multiple sites that can be manipulated to regulate the flow of ions through the channel (Fig. 4). In addition, a number of selective and relatively potent antagonists have been available for this receptor for almost a decade. Phosphonate-containing analogs of glutamate, including D-AP5, CPP, and D-AP7, are specific and competitive antagonists at the site that binds glutamate. A group of compounds, including known psychotomimetics (drugs that can pro-

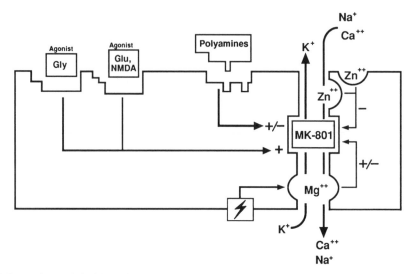

FIG. 4. Schematic model of the NMDA receptor. The flow of ions through the channel of the NMDA receptor can be regulated by a variety of factors. Glycine (Gly) and glutamate (Glu) must both bind to the NMDA receptor to cause opening of the ion channel. Polyamines bind to a distinct recognition site on the receptor to regulate the opening of the ion channel. Compounds such as MK-801 appear to bind in the open channel. At physiological concentrations of Mg^{++}, the channel is blocked unless the membrane is depolarized. Zn^{++} also regulates the opening of the ion channel. Adapted from Williams K, Romano C, Dichter MA and Molinoff PB. *Life Sci.* 1991;48:469–498.

duce manifestations resembling those of a psychosis) interact with the open channel to prevent the flow of ions through the channel and are selective blockers of the NMDA receptor. It is not clear whether the psychotomimetic effects of these compounds are mediated by interaction with the NMDA receptor or by interaction with other sites in the CNS. These compounds include phencyclidine (PCP, angel dust), *N*-allylnormetazocine (SKF 10047), ketamine (a dissociative anesthetic), (+)-5-methyl-10,11-dihydro-5*H*-dibenzocyclohepten-5,10-imine maleate (MK-801, an anticonvulsant), and dextromethorphan (the active compound in cough syrup). This receptor is also blocked by the divalent cation Mg^{++}. The extent of this blockade is dependent on the transmembrane potential; as the membrane is depolarized, the magnitude of the block is reduced, and ions can flow through the channel. Glycine, zinc, and polyamines also regulate the NMDA receptor. Although the properties of the sites for each of these regulators and the physiological relevance of the interactions are still under investigation, it is clear that there is a require-

ment for glycine such that glutamate (or NMDA) does not cause opening of the ion channel in the absence of glycine. Therefore, it is appropriate to call glycine a cotransmitter. Depolarization induced by the opening of the channel is the result of an influx of Na^+ and Ca^{++} ions. The permeability to Ca^{++} and the voltage-dependent block by Mg^{++} differentiates this receptor from the other EAA receptors that are impermeable to Ca^{++} and not blocked by Mg^{++}.

The localization of NMDA receptors has been examined using many of the compounds described above. They are found in various brain regions, including the hippocampus, which has one of the highest densities of NMDA receptors. Agents that block the NMDA receptor generally do not block rapid synaptic responses in the hippocampus or elsewhere. This suggests that the NMDA receptor does not mediate rapid synaptic responses. When a neuron is partially depolarized, however, the block by Mg^{++} is alleviated and ions can flow through the channel.

In the early 1970s, Bliss and his colleagues demonstrated that a single stimulus delivered to the inputs to area CA1 in the hippocampus causes a larger postsynaptic depolarization after repetitive stimulation of the inputs (Fig. 5). This increase in the efficacy of synaptic transmission lasted for up to 72 hr and is called *long-term potentiation* (LTP). In the mid 1980s, Collingridge and his colleagues demonstrated that NMDA receptor antagonists can prevent the induction of LTP. More recently, it was demonstrated that NMDA can increase the efficacy of synaptic transmission. Although the biochemical mechanisms involved in the process have not been resolved, it appears that repetitive stimulation of the inputs depolarizes postsynaptic neurons and removes or reduces the block of the NMDA receptor by Mg^{++}. The influx of Ca^{++} through the NMDA receptor is presumed to result in activation of Ca^{++}-dependent processes, possibly including Ca^{++}-dependent protein kinases, which can specifically phosphorylate proteins. After repetitive stimulation, there may be changes in the presynaptic terminal that lead to an increase in release of EAAs and changes in the postsynaptic terminal that result in increases in the amount of current that will go through non-NMDA receptor channels (Fig. 5). Because the hippocampus is thought to be involved in the consolidation of memory (see Chapters 1 and 15) it is hypothesized that LTP is a physiological correlate of memory. In fact, NMDA receptor antagonists can block the acquisition of memory in rodents.

Molecular Cloning of EAA Receptors That Are Coupled to Ion Channels

Since 1989, a number of cDNA clones have been isolated that can be used to express func-

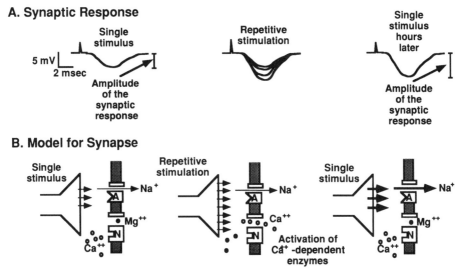

FIG. 5. Schematic illustration of LTP and the hypothesized role of the NMDA receptor in LTP. **A:** When a single stimulus is applied to the inputs of the CA1 pyramidal cells in the hippocampus, the cells are depolarized. If the inputs are repetitively stimulated, the amplitude of the postsynaptic depolarization increases. If the inputs to area CA1 are activated by a single stimulus after the repetitive stimulation, the size of the postsynaptic response is larger than the response observed before repetitive stimulation. **B:** With a single stimulus, the AMPA/kainate receptors (A) are activated and the postsynaptic neuron is depolarized. The NMDA receptors (N) are blocked by Mg^{++}. With repetitive stimulation, both the NMDA and the non-NMDA receptors are activated. The influx of Ca^{++} through the NMDA receptor may activate Ca^{++}-dependent enzymes including protein kinases that may regulate both presynaptic and postsynaptic components of synaptic transmission. If a single stimulus is applied to the inputs after repetitive stimulation, the amount of neurotransmitter released and the flow of ions though the non-NMDA receptors are thought to increase, causing a larger synaptic response.

tional EAA receptors coupled to ion channels. To date, at least nine distinct cDNAs have been isolated that express non-NMDA receptors. At least two different nomenclatures are being used to describe these clones. The two most frequently used define the cDNAs as GluR1, GluR2, . . . through GluR7 or GluRA, GluRB, . . . through GluRF. In addition, there are receptors known as KA-1 and KA-2 receptors. The sequences of the first four cDNAs in these series are highly similar. Because the proteins expressed from these cDNAs have a higher affinity for AMPA and quisqualate than for kainate, they are generally thought to represent AMPA receptor subunits. Two variants of each of these first four cDNAs have been isolated that differ by only 38 amino acids. Therefore, each subunit mRNA can be alternatively spliced to produce variants that have been called flip and flop (e.g., GluR1flip or flop, GluR2flip or flop, etc.). The sequences of GluR5, GluR6, and GluR7 have less similarity to GluR1 through 4 than GluR1 through 4 have to each other. GluR5 expresses a protein that binds radioactive kainate, but the protein is not active in electrophysiological assays. It is possible that GluR5 requires other subunits to form a functional ion channel. GluR6 expresses a protein that, in electrophysiological experiments, responds to kainate but not to AMPA, and the DNA is transcribed in brain regions that express kainate receptors. These observations suggest that this cDNA represents a subunit of the kainate receptor. None of these subunits display the properties of the NMDA receptor. Several groups have isolated cDNA clones that lead to expression of a receptor that displays many of the properties of the NMDA receptor that is expressed in brain; these are called NMDAR1 and NMDAR2A through NMDAR2D. The mRNA for the NMDAR1 receptor can be alternatively spliced to produce seven different splice variants that are called NMDAR1A, NMDAR1B, . . . through NMDAR1G. It is generally assumed that combinations of NMDAR1 with NMDAR2 subunits form functional receptors in vivo.

Most of the functional studies of these clones have been carried out by expressing a single subunit in a cell that does not normally express these EAA receptors. These are called homomeric receptors. Based on studies of other receptors that are coupled to ion channels, such as those for ACh, glycine, and GABA, it is generally thought that the EAA receptors are made up of combinations of subunits. It is not known how the subunits for the EAA receptors are assembled in vivo. The subunits and the splice variants of each subunit are expressed at different times during development and are differentially distributed in regions of the CNS. It is anticipated that during the next few years more subunits will be isolated, and that a variety of approaches will be used to define the combinations of subunits that are assembled in vivo.

Receptors Coupled to Second-Messenger Systems: Metabotropic Receptors

Receptors for EAAs are also coupled to second-messenger systems and are called metabotropic receptors. Some of these receptors are coupled to increased activity of phospholipase C, which hydrolyzes phosphatidylinositol-4,5-bisphosphate. One of the products of phosphatidylinositol4,5-bisphosphate hydrolysis, inositol-1,4,5-trisphosphate, mobilizes Ca^{++} from intracellular stores. The other product, diacylglycerol, activates protein kinase C, which phosphorylates proteins. Another group of EAA receptors is negatively coupled to adenylyl cyclase activity. Adenylyl cyclase converts ATP into cAMP, which leads to activation of protein kinase A. Both of these biochemical cascades can regulate many intracellular events. Recently, Nakanishi and his colleagues isolated cDNA clones that express these activities. These clones have been called $mGluR1_{\alpha}$, $mGluR1_{\beta}$, and mGluR2, . . . through mGluR6. Both forms of mGluR1 are coupled to increased hydrolysis of phosphatidylinositol-4,5-bisphosphate and are produced from alternative slicing of mRNA. mGluR2, mGluR3, mGluR4, and mGluR6 are negatively coupled to adenylyl cyclase. The pharmacology of the metabotropic EAA receptors has not been well characterized, although it is known that the receptor coupled to hydrolysis of phosphatidylinositol-4,5-bisphosphate is activated by quisqualate. The lack of an adequate pharmacological characterization of these receptors has precluded examination of their distribution and limited the characterization of their physiological role.

Neuronal Pathways That Use EAAs as Neurotransmitters

Most of the rapid depolarizing responses in the CNS are mediated by EAAs. Amino acids are thought to be the primary mediators of most of the rapid depolarizing synaptic responses in the mammalian CNS. They have not, however, met all of the criteria to be called neurotransmitters. Potent and specific antagonists are still lacking for some of the EAA receptor subtypes, and questions remain about the metabolic compartmentalization of transmitter pools of glutamate and aspartate. Support for the role of these amino acids as neurotransmitters in specific neuronal pathways has come from several approaches: (1) demonstration of release and uptake of these amino acids, (2) comparison of the actions of the endogenous transmitter to the effects of applied glutamate or aspartate, (3) examination of the effects of the EAA antagonists on synaptic transmission, (4) localization of glutamate- and aspartate-like immunoreactivity, and (5) localization of receptors for the EAAs. These criteria supply evidence for a role for glutamate and/or aspartate as neurotransmitters in numerous projection pathways in the CNS (Fig. 6) that carry neuronal signals from the somatosensory systems touch, pain, vision, sound, smell, and taste into the CNS, and transmit signals that lead to the initiation of muscle contraction. In the mammalian nervous system, they do not mediate the rapid depolariz-

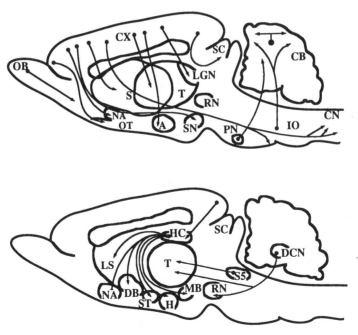

FIG. 6. Proposed pathways that use acidic amino acid transmitters in the mammalian brain: A, amygdala; CB, cerebellum; CN, cuneate nucleus; CX, cerebral cortex; DB, nucleus of the diagonal band; DCN, deep cerebellar nuclei; H, hypothalamus; HC, hippocampus; IO, inferior olive; LGN, lateral geniculate nucleus; LS, lateral septum; MB, mammillary body; NA, nucleus accumbens; OB, olfactory bulb; OT, olfactory tubercle; PN, pontine nuclei; RN, red nucleus; S, striatum; SC, superior colliculus; SN, substantia nigra; ST, bed nucleus of the stria terminalis; S5, spinal nucleus of nerve 5; T, thalamus.

ing signals that cause muscle contraction at the neuromuscular junction. At present, it is impossible to distinguish between pathways that use glutamate or aspartate as neurotransmitters.

INHIBITORY AMINO ACIDS

The amino acids GABA and glycine are the predominant inhibitory neurotransmitters in the mammalian CNS. The identification of GABA as an inhibitory neurotransmitter occurred much earlier than the acceptance of the EAA neurotransmitters. GABA was first isolated from nervous tissue in the early 1950s, although its role was unclear. A few years later a factor was isolated from brain that inhibited the stretch receptor neuron of the crayfish. In 1957, this factor was identified as GABA. In the 1960s and early 1970s, convincing evidence was developed to support a role for GABA as the predominant inhibitory neurotransmitter in the mammalian CNS.

The amino acid glycine is also thought to mediate hyperpolarizing responses in the CNS, but its effects are not as widespread as those of GABA. In the 1960s, glycine was identified as an inhibitory neurotransmitter in the spinal cord. Its effects were blocked by strychnine, a compound that does not affect hyperpolarizing responses to GABA. Thus, in contrast to our current understanding that glutamate and aspartate do not appear to preferentially activate different receptors, GABA and glycine act at separate populations of receptors.

Localization and Synthesis

GABA and glycine are present in the CNS at very high levels. The levels of GABA are several hundredfold higher than those of many established neurotransmitters, approaching the levels of glutamate and aspartate. GABA is essentially restricted to neural tissues, although very low levels are found in the periphery. Some regional variation, up to

fivefold, exists, but it is less than with neurotransmitters such as dopamine and ACh. GABA has been localized to synaptic vesicles, suggesting a neurotransmitter role for this amino acid. Many of the enzymes that regulate the levels of GABA have been extensively characterized.

Ironically, glutamate, one of the major excitatory neurotransmitters, is the only known precursor for GABA. The glutamate that serves as a precursor for the synthesis of GABA comes from both α-ketoglutarate and glutamine. The levels of GABA are maintained by a cycle that continuously supplies glutamate for GABA synthesis. This cycle, the GABA shunt (Fig. 7), bypasses part of the tricarboxylic acid and involves both glial cells and presynaptic terminals. In this cycle, the GABA that is transported into glial cells is metabolized to succinate semialdehyde by GABA - α - oxoglutarate transaminase (GABA-T), an enzyme that converts α-ketoglutarate to glutamate. The glutamate is then metabolized to glutamine, which can be exported back to the neuron. In the neuron, glutamine is converted back to glutamate by glutaminase. Glutamate decarboxylase (GAD) converts glutamate to GABA (step 5 in Fig. 7). It is generally assumed that modulation of GAD activity controls the synthesis of GABA, since GAD is regulated by glutamate, adenine nucleotides, and chloride. Most of the enzymes involved in the regulation of the synthesis and degradation of GABA have been purified to homogeneity and used in the development of antibodies for immunocytochemistry. Antibodies have also been raised against GABA itself.

The amino acid glycine is the other major inhibitory neurotransmitter in the mammalian CNS. Glycine is a nonessential amino acid that makes up 1% to 5% of the protein consumed in an average diet. As a common amino acid, it serves multiple functions in the CNS. It is a precursor for the synthesis of nucleic acids, it is incorporated into proteins, and it is a precursor for the synthesis of porphyrins and bile salts. Glycine is also required for activation of NMDA receptors

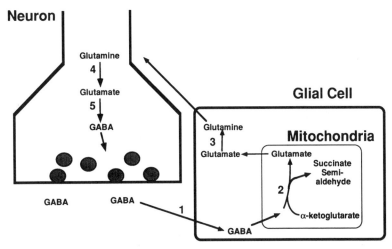

FIG. 7. Compartmentalization of GABA metabolism in the brain: the GABA shunt. After release from the presynaptic terminal, GABA is transported into glial cells by a sodium-dependent high-affinity transport process (1). The GABA is converted to glutamate by GABA-α-oxoglutarate transaminase (2), and the glutamate is converted to glutamine by glutamine synthetase (3). The glutamine in the presynaptic terminal is converted to glutamate by glutaminase (4), and the glutamate is converted to GABA by glutamic acid decarboxylase (5).

(see section on EAA transmitters). Therefore, it is involved in both inhibitory and excitatory responses in the CNS. Although glycine can cross the blood–brain barrier, it can also be synthesized from serine by the enzyme serine hydroxymethyltransferase. However, the distribution of this enzyme does not correlate with other markers for neurons that are thought to use glycine as a neurotransmitter. Therefore, it is not clear that this enzyme specifically regulates the synthesis of the glycine that is used as a neurotransmitter.

Release and Inactivation

GABA and glycine are released upon depolarization and are inactivated by uptake mechanisms. GABA and glycine are released from preparations of nerve terminals (synaptosomes) or from brain/spinal cord preparations by a Ca^{++}-dependent process. Furthermore, because this release can be reduced by prior lesioning of defined neuronal pathways, the lesioned pathways are thought to be the source of the release.

GABA and glycine are cleared from the synapse by sodium-dependent transport processes, not by metabolism to inactive metabolites. A transmembrane sodium gradient provides the energy to transport glycine and GABA against their concentration gradients. Unlike the uptake of glutamate and aspartate, which are accumulated by the same carrier, glycine and GABA are accumulated by distinct transporters. GABA is transported into both glia and neurons. The uptake of GABA into neurons and glia has been differentiated in studies with selective inhibitors, suggesting that the transporters expressed by glial cells are different from the transporters expressed by neurons. A GABA transporter was biochemically purified to homogeneity in the mid-1980s by Kanner and his colleagues. The sequence of this protein was used to isolate a cDNA that leads to expression of GABA transport activity. cDNAs for several additional sodium-dependent GABA transporters have been isolated. The amino acid sequences of all of these GABA transporters are similar to the sequences for the sodium-dependent transporters for norepinephrine, serotonin, dopamine, and GABA. All of these transporters are predicted to span the plasma membrane 12 times.

Receptors for GABA and Glycine

GABA and glycine hyperpolarize neurons by interacting with different receptors. In many synaptic pathways thought to use glycine or GABA as the neurotransmitter, the postsynaptic neuron is rapidly hyperpolarized after stimulation of the presynaptic fiber. Application of either GABA or glycine results in a rapid onset hyperpolarization that is of short duration and results from an increase in membrane permeability to chloride ions. Unlike the excitatory neurotransmitters, which do not appear to show significant specificity for receptor subtypes, GABA and glycine act at distinct receptor sites with uneven regional distributions. Bicuculline blocks the hyperpolarization induced by GABA without affecting the actions of glycine. Strychnine shows the opposite specificity. Glycine appears to be an inhibitory neurotransmitter in the caudal parts of the CNS, including the spinal cord and brain stem. GABA, the predominant inhibitory neurotransmitter in the rostral parts of the CNS, also mediates some of the inhibitory responses in the spinal cord and brain stem.

GABA Receptors

There are two types of GABA receptors, $GABA_A$ and $GABA_B$, with the former coupled to ion channels that are permeable to chloride and the latter coupled to second-messenger systems. The $GABA_A$ receptor is regulated by agents that interact with distinct modulatory sites on the receptor–channel complex (Fig. 8). Bicuculline competitively blocks the receptor acting at the recognition site for GABA. Picrotoxin blocks the $GABA_A$ receptor noncompetitively by preventing the flow of ions through the channel. Barbiturates and benzodiazepines interact with the $GABA_A$ receptor. Benzodiazepines, which include anxiolytics like diazepam (Valium), allosterically increase the binding of GABA to the receptor. These compounds augment the action of GABA at the receptor by increasing the frequency of channel opening. Barbiturates potentiate the effects of GABA, although at a site different from those utilized by benzodiazepine-like compounds. Barbiturates increase the time that the channel stays open in the presence of GABA instead of increasing the frequency of channel opening. There is also evidence that steroids and ethanol can augment the action of GABA at this receptor. The $GABA_A$ receptor is linked to a channel permeable to monovalent anions.

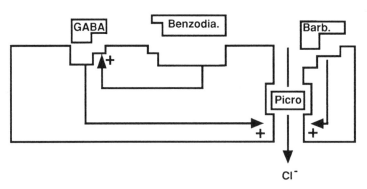

FIG. 8. Schematic model of the $GABA_A$ receptor. The receptor spans the cell membrane. GABA binds to the outside of the receptor, causing an influx of Cl^- ions through the channel. Benzodiazepines and barbiturates interact with different recognition sites on the receptor and increase the effectiveness of GABA. Steroids and ethanol may also interact with the receptor to increase the effectiveness of GABAergic transmission.

This receptor is generally modeled like a barrel with several staves that surround an opening that is thought to form the ion channel. This model is primarily derived from detailed molecular studies of the nicotinic ACh receptor (see Chapter 6). The binding of GABA to its recognition site results in an opening of the pore and an influx of chloride. The chloride hyperpolarizes the neuron, which decreases the probability of initiation of an action potential.

Until recently, it was thought that the GABA$_A$ receptor was a single molecular entity composed of multiple subunits. The application of gene-cloning techniques has demonstrated that this receptor actually represents a family of receptors with similar properties. Compounds with a high affinity for the GABA receptor complex were used as tools for purification of a receptor complex composed of four or five different subunits. The amino acid sequences from these proteins were used to isolate cDNAs that led to expression of an ion channel activated by GABA. These cDNAs were used to isolate other cDNAs with similar sequences. With this technique, α, β, γ, δ, and ρ subunits were isolated, and these subunits were used to isolate additional related cDNA sequences. To date, six α, three β, three γ, one δ, and two ρ subunits have been isolated. Given the existence of so many subunits, there are an enormous number of possible combinations of subunits that could lead to assembly of receptors in vivo. It is not known which of the specific combinations are expressed in vivo, but it is generally assumed that different subunits are assembled to form heteromeric receptors. Different α subunits are selectively expressed in different brain regions and at different times during development. This raises the possibility that selective drugs may be developed to alter GABAergic function in selected brain regions. It also explains why neonates and adults may respond differently to GABAergic drugs.

GABA$_B$ receptors are differentiated from GABA$_A$ receptors on the basis of insensitivity to bicuculline and sensitivity to β-(p-chlorophenyl) GABA, also known as baclofen or lioresal. Activation of these receptors causes a decrease in the release of other neurotransmitters, including catecholamines and glutamate, and results in opening of potassium channels.

Glycine Receptors

The glycine receptor, like the GABA$_A$ receptor, is generally thought to be coupled to a channel permeable to chloride. Activation of this receptor results in hyperpolarization of neurons. The action of glycine at this receptor is competitively blocked by strychnine and is insensitive to the GABA$_A$ receptor antagonist bicuculline. Activation of glycine receptors is not affected by benzodiazepines or barbiturates. The glycine receptor has been purified to homogeneity, and cDNAs that lead to the expression of functional glycine receptors have been isolated. Comparison of the amino acid sequences of GABA and glycine receptors shows that there is 70% homology of the portions of the protein thought to span the lipid bilayer and therefore form the ion channel. As with the GABA$_A$ receptor, many different subunits with similar sequences have been isolated. There is evidence to suggest that the expression of the different subunits is developmentally regulated.

Neuronal Pathways That Use Inhibitory Amino Acids as Neurotransmitters

While GABA is generally thought to hyperpolarize neurons throughout the CNS, the actions of glycine tend to be restricted to caudal areas of the CNS. As might be predicted for the major neurotransmitter for inhibitory interneurons, GABA is widely distributed throughout the CNS. The synaptic pathways that use GABA as a neurotransmitter have not been completely identified. At many synapses, both the endogenous neurotransmitter and GABA hyperpolarize postsynaptic neurons. Both responses are blocked by bicuculline and picrotoxin, but not by strychnine.

The synthetic and degradative enzymes for GABA, glutamate decarboxylase, and GABA-T have been purified to homogeneity and used to elicit antibodies. Antibodies have also been raised against GABA after conjugation to a carrier protein. Both types of antibodies have been used for localization of GABAergic pathways. The benzodiazepines and other compounds that have a high affinity for the GABA receptor have been used to define the distribution of GABA receptors by autoradiography. Pathways thought to use GABA as the neurotransmitter include both somatosensory systems and motor systems distributed throughout the CNS.

Although glycine is found throughout the CNS, it is enriched in the spinal cord, the medulla-pons, and the retina. These same brain regions are also enriched in sodium-dependent uptake sites for glycine, binding sites for strychnine, and glycine-like immunoreactivity. On the basis of these observations it is thought that although other pathways may use glycine, these are the major areas of the CNS that use glycine as a neurotransmitter.

OTHER NEUROTRANSMITTER CANDIDATES

Although glutamate, aspartate, GABA, and glycine are the predominant neurotransmitters mediating rapid hyperpolarizing and depolarizing responses in the CNS, other amino acids may mediate these responses in some areas of the brain. Quinolinic acid, L-cysteic acid, and L-homocysteic acid are found in the brain and are able to depolarize neurons. In some cases, these amino acids are taken up by a sodium-dependent transport system and are released upon depolarization. Taurine, found in very high concentrations in the CNS, mimics the inhibitory neurotransmitters and is transported by a sodium-dependent carrier. Peptide analogs of glutamate such as N-acetylaspartylglutamate, found in high concentrations in the CNS, may mimic some of the actions of glutamate and aspartate. Many investigators are pursuing the possibility that these compounds are either excitatory or inhibitory neurotransmitters.

AMINO ACID NEUROTRANSMITTERS AND DISEASE

The amino acid transmitter systems have been implicated in a wide range of neurodegenerative and psychiatric disorders. The neurotoxic effects of glutamate were first reported in the late 1950s when it was demonstrated that retinal neurons were damaged by glutamate. Neurons in the hypothalamus and circumventricular organs, regions of the CNS not well protected by the blood–brain barrier during the neonatal period, were also damaged by glutamate. Cytopathological examination revealed an acute swelling of neuronal cell bodies followed by irreversible cytotoxicity. Neurons seem to be selectively vulnerable to EAA agonists; glial cells or axons passing through the region are spared. Most of the compounds that activate EAA receptors cause neuronal degeneration in vivo. The potency of compounds for activating glutamate receptors correlates with their cytotoxic potency, and the degeneration can be blocked by EAA receptor antagonists. Based on these observations, it is hypothesized that cell death is the result of persistent activation of receptors for EAAs. These compounds are therefore called *excitotoxins.*

Persistent activation of receptors for the EAAs has been implicated in both acute and chronic insults that result in neuronal degeneration in the CNS. Conditions involving neuronal degeneration include Alzheimer's disease, Huntington's disease, olivopontocerebellar atrophy, hypoxia/ischemia (inadequate oxygenation or blood flow, respectively, to the CNS), and head trauma. Three lines of evidence support a role for EAAs in neurodegeneration. The patterns of neuronal vulnerability parallel the patterns predicted by injection of exogenous EAAs. For example, Huntington's disease is characterized by neuronal degeneration in the striatum with selective sparing of neurons that contain somatostatin and neuropeptide Y. The same populations of neurons are spared upon injection of NMDA receptor agonists into the striatum of rodents. During many of the acute insults it has been possible to measure increases in the extracellular concentrations of glutamate and aspartate. In some cases, antagonists of NMDA receptors have been shown to reduce the extent of the damage that would otherwise be induced by an acute insult to the CNS. While it is unlikely that EAAs are the sole toxins in these insults, it is probable that this system plays a part in the neuronal degeneration observed under these conditions.

At least three possible mechanisms have been proposed for the excitotoxicity of these amino acids (Fig. 9). One of the original hypotheses was that these amino acids deplete energy stores by causing persistent activation of ion channels. The sodium-potassium ATPase, which maintains the transmembrane gradient of sodium, would continue to catalyze ATP hydrolysis in an attempt to maintain normal transmembrane gradients of sodium and potassium until the cell runs out of energy (ATP) and dies. Another hypothesis is that the influx of ions through the ion channel results in an osmotic influx of water into neurons and that the neurons swell and burst like overinflated balloons. This would explain the neuronal swelling that is observed initially. The third hypothesis is that the toxicity is a result of activation of the NMDA receptor, which allows an influx of calcium. The rise in intracellular calcium is hypothesized to activate calcium-dependent proteases and oxygenases that kill the neurons. Currently, there is evidence to suggest that all three of these mechanisms contribute to excitotoxicity.

Seizure Disorders

Seizure activity can generally be thought of as the result of an imbalance between the excitatory and inhibitory amino acid systems (see Chapter 22). As would be predicted, seizure activity can be induced by blocking inhibitory amino acid receptors or by persistently activating EAA receptors. Current therapies for seizure disorders focus on in-

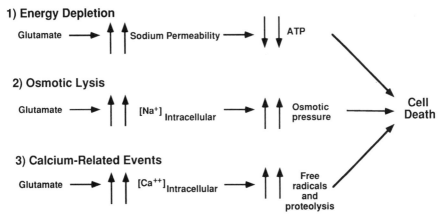

FIG. 9. Proposed mechanisms of glutamate-induced toxicity. At least three separate mechanisms have been proposed for glutamate neurotoxicity. (1) The influx of sodium through the ion channels may deplete cellular ATP levels and cause cell death. The Na^+-K^+-ATPase would require more energy to maintain the transmembrane gradients of these ions. (2) The influx of Na^+ ions may cause an osmotic influx of water that could cause the cell to swell and burst. (3) The influx of Ca^{++} through NMDA receptors may cause excessive activation of Ca^{++}-dependent enzymes, including proteases and lipoxygenases. The proteases could abnormally digest the cellular protein and the lipoxygenases can produce free radicals. These events could cause cell death.

creasing the effectiveness of the inhibitory transmitters. As antagonists of the EAA receptors are developed, these agents will probably be used to modify seizure activity.

Psychiatric Disorders

Many anxiolytics (compounds that reduce anxiety) act directly on the GABA$_A$ receptor. Anxiolytics, such as opiates, barbiturates, ethanol, and benzodiazepines, reduce anxiety, induce sleep, reduce seizure activity, and relax muscles. Of these compounds, benzodiazepines are the most commonly employed in clinical practice. The potential of different benzodiazepines to reduce anxiety (see Chapter 19) is correlated with their affinity for the GABA$_A$ receptor, suggesting that these compounds reduce anxiety by direct interaction with this receptor. Although anxiety can be reduced by drugs that increase GABAergic transmission, it is not clear that anxiety is induced by a biochemical imbalance in the GABAergic system.

SUMMARY

The amino acids—glutamate, aspartate, GABA, and glycine—mediate most of the rapid hyperpolarizing and depolarizing responses in the mammalian CNS. If a neuron is exposed to an EAA, the transmembrane potential can be lowered sufficiently to initiate an action potential that is propagated to the next neuron. If a neuron is exposed to an inhibitory amino acid, the opposite reaction occurs. Therefore, these two systems tend to balance one another and control integration of information processing in the CNS. Over the last three decades, our understanding of the mechanisms that regulate the responses mediated by this class of neurotransmitters has increased dramatically. The development of agonists and antagonists that affect these systems has led to the identification of subtypes of receptors that mediate the actions of these amino acids. Numerous studies now

provide strong evidence that these systems are involved in both normal and abnormal brain function. Gene-cloning techniques have identified subtypes of receptors that had not been differentiated pharmacologically. Considerable evidence suggests that pharmacological agents that interact with these systems will be useful in treating a wide array of psychiatric and neurodegenerative disorders.

BIBLIOGRAPHY

Original Articles

Beal MF, Kowall NW, Ellison DW, Mazurek MF, Swartz KJ, Martin JB. Replication of the neurochemical characteristics of Huntington's disease by quinolinic acid. *Nature* 1986;321:168–171.

Choi DW, Maulucci-Gedde M, Kriegstein AR. Glutamate neurotoxicity in cortical cell culture. *J Neurosci* 1987;7:357–368.

Egebjerg J, Bettler B, Hermans-Borgmeyer I, Heinemann S. Cloning of a cDNA for a glutamate receptor subunit activated by kainate but not AMPA. *Nature* 1991;351:745–748.

Guastella J, Nelson N, Nelson H, Czyzyk L, Keynan S, Miedel MC, et al. Cloning and expression of a rat brain GABA transporter. *Science* 1990;249:1303–1306.

Herron CE, Lester RAJ, Coan EJ, Collingridge GL. Frequency-dependent involvement of NMDA receptors in the hippocampus: a novel synaptic mechanism. *Nature* 1986;322:265–268.

Hollmann M, O'Shea-Greenfield A, Rogers SW, Heinemann S. Cloning by functional expression of a member of the glutamate receptor family. *Nature* 1989;342:643–648.

Johnson JW, Ascher P. Glycine potentiates the NMDA response in cultured mouse brain neurons. *Nature* 1987;325:529–531.

Kauer JA, Malenka RC, Nicoll RA. NMDA application potentiates synaptic transmission in the hippocampus. *Nature* 1988;334:250–252.

Kleckner NW, Dingledine R. Requirement for glycine in activation of NMDA-receptors expressed in *Xenopus* oocytes. *Science* 1988;241:835–837.

Moriyoshi K, Masu M, Ishii T, Shigemoto R, Mizuno N, Nakanishi S. Molecular cloning and characterization of the rat NMDA receptor. *Nature* 1991;354:31–37.

Morris RGM, Anderson E, Lynch GS, Baudry M. Selective impairment of learning and blockade of long-term potentiation by an N-methyl-D-aspartate receptor antagonist, AP5. *Nature* 1986;319:774–776.

Pines G, Danbolt NC, Bjørås M, Zhang Y, Bendahan A, Eide L, et al. Cloning and expression of a rat brain L-glutamate transporter. *Nature* 1992;360:464–467.

Pritchett DB, Lüddens H, Seeburg PH. Type I and type II GABA$_A$–benzodiazepine receptors produced in transfected cells. *Science* 1989;245:1389–1392.

Sommer B, Keinänen K, Verdoorn TA, Wisden W, Burnashev N, Herb A, et al. Flip and flop: a cell-specific functional switch in glutamate-operated channels of the CNS. *Science* 1990;249:1580–1585.

Tanabe Y, Masu M, Ishii T, Shigemoto R, Nakanishi S. A family of metabotropic glutamate receptors. *Neuron* 1992;8:169–179.

Williams K, Dawson VL, Romano C, Dichter MA, Molinoff PB. Characterization of polyamines having agonist, antagonist, and inverse agonist effects at the polyamine recognition site of the NMDA receptor. *Neuron* 1990;5:199–208.

Books and Reviews

Choi DW. Glutamate neurotoxicity and diseases of the nervous system. *Neuron* 1988;1:623–634.

DeLorey TM, Olsen RW. GABA and glycine. In: Siegel GJ, Agranoff BW, Albers RW, Molinoff PB, eds. *Basic neurochemistry,* 5th ed. New York: Raven Press; 1994 (in press).

Dingledine R, McBain CI. Excitatory amino acid transmitters. In: Siegel GJ, Agranoff BW, Albers RW, Molinoff PB, eds. *Basic neurochemistry,* 5th ed. New York: Raven Press; 1994 (in press).

Fagg GE, Foster AC. Amino acid neurotransmitters and their pathways in the mammalian central nervous system. *Neuroscience* 1983;9:701–719.

Mayer ML, Westbrook GL. The physiology of excitatory amino acids in the vertebrate central nervous system. *Progr Neurobiol* 1987;28:197–276.

McGeer PL, Eccles JC, McGeer EG. Inhibitory amino acid neurotransmitters. In: *Molecular neurobiology of the mammalian brain.* 2nd Ed. New York: Plenum Press; 1987:197–234.

McGeer PL, Eccles JC, McGeer EG. Putative excitatory neurons: glutamate and aspartate. In: *Molecular neurobiology of the mammalian brain.* 2nd Ed. New York: Plenum Press; 1987:175–196.

McGeer PL, McGeer EG. Amino acid neurotransmitters. In: Siegel GJ, Agranoff BW, Albers RW, Molinoff PB, eds. *Basic neurochemistry.* 5th Ed. New York: Raven Press; 1994 (in press).

Nakanishi S. Molecular diversity of glutamate receptors and implications for brain function. *Science* 1992;258:597–603.

Robinson, MB, Coyle JT. Glutamate and related acidic excitatory neurotransmitters: from basic science to clinical application. *FASEB J* 1987;1:446–455.

Watkins JC, Evans RH. Excitatory amino acid transmitters. *Annu Rev Pharmacol Toxicol* 1981;21:165–204.

Synaptic Transmission
Peptides

Terry D. Reisine

In view of the correspondence between the natural and synthetic peptides in terms of their biological potencies, their mass spectra and electrophoretic mobilities, we conclude that our assigned structures for the two peptides comprising natural enkephalin are correct. . . .

The discovery in the brain of two endogenous pentapeptides with potent opiate agonist activity raises a number of pertinent questions which cannot be adequately dealt with in this paper. It will now be possible, however, to test the hypothesis that these peptides act as neurotransmitters or neuromodulators at synaptic junctions.

J. Hughes, T. W. Smith, H. W. Kosterlitz, L. A. Fothergill,
B. A. Morgan, and H. R. Morris,
Identification of two related pentapeptides from the brain with potent opiate agonist activity.
Nature 1975;258:577–579, p. 579

- The enkephalins are endogenous opiate-like peptides.

- Enkephalin is widely distributed in the nervous system.

- The opiate alkaloids and endogenous opiates are potent analgesic agents.

- A major pharmacological action of opiate alkaloids, and the major side effect of their clinical use, is the induction of tolerance and physical dependence.

- Somatostatin is heterogeneously distributed in neurons in the brain, and is believed to be a neurotransmitter or neuromodulator.

- Somatostatin has been shown to induce diverse actions in the CNS.

- One of the best-established biological actions of somatostatin in the brain is the facilitation of dopamine transmission in the striatum.

- One of the first peptides identified as a potential neurotransmitter, substance P, is present in sensory neurons and in the CNS.

- Substance P plays an important role in the perception of pain.

- Cholecystokinin (CCK) has been shown to be expressed in neurons in the brain and is distributed heterogeneously in the CNS.

- Some of the actions of CCK on mesolimbic dopamine neurons are similar to those of antipsychotic agents.

- CCK has a major role in the regulation of food intake.

- Neurotensin is widely distributed in the CNS where it may act as either a neurotransmitter or a neuromodulator.

This chapter reviews our understanding of peptides acting in the nervous system. A few examples of peptides that have been extensively investigated are described in the following sections. Specifically covered are synthesis, release and inactivation, receptor interactions, as well as biological effects and mechanisms of action.

Peptides are a class of endogenous compounds that can act as neurotransmitters or neuromodulators in the nervous system. They differ in many respects from classical transmitters such as acetylcholine or norepinephrine. The mechanisms by which peptides are synthesized and inactivated are different from those of classical transmitters. The synthesis of peptides is directed by genes controlling the expression of mRNA that encodes peptide prohormones (Fig. 1). Prohormones are biologically inert, and mature peptide transmitters are synthesized from prohormones by proteolytic processing events. The processing of the prohormone to the biologically active peptide can involve the actions of multiple proteolytic enzymes located in diverse regions of neurons. Peptide synthesis is initiated in the cell body of neurons since that is where the genes encoding the peptides are located, whereas the synthesis of classical transmitters can take place in both the cell body and the nerve terminal. Once released from neurons, peptides are inactivated by peptidases within the synapse. In contrast, classical neurotransmitters may be taken up into neurons and reutilized. No peptide has been reported to be selectively taken up into neurons via an active process.

While peptides differ from classical transmitters, they also have many similar characteristics. Some of the characteristics that peptides share with classical neurotransmitters are as follows: Peptides are released from neurons via an active, calcium-dependent mechanism. They stimulate membrane-bound receptors to regulate the activity of neurons. Furthermore, a large number of peptides have been shown to be biologically active in the nervous system, exerting diverse functions and playing important roles in the generation of a number of behaviors in animals. Alterations in peptide neurotransmission in humans may lead to the abnormal behaviors associated with many neuropsychiatric disorders.

ENKEPHALINS

The enkephalins are endogenous opiate-like peptides. Methionine-enkephalin and leucine-enkephalin are the predominant biologically active enkephalins in the nervous system (see Fig. 2 for structures). They were identified, purified, and characterized in the early 1970s. Their discovery was the result of many years of intensive effort to find endogenous substances that acted on the "morphine receptor." Morphine is an alkaloid present in opium poppies that had been known for many years to exert potent and dramatic pharmacological effects in animals. Snyder and associates showed that morphine and other opiate alkaloids bound selectively and with high affinity to receptors in the nervous system to induce their pharmacological effects. The enkephalins are endogenous substances that bind to morphine receptors.

Enkephalins are derived from the larger precursor molecule preproenkephalin. Both preproenkephalin and the gene that encodes it have been extensively characterized. Preproenkephalin contains four methionine-

Biological Bases of Brain Function and Disease, edited by Alan Frazer, Perry B. Molinoff, and Andrew Winokur. Raven Press, Ltd., New York © 1994.

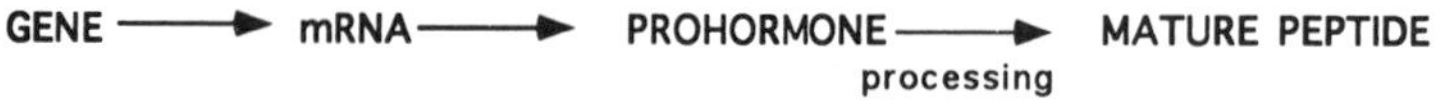

GENE ⟶ mRNA ⟶ PROHORMONE ⟶ MATURE PEPTIDE
processing

FIG. 1. Gene expression.

enkephalin molecules and one leucine-enkephalin molecule (Fig. 2). Each enkephalin molecule is flanked by pairs of dibasic amino acid residues. These basic amino acid residues serve as signals for the processing of proenkephalin to the mature peptide. Only one processing enzyme for proenkephalin has been clearly identified and characterized and that enzyme is referred to as carboxypeptidase H. This processing enzyme has been purified to homogeneity, cloned, and fully sequenced. It is present in secretory granules where part, if not all, of proenkephalin processing occurs. Carboxypeptidase H is not selective for proenkephalin but is also involved in the processing of other neuroactive peptides.

Both methionine- and leucine-enkephalin have been shown to be released from central and peripheral neurons in a calcium-dependent manner. The release is dependent on neuronal activity and is also regulated at the presynaptic level by neurotransmitters. Once released from neurons, enkephalin is inactivated by an enzyme called enkephalinase. This enzyme has been characterized extensively, and a number of attempts have been made to develop inhibitors of this enzyme that could prolong the actions of enkephalins. The extension of the biological lifetime of enkephalins has been speculated to be useful in the treatment of chronic pain since enkephalin is an analgesic. Several years ago a highly potent enkephalinase inhibitor, thiorphan, was developed; it has been shown to prolong the actions of enkephalin in the nervous system.

Enkephalin is widely distributed in the nervous system. Among their many locations in the nervous system, enkephalin-containing

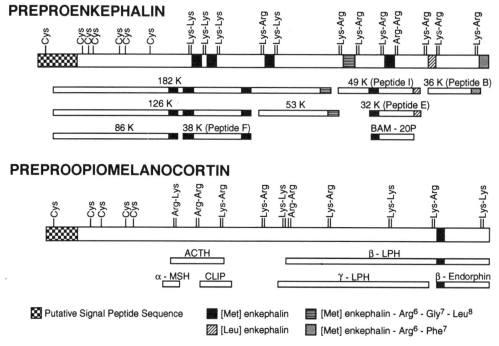

FIG. 2. Opiate preprohormones.

interneurons have been identified in the dorsal horn of the spinal cord and are believed to play a role in the body's ability to recognize painful stimuli. Enkephalin is present in relatively high concentrations in the striatum, and an enkephalinergic pathway has been described which has cell bodies in the caudate putamen and terminals in the globus pallidus. It has been suggested that these neurons have a role in the control of movement. Numerous enkephalin-containing neurons are expressed throughout the limbic system and are believed to have an influence on mood and other affective behaviors. Furthermore, high levels of enkephalin are present in the nucleus tractus solitarii, a brain region involved in the regulation of respiration. The presence of enkephalin in this nucleus is consistent with the known respiratory depressant effects of opiates. Interestingly, enkephalinergic neurons have a regional distribution in the central nervous system (CNS) different from that of neurons containing the other known endogenous opiates, β-endorphin and dynorphin. The latter opiates contain the enkephalin sequences in their structure and for some time were believed to function solely as precursors of enkephalin. The differential distribution of enkephalin, β-endorphin, and dynorphin in brain is consistent with recent findings that the endogenous opiates are a family of peptides encoded by different genes and processed from different precursors, and therefore represent distinct neurotransmitters or neuromodulators.

Enkephalins induce their biological effects by stimulating membrane-bound receptors. Pharmacologically distinct subtypes of opiate receptors are expressed in the nervous system (Table 1). The μ-opiate receptor expresses high affinity for morphine and other opiate alkaloids as well as the opiate antagonist naloxone, but relatively lower affinity for enkephalins. Enkephalins, in contrast, bind with high affinity to δ-opiate receptors. The δ-opiate receptors have lower affinity for morphine and naloxone than do μ receptors. A third subtype of opiate receptor is the κ receptor. This receptor has high affinity for the synthetic compounds ethylketocyclazocine and naloxone but relatively low affinity for enkephalins, and it exhibits a high affinity for the endogenous opiate dynorphin.

The δ receptors are the predominant opiate receptors that mediate the actions of enkephalins in the nervous system. Interestingly, an endogenous substance that acts on μ receptors is not known, despite the fact that the μ-opiate receptors were the first class of opiate binding sites identified in the body, and their discovery led to extensive research on endogenous opiates and the eventual purification of endogenous opiate peptides. The μ-opiate receptors are distinct from δ-opiate receptors. Not only do they have a different regional distribution in the body, but the molecular properties of μ- and δ-opiate receptors are different. Furthermore, a number of studies have shown that these two classes of opiate receptors can be differentially regulated by opiate agonists that selectively bind to each receptor subtype.

The cellular mechanisms through which enkephalins induce their biological effects have been examined using both biochemical and electrophysiological techniques. The δ-opiate receptors are coupled to GTP-binding (G) proteins (see Chapter 4). The G proteins

TABLE 1. *Subtypes of opiate receptors*

Name	μ	δ	κ
Potency order	BE > Dy > EN	BE = EN > Dy	Dy $\gg$ BE $\gg$ EN
Selective agonists	DAMGO	DPDPE, DADLE	U69593
Selective antagonists	CTAP	ICI 174864	Norbinaltorphimine
Effector	Inhibits cAMP; increases K^+ channel	Inhibits cAMP; increases K^+ channel	Inhibits Ca^{++} channel

BE, β-endorphin; Dy, dynorphin A; EN, enkephalin.

link a number of neurotransmitter receptors to second messengers or cellular effector systems and are a critical component in the signal transduction process. δ-Opiate receptors are coupled to a subspecies of G protein that is inhibited by pertussis toxin. Pertussis toxin can enter cells and catalyze the ADP ribosylation of the G proteins G_i and G_o, thereby inactivating the G proteins and breaking the link between the receptors and the cellular effector systems they modulate. G_i couples δ-opiate receptors to the catalytic subunit of adenylyl cyclase, and enkephalin is a potent inhibitor of cAMP formation in neurons. G proteins also link δ-opiate receptors to ionic conductance channels. Enkephalin and enkephalin analogs have been shown to inhibit calcium (Ca^{++}) currents in both central and peripheral neurons to reduce Ca^{++} influx. The blockade of Ca^{++} influx may be an underlying mechanism that explains the inhibition of neurotransmitter release by enkephalins in spinal cord neurons. Enkephalins also hyperpolarize neurons by stimulating K^+ currents. The stimulation of K^+ conductance appears to be the mechanism through which enkephalins inhibit the firing activity of both central and peripheral neurons. G proteins couple enkephalin receptors to both Ca^{++} channels and K^+ channels. Interestingly, a family of pertussis toxin–sensitive G proteins, including at least three forms of G_i and two of G_o, are expressed in the nervous system. These different G proteins may be responsible for coupling δ-opiate receptors to different cellular effector systems.

The opiate alkaloids and endogenous opiates are potent analgesic agents. Among the opiates' various physiological and pharmacological effects is the induction of analgesia at multiple sites of action. The μ- and δ-opiate receptors have been most closely associated with the pain-relieving actions of morphine and endogenous opiates. Both μ- and δ-opiate receptors are expressed in the dorsal horn of the spinal cord, and enkephalins, present in interneurons, are also localized to this region. Opiates may induce anal-

gesia in the spinal cord by inhibiting the release of the peptide, substance P. Substance P is found in sensory afferents that are responsible for carrying the sensation of pain from the periphery to brain. Enkephalins and morphine were shown to reduce electrically evoked substance P release from slices of the spinal cord. Furthermore, opiate receptors may be localized to sensory afferent terminals. This is suggested from studies in which transection of the sensory input to the spinal cord or chemical lesions of sensory neurons with capsaicin greatly reduced the density of opiate receptors in the dorsal horn of the spinal cord. These findings indicate that opiates may inhibit release of substance P at a presynaptic level. Since opiates are known to reduce Ca^{++} conductance in neurons, they could block release of substance P by reducing Ca^{++} influx into substance P–containing nerve terminals. Opiates most likely act through other mechanisms to reduce pain perception. In particular, they may directly inhibit the activity of spinal afferents to brain. Furthermore, intracerebroventricular injection of enkephalins and other endogenous opiates induces potent analgesic actions, indicating that opiates can act in brain to induce analgesia.

A major pharmacological action of opiate alkaloids, and the major side effect of their clinical use, is the induction of tolerance and physical dependence. The opiate alkaloids have been known for many years to be addictive (see Chapter 20). Tolerance is a phenomenon that occurs with repeated use of opiates and necessitates the administration of increasing doses of the opiate to induce the same apparent biological response. Repeated administration of opiates can induce a physical and psychological requirement for the compound such that the absence of exogenous opiates in the body can trigger severe physiological responses. These withdrawal responses can be life threatening.

Opiate addiction can be treated by gradually reducing the intake of opiates to the addict. Recent experimental therapies for the treatment of opiate addiction have involved the use of α_2-adrenergic agonists like clonidine. This therapy is based on the hypothesis that opiates and norepinephrine acting through α_2-adrenergic receptors can induce similar biological effects in brain and that by giving an addict clonidine it is possible to quickly remove opiates from the patient without precipitating withdrawal symptoms. Since clonidine is much less addictive than opiates, it is possible to rapidly relieve the opiate addiction without inducing clonidine addiction. This therapy is still experimental and has not been established as an effective and practical treatment of opiate addiction. More effective therapies for opiate addiction may become available as more is known about the cellular mechanisms associated with opiate addiction (see Chapter 20).

SOMATOSTATIN

Somatostatin is heterogeneously distributed in neurons in the brain, and is believed to be a neurotransmitter or neuromodulator. This 14-amino-acid peptide (Fig. 3) was first purified from the hypothalamus and characterized as a physiological inhibitor of growth hormone secretion from the anterior pituitary. Somatostatin is present in hypothalamic neurons that innervate the median eminence. It is released from these neurons and gains entrance to a portal blood supply that transports the peptide to somatotrophs in the pituitary. Somatostatin is known to be a major factor in the generation of the pulsatile pattern of growth hormone secretion from the anterior pituitary and is itself released in a pulsatile manner (Fig. 4). It is known to have a number of other physiological actions in peripheral tissues. It blocks release of prolactin and thyrotropin-stimulating hormone from the anterior pituitary. Furthermore, somatostatin released from δ cells in the pancreas is a physiological inhibitor of glucagon and insulin secretion from pancreatic islets.

Like other neuropeptides, somatostatin is derived from a precursor, preprosomatostatin (Fig. 3). The gene encoding preprosomatostatin was identified several years ago. This gene is expressed in discrete neurons in brain. Neurotransmitters that stimulate cAMP production and cAMP-dependent protein kinase activity in somatostatin-containing neurons have been shown to activate the soma-

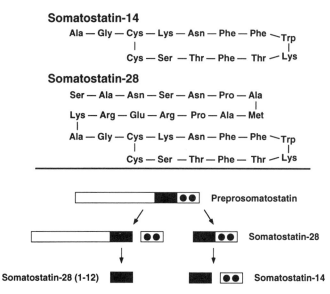

FIG. 3. Structures of somatostatin and its precursors.

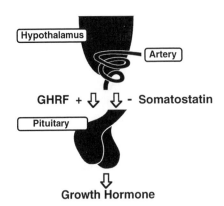

FIG. 4. Regulation of growth hormone release by somatostatin. GHRF, growth hormone–releasing factor.

tostatin gene. This activation involves stimulation of somatostatin gene transcription. Using molecular biological techniques, the region upstream from the initiation site of transcription in the somatostatin gene that mediates cAMP stimulation of transcription was identified. A small DNA fragment of this cAMP-responsive element of the prosomatostatin gene was used to purify a nuclear protein named cAMP-responsive element-binding protein (CREB), which mediates stimulation of somatostatin gene activity by cAMP. This transactivating factor is a substrate for cAMP-dependent protein kinase and was shown to bind to the somatostatin gene to stimulate transcription. This was one of the first cases of a link being established between second messengers such as cAMP and the control of neuropeptide gene activity. Since the DNA sequence in the somatostatin gene that binds CREB is found in other peptide genes, CREB or CREB-like proteins may mediate the actions of a number of hormones or transmitters in controlling the synthesis of neuroactive peptides.

Somatostatin is derived from preprosomatostatin through several processing pathways (Fig. 3). Two basic amino acid residues (arginine-lysine) that are an amino terminal extension of somatostatin can serve as a signal for the cleavage of somatostatin from prosomatostatin. Interestingly, there is another

biologically active prosomatostatin peptide, somatostatin-28, that contains somatostatin within its C-terminal region (Fig. 3). Somatostatin-28 is also generated from the processing of prosomatostatin and can then be further cleaved to yield somatostatin-14. Some evidence exists that somatostatin-28 is not simply a precursor of somatostatin-14 but may act as a distinct neurotransmitter or modulator. The tissue distributions of somatostatin-14 and somatostatin-28 are different. Somatostatin-28 is the predominant prosomatostatin cleavage product in the gut whereas very little somatostatin-28 is expressed in the pancreatic islets where somatostatin-14 pre-dominates. Somatostatin-14, rather than somatostatin-28, is the predominant form of somatostatin in the brain, although some brain regions express both prosomatostatin-derived peptides.

Somatostatin-28 and somatostatin-14 may have different actions in the pancreas. Somatostatin-28 is much more potent than somatostatin-14 in blocking insulin release. This difference in potencies allows somatostatin-28 to be a physiological regulator of insulin release despite the low levels of this peptide in the islets. In contrast to insulin release, somatostatin-14 is much more potent in blocking glucagon release than somatostatin-28. This finding suggests that the two prosomatostatin by-products may have different physiological roles in regulating pancreatic hormone release. Furthermore, somatostatin-14 and somatostatin-28 may have different actions in the brain. Recent electrophysiological studies have shown that somatostatin-14 can stimulate a delayed rectifier K^+ current in brain neurons whereas somatostatin-28 inhibits this same ionic current.

Both somatostatin-14 and somatostatin-28 are released from neurons in brain, and this release is Ca^{++}-dependent. No specific degrading enzyme has been identified for somatostatin. However, the biological half-life of somatostatin in the brain is very short, most likely due to the actions of nonselective peptidases. The prosomatostatin-derived peptides are mainly localized to interneurons in cerebral cortex, striatum, hippocampus, and hypothalamus. Somatostatin has been shown to be colocalized with the classical transmitter γ-aminobutyric acid (GABA) in the hippocampus and cerebral cortex, and there is some evidence that somatostatin and GABA may interact in these brain regions. Interestingly, somatostatin is not localized to GABA neurons in the striatum. However, it is present in neuropeptide Y–containing neurons in this brain region.

Somatostatin has been shown to induce diverse actions in the CNS. The actions of somatostatin are mediated by membrane-bound receptors. Evidence exists that multiple subtypes of somatostatin receptors are expressed in the nervous system and in peripheral organs. Results of biochemical studies have revealed that the sizes of brain and pancreatic somatostatin receptors are different, suggesting that different genes or mRNAs may encode different somatostatin receptors. The pharmacological characteristics of brain and pituitary somatostatin receptors also differ, suggesting that somatostatin receptor subtypes may be expressed in these tissues. Furthermore, biochemical and pharmacological evidence suggests that different somatostatin receptors are expressed in different regions of the brain.

The subtypes of somatostatin receptors may mediate some of the diverse cellular actions of somatostatin in the CNS. Somatostatin inhibits adenylyl cyclase activity and cAMP formation in brain, and G proteins have been shown to couple somatostatin receptors to the catalytic subunit of adenylyl cyclase. Somatostatin also inhibits Ca^{++} currents and stimulates K^+ currents in central neurons; these effects are also mediated by G proteins. Conceivably, distinct subsets of G proteins couple somatostatin receptors to different cellular effector systems.

One of the best-established biological actions of somatostatin in the brain is the facilitation of dopamine transmission in the striatum. Somatostatin has been shown to stimulate dopamine release and dopamine turnover in the striatum. Furthermore, somatostatin facilitates dopamine-induced locomotor behavior and stereotypy. Most likely, somatostatin stimulates dopamine release via an indirect mechanism involving striatal interneurons since its effects on dopamine release are prevented by tetrodotoxin, which blocks sodium channels and inhibits the firing of striatal interneurons. Furthermore, the stimulatory actions of somatostatin on dopamine release can be observed in slices of striatum in which all extrastriatal afferents have been destroyed. The identity of the striatal interneurons or secondary neurons mediating somatostatin actions are not known but they may include neurons containing GABA, acetylcholine, or glutamate, all of which have been reported to stimulate striatal dopamine release via a direct tetrodotoxin-insensitive mechanism.

It has been shown that somatostatin neurons and somatostatin neurotransmission are abnormal in a neuropsychiatric disorder associated with aging. In Alzheimer's disease (see Chapter 23), which is characterized by a loss of short-term memory as well as other cognitive deficits, a major decrease in the number of somatostatin-expressing neurons has been reported. However, most somatostatin receptors in limbic regions are not altered. This information, together with the findings of behavioral studies showing that somatostatin inhibits the extinction of active avoidance behavior, has led to the suggestion that somatostatin may facilitate various cognitive functions. Therefore, the development of agonists at somatostatin receptors that can cross the blood–brain barrier might be useful in the treatment of this severe degenerative disorder.

Recent advances in the pharmacology of somatostatin have led to the development of peptides that are clinically useful agonists at somatostatin receptors. Since somatostatin is rapidly degraded in biological tissues, it has been relatively useless as a pharmacological agent. However, a peptide, SMS-201-995 (Sandostatin), has been developed that is stable in biological tissues, and it has been shown to be effective in the treatment of acromegaly, which is a severe pituitary disorder associated with excess growth hormone secretion. Sandostatin has also been reported to reduce tumor size in insulinomas as well as some metastatic cancers of the gut. Since subtypes of somatostatin receptors may mediate distinct physiological actions of prosomatostatin-derived peptides, development of stable receptor subtype-selective agonists or antagonists could greatly increase the therapeutic usefulness of somatostatin in the treatment of endocrine and exocrine diseases.

SUBSTANCE P

One of the first peptides identified as a potential neurotransmitter, substance P, is present in sensory neurons and in the CNS. In the 1930s, von Euler and Gaddum identified an activity in a brain extract that had a pronounced vasopressor effect. A number of years later, the active ingredient of this extract, substance P, was purified. Substance P is an 11-amino-acid peptide that is part of the tachykinin family of peptides (Fig. 5). The peptides in this family, which include eledoisin, physalaemin, and substance K, share substantial sequence homology. Each has the same three amino acids at its C terminus, which are necessary for biological activity. Furthermore, each of these peptides is able to induce similar biological effects despite different rank orders of potencies for different responses. Both substance P and substance K are expressed in the mammalian nervous system. The preprotachykinin gene that encodes substance P and substance K has been identi-

fied and contains seven exons (Fig. 6). At least two species of mRNA are transcribed from the preprotachykinin gene. One mRNA encodes only substance P while the other encodes both substance P and substance K (Fig. 6). The two mRNAs result from alternative splicing of exon 6, which encodes substance K. Substance P is encoded by exon 3 (see Chapter 5). Because of this splicing, some tissues express only substance P, while others produce both tachykinins.

Different receptors mediate the biological effects of substance P and substance K although both peptides, as well as other tachykinins, can interact with each receptor to varying degrees. Both receptors have been cloned; while sharing substantial sequence homology, they show significant regions of structural variations. Both receptors appear to be linked to G proteins, and their activation leads to stimulation of phospholipase C and protein kinase C, which results in increased intracellular Ca^{++}.

Substance P plays an important role in the perception of pain. Substance P is present in high concentrations in sensory neurons such as the dorsal root ganglia and is involved in pain perception. Dorsal root ganglia neurons terminate in the dorsal horn of the spinal cord, and stimulation of these neurons causes release of substance P. Substance P applied iontophoretically to dorsal horn neurons induces neuronal excitation and depolarizes second-order neurons of the spinothalamic tract involved in pain transmission. Transection of the dorsal root ganglia reduces substance P levels in the dorsal horn. Furthermore, administration of the compound capsaicin, a major ingredient of red peppers, depletes substance P from the dorsal root ganglia afferents and reduces behavioral responses to painful, noxious stimuli. Capsaicin is believed to act by causing the degeneration of sensory neurons containing substance P.

Substance P is also present in the CNS. A major substance P-containing pathway originates in the striatum and projects to the substantia nigra. Striatal substance P neurons

Substance P	Arg-Pro-Lys-Pro-Gln-Gln-Phe-Phe-**Gly-Leu-Met**
Substance K	His-Lys-Thr-Asp-Ser-Phe-Val-**Gly-Leu-Met**
Eledoisin	Glu-Pro-Ser-Lys-Asp-Ala-Phe-Ile-**Gly-Leu-Met**
Physalaemin	Glu-Ala-Asp-Pro-Asn-Lys-Phe-Tyr-**Gly-Leu-Met**

FIG. 5. Amino acid sequences of the tachykinins.

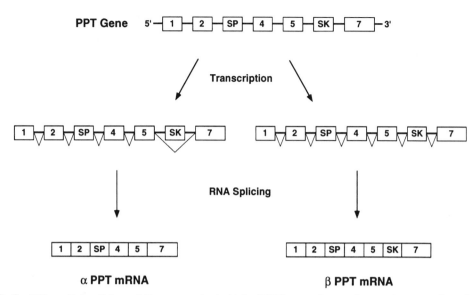

FIG. 6. Differential splicing of the preprotachykinin (PPT) gene to produce substance P and substance K.

also coexpress GABA and dynorphin. These neurons have been shown to degenerate in Huntington's disease, which is a neurological disorder characterized by severe movement abnormalities (see Chapter 23). While the substantia nigra receives a large substance P neuronal input and contains the highest amounts of substance P in the brain, substance P receptors are expressed at a very low density in this brain region. This mismatch between transmitter level and receptor density, which has been reported for other peptide transmitter systems (e.g., the enkephalins), was clarified by results of recent studies showing that relatively high levels of substance K receptors are expressed in the substantia nigra. These findings suggest that substance K, rather than substance P, may be the predominant biologically active preprotachykinin in the substantia nigra.

CHOLECYSTOKININ

Cholecystokinin (CCK) is a linear octapeptide that was originally characterized in terms of its ability to control gallbladder contraction. It is expressed in high concentrations in the gut and pancreas, where it has an important role in the stimulation of amylase secretion. Its presence in brain was first demonstrated through the use of antisera generated against the gut peptide gastrin. Gastrin, CCK, and the frog peptide caerulein have similar structures and biological activities (Fig. 7). However, caerulein is expressed only in frogs, and gastrin is found predominantly in the gut of mammals. These peptides have a unique characteristic in that they all have a sulfate group attached to a tyrosine residue, which is necessary for the biological activity of the peptides. The sulfation occurs as an early post-translational processing event since preprocholecystokinin is already sulfated. The sulfation is catalyzed by a specific sulfotransferase that transfers sulfate from adenosine-3'-phosphate-5'-sulfatophosphate to CCK.

CCK is derived from preprocholecysto-

Cholecystokinin	Asp-Arg-Asp-Tyr*-Met-Gly-Trp-Met-Asp-Phe
Caerulein	Glu-Gln-Asp-Tyr*-Thr-Gly-Trp-Met-Asp-Phe
Gastrin	Glu-Glu-Glu-Ala-Tyr*-Gly-Trp-Met-Asp-Phe

FIG. 7. Amino acid sequences of cholecystokinin and related peptides. *, Sulfated.

kinin. The gene encoding CCK has been identified and contains three exons, with exons 2 and 3 encoding preprocholecystokinin. There are multiple biologically active forms of CCK, including CCK-33, CCK-39, and CCK-58. All of these larger forms contain CCK in their C-terminal region and are probably processing intermediates of mature CCK.

Cholecystokinin (CCK) has been shown to be expressed in neurons in the brain and is distributed heterogeneously in the CNS. CCK is present in cell bodies in the cerebral cortex as well as in limbic regions such as the hippocampus and amygdala. In the hypothalamus, CCK is present in both the magnocellular neurons that project to the posterior pituitary and the parvocellular region of the paraventricular nucleus. The parvocellular neurons project to the median eminence, and CCK released from these neurons may control the release of anterior pituitary hormones such as adrenocorticotropin. CCK is found in high levels in the midbrain, particularly in the substantia nigra and ventral tegmental area. The CCK in the ventral tegmental area is believed to be colocalized with dopamine in neurons projecting to the nucleus accumbens. This is suggested from immunocytochemical studies as well as from the finding that lesioning of the dopamine neurons in the ventral tegmental area–nucleus accumbens pathway with 6-hydroxydopamine resulted in a major reduction in CCK in the nucleus accumbens and A10 region. CCK is also present in some neurons in the substantia nigra. However, there is little if any CCK projection to the caudate nucleus from the substantia nigra.

Substantial evidence exists that CCK and dopamine released from ventral tegmental area neurons interact in the nucleus accumbens. CCK has been shown to potentiate the ability of the dopamine agonist apomorphine to inhibit firing of nucleus accumbens neurons. Furthermore, CCK microinjected into the nucleus accumbens can potentiate dopamine-induced locomotor activity and stereotypy. CCK does not induce these behaviors by itself and does not modulate dopamine-mediated behaviors in the striatum.

CCK applied iontophoretically to either ventral tegmental area or substantia nigra dopamine neurons depolarizes the neurons and greatly increases their firing rate. Continuous application of CCK to midbrain dopamine neurons overexcites the cells such that depolarization blockade occurs and the neurons become quiescent. This effect is specific since it is blocked by the CCK receptor antagonist proglumide. Presumably, CCK released from ventral tegmental neurons can act on dopamine-containing cell bodies or dendrites to stimulate firing activity.

CCK also potentiates the inhibition by dopamine of ventral tegmental area and substantia nigra firing activity, and this effect is also blocked by proglumide. The mechanism by which CCK potentiates dopamine inhibition of midbrain neuronal firing activity is not known. Conceivably, the direct stimulatory action of CCK and its potentiation of the effects of dopamine are mediated via distinct cellular mechanisms, possibly involving different CCK receptor subtypes.

Some of the actions of CCK on mesolimbic dopamine neurons are similar to those of antipsychotic agents. Dopamine receptor antagonists such as haloperidol increase the firing activity of ventral tegmental area and substantia nigra dopamine neurons, presumably by blocking the feedback inhibitory actions of dopamine on autoreceptors localized to dopamine cell bodies and/or dendrites. Similarly, CCK applied to these neurons increases firing activity. Chronic administration of haloperidol to rats induces a depolarizing block of ventral tegmental area and substantia nigra dopamine neurons, much like the continuous microiontophoretic application of CCK to midbrain neurons. Depolarization-induced blockade of neuronal activity of nigrostriatal dopamine neurons may be responsible for some of the motor side effects of neuroleptics. Administration of the CCK antagonist proglumide to animals chronically pretreated with haloperidol overcomes the blockade of nigrostriatal dopamine neurons and results in an increase in the firing activity of these midbrain dopamine neurons. Thus, selective central CCK receptor antagonists may be useful in attenuating some of the harmful side effects of the use of neuroleptics in the treatment of schizophrenia. Results of these electrophysiological studies have led to the suggestion that CCK may act as an endogenous neuroleptic. As a result, a number of investigators have proposed that abnormalities in CCK transmission in the mesolimbic dopamine pathway may be involved in the pathophysiology of schizophrenia.

CCK has a major role in the regulation of food intake. CCK can act both peripherally and centrally to control eating (see Chapter 21). It can modulate the rate of gastric emptying by regulating the activity of the pyloric sphincter. Furthermore, central administration of CCK inhibits eating in animals. Abnormalities in CCK transmission have been implicated in eating disorders such as anorexia nervosa and obesity and have led to intensive efforts to develop CCK receptor antagonists to investigate the role of CCK in these diseases and as potential therapeutic agents. Proglumide and benzotript are compounds that have been shown to antagonize biological actions of CCK both in peripheral tissues and in brain. More recently, however, the compound asperlicin (L-363718) was shown to be a powerful inhibitor of CCK's actions in peripheral tissues. Interestingly, asperlicin has little effect on brain CCK receptors; this suggests that CCK receptors in brain and peripheral tissues are different.

The cellular mechanisms of action of CCK are mediated by membrane-bound receptors. These receptors are coupled to the enzyme phospholipase C, and CCK is known to stimulate phosphatidylinositol turnover to induce its biological effects. The increase in phosphatidylinositol turnover leads to increases in Ca^{++} mobilization in cells as well as an increase in diacylglycerol formation and activation of protein kinase C activity. These cellular mechanisms of action of CCK have been most clearly identified in pancreatic acinar cells where CCK is known to stimulate amylase secretion. The precise cellular mechanism of action of CCK in brain is not known.

NEUROTENSIN

Neurotensin is widely distributed in the CNS where it may act as either a neurotransmitter or a neuromodulator. Neurotensin is a 13-amino-acid-containing peptide that was originally isolated from hypothalamus (Fig. 8). It has a powerful hypotensive effect and also induces hypothermia.

Neurotensin is derived from preproneurotensin, which is 170 amino acids in length. The gene encoding neurotensin has four exons and three introns with exon 4 encoding neurotensin as well as the neurotensin-related peptide neuromedin N. Neuromedin N and neurotensin have similar C-terminal regions. Two mRNAs with widely differing distributions in brain are encoded by the neurotensin gene.

Neurotensin concentrations are particularly high in several limbic and mesolimbic brain regions such as the amygdala, hippocampus, and nucleus accumbens. Neurotensin immunoreactivity has also been localized to the ventral tegmental area, and these neurotensin-containing neurons have been proposed to project to the nucleus accumbens. Immunohistochemical studies have suggested that neurotensin is colocalized with dopamine in ventral tegmental area neurons. In fact, a population of ventral tegmental area neurons coexpresses not only dopamine and neurotensin but also CCK.

An association of neurotensin with dopamine in the ventral tegmental area is also supported by the results of studies that have shown that neurotensin microinjected into the ventral tegmental area stimulates locomotor activity and increases dopamine turnover in the nucleus accumbens. These find-

Neurotensin   Glu-Leu-Tyr-Glu-Asn-Lys-Pro-Arg-Arg-Pro-Tyr-Ile-Leu

FIG. 8. Amino acid sequence of neurotensin.

ings indicate that neurotensin, released from ventral tegmental area dopamine neurons, stimulates dopamine neurons, possibly through autoreceptors that increase neuronal activity and subsequently increase the release of dopamine from nerve terminals in the nucleus accumbens.

Neurotensin antagonizes the actions of dopamine in the nucleus accumbens since microinjection of neurotensin into the nucleus accumbens inhibits dopamine-induced locomotor activity. The mechanism of this inhibition is not known, but may involve either an attenuation of dopamine release via a presynaptic mechanism at dopamine nerve terminals or a modulation of the postsynaptic actions of dopamine via an alteration in dopamine receptor function.

One of the highest densities of neurotensin receptors in brain is in the substantia nigra, an area that also has a high level of neurotensin. Lesions of the nigrostriatal dopamine pathway produced with 6-hydroxydopamine greatly reduce neurotensin receptor binding in the substantia nigra, suggesting that neurotensin receptors are localized to dopamine neurons. Furthermore, results of electron microscopic studies have led to the suggestion that neurotensin binding sites are localized to dopamine neurons in the substantia nigra. However, neurotensin microinjected into the substantia nigra does not modify locomotor activity, suggesting that it does not serve the same regulatory role on dopamine neurons in the substantia nigra as it does in the ventral tegmental area.

Because it induces responses similar to those of dopamine receptor antagonists (i.e., it increases dopamine turnover in mesolimbic neurons and blocks the postsynaptic actions of dopamine in the nucleus accumbens), neurotensin has been suggested to be an endogenous neuroleptic-like compound. Neurotensin's actions on dopamine transmission appear to be selective for mesolimbic dopamine neurons. Thus, selective neurotensin agonists that cross the blood–brain barrier could be useful antipsychotic agents.

SUMMARY

A large number of peptides have been identified in the CNS and have been postulated to be neurotransmitters or neuromodulators. Peptides are expressed in much lower concentrations in the brain than are classical transmitters, and their mechanisms of biosynthesis are more complicated. The control of peptide synthesis can involve changes in gene activity, gene splicing, mRNA processing, and translation and prohormone processing. Sophisticated molecular biological and protein chemistry techniques had to be developed just to investigate the most basic aspects of peptide biosynthesis (see Chapter 5). As a result, progress in our understanding of the expression and role of peptides in the nervous system has lagged considerably behind our understanding of the roles of the classical transmitters.

Evidence obtained over the last decade has revealed that families of peptides are expressed in the nervous system. The peptides within each family share some similarities, such as common amino acid sequences. This allows peptides within families to bind, with varying potencies, to the same receptors to induce the same biological responses. Furthermore, peptides within families may be encoded by the same gene or family of genes and share common biosynthetic pathways. However, peptides within families may also show striking differences. While some portions of their sequences are common, other regions can be very different in sequence. These structural differences allow members of peptide families to have high-affinity interactions with distinct receptor subclasses. If peptide family members are encoded by different genes or mRNAs, they can be differentially expressed in the nervous system. These differences among members of peptide families greatly increase the diversity of action of the peptide family of neurotransmitters and neuromodulators.

Our understanding of how peptides act in the CNS has been hindered by the lack of pharmacological agents that either mimic or antagonize their actions. Furthermore, few peptide analogs gain entrance to the brain since peptides are charged and do not generally cross the blood–brain barrier. Since peptides play a critical role in a number of neuropsychiatric disorders, development of stable peptide agonists and antagonists that gain access to the brain may be useful in the treatment of some psychiatric diseases.

BIBLIOGRAPHY

Original Articles

Hershey AD, Krause JE. Molecular characterization of a functional cDNA encoding the rat substance P receptor. *Science* 1990;247:958–962.

Hughes J, Smith TW, Kosterlitz HW, Fothergill LA, Morgan BA, Morris HR. Identification of two related pentapeptides from the brain with potent opiate agonist activity. *Nature* 1975;258:577–579.

Jessel TM, Womack MD. Substance P and the novel mammalian tachykinins: a diversity of receptors and cellular actions. *Trends Neurosci* 1985;8:43–45.

Mudge AW, Leeman SE, Fischbach GD. Enkephalin inhibits release of substance P from sensory neurons in culture and decreases action potential duration. *Proc Natl Acad Sci USA* 1979;76:526–530.

White FJ, Wang RY. Interactions of cholecystokinin octapeptide and dopamine on nucleus accumbens neurons. *Brain Res* 1984;300:161–166.

Yamada Y, Post SR, Wang K, Tager HS, Bell GI, Seino S. Cloning and functional characterization of a family of human and mouse somatostatin receptors expressed in brain, gastrointestinal tract and kidney. *Proc Natl Acad Sci USA* 1992;89:251–255.

Books and Reviews

Bloom, F. The endorphins: a growing family of pharmacologically pertinent peptides. *Annu Rev Pharmacol Toxicol* 1983;23:151–170.

Brownstein MJ. Neuropeptides. In: Siegel GJ, Agranoff BW, Albers RW, Molinoff PB, eds. *Basic neurochemistry,* 5th ed. New York: Raven Press; 1994 (in press).

Epelbaum J. Somatostatin in the central nervous system: physiology and pathological modifications. *Progr Neurobiol* 1986;27:63–100.

Hökfelt T, Johansson O, Ljungdahl A, Lundberg JM, Schultzberg M. Peptidergic neurons. *Nature* 1980;248:515–521.

Krieger DT, Brownstein MJ, Martin JB. *Brain peptides.* New York: Wiley; 1983.

Martin JB, Reichlin S. *Clinical neuroendocrinology.* 2nd Ed. Philadelphia: FA Davis; 1987.

Simon EJ, Hiller JM. Opioid peptides and opioid receptors. In: Siegel GJ, Agranoff BW, Albers RW, Molinoff PB, eds. *Basic neurochemistry,* 5th ed. New York: Raven Press; 1994 (in press).

Vanderhaeghen JJ, Crawley JN. *Neuronal cholecystokinin.* New York: New York Academy of Sciences; 1985.

Neuroendocrinology

Peter C. Whybrow

Her pure and eloquent blood
Spoke in her cheeks, and so distinctly wrought
That one might almost say, her body thought.

John Donne,
Of the Progress of the Soul; Second Anniversary, 1612

- The purpose of cellular communication is to sustain an internal balance that provides optimum adaptation to the environment.

- Neuroregulatory mechanisms are the key to successful adaptation through endocrine signaling.

- The pituitary gland is the key linkage between the brain and the peripheral endocrine glands with both a neural and a glandular portion.

- The neuroendocrine system provides for both acute response and long-term adaptation.

- When there is over- or underproduction of peripheral gland hormones, endocrinopathies result.

- The peripheral hormones sustain the fundamental processes of life including growth, salt and water metabolism, energy production, and reproduction.

- The brain-thyroid axis and its disorders provide an excellent illustration of how our understanding of neuroendocrinology has progressed over the past century.

- Diagnostic methods have improved with our clinical understanding of the dynamic regulation of neuroendocrine systems and basic research into the measurement and synthesis of the individual axis hormones.

- Clinical and basic science research have provided insights into the other fundamental life processes that are under neuroendocrine regulation: hormones of growth (growth hormone), control of reproduction (sex hormones), and hormones of salt and water metabolism and stress (corticosteroids).

- In the research on stress and adaptation, the novelty of the stressor and the control that could be exerted by the individual over the stressful situation emerged as key issues determining the stress response.

- In social animals, such as primates and ourselves, the social order is a major determinant of neuroendocrine arousal.

- An intimate relationship exists between the brain, the neuroendocrine system, and immune function.

- In all persons, but particularly in those disposed through genetic or early experience, chronic stress can lead to profound clinical depression.

- As in chronic stress, the HPA axis is profoundly disturbed in many depressed individuals, both in its circadian rhythmicity and in its regulation.

- The feedback of the neuroendocrine messengers to the brain may play an important role in the modulation of brain function and normal behavior.

- Thyroid hormones appear to be of particular importance in the expression and treatment of manic-depressive disease.

This chapter summarizes the anatomy and physiology of neurochemical systems in brain that regulate endocrine function. The hierarchical organization of the endocrine system is reviewed, with an emphasis on hormone abnormalities that result from defects in regulation. Finally, the importance of the neuroendocrine system in behavioral adaptation and its linkage with the immune system are discussed.

Signaling, the accurate and orderly transfer of information between cells, is essential to the survival of all multicellular organisms. Endocrine signaling systems appear early in evolution. A chemical substance or messenger is released from one cell into the bloodstream and upon arrival at the surface of a second it modifies the latter's behavior. The brain and the nervous system in general can be viewed simply as a highly adaptive group of cells in which this same principle holds. Specialized evolution of the neuron with its many dendritic connections and elongated axon has facilitated close physical contact and therefore a more direct and rapid transmission of the necessary information. However, the passage of that information between the two cells still depends on the release of the chemical substance which now passes across a very small gap called a synapse rather than by way of the bloodstream.

In higher animals the neuroendocrine system provides a vital link between brain, the command center of behavior, and peripheral organs and cells. Through a system of messengers communicating with specialized organs responsible for the control of reproduction, growth, salt and water and energy metabolism, for example, the brain is able to promote and orchestrate optimum adaptation.

There is also increasing evidence that the immune system, in conjunction with the central nervous system (CNS) and the endocrine system, constitutes the third major system of communication using many of the same principles that have been presented in earlier chapters. With characteristic parsimony, nature has conserved on the number of messengers used in these communication systems, and so we find transmitters in the nervous system (neurotransmitters) sometimes identical to those messengers (now called hormones) that are used in the endocrine system. Indeed, because systems of chemical communication and control are widespread throughout the animal and plant world, hormones and peptides that occur in humans and vertebrates appear also in plants. Hence the chemical structure of steroids, which are very important signaling hormones in vertebrates, is found in plants in combination with carbohydrates where they are called glycosides. Digitalis, an ancient remedy still used today in heart disease, is an example of such a combination. Similarly, the so-called endorphins, small peptides found naturally in the CNS (see Chapter 8), are analogs of the opiates found in many plants, which may explain why opiates are so effective in the control of pain and so addicting (see Chapter 20).

During the course of evolution, serial adaptation has exploited many of these simple messengers to good advantage. Again, the steroids provide an excellent example. In mammals, corticosteroids play a major part in the maintenance of the body's electrolyte balance; in fish, they discharge the same responsibility as the exchange of ions and water within the gills of the fish is under corticoste-

Biological Bases of Brain Function and Disease, edited by Alan Frazer, Perry B. Molinoff, and Andrew Winokur. Raven Press, Ltd., New York © 1994.

roid control. The transmission of sodium through the highly permeable skin of the frog, and the production of tears (avian dewdrops) by marine birds who must live for many days without fresh water, are similarly controlled. Indeed, we retain vestiges of such functions in our own salty tears and in the capability of the sweat glands to move sodium out of the body during perspiration.

PRINCIPLES OF NEUROENDOCRINE REGULATION

The purpose of cellular communication is to sustain an internal balance that provides optimum adaptation to the environment. All three of the major communication systems in the body—CNS, endocrine system, and immune system—have but one general purpose: to sustain an internal balance of metabolic function that will afford response to an external environment that is forever changing—in short, to provide adaptive advantage through autonomy. It is this capacity to sustain autonomy from the environment, to remain stable in the face of low entropy, that is the quintessence of life.

The nineteenth-century French physiologist Claude Bernard first pointed out that such stability is only possible through complex regulatory mechanisms that are capable of adaptation to the continuous change in the internal and external environments of the cell and the individual. Bernard's original work on the mechanisms surrounding the storage and release of glycogen in the body led to his formulation of the famous principle of the "milieu interieur" and the concept of regulatory control of physiological processes. Life, in fact, is based on a paradox. Stability of function is possible only through constant and adaptive change. However, to be adaptive the change must be both appropriate and precise. Indeed, it must be highly regulated.

Neuroregulatory mechanisms are the key to successful adaptation through endocrine signaling. Neuroendocrine regulatory mechanisms have certain principles in common

with all other neurobiological control systems. The most important is the closed homeostatic loop. Here the controlled variable determines the rate of its own manufacture; most common is that the output of the sys-

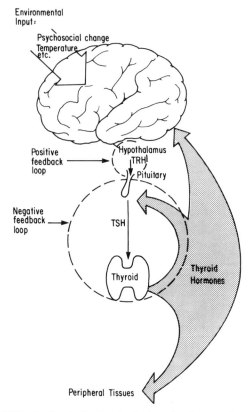

FIG. 1. Control of a typical endocrine system: The brain–thyroid axis. The cascade of thyroid hormone secretion is initiated by secretion of thyrotropin-releasing hormone (TRH) in the hypothalamus. The production of thyroid hormone inhibits thyroid-stimulating hormone (TSH) secretion and reduces the stimulus to further thyroid hormone production and release. It is probable that a positive feedback loop also operates when a rising output accelerates production. The time frame of response for the two mechanisms is different, however, with the positive loop having a shorter period than the negative one. This positive feedback then serves to maximize acute production, which is ultimately inhibited through negative feedback to both the pituitary and the hypothalamus as peripheral levels of the hormone rise. From Whybrow PC, Akiskal HS, McKinney WT. *Mood disorders: toward a new psychobiology.* New York: Plenum Press; 1984.

tem inhibits production. Hence, increasing levels of hormone in the bloodstream inhibit those neurons and secretory cells that initiate the cascade of signals to produce the peripheral hormone. This is known as a negative feedback system.

The nervous system and the endocrine system (the neuroendocrine system) are integrated in the hypothalamus where cells that produce the peptides that initiate the cascade of peripheral endocrine activity are located. The mediator and sentinel of this cascade is the pituitary gland, which produces the messengers that activate the target endocrine organs. In turn, the peripheral hormones produced by these targeted endocrine glands feed back on the neurons of the pituitary and the brain, influencing not only the further release of hormones but also the modifying function of the brain itself. The brain is thus both an end organ of hormone influence and the regulator of hormone action (Fig. 1).

ANATOMY AND PHYSIOLOGY OF NEUROENDOCRINE REGULATION

The pituitary gland is the key linkage between the brain and the peripheral endocrine glands, with both a neural and a glandular portion. The pituitary, once termed the master gland of the endocrine system, is actually closer to a sentinel since it sits at the interface between the brain and the peripheral endocrine organs. Embryologically, the pituitary originates from the brain and the gut.

The *posterior pituitary* (or neurohypophysis) is a continuous outgrowth of the diencephalon and contains terminals from axons that have their cell bodies in the hypothalamus. It produces oxytocin, which causes contraction of smooth muscle in both the uterus and breast, and vasopressin, which acts on the kidney to promote water retention. Vasopressin also increases blood pressure by its effects on the smooth muscle of arterioles. The release of both of these hormones is controlled by hypothalamic neurons.

The glandular or *anterior pituitary* gland is called the adenohypophysis. This portion of the pituitary originates from the pharynx and, while not directly linked to the brain itself, is connected through a complex of blood vessels called the hypophyseal-portal tract. These portal veins carry releasing factors from where they are manufactured in the hypothalamus to the cells of the pituitary. The importance of this special portal system is that the releasing factors arrive at the pituitary relatively undiluted. The portal system is a fine example of a special anatomic modification to facilitate the precise transfer of information by chemical messenger from one cell to the next. In turn, the anterior pituitary orchestrates the remaining target glands that make up the peripheral endocrine system (Fig. 2).

Our modern understanding of the neuroendocrine system owes much to the interaction of clinical endocrinology and neuroscience research. Our knowledge of the cellular action of the peripheral endocrine hormones and their general influence on the body has been greatly enhanced by the study of endocrine diseases such as Addison's and Cushing's (both diseases of the adrenal glands) and hyper- and hypothyroidism. Some of these disorders are discussed later in this chapter. However, it was only recognized in 1955, through the work of the English endocrinologist Jeffrey Harris, that the initiation of endocrine release actually begins in the hypothalamus.

Since then, the hunt for the releasing factors in the hypothalamus has been intense and fascinating and is still not complete. Most of these factors are small peptides and many probably have neurotransmitter functions in addition to their activity as endocrine system releasing hormones. They are present only in very small amounts in the brain, and this is in part why they have been hard to detect. For example, during the initial identification and purification of thyrotropin-releasing hormone (TRH), it took 300,000 sheep hypothalami to generate 1 mg of TRH. As the releasing factors have been discovered,

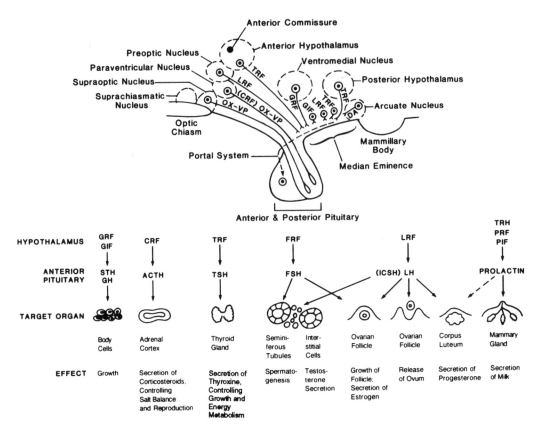

FIG. 2. Hypothalamic–pituitary system for neuroendocrine control in the mammal. ACTH, adrenocorticotrophic hormone; CRF, corticotropin-releasing factor; FRF, follicle-stimulating hormone–releasing factor; FSH, follicle-stimulating hormone; GIF, growth hormone release–inhibiting factor (somatostatin); GH, growth hormone; GRF, growth hormone–releasing factor; ICSH, interstitial cell–stimulating hormone; LH, luteinizing hormone; LRF, luteinizing hormone–releasing factor (also called LHRH, luteinizing hormone–releasing hormone); PIF, prolactin release–inhibiting factor; PRF, prolactin-releasing factor; STH, somatotropic hormone; TRF, thyroid hormone–releasing factor, TSH, thyroid-stimulating hormone. From Shepherd GM. *Neurobiology.* New York: Oxford University Press; 1983.

however, they have become valuable tools not only in research but also for testing the dynamic integrity of the endocrine system in a clinical setting.

The neuroendocrine system provides for both acute response and long-term adaptation. Through its connections to the rest of the CNS the hypothalamus is intimately linked to the surrounding environment and capable of acute response in an emergency. Much of our immediate response to an acute fright is mediated through the autonomic nervous system, but the endocrine system is also capable of rapid signaling. This particular acute response is called *feedforward* to distinguish it from *feedback,* which, as we have learned, will return the system to its homeostatic *set point.* The acute changes occurring in the neuroendocrine system when under challenge are called the *stress response.* In addition, the neuroendocrine system must be capable of managing those longer term periodic challenges in the environment that result from our living on a rapidly rotating planet that spins at an angle to the source of life's energy—the sun.

The ongoing regulation of the neuroendocrine system is largely of the negative feedback variety. Furthermore, the system must be able to accommodate both short-term stress and the longer term demands at the same time. Here the concept of set point is very important. Feedback regulation occurs both at the level of the pituitary gland and within the brain itself, especially in the hypothalamus. If feedback occurred only at the level of the pituitary gland, it would be difficult to change the overall set point at the same time the system remained responsive to acute emergencies. The amount of hormone produced by the adrenal and thyroid glands helps determine the brain's set point. If a large amount of hormone is produced, then not all of it is bound by protein carriers in the bloodstream and more free hormone is available to cross the blood–brain barrier into the brain. Through mechanisms that we do not entirely understand, the pituitary and the brain balance each other such that long-term changes in set points do occur, but at the same time the neuroendocrine system remains responsive to acute disturbance. The acute response to a stressor is discussed in a later part of this chapter when adaptation is considered in detail.

Adaptation to recurrent changes in the planetary environment is also very important to the animal and underpins various complex cycles of behavior, particularly reproduction. In many higher animals including human beings, reproductive behaviors are orchestrated through clocks that have been developed over evolutionary time and are now indigenous functions of the CNS. For example, the photic period (the balance of light to dark in a 24-hr period), which changes in temperate climates depending on the season of the year, triggers such behaviors as hibernation and the timing of pregnancy. Most of these mechanisms are orchestrated by the neuroendocrine system. One good example is that of the deer herd where mating occurs in the fall and the young are born in the spring. This animal cycle, which is well marked by mating behaviors and the growth and loss of antlers by the male, is under the control of the sex hormones. Gonadal activity is in turn modulated by melatonin, which is a hormone produced by the pineal gland and inhibited by sunlight. During the long sunny days of summer, light impinging on the eye decreases the production of melatonin; sexual hormones and sexual activity increase and by fall most of the does are pregnant. The long 8-month pregnancy ensures that most of the young are born in the spring when they have the greatest chance for survival.

Daily (or circadian) endocrine cycles are also important to normal behavioral function. Many of these rhythms are orchestrated by a master clock in the anterior hypothalamus. This master clock is a tightly knit collection of neurons called the suprachiasmatic nucleus because it lies above the crossing of the optic nerves (see Chapter 11). The internal clocks that control body temperature, sleep, alertness, hormone levels, and so forth, run at a slightly longer period than 24 hr and are resynchronized each day by the morning light and many social cues. We are probably most aware of the presence of these clocks when some rapid change in the external environment occurs, such as flying across time zones. Suddenly our internal clock is at variance with the environmental time clues of our new habitat. We become very aware of the difference when our body demands sleep and food at what appear to be environmentally inappropriate times! That the internal clock has a somewhat longer period than 24 hr and by preference slows down is one explanation of why it is easier to fly west than east.

These rhythms, which are very important in the orchestration of normal behavior, become disturbed in many behavioral disorders. Hence the depressed person wakes up early, has no appetite, loses the rhythm of bowel function, and has definite changes in the circadian parameters of many endocrine variables, including adrenocorticol and thyroid hormones. Some of these elements are mentioned later in this chapter when specific aspects of behavioral disorders and endocrinology are discussed.

ACTIONS OF PERIPHERAL HORMONES

When there is over- or underproduction of peripheral gland hormones, endocrinopathies result. Students of the history of science may recognize in modern endocrinology some of the vestiges of the humoral theories of Hippocrates. It was thought that the three Hippocratic stages of disease (irritation, coction, and crisis) were dependent on glandular secretions. Theophile de Bordeu, physician to Louis XV, suggested that the behavioral differences between eunuchs and noncastrated men were explained by the loss of internal secretion by the male organs. In a classic experiment in 1849, Bertold confirmed Bordeu's observations, showing that the capon characteristics that emerge after a cockerel is castrated could be prevented by transplanting the testes into the abdomen. Furthermore, on examining the birds postmortem, it was found that the testes had attached to very vascular parts of the bowel; Bertold postulated that the testes continued to provide a male hormone that was distributed via the bloodstream.

Over the past 100 years these classic experiments have been paralleled by clinical observation and research into the *endocrinopathies,* conditions when excess or deficiency of peripheral hormones (because of disease) produce gross changes in many bodily functions including behavior. It was from careful analyses of these syndromes, first by clinical observation and anatomic pathology, and later as individual hormones and the hypothalamic and pituitary releasing factors were identified through experiments in clinical populations, that we have gained our modern understanding of endocrinology.

The peripheral hormones sustain the fundamental processes of life including growth, salt and water metabolism, energy production, and reproduction. A careful review of Fig. 2 will quickly summarize for the reader the fundamental nature of the processes controlled by the endocrine glands. The control of reproductive function represents a major focus of activity; there is interlacing of hormonal function and common use of many hormones in both male and female reproduction. Other fundamental processes controlled are the growth and development of the individual through growth hormone secretion, the processes of energy metabolism (the thyroid gland), and salt and water metabolism and stress (the adrenal cortex). There is metabolic overlap among the endocrine systems so that a major disturbance of one will influence the activity of the other systems. Through this interdependence they serve a vital background function to the housekeeping of adaptation and survival.

Thyroid Hormone

The brain–thyroid axis and its disorders provide an excellent illustration of how our understanding of neuroendocrinology has progressed over the past century. The profound metabolic effects of disorders of the thyroid gland were among the first to be described. Indeed, when *thyrotoxicosis* (an excess of circulating thyroid hormone) was first described in the early 1800s, it was thought to be a disease of the nervous system because commonly it appeared to be precipitated by fright and stressful situations. Furthermore, the effects of the disorder—tremulousness, weight loss, irritability, and anxiety—mimicked a syndrome of nervous dysfunction. Similarly, when the syndrome of inadequate circulating thyroid hormone was recognized later in the century as the cause of adult dementia and of cretinism occurring in young children, the profound disturbance again appeared to be in the brain. However, careful review of these early descriptions of excessive and deficient thyroid hormone clearly indicates the metabolic effects of thyroid hormone in many organ systems.

The peripheral signs and symptoms of *hypothyroidism* (too little circulating thyroid hormone) are the effects of deceleration of cellular metabolic processes and the accumulation of mucopolysaccharide in the vocal chords and subcutaneous tissue. It is this abnormality that gives hypothyroidism its other name of *myxedema*. Weakness, fatigue, lethargy, and vague psychiatric disturbances such as irritability and apathy predominate early in the disorder and may go unnoticed until other symptoms begin to emerge. Soon a coarse, dry skin develops with decreased body and scalp hair especially evident in thinning of the outer third of the eyebrows. The myxedema appears as a puffy, nonpitting swelling of the skin and is especially noticed around the eyes and on the shins. The skin becomes yellow because of carotene (vitamin A) accumulation, and the voice becomes husky because of thickening of the vocal chords. Hearing diminishes acutely; we know from modern experiments that the thyroid hormones are particularly important to the maintenance of the auditory pathways in the brain. Other changes in neurological function appear, particularly a delayed relaxation phase of the deep tendon reflexes; a painful wrist affliction called the carpal tunnel syndrome and peripheral neuropathies may occur. The individual becomes intolerant to cold, gains modestly in weight, is constipated, and complains of muscle cramps. Changes in the heart muscle also occur with slowing of the heart rate and a lower voltage and extension in time of the waveform on the electrocardiogram. Menstrual irregularities and disturbances of the liver enzymes plus anemias complete the picture.

Thyrotoxicosis, in which a sustained elevation of plasma levels of unbound thyroid hormones appears in the bloodstream, paints the opposite clinical picture. Individuals with this condition have an increased metabolic rate with heat intolerance, raised heart rate, excessive sweating, weight loss despite increased appetite, increased bowel movements, and an inability to concentrate or sit still. Sometimes nervous complaints such as anxiety predominate; in other individuals, cardiovascular symptoms are the most common with a racing pulse, arrhythmias, and enlargement of the heart secondary to the increased pumping of blood throughout the body required by the raised metabolism. Muscle wasting occurs as the protein metabolism of the individual is disturbed to provide increased energy. The limb and girdle muscles are especially affected, and the deep tendon reflexes are hyperactive. The skin becomes moist, velvety, and warm to the touch; the hair is thin and fine; and sometimes the eyes are changed with staring, infrequent blinking and widened gaze resulting from stimulation of the sympathetic nervous system. This so-called *exophthalmos* is due to an infiltration of the eye socket with the same type of myxedema that is found in hypothyroidism. The person complains of tension and dysphoria (being subjectively uncomfortable), and the syndrome is sometimes confused with anxiety. In certain types of thyrotoxicosis the thyroid gland not only produces increased thyroid hormone but itself enlarges; this is given the name *goiter*.

Diagnostic methods have improved with our clinical understanding of the dynamic regulation of neuroendocrine systems and basic research into the measurement and synthesis of the individual axis hormones. Initially, the thyroid endocrinopathies were diagnosed entirely by a physician's investigation of clinical signs and symptoms. The treatment for these disorders was either the removal of the thyroid gland to reduce the production of thyroxine in thyrotoxicosis or the administration of ground-up thyroid glands of sheep for those hypothyroid persons who did not produce enough thyroxine of their own.

Laboratory research over the years has been able to establish accurate measurement of thyroxine (T_4) and its metabolic derivatives including the most active hormone, triiodothyronine (T_3) (Fig. 3). T_4 is the predominant hormone secreted by the gland; T_3 is the hormone that "turns on" the metabolic processes of the cell. Complex systems of metabolic balance maintain optimum levels of available T_3 to all cells including the pituitary gland and brain, where the level of T_3 controls the release of TRH in the hypothalamus and thyroid-stimulating hormone (TSH) in the pituitary. Together this cascade regulates

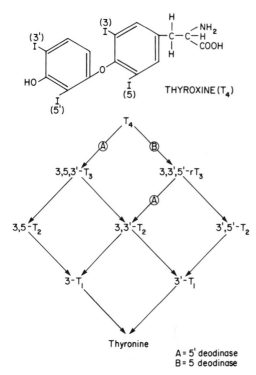

A = 5' deodinase
B = 5 deodinase

FIG. 3. Thyroxine and its metabolic pathways. There is a dynamic balance between the deiodinase enzymes (A and B in the diagram) which modulate metabolic activity. For example, under conditions of starvation, more reverse T_3, a relatively inert thyroid hormone, is manufactured and T_3, the most metabolically active hormone, is reduced.

the supply of thyroid hormone in a normal situation.

The syndromes of excess and deficient thyroid hormone are frequently linked by an autoimmune process that may have a genetic basis. In this illness, termed Hashimoto's disease (after the Japanese physician who first described it), the thyroid gland is slowly destroyed by *auto*antibodies developed by the immune system. The cell damage in the thyroid gland may initially cause a release of hormone, sometimes to excess (thyrotoxicosis), but subsequently, as the thyroid gland dies, there is a deficiency of hormone-producing cells and hypothyroidism results. Thus, the natural history for many individuals who suffer the disease is that first they

have thyrotoxicosis (which is treated) and then subsequently develop hypothyroidism.

The change in the capacity to produce thyroid hormone occurs slowly during the illness, and it is now recognized that thyroid disease is a graded phenomenon. Clinical symptoms alone are not always a reliable way to make a diagnosis. Hence, testing the brain–thyroid axis by peripheral hormone measurement and hormone challenge becomes very important in the endocrine clinic. This accurate assessment of the brain–thyroid axis has also been made possible by advances in neuroendocrine research that permit measurement of TSH, T_4, T_3, and antibodies to the thyroid gland in the bloodstream. Also, by using TRH as a challenge hormone, measurement of the sensitivity of the axis to perturbation can be carried out. This in combination with the levels of hormone found in the bloodstream permits an accurate diagnosis of the prevailing state of thyroid metabolism and whether hyper- or hypothyroidism is present.

TRH was the first releasing hormone to be identified. Its identification and synthesis in biologically active form were accomplished independently by Roger Guillemin and Andrew Schally in 1969; they shared a Nobel Prize for this work in 1977. The principle of the TRH challenge test (Fig. 4) is based on our understanding of feedback control. When, for example, there is an excess of thyroid hormone in the bloodstream, the pituitary receptors to TRH will be dampened by the increased level of T_3 arriving at the pituitary, and a standard dose of TRH will fail to increase the production and secretion of TSH. Thus, in the 90 min after injection of TRH, there will be a flattened TSH response. In contrast, when hypothyroidism exists, there will be an exaggerated rise of TSH in response to TRH because the TRH receptor is more sensitive and will instruct the pituitary to release TSH.

Thus, through a combination of clinical observation and conceptual understanding plus neuroendocrine research and application of that research in the clinic, we are now

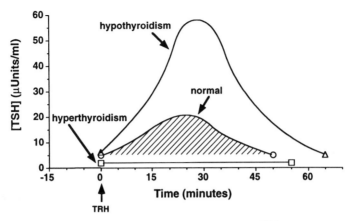

FIG. 4. TRH challenge test. When thyrotropin-releasing hormone (TRH) receptors in the pituitary are exposed to a normal circulating level of thyroid hormone, the challenge with injected TRH produces a modest increase in thyroid-stimulating hormone (TSH) production (normal curve, 0). When hypothyroidism is present, there is an exaggerated response (△) because of the lack of feedback inhibition of peripheral thyroid hormones (T_3 and T_4) on the pituitary cells which secrete TSH. Challenge with TRH in hyperthyroidism is associated with a flattened response (□) because the TRH receptor is already down-regulated by the excessive thyroid hormone circulating in the body.

able to diagnose thyroid disorders with great accuracy. This has helped both in early diagnosis, when clinical symptoms and signs are not definitive, and in the construction of appropriate and early treatment interventions.

Growth and Sex Hormones, and Corticosteroids

Clinical and basic science research have provided insights into the other fundamental life processes that are under neuroendocrine regulation: hormones of growth (growth hormone), control of reproduction (sex hormones), and hormones of salt and water metabolism and stress (corticosteroids).

Growth Hormone

In adults the excess production of growth hormone produces an enlargement of the facial features and the hands and feet, a syndrome known as *acromegaly;* in children such excess of hormone results in *gigantism.* The difference in symptoms exists because after puberty the growth of the long bones is

constrained by the growth plate or epiphysis, which has calcified and closed; thus, in adults when excess growth hormone is circulating, enlargement occurs only in bones that can continue to grow, such as the jaw, the hands, and the feet. Soft-tissue changes also occur, with thickening of the skin and an increase in the subcutaneous tissue. In some individuals, the major organs of the body (lungs, heart, liver, and kidneys) also enlarge with a resulting grotesque bodily deformation as the illness progresses. Almost all of the cases of acromegaly are associated with tumors of the anterior pituitary, the adenohypophysis. Whether these tumors occur spontaneously or are stimulated by an excessive production of releasing hormone from the hypothalamus is still a subject of debate. There is evidence on both sides of the issue, which ultimately will be decided by further research. An initial diagnosis of acromegaly or gigantism is made even today on the basis of the clinical presentation, but it can be confirmed by measuring serum growth hormone levels at a much earlier stage of the illness.

Inadequate production of growth hormone, especially in children, can have very deleterious effects leading to dwarfism. If not corrected by administration of the synthetic hormone before adolescence, this can result in deformities for life. Any child who falls below the normal growth charts for age and sex must be considered a candidate for dwarfism. Some investigators estimate that growth hormone deficiency may be as frequent as 1 in 4,000 children; however, other studies put it as infrequent as 1 in 80,000.

Sex Hormones

The neuroendocrine control of sexual behavior and reproduction is of manifest complexity. While Theophile de Bordeu drew a valid comparison between the different behavior of the eunuchs and the courtiers of the court of Louis XV, on close questioning he would surely have admitted that there was a wide variation among individuals. Eunuchs frequently indulged in sexual behavior and some were even married! While sexual potency and interest decline after castration in both animals and humans, it is also clear that sexual behavior cannot be exclusively predicted from the prevailing levels of testosterone or estrogen. Rather, it is a complex interaction of stimulus and response. The brain and the pituitary–gonadal axis work in a truly integrated fashion; the releasing factors of the hypothalamus can only initiate the cascade of neuroendocrine activity that initiates sexual and reproductive behavior when the neuronal structures are appropriately primed by gonadal hormone secretion. This neuronal priming begins in utero. Basically, every brain begins as female and remains so unless exposed to male gonadal hormones at a critical period in embryonic development.

In humans this process occurs before birth. In the rat, however, it occurs postnatally, thus permitting experimental manipulation of the brain's "sexual identity." It appears that androgenic influence is essential during this critical postnatal period for male sexual behavior and reproductive function to be normal later in life.

Thus, in the adult male, gonadal hormones act on a nervous system that has been primed in the very early stages of the individual's life. However, the releasing factors and the trophic hormones that drive the system are common to both male and female; only the peripheral sex hormones are at variance. Hence, referring again to Fig. 2, follicle-stimulating hormone (FSH) is responsible not only for the secretion of estrogen from the female ovary but also for spermatogenesis in the testes. Similarly, luteinizing hormone (LH) initiates ovulation as well as testosterone secretion.

In the female there exists a pattern of cyclic change, not present in the male, that determines sexual receptivity and reproductive ability. This complex interaction of brain, pituitary, and ovary can be seen particularly clearly in the estrous cycle of the female rat (Fig. 5). Lasting 5 days, the cycle begins as estrogen levels rise and release the hypothalamic hormone gonadotropin-releasing hormone (GnRH). With GnRH release, sexual behavior begins and at the same time LH secreted by the pituitary under the stimulation of GnRH induces ovulation in the ovary. The subsequent rise of progesterone, coinciding with the fall in estrogen production, is associated with sexual receptivity to the male.

In primates and humans, the cycle is basically the same. However, there is even greater CNS control by anatomic structures above the hypothalamus. Social factors become extremely important in courtship, sexual behavior, and the choice of sexual partner. Female rhesus monkeys, for example, have a 28-day cycle and they will show receptivity to different males depending on social preference at the time of ovulation. In males, testosterone levels and sexual activity relate in large part to their social dominance. Thus, in higher primates including humans, disturbances of the hormonally driven patterns of sexual behavior occur frequently and are predominantly determined at the level of cortical function and not at the hypothalamus! It is well recognized in human beings that psychological stress and many psychiatric disorders,

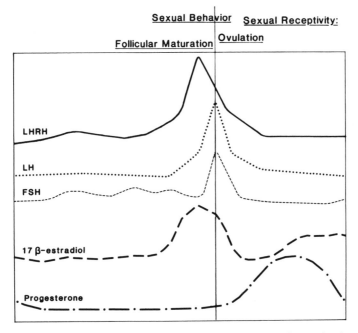

FIG. 5. Estrous cycle in the female rat. Estrogen levels rise to initiate the cycle; the orchestration of the releasing hormones and progesterone determines the timing of sexual behavior, ovulation, and mating with the male.

particularly such disturbances as anorexia nervosa and depression, will profoundly affect the menstrual cycle and disturb sexual interest and drive in both sexes. Conversely, in some disorders such as mania, sexual interest may be increased.

Corticosteroids

The *adrenocortical steroids* are protean in their action, influencing many cellular processes including the expression of fundamental genetic messengers within the cell. In this action they are essential to life, specifically to adaptation and to the individual's response to stress.

The syndromes of excess and deficiency of the adrenocortical hormones, like the syndromes of thyroid abnormality, have been described for many years. Cushing's disease, named after the great American neurosurgeon Harvey Cushing, is caused by a sustained and increased production of corticosteroids from the adrenal glands. In most cases

this is secondary to excessive production of adrenocorticotrophic hormone (ACTH) from the pituitary gland because of a tumor of the adenohypophysis. Such tumors account for approximately 65% of individuals with hypercortisolism. In keeping with the pervasive actions of corticosteroids in the body, the physical signs and symptoms of Cushing's disease involve almost every organ system including the brain. Some of the same symptoms emerge in individuals who receive high doses of corticosteroids over a prolonged period of time for inflammatory disease. The typical "moon face," rounded and soft, occurs as a consequence of fatty deposits. Abnormal collections of fatty deposits are also found in the shoulders and trunk of subjects with Cushing's disease. The muscles of the body become thin and wasted, as does the skin, which is easily bruised. Changes can be detected in sugar metabolism and also in salt and water metabolism. Hirsutism (abnormal hairiness), acne, and amenorrhea (absence or abnormal stoppage of menses) may occur as the illness progresses, secondary to the production of less potent androgens by the adrenal cortex.

Profound mental changes occur in Cushing's disease, particularly cognitive impairment, depression, and fatigue. Similar symptoms are present in psychiatric depression where enlargement of the adrenal cortex and increased secretion of cortisol also occur. If the illness progresses untreated, psychosis may develop which, together with the intellectual clouding noted earlier, marks a deteriorating delerium or organic brain syndrome, induced by the increased level of steroid production. Similar changes will sometimes by seen in individuals who are given high doses of the glucocorticoid hormone prednisone for inflammatory illness, especially when there is a family history of psychiatric disturbance.

The opposite syndrome, that of Addison's disease, results from levels of steroid hormones falling below the body's requirements. Sometimes it is secondary to pituitary failure, in which case it is associated with the failure of other endocrine systems such as the thyroid and the gonads. More commonly it is an autoimmune process, hemorrhage, or infection that destroys the adrenal gland itself. Tuberculosis was the most common cause of destruction of the adrenal gland, prior to its modern treatment. The adrenal insufficiency may emerge slowly or have an acute onset; sometimes the latter is precipitated by an increased demand for steroid hormones such as infection or trauma. The classical picture is one of weakness, fatigue, anorexia, and weight loss together with nausea and vomiting, salt craving, and skin pigmentation. Arterial hypertension is common, and shock may develop, with stupor and coma in the acute syndrome. Mental changes again are common with florid psychoses and confusion.

Adrenocorticol production increases during environmental challenge. The Hungarian endocrinologist Hans Selye was the first to demonstrate that chronic stress has a profound effect on the hypothalamic–pituitary–adrenal (HPA) axis. Indeed, for years he postulated that excess steroid production was the cause of many stress-related diseases. This idea was shattered, however, in the 1950s when it was shown that high doses of administered steroids could be therapeutic in many "stress disorders" such as arthritis and asthma. It is now recognized, although the details are not well understood, that the corticosteroids function as mediators in the complex immune response preventing excessive response to foreign agents. Through this new work and a rapidly advancing understanding of the immune system, it is now recognized that the brain, the endocrine system, and the immune system are tied together inextricably.

NEUROENDOCRINOLOGY AND BEHAVIOR

The Dynamics of Adaptation

The neuroendocrine system plays a fundamental role in adaptation to environmental challenge. Fear, the almost instantaneous subjective awareness that danger is at hand, is mediated through the autonomic nervous system, but simultaneously there begins a flush of epinephrine and corticosteroid secretion from the adrenal glands. In his paper of 1914, "The Emergency Function of Adrenal Medulla in Pain and Major Emotions," the American physiologist Walter Cannon documented the rise in catecholamines in the blood of a cat frightened by a barking dog. His work marked the beginning of research on the physiology and chemistry of emotion and stress. Experience during the two world wars heightened scientific and public awareness of the destructive challenge of chronic stress. When Selye outlined his concept of the "general adaptation syndrome" in his book *The Physiology and Pathology of Exposure to Stress,* further interest was stimulated in understanding the body's reactions to stress.

Also, technical advances were making it increasingly possible to accurately measure steroid levels in human blood. This led to a concentrated period of research on the chemistry of the stress response. Harvard oarsmen, parachutists, individuals visiting dentists, and those taking exams or having surgical operations were all found to have elevated levels of circulating 17-hydroxycorticosteroids (i.e., glucocorticoids). Furthermore, as the research progressed, some very interesting points began to emerge that link higher cortical function to the active response to challenge.

In the research on stress and adaptation, the novelty of the stressor and the control that could be exerted by the individual over the stressful situation emerged as key issues determining the stress response. While situations that were novel to the individual or demanded great physical exertion increased corticosteroid production (and also increased epinephrine and norepinephrine secretion from the adrenal medulla), it was when the individual was called on to make complex decisions within certain time constraints (such as landing an aircraft on a carrier deck) that the highest levels of steroid excretion occurred. Subsequently, in studies of men in combat, it was found that 24-hr urinary excretion of corticosteroids was far higher in the officers, those held responsible for the success and safety of the group of soldiers, than in the fighting men themselves. The degree of control that an individual could exert over the situation and the personal meaning of the challenge emerged as critical variables in determining arousal and the neuroendocrine response. The conclusion from such results is that neuroendocrine function is not a closed system but one open to higher cortical control above the hypothalamus.

Animal experiments have helped us to understand the sequence of events occurring in such stressful situations. In rodents exposed to a cold swim, there is a consistent rise of ACTH and a decrease in secretion of growth hormone and the gonadatropic hormones—indeed, an orchestration of neuroendocrine activity designed to maximize adaptation. Corticotropin-releasing factor (CRF), the hypothalamic-releasing hormone that regulates the secretion of ACTH, appears to play a key role in this process, promoting the release of epinephrine and norepinephrine which in turn elevate blood pressure, heart rate, and blood sugar levels. Continuing this challenge lowers brain norepinephrine, increases the reuptake of labeled norepinephrine by the neuron, and produces a hypoactive behavioral syndrome for as long as 24 hr. In rats that swim to exhaustion, brain norepinephrine levels are reduced by 20% and brain serotonin is elevated. If the perturbing events persist or escape from behavioral control, the HPA axis changes persist, and increased release of thyroid hormone also begins to occur. Testosterone and estrogen fall, with consequent inhibition of sexual behavior and the ovulatory cycle.

In social animals, such as primates and ourselves, the social order is a major determinant of neuroendocrine arousal. Studies of primates in groups emphasize just how sensitive these neuroendocrine responses are to social order. The challenge for food, territory, or sexual partner is frequently imbedded in the context of social hierarchy. Dominance and status are settled by threat and by fighting among the contenders. When monkeys are placed in a competitive social situation, peripheral levels of epinephrine and norepinephrine rise together with the steroids. However, as the outcome of the competition is decided, the neuroendocrine patterns of the dominant and nondominant animals diverge significantly. In the defeated animal, corticosteroids remain high, indeed may climb higher, whereas for the victor there is a rapid decline. Similar changes occur in the adrenosympathetic system. Arousal continues in the subordinate animal who withdraws and no longer seeks to fight. In females under challenge, steroids also rise but fall precipitously if they come under the protection of a dominant male.

Such physiological changes, when placed in the context of social behavior, have obvious adaptive value for the group as a whole. After initial struggles, when a hierarchy has been established a period of relative calm and cooperation usually develops. However, what of the animal that is driven beyond its capacity to adapt and loses its place in the dominance hierarchy? Evidence suggests that this will lead to continued high levels of steroid hormones but a decline in growth hormone, the biogenic amines (norepinephrine and epinephrine), and the sex hormones. The animal withdraws from the group, and exploratory behavior virtually ceases. Indeed, in some instances the animal may become ill and eventually die. Such an outcome reminds us not only of human depression but also of the connections noted earlier between the neuroendocrine axis and the regulation of the immune system.

An intimate relationship exists between the brain, the neuroendocrine system, and immune function. Of late there has been an enormous increase in our knowledge regarding how the immune system is regulated. It is clear that a reciprocal relationship exists be-

tween immune defense and neuroendocrine function. Again, the HPA axis plays an important role.

The immunologically reactive cells of the immune system include macrophages, neutrophils, lymphocytes, and natural killer cells (Fig. 6). Immunity can be broken down to an analysis of the cell biology of immune responses and the biological activities of cell-derived molecules. A large number of these effector molecules are biologically active peptides. Of these, interleukin-1 (IL-1), a peptide produced by macrophages, appears to be an important messenger between the immune system and the HPA axis. The presence of a foreign protein in the body will quickly lead to increased production of IL-1, which appears to have two sites of action, one of which is the hypothalamus. Despite the large size of the molecule, it presumably penetrates through gaps in the blood–brain barrier that include the organ vasculosium of the lamina terminus of the hypothalamus. Exactly how

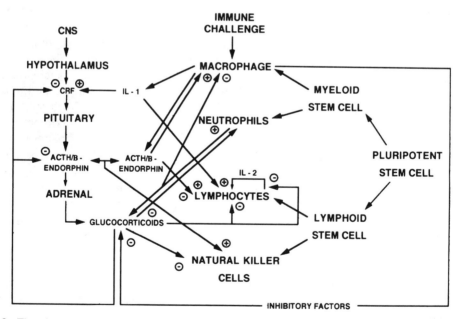

FIG. 6. The close connections between the immune system and the corticosteroid brain axis. Upon immune challenge the macrophage releases interleukin-1 (IL-1) that stimulates both lymphocyte production and corticotropin-releasing factor (CRF) production at the same time. As the immune reaction develops, glucocorticoids increase. These act as a moderating influence on the immune reaction, preventing it from going out of control. After Bateman A, et al. *Endocr Rev* 1989;10:92–112.

IL-1 works is not clear but one theory is that it sensitizes neurons that contain CRF to the effects of norepinephrine and leads to an outpouring of ACTH from the pituitary gland and subsequently 17-hydroxycorticosteroids from the adrenal cortex. This increased activity in the HPA axis damps down the immunological reaction of the body, thus completing a classic feedback system similar to the one described earlier in reviewing the brain–hypothalamic–endocrine gland axes of the neuroendocrine system.

Hence, the HPA axis is capable of regulating immunological activity and vice versa. When the immune system is stimulated by a foreign antigen, rapid stimulation of hypothalamic CRF and the cascade occurs resulting in steroid production. The details of this enormously complex intertwining have yet to be worked out but the implications are already clear. In a situation of chronic psychological stress, perhaps due to social disruption or bereavement, high levels of circulating steroids will dampen the immune response and make an individual animal much more prone to infection. The implications of this will become more apparent as the neuroendocrine dynamics of human depression are reviewed.

DEPRESSION, ADAPTIVE FAILURE, AND THE HPA AXIS

In all persons, but particularly in those predisposed through genetic or early experience, chronic stress can lead to profound clinical depression. Sadness is a ubiquitous human experience, frequently associated with grief and the loss of an important person or ideal. One might argue that it is the price paid for attachment and a sense of purpose. For most individuals, the episode lasts days or weeks and spontaneous recovery occurs. However, for some, approximately 10% of the population, the syndrome will progress to a severe clinical depression at some point in their lifetime, as described in detail in Chapter 17. Very often, these individuals have a history of family members with the same disorder.

Also, under stress, the illness may reappear after intervals of health, suggesting an underlying pathophysiology that is genetically predisposed or related to previous psychological or biological experience.

The depressed individual develops a pervasive sense of hopelessness and sadness whereby the world is diminished in all its elements: relationships with other people become impoverished; sleep is disturbed and appetite is lost; there is difficulty in concentrating and making decisions. The usual rhythm of sleep is impaired; energy drains away, and the individual becomes preoccupied with ruminative, negative thoughts. Many of these symptoms suggest a drive disturbance of the diencephalon, particularly of hypothalamic regulation.

On close clinical investigation it emerges that there is considerable evidence for such a disturbance. Changes in the circadian pattern of sleep, growth hormone, prolactin production, thyroid hormones, and particularly in the corticosteroid axis are all very apparent.

As in chronic stress, the HPA axis is profoundly disturbed in many depressed individuals, both in its circadian rhythmicity and in its regulation. The production of corticosteroids is frequently greatly increased in those who are depressed. This finding, which was established nearly a quarter of a century ago, has been replicated by many workers. Not only are the levels elevated but the usual circadian profile, with cortisol levels highest in the early morning and diminished through the day, is flattened and advanced in phase (i.e., it occurs earlier than normal in the 24-hr cycle). This correlates with other evidence in depressives of "phase advance," of the timing of the first REM sleep period, the rise in nocturnal melatonin, and the change in body temperature rhythm. In a nondepressed individual the usual morning rise of cortisol can be suppressed by giving a synthetic steroid (dexamethasone) at midnight. This fools the pituitary into thinking that high levels of circulating steroid already exist; the morning surge of ACTH is precluded and with it the early morning increase in cortisol. This dexamethasone suppression test, however, is abnormal in a considerable number of depressed patients, who fail to suppress circulating steroids so as to have higher than normal circulating levels of cortisol in the morning after the administration of dexamethasone the night before. While not highly specific or correlated precisely with the severity of the depression, the abnormal dexamethasone suppression test is present frequently enough to clearly indicate that abnormalities of HPA regulation in depression are similar to those in chronic stress.

The production of CRF seems to be of cardinal importance in the depressive syndrome. As technical advances have made it possible to more accurately measure ACTH and corticosteroids, it has become apparent that there is an increased ACTH secretion in depressed patients compared to controls and that the adrenal gland itself is frequently enlarged. CRF was first identified in 1955 but it took 25 years for the peptide to be sequenced and manufactured. Since then, its availability has allowed us to probe pituitary–adrenal function (as a neuroendocrine challenge) in patients as well as in animal studies. One hypothesis to explain clinical depression is that because of chronic stress and brain arousal secondary to insurmountable environmental challenge or loss in predisposed individuals, CRF will be chronically increased and this will in turn drive the HPA axis to sustained hyperactivity. This hypothesis has been tested by administration of CRF to depressed patients. It was found that the depressives had a blunted ACTH response but a normal cortisol response compared to controls. This suggested that the ACTH blunting was secondary to decreased sensitivity of the receptor on the corticotroph (the cell that produces ACTH) because of chronic CRF hypersecretion. One way of testing this suggestion would be to measure CRF in the brain itself but for obvious reasons that cannot be done in human beings. An alternative, although it is at best a crude marker of brain activity, is to measure CRF in cerebrospinal fluid. Of the studies that have been conducted to date in depressed persons, most demonstrate ele-

vation of CRF, although this is not a consistent finding.

Support for the hypothesis that overproduction of CRF is an important element in the pathophysiology of depression is also derived from animal studies. When administered directly to the brain of laboratory animals, CRF decreases sexual activity, disturbs sleep, diminishes appetite, and increases "emotionality"—symptoms all very reminiscent of the human syndrome of depression.

Taken together, clinical and basic science investigations over the past 25 years suggest that in depression there is a chronic secretion of corticosteroids secondary to increased arousal and CRF production in the hypothalamus. This is in marked distinction to Cushing's syndrome, where the hypersecretion of ACTH and cortisol is usually secondary to a tumor within the pituitary gland itself (Fig. 7).

THYROID HORMONES, DEPRESSION, AND THE MODULATION OF MANIC-DEPRESSIVE DISEASE

The feedback of neuroendocrine messengers to the brain may play an important role in the modulation of brain function and normal behavior. As discussed earlier in this chapter, a profound lack of thyroid hormone (hypothyroidism) is frequently associated with depressed mood. The reciprocal possibility, that individuals who are depressed may have a disturbance of their thyroid function, has intrigued clinicians for many decades. Approximately 20 years ago it was shown that thyroid hormones can help speed the recovery of some individuals, particularly women, from depressive illness. This implied not only that thyroid hormones could modulate mood, but that adequate supplies of thyroid hormone available to brain were an adaptive advantage. In the neuroendocrine evaluation of depressed patients, those individuals with an elevated level of circulating thyroid hormone appear to be those who do well with antidepressant treatment. Others (about

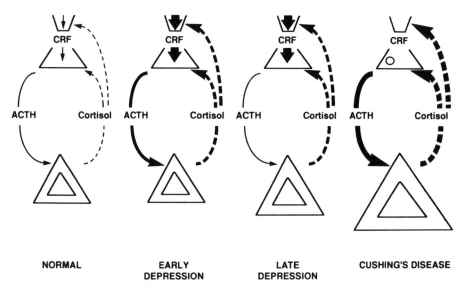

FIG. 7. Depression as a response to stress and overproduction of corticotropin-releasing factor (CRF). Under environmental challenge, CRF is elevated and because of chronic stress remains elevated, increasing adrenocorticotrophic hormone (ACTH), which in turn leads to sustained increase in cortisol and adrenal gland hypertrophy. Subsequently, ACTH falls with down-regulation of the pituitary corticotroph receptor, but because of adenocortical increase in sensitivity and size the level of cortisol remains high in chronic depression. This is in contrast to Cushing's disease where CRF production is normal or suppressed and ACTH is elevated because of the presence of a pituitary tumor. After Gold PW, Chrousos GP. *Psychoneuroendocrinology* 1983;10:401–419.

10%) who have diminished supplies of thyroid hormone frequently need thyroid hormone supplementation to recover from their depression.

Thyroid hormones appear to be of particular importance in the expression and treatment of manic-depressive disease. Some individuals who suffer from depression are genetically also predisposed to episodes of excitement (see Chapter 16). In these periods when energy is increased, euphoria or irritability is the predominant mood and the individuals sleep little; this can lead to considerable disorganization and even psychosis. Such persons frequently have a strong family history over several generations of a similar disorder, which is called *manic-depressive disease* or *bipolar illness.*

Lithium is a very effective treatment for this illness (see Chapter 17). Lithium carbonate, however, turns out to be a significant antithyroid agent, and it was soon reported that individuals taking lithium could develop hypothyroidism. Subsequently, as the number of people treated with lithium increased, a small group of patients was found to have a variant of the illness, one in which very frequent episodes of illness occur (by definition greater than four times a year). These individuals not only were resistant to treatment with lithium, but also had this malignant variant of rapid cycles as part of their illness.

Subsequent studies determined that this same group had a much higher incidence of thyroid disease than other bipolar individuals taking lithium, which suggested that this particular group of patients had a greater predisposition to the development of thyroid disturbance. In addition, the use of tricyclic antidepressants appeared to increase the risk for rapid cycling. Tricyclic drugs increase the availability of biogenic amines in the synaptic cleft by preventing their reuptake into the neuron (see Chapter 17). Further research has shown that such drugs, particularly the noradrenergic reuptake–inhibiting ones, will inhibit the uptake of thyroxine into the neuron as well.

The brain is particularly dependent on thyroxine, preferring to convert its own T_3 from T_4 taken up into the neuron rather than gathering T_3 directly from the bloodstream as do most organs in the body. Lithium itself impairs the deiodination of T_4 to T_3 both in the pituitary and in the brain. Hence, when used in combination, lithium and tricyclic antidepressants may burden the thyroid economy of the brain in a predisposed individual, potentially creating a relative thyroid hormone deficiency in the neuron. This disturbed neuroendocrine function worsens the manic-depressive illness, making it resistant to the usual therapeutic intervention and fostering the development of illness called *rapid cycling.*

If this hypothesis is correct, then changing thyroid status and increasing the availability of thyroid hormone to brain should reverse the syndrome. Indeed, this seems to be the case. High doses of thyroxine given to people with rapid-cycling manic-depressive disease in combination with the usual psychotropic agents for the treatment of bipolar illness reduce the malignant cycling in a significant number of persons and, in some, induce a complete eradication of the symptomatology. This suggests that thyroid hormone availability to brain may play an important role in modifying the phenotypic expression of manic-depressive pathophysiology.

SUMMARY

Neuroendocrine research has offered a type of "window to the brain" and permitted the development of knowledge about how communication systems are regulated between living cells. It has also confirmed that the brain is ultimately connected through a complex series of feedback loops with all adaptive functions that sustain the higher living organism. As we advance further in neuroscience, the regulatory principles of neuroendocrinology will be further illuminated by our knowledge of molecular and cellular processes. This will enhance our spectrum of understanding of behavior including that of the whole animal. As such, neuroendocrinology will remain as it began—a bridging science about how living creatures really work.

BIBLIOGRAPHY

Original Articles

Bauer MS, Whybrow PC. The effect of changing thyroid function on cyclic affective illness in a human subject. *Am J Psychiatry* 1986;143:633–636.

Gold PW, Chrousos GP. Clinical studies with corticotropin releasing factor: implications for the diagnosis and pathophysiology of depression, Cushing's disease, and adrenal insufficiency. *Psychoneuroendocrinology* 1985;10:401–419.

Books and Reviews

Athanassenas G, Wolters CL. Sleep after transmeridian flights. In: Reinberg A, Vieux N, Andlauer P, eds. *Night and shift work: biological and social aspects.* New York: Pergamon Press; 1981:139–147.

Bateman A, Singh A, Kral T, Solomon S. The immune–hypothalamic–pituitary–adrenal axis. *Endocr Rev* 1989;10:92–112.

Bauer MS, Whybrow PC. Rapid cycling bipolar disorder: clinical features, treatment and etiology. In: Amsterdam JD, ed. *Refractory depression.* New York: Raven Press; 1991:191–208.

Droba M, Whybrow PC. Endocrine and metabolic disorders. In: Kaplan HI, Sadock BJ, eds. *Comprehensive textbook of psychiatry.* 5th Ed. Baltimore: Williams & Wilkins; 1989:1209–1221.

Goss RS, Dinsmore CE, Grimes LN, Rosen LK. Expression and suppression of circannual antler growth cycle in deer. In: Pengelley ET, ed. *Circannual clocks: annual biological rhythms.* New York: Academic Press; 1974:393–492.

McEwen BS. Endocrine effects on the brain and their relationships to behavior. In: Siegel GJ, Agranoff BW, Albers RW, Molinoff PB, eds. *Basic neurochemistry,* 5th ed. New York: Raven Press; 1994 (in press).

Munck A, Guyre PM, Holbrook NJ. Physiological functions of glucocorticoids in stress and their relation to pharmacological actions. *Endocr Rev* 1984;5:25–44.

Sapolsky RM, Krey LC, McEwen BS. The neuroendocrinology of stress and aging: the glucocorticoid cascade hypothesis. *Endocr Rev* 1986;7:284–301.

Shepherd GM. *Neurobiology.* New York: Oxford University Press; 1983.

Whybrow PC. Hyperthyroidism: behavioral and psychiatric aspects. In: Braverman LE, Ingbar SH, eds. *The thyroid.* 6th Ed. Philadelphia: JB Lippincott; 1991:863–870.

Whybrow PC. Hypothyroidism: behavioral and psychiatric aspects. In: Braverman LE, Ingbar SH, eds. *The thyroid.* 6th Ed. Philadelphia: JB Lippincott; 1991:1078–1083.

10

The Sleep Cycle

William A. Ball, Adrian R. Morrison, and Richard J. Ross

O soft embalmer of the still midnight,
*   Shutting, with careful fingers and benign,*
Our gloom-pleased eyes, embowered from the light,
*   Enshaded in forgetfulness divine;*
O soothest Sleep! if so it please thee, close
*   In the midst of this thine hymn my willing eyes,*
Or wait the amen, ere the poppy throws
*   Around my bed its lulling charities;*
Then save me, or the passed day will shine
Upon my pillow, breeding many woes;
*   Save me from curious conscience, that still lords*
Its strength for darkness, burrowing like a mole;
*   Turn the key deftly in the oiled wards,*
And seal the hushed casket of my soul.

John Keats,
To Sleep, 1819

- The recognition of rapid eye movement sleep (REMS) and non-REMS (NREMS) was a major breakthrough in our understanding of sleep and its disorders.

- In a sleeping period there are shifts from NREMS to REMS and back again.

- Although considerable agreement exists about the criteria for defining the stages of sleep, there is little consensus about the function of sleep.

- Multiple brain sites influence the onset of sleep.

- The lower brain stem is a critical site of sleep regulation.

- Control of breathing, brain temperature, and heart activity changes across the sleep cycle.

- Brain mechanisms that are active when an animal responds to stimuli while awake also characterize the neural activity of REMS.

- Sleep disorders are widespread.

- A systematic classification of sleep disorders delineates the variety of ways that sleep can be disturbed.

- Apnea is a cessation or an interruption of breathing.

- Some sleep disorders involve partial arousal from different stages of sleep or arise within specific states of sleep.

- Sleep is commonly disturbed in a variety of psychiatric conditions including depression and post-traumatic stress disorder.

The purpose of this chapter is to impart an understanding of how early discoveries in sleep research continue to provide a framework for clinical and basic investigations. The chapter discusses the two fundamental varieties of sleep—rapid eye movement sleep (REMS) and non-REMS (NREMS). The stages within NREMS are also described. Theories of how sleep is generated are outlined within the context of the notion of sleep state. Mechanisms of sleep and changes in the regulation of basic physiological activities across the sleep cycle are discussed. Finally, some common disorders of sleep and selected psychiatric disorders that affect sleep are described.

In a room quiet enough for someone to hear a pin drop, a cat lies quietly. A pin drops. The cat turns its head, directs its ears toward the source of the sound, and stares intently. During this orienting response, its heart rate slows, then quickens. The cat gets up and goes over to the pin, sniffs, and returns to lie quietly and fall asleep. Paradoxically, these active, waking behaviors provide a basis for understanding some of the mechanisms that underlie sleep. The alerting response to unexpected or new stimuli occurs many times a day, and the cat frequently exhibits behavioral quiescence, drowsiness, then characteristic phases of sleep. During sleep, the body is normally relatively inactive, but this inactivity belies both the active inhibition of some neural activity and the release of other neural activity within the central nervous system (CNS). Autonomic changes manifest themselves as shifting patterns of control of body temperature, heart rate, and respiration that are interwoven with a change in the regulation of mechanisms that in waking produce alerting to intense or unexpected stimuli. The sleeping brain is far from an inactive one; and, indeed, one phase of sleep includes many of the characteristics of alert wakefulness despite virtual total paralysis of the skeletal muscles. One of the central themes of this

chapter is that mechanisms of alerting are precisely those that produce some neurophysiological characteristics of sleep.

REM SLEEP

The recognition of REMS and non-REMS was a major breakthrough in our understanding of sleep and its disorders. Sleep as a subject for study was largely ignored by biomedical scientists until approximately 35 years ago even though humans spend about 30% of their time asleep and well-fed predators, such as laboratory cats, more than 50%. This neglect reflected the prevailing opinion that sleep was an "uninteresting" period of withdrawal from the world: waking proceeded into sleep as gradually diminishing neural activity in sensory pathways resulted in decreased central brain activity. This *passive* theory of sleep was held by almost all of the neuroscientists of the day until the discovery of REMS in 1953 by the American neurophysiologists Eugene Aserinsky and Nathaniel Kleitman. REMS was first recognized in human infants because of the rapid, jerking eye movements that have given this state of sleep its name. What had been recognized as sleep on the basis of behavioral attributes and a distinctly different brain wave pattern recorded on the electroencephalogram (EEG) then became known as non-REMS. Thus, rather than rely on behavioral observations alone to determine the sleep state, the sleep

Biological Bases of Brain Function and Disease, edited by Alan Frazer, Perry B. Molinoff, and Andrew Winokur. Raven Press, Ltd., New York © 1994.

researcher now generally uses EEG recordings obtained from surface electrodes in humans and chronically implanted stainless steel screw and wire electrodes in animals. The description of REMS triggered an avalanche of studies that led to the development of the new clinical specialty of sleep disorders medicine.

In a sleeping period there are shifts from NREMS to REMS and back again. Recognition of REMS as a distinct state with recorded characteristics that differed markedly from those previously associated with sleep forced investigators to rethink the idea that sleep results from a simple passive withdrawal of sensory input. Sleep had to be regarded as an active process. "Classical" sleep (i.e., NREMS) had been recognized by the

appearance of larger amplitude, lower frequency waves recorded on the EEG when compared with the low-amplitude, high-frequency waves of waking. Only careful observation could detect that sleep was not uniform in character. What came to be understood was that during a sleeping period an animal periodically shifts from NREMS to REMS and then back to NREMS several times, each pairing being called a *sleep cycle*. As already noted, rapid eye movements are characteristic of REMS and provide a convenient name for this state. In addition to the twitching of peripheral body muscles and eye movements during REMS, the keen observer will see an animal literally "melt" before his eyes because the skeletal muscles become paralyzed. The active inhibition of the motor

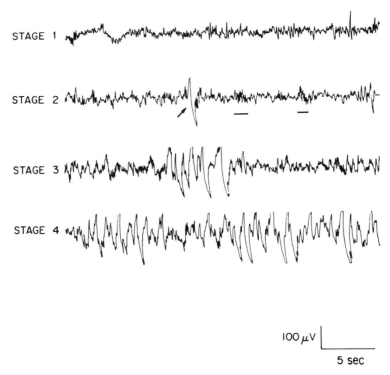

FIG. 1. Sleep stages in humans. The progression of sleep stages illustrates the increased amplitude and decreased frequency of waveforms that characterize NREMS in humans. Stage 2 marks the appearance of sleep spindles (underlined waves), which are 12- to 14-Hz (cycles/sec) clusters of waveforms, and K complexes (arrow), which are large spike-like waves. Stages 3 and 4 have an increasing percentage of large, slow (4–5 Hz) waveforms. Humans typically enter REMS from stage 2. From Carskadon MA, Dement W. *Principles and practices of sleep medicine,* Chap. 1. Philadelphia: WB Saunders; 1989.

neurons that innervate these muscles is only briefly interrupted when excitatory barrages from the brain stem lead to peripheral muscle twitches.

In humans and other mammals such as cats, normal sleep begins with a period of NREMS followed by a shift to REMS, with an EEG pattern similar to that of active waking. Within NREMS different stages of sleep recur regularly, the progression being from stage 1 to stage 4 in the human (Fig. 1). Sleep spindles, bursts of 12- to 14-Hz (cycles/sec) waveforms, characterize stage 2 of NREMS in humans (Fig. 1, underlined waveforms) and are typical of NREMS in cats (Fig. 2B).

Large-amplitude, low-frequency (1 to 3 Hz) waves known as δ waves emerge in stages 3 and 4 in humans (Fig. 1) and are prominent in deep NREMS in cats (Fig. 2B and C).

In addition to the characteristic low-voltage, fast EEG activity, the hippocampal rhythm of approximately 7 cycles/sec (θ rhythm) during REMS is also characteristic of alert waking. Another waveform, the ponto-geniculo-occipital (PGO) wave (Fig. 1C and D), discussed in detail later, appears spontaneously in REMS of cats. It can be recorded from widespread areas of the brain, including the pons, lateral geniculate body, and occipital (visual) cortex. Brain tempera-

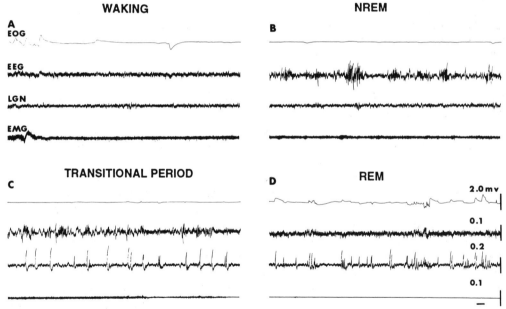

FIG. 2. Sleep stages of the cat. **A:** Waking. The electro-oculogram (EOG) shows moderate activity typical of waking. The EEG tracing represents the low-voltage, fast activity of active waking. No spiking activity is observed in the lateral geniculate nucleus (LGN). The dense tracing of the electromyogram (EMG) reflects the active muscle tone of waking. **B:** NREMS. The EOG shows no activity. The EEG displays larger amplitude waves with sleep spindles (clusters of large-amplitude waves). No activity is observed in the LGN, and the EMG shows only a slight decrement in muscle tone. **C:** Transitional period. This state represents a bridge between NREMS and REMS. Eye movement activity remains low, and waves on the EEG remain large. LGN activity now includes spike-like waves called ponto-geniculo-occipital (PGO) waves, and the muscle tone of the EMG begins to decline. **D:** REMS. The EOG tracing exhibits marked activity representing eye movements, and the EEG tracing resembles that of waking in the low-voltage, fast pattern. PGO waves are consistently present on the LGN tracing. The EMG exhibits essentially no activity, consistent with the virtually complete loss of muscle tone (atonia) characteristic of REMS. From Morrison AR. *Progress in psychobiology and physiological psychology.* New York: Academic Press; 1979.

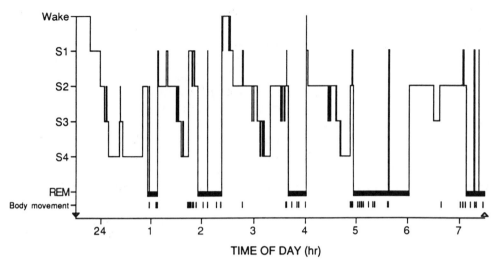

TIME OF DAY (hr)

FIG. 3. A sleep histogram demonstrating the typical progression of human sleep stages 1 through 4 (S1–S4) of NREMS and REMS. The width of each horizontal line represents the amount of time spent in a particular stage of sleep. Note that the amount of time spent in REMS increases from midnight (24) through early morning (7 A.M.) while the amount of time in S3 and S4 (the deeper stage of NREMS) declines. From Carskadon MA, Dement W. *Principles and practices of sleep medicine,* Chap. 1. Philadelphia: WB Saunders; 1989.

ture, which falls in NREMS, rises again in REMS. Recordings from single neurons—primarily done in cats—reveal similar rates of spontaneous firing in many regions in both waking and REMS. In most instances, firing frequency is lower in NREMS. The sequence of NREMS and REMS repeats itself roughly every 90 min in humans and more frequently in small animals. The human sleep cycle is characterized by a greater percentage of NREMS during the early part of the night followed by a gradual increase in the amount of REMS (Fig. 3). The more vivid and visually striking types of human dreams and nightmares arise during REMS and therefore are more common later in the night. The rapid back-and-forth eye movements (Fig. 2D) of REMS have prompted some investigators to speculate that in humans the eye movements are appropriate to the dream imagery. REMS has sometimes been called *paradoxical sleep* because of the seeming incongruity of an active brain and dreaming in humans coupled with an essentially paralyzed sleeper.

STAGES AND FUNCTION OF SLEEP

After the discovery of REMS, the important steps of standardizing the definition of sleep stages were accentuated. A state refers to a set of behavioral and physiological parameters that change through the sleep/wake cycle. Sleep-related behavior generally includes cessation of movement and the assumption of species-specific postures. Overt responses to stimuli diminish, muscle tone declines somewhat in the beginning of NREMS (note the EMG in Fig. 2B), and sleep progresses through the various stages typical of the EEG recordings. The EEG recordings of the stages of sleep are illustrated in Figs. 1 and 2 for humans and cats, respectively. The similarity of the low-voltage, fast EEG activity of REMS and waking is clearly illustrated in Fig. 2A and D, an observation that holds across species. Nonocular muscles are nearly paralyzed during REMS (Fig. 2D) except for brief twitches of the extremities and the diaphragmatic muscle of breathing.

Although considerable agreement exists

about the criteria for defining the stages of sleep, there is little consensus about the function of sleep. In terms of its function, some investigators have maintained that sleep extends scarce resources of food and water through a period of behavioral quiescence that reduces energy consumption. Other researchers have contended that regulation of brain temperature is a key function of NREMS, the regular decline in temperature during NREMS serving to compensate for relative elevation during waking. In this view, maintaining optimum brain temperature may be important for efficient functioning of the CNS. Still other investigators have argued that, although the brain as a whole remains active during sleep, different regions show differential activity. The net result may be that any decline in sensitivity of some neuronal systems to a given neurotransmitter such as norepinephrine can be reversed by a period of neuronal inactivity. Why sleep comes in two varieties has also remained a mystery. REMS has been thought to (1) prevent terminal lapse into coma by periodic activation of the brain in the middle of sleep; (2) promote neuronal development during the high percentage of REMS time early in life; or (3) facilitate consolidation of memories stored during waking. The progression of the sleep/wake cycle remains without a recognized function.

While the search for the function of sleep continues to motivate considerable research, the study of the mechanisms underlying sleep and the physiological changes across the sleep/wake cycle has made great progress. The rest of this chapter focuses on the following major themes:

1. The two states of sleep, REMS and NREMS, differ fundamentally in their regulation of homeostasis.
2. REMS is a state in which the brain functions in some respects as if it were in an active waking state: some CNS mechanisms that become active in waking when an animal is alerted by stimuli (e.g., ori-

ents to or shifts attention to a stimulus) also become active during REMS even in the absence of external stimuli.
3. The regulation of sleep involves the interaction of populations of neurons, not the mere turning on and off of a single "sleep center."
4. The shifting regulation of basic homeostatic mechanisms across sleep states and the concept of REMS as a state of paradoxical hyperalerting both have implications for the understanding of certain human illnesses.

SLEEP MECHANISMS

Initiation

Multiple brain sites influence the onset of sleep. It is not yet clear how sleep is initiated. Investigators have attempted to identify populations of neurons with activity that closely correlates with the beginning and end of NREMS or REMS. Surgical isolation of the brain rostral to the caudal pons from the rest of the CNS in cats leads to continual wakefulness as indicated by the EEG, a finding that implicates caudal brain stem structures in the initiation of sleep. Also, activity in neurons in the basal forebrain preoptic area that correlates strongly with NREMS onset has been described. Lesions in this area tend to promote wakefulness. Thalamic regions are the generator sites of the sleep spindles characteristic of NREMS, and frontal cortical regions have also been found to promote sleep. Thus the onset and maintenance of sleep seem to involve a set of different neural populations rather than a single, central "switch."

Some researchers focus on the identification of biochemical *sleep factors,* endogenous substances generated either in the CNS or the periphery, that would "prime" the nervous system to enter a state of sleep. Experiments have shown that if spinal fluid from sleepy animals is injected into alert animals, the latter may fall asleep. An intriguing hypothesis is that a circulating factor or factors may derive from substances resembling those found in the cell walls of intestinal bacteria; similar substances may induce fever and sleepiness during infections. Circulating factors may affect more purely neural mechanisms in the regulation of the sleep cycle. Because REMS almost invariably follows NREMS, reorganization during NREMS must occur in the brain regulators, such as the hypothalamus, to allow the emergence of REMS.

The lower brain stem is a critical site of sleep regulation. Although multiple brain sites influence the onset of sleep, the lower brain stem (see Chapter 1) has been a major focus of research on the brain mechanisms underlying sleep, particularly REMS, since the early 1960s. This derives largely from the work of the French neurophysiologist Michel Jouvet, who demonstrated that a REMS-like state still appeared in cats in which the pons and medulla had been surgically isolated from the rest of the brain. These cats periodically exhibited a collapse of muscle tone with superimposed muscle twitches just as in normal REMS. Some neurons in the pons become selectively active during REMS, and the importance of brain stem influences on REMS seems well established.

The initiation of REMS probably includes activation of cholinergic neurons. Administration of agents that directly or indirectly stimulate receptors for acetylcholine in the dorsal pons of intact and decerebrate cats can induce a REMS-like state. Thus, injection of carbachol directly into the dorsal pons can within minutes induce a state with all the usual electrophysiological and peripheral signs of REMS. The normal source of this stimulation is likely to be the many acetylcholine-containing neurons at the boundary of the mesencephalic and pontine tegmenta. These neurons excite medullary neurons either directly or indirectly via the pons, and medullary neurons in turn excite glycinergic inhibitory interneurons in the spinal cord. Flaccid paralysis (very low muscle tone, termed *atonia*) of skeletal muscles results.

Norepinephrine appears to play a permissive role in REMS generation. Both noradrenergic neurons of the pontine locus coeruleus and serotonergic neurons of the dorsal raphe nucleus become increasingly inactive through NREMS and are virtually inactive (or "silent") during REMS. Although serotonergic neurons of the mesencephalic dorsal raphe nucleus do stop firing during REMS, some work suggests that this silence depends on the motor inhibition of REMS and may not play the same role as norepinephrine in the actual generation of REMS.

One theory about the neural regulation of the sleep cycle holds that alternation of NREMS and REMS is not merely accompanied by changes in the activity of cholinergic, noradrenergic, and serotonergic neurons but is actually the product of reciprocal interactions among them. In rough outline, activity in cholinergic neurons would tend to promote the onset of REMS while activity in noradrenergic and serotonergic neurons would tend to inhibit the effects of the cholinergic REMS generators. Endogenous pacemaker activity in unidentified neurons would slowly overcome this inhibition such that the level of activity in cholinergic neurons increases to a critical level, and noradrenergic and serotonergic neurons would in turn be inhibited by the cholinergic neurons. Although an intriguing preliminary hypothesis, it does not explain how REMS ends, how the length of the NREMS period is regulated, or how fundamental changes in hypothalamic influences on homeostasis are initiated.

In normal humans and animals sleep occurs according to a circadian rhythm that can be entrained to occur at the same time each day by the light/dark cycle (see Chapter 11). Sleep will maintain a regular but drifting pattern (as do all such rhythms) in the absence of light cues as long as the suprachiasmatic nucleus of the hypothalamus is intact. Destruction of this hypothalamic nucleus alters the normal distribution of sleep in the 24-hr period but not the total amount. Work with primates and rodents has revealed that the tendency to enter REMS at various points in the 24-hr period (so-called ultradian rhythm) depends for its timing on another, unknown region, not the well-localized suprachiasmatic nucleus. Perhaps activity in both the hypothalamus and the caudal brain stem is required because REMS is tightly linked to the body temperature rhythm, which in turn is greatly influenced by the hypothalamus.

Homeostasis

Control of breathing, brain temperature, and heart activity changes across the sleep cycle. Homeostasis refers to the regulation of the basic processes that maintain the internal milieu, the internal conditions that allow the body and the nervous system to function. Sleep poses a special problem for homeostasis because the usual behavioral mechanisms regulating eating, drinking, and avoidance of predators are suspended. There are changes in the regulation of breathing, heart rate, and brain temperature as well.

Despite the similarities between REMS and alert waking, the two states are of course very different. Reduced responsiveness and paralysis in REMS are the two most obvious distinguishing features. Waking involves autonomic regulation of such basic functions as temperature control as well as behaviors that enhance these functions, such as choosing a shady place to nap on a hot, sunny day (Fig. 4). The reduced responsiveness during sleep clearly makes an individual vulnerable to threats (such as predators), but another feature greatly accentuates this vulnerability. Homeothermic animals experience a modification of the very tight homeostatic regulation that so characterizes the rest of their lives. Activity of the sympathetic nervous system (tending, for example, to increase heart rate) is depressed in REMS except for periodic bursts of activity. In contrast, activity of the parasympathetic nervous system (e.g., slowing heart rate) increases in both sleep phases. A central region mediating the

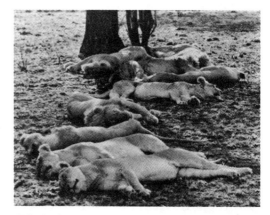

FIG. 4. Sleeping lions. Temperature regulation in waking includes behavior such as choosing an appropriate place to sleep. These lions take a relatively cool nap shaded from the African sun. Reproduced with permission of George Schaller.

autonomic nervous system (both sympathetic and parasympathetic divisions) is the hypothalamus. In NREMS homeostatic regulation continues, but in REMS the hypothalamus does not respond to signals that ordinarily elicit the correcting responses that keep the functioning of the various body systems within narrow limits. For example, during REMS many hypothalamic thermosensitive units no longer react to hypothalamic cooling or warming as part of the mechanisms that maintain temperature during waking within rather narrow limits. Gross temperature changes will arouse an animal from REMS or prevent it from entering the state, but subtle, autonomic heat loss mechanisms do not operate as they would in waking in addition to the decline in behavioral adjustment to ambient conditions. Heating of the hypothalamus that induces panting in cats in wakefulness and NREMS does not do so in REMS.

Very young mammalian infants spend a great proportion of their time in REMS, as high as 90% of a 24-hr period in some species, which would put them at a distinct disadvantage without maternal warming. With maturation to childhood, animals spend about 25% of total sleep time in REMS, a figure that remains essentially the same throughout life. Homeostatic regulation of temperature across the sleep cycle develops in parallel with the maturation of sleep patterns. As the amount of time spent in REMS declines, tighter control of temperature is achieved overall but REMS retains a more "infantile" form of homeostatic regulation.

In the cardiovascular system, great regularity and a reduced heart rate characterize NREMS. Respiration is slow and even in NREMS, with only a moderately reduced sensitivity to oxygen and carbon dioxide. REMS, however, is marked by respiratory irregularity and depression of reflexes such that the sensitivity to changes in the level of oxygen or carbon dioxide may be reduced. Arousal to wakefulness in response to these irregularities is increased compared with NREMS. The sleeper may literally wake up in order to breathe adequately. Although the diaphragm continues to contract, the nearly total loss of tone (atonia) in other muscles of respiration (intercostal and upper airway) makes breathing more burdensome in REMS.

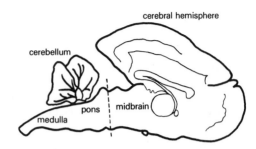

FIG. 5. A saggital section of the brain of the cat. The dotted line represents the junction of the pons and the midbrain. The dorsal part of this junction (i.e., in the direction of the cerebellum) is a key area for generating REMS and some of its phenomena such as the ponto-geniculo-occipital wave. Reproduced with permission of Adrian R. Morrison.

REMS as a State of Paradoxical Alerting

Brain mechanisms that are active when an animal responds to stimuli while awake also characterize the neural activity of REMS. Another unifying description of REMS is that of a state marked by brain stem activity that is also prominent when a *waking* animal or human is alerted by, orients to, or shifts its attention to a stimulus. REMS may be akin to a state in which the sleeper is essentially paralyzed during intense activity of the brain in an "alerting mode." Just as REMS is a state in which homeostatic regulation is loosened, it may also be described as a state in which the central correlates of alerting are spontaneously active when motor behavior is, paradoxically, markedly reduced.

An illustration of this concept of REMS comes from observations of cats with bilateral thermal lesions in the pons (Fig. 5); such lesions eliminate the normal muscle paralysis (atonia) but leave other electrophysiological and temperature changes of REMS intact. These lesioned animals display behavior ranging from exaggerated phasic movements such as twitches to head lifting to walking on all fours (Fig. 6), depending on the size and location of the lesion. With the ability to move, such cats spontaneously exhibit behaviors associated with a wakeful cat: orienting, searching, pouncing, and exhibiting undirected startle. Some cats will rise and walk around the cage, then stop and appear to stare at stimuli not seen by the experimenters (Fig. 6). Some animals will actually "pounce" on unseen targets.

Observations of normal cats with standard sleep recording electrodes in place also provide evidence that REMS resembles active waking. Waves resembling spontaneous PGO waves of REMS can be observed during waking in the lateral geniculate body of the thalamus and the occipital cortex. Such waveforms often occur when the eyes move and hence are sometimes called *eye movement potentials.* These PGO-like waves thus have a close association with activity involved in the acquisition of sensory information. Animals presented with a variety of visual, auditory, or olfactory stimuli typically turn their head and eyes toward the source of the stimulus. This orienting behavior is widespread among

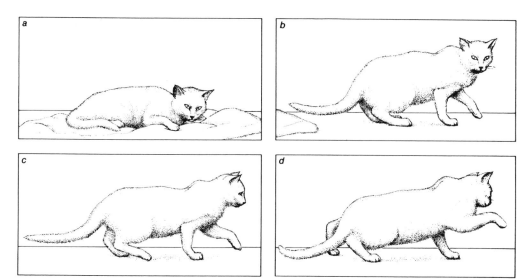

FIG. 6. Schematic illustration of a cat with lesions of the dorsal pons. The cat is actually in a variant of REMS, known as REMS without atonia. The usual absence of muscle tone in REMS is abolished by the lesion. The EEG and lateral geniculate nucleus (LGN) resemble those of panel D in Fig. 2. The curved posture of the cat's back betrays the abnormal motor control induced by the lesion, and such animals can be electrophysiologically in a state of sleep while exhibiting behavior including orienting to and staring at unseen objects. **a:** A sleeping cat begins to raise its head. **b:** The still sleeping cat rises. **c:** The cat remains in REMS while walking. **d:** REMS persists while the cat paws an unseen object. From Morrison AR. A window on the sleeping brain. Copyright April 1983, by Scientific American, Inc.

mammals including humans. During the initial presentations of the stimuli, PGO-like waves similar to the PGO wave of REMS are typically observed in the lateral geniculate bodies or visual cortex. PGO-like waves are thus closely associated with the first, overt responses to new, unexpected, or intense stimuli. Because spontaneous PGO waves are characteristic of REMS, the existence of similar waves associated during waking with an orienting response to external stimuli suggests that normal REMS itself might involve activation of neural mechanisms underlying orienting.

The classic reticular activating system believed to underlie cortical low-voltage, high-frequency activity of waking (*desynchronization*) also has brain stem origins. Mechanisms that desynchronize the cortex in waking and REM are partially localizable to the dorsal pons near the midbrain. This is a region that seems to generate PGO waves as well. Output cholinergic neurons between the pons and the midbrain are responsible for

the generation of PGO waves. The brain stem thus is one of the sources of an active, alert cortex as well as events such as the PGO wave that seem to accompany orienting during waking.

CLINICAL IMPLICATIONS

Sleep disorders are widespread. The comment "I slept terribly" is universal at some point in an individual's life. People feel irritable, out of sorts, tired, and even depressed when sleep is poor. Some sleep research wags have argued that a good night's sleep is that which one needs to remain in a good mood on a Monday morning work day! Patients often enter a doctor's office complaining of a pattern of fatigue and difficulty in falling or staying asleep. Confronted with these complaints, a clinician must consider a variety of conditions that affect sleep, ranging from medical problems such as chronic pain to psychiatric disorders such as depression or anxiety. One result of the interest in the basic mechanisms of human and animal sleep has been the emergence of an entire field, the evaluation of sleep disorders.

Techniques of recording the EEG, muscle activity, heart rate, respiration, and eye movements in the animal laboratory have been adapted to sleep recordings of people with sleep problems. These data comprise the polysomnogram. Electrodes are placed on the scalp for the EEG, on the chin for muscle activity, and near the eyes to detect eye movements. Thermistors are placed in front of the nose and mouth to measure breathing.

The prevalence of sleep problems and the emergence of standardized criteria for describing the amount of NREMS and REMS have prompted more systematic clinical descriptions of sleep disorders. The latter are generally classified as disorders of initiating and maintaining sleep (DIMS), sleep/wake schedule disorders, disorders of excessive somnolence (DOES), and parasomnias.

DIMS, Sleep/Wake Schedule Disorders, and DOES

A systematic classification of sleep disorders delineates the variety of ways that sleep can be disturbed. Sleep disturbances often accompany underlying psychiatric disorders such as depression, in which patients have trouble falling asleep, or wake up in the middle of the night, or wake up very early in the morning. Other individuals have a form of DIMS in which they have trouble falling asleep in the absence of any obvious medical or psychiatric disorder. Often the cause for such "psychophysiological" insomnia remains unclear. It may represent a learned pattern of behavior in which the individual becomes negatively conditioned to unsuccessful attempts at falling asleep. The bedroom, thoughts of sleep, and preparations for sleep such as changing into pajamas all may arouse anxiety and worry about being able to fall asleep. A cycle is created in which the erstwhile sleeper anticipates difficulty in fall-

ing asleep; and the negative prophecy is fulfilled, reinforcing the pattern of worry and poor sleep. Treatment usually includes the judicious use of medications and behavioral modification.

A so-called *sleep/wake schedule* disorder often reflects the natural tendency for an individual's biological clock to run slightly longer than the 24-hr day (see Chapter 11). The tendency for most individuals is therefore to fall asleep increasingly later and to awaken later. This common affliction of students can result from a lack of consistent waking times. One radical cure has sometimes included the scheduling of five consecutive early-morning undergraduate classes in a week, but most individuals with the disorder do not spontaneously adopt such a strategy. Some individuals suffer from such disorganized schedules that sleep is irregular. Workers with frequently and erratically changing shift schedules are particularly prone to sleep/wake schedule disorders. Behavioral interventions to regulate sleep schedules are often effective in improving sleep/wake schedule disorders.

Other sleep disorders also have marked effects on daytime performance and tendency to sleep. There are several varieties of DOES. Nocturnal myoclonus is a condition of repetitive leg movements that may continually arouse the sleeper, leading to excessive fatigue during the day. Sedative medications such as clonazepam, a benzodiazepine, may be helpful (see Chapter 19).

Narcolepsy is an often disabling form of DOES in which the individual experiences sometimes dangerous sleep attacks in places not usually associated with sleep, such as the bathroom, or during routine activities such as driving a car. Individuals suffering from the disorder are subject to a potentially dangerous condition known as *cataplexy* (loss of muscle tone). Strong emotions such as laughter and startling stimuli may produce cataplexy in which the person loses muscle tone and falls. Narcoleptic patients may also experience sleep paralysis during which they are awake at night, unable to move but still "seeing" an ongoing dream. Patients studied in the sleep laboratory typically enter REMS within minutes when taking a nap during the day or falling asleep at night. Narcolepsy is often considered a disorder in which mechanisms underlying REMS are activated at inappropriate times. The cataplectic loss of muscle tone is reminiscent of the muscle paralysis associated with normal REMS, and the sleep paralysis and dreams in an otherwise alert individual further suggest that the mechanisms governing the timing of REMS are disturbed in narcolepsy.

Apnea is a cessation or an interruption of breathing. Other DOES reflect a potentially dangerous worsening of the already loosened regulation of respiration during REMS, especially for individuals with cardiac or pulmonary illnesses. Some adults experience a pattern of interrupted breathing, called *apnea,* during the night. As breathing is interrupted and the oxygen content of the blood declines, the individual tends to rouse either into waking briefly or into lighter stages of NREMS in order to breathe. The net result is poor-quality sleep, excessive sleepiness during the day, and disturbances in mood and concentration. As described earlier, the burden of respiration increases during REMS due to atonia of some of the muscles of respiration. The decreased tone of airway muscles during REMS atonia narrows the passages of air exchange, and a sleeper essentially tries to breathe past what amounts to a closed valve. Apnea is typically exacerbated in obese individuals, and it is possible that the additional weight of fatty tissue on airway muscles increases the tendency for the airway to collapse. Central apnea involves a decrease in CNS-mediated respiratory drive rather than a blockage of the air passages; central apnea may become worse during the irregular respiratory control of REMS.

Some young infants for unknown reasons fall victim to a disorder called *sudden infant death syndrome* (SIDS). We speculate that, coupled with a normal decline in responsiveness to carbon dioxide or oxygen characteristic of REMS, a vulnerable infant's decreased muscle tone in the airway during REMS might impair respiration to the point of death. Cat models may provide further understanding of how REMS mechanisms of muscle atonia and intrinsic vulnerability to irregular respiratory activity during REMS produce adult sleep apnea or SIDS.

Parasomnias

Some sleep disorders involve partial arousal from different stages of sleep or arise within specific states of sleep. Parasomnias are disorders that include partial arousals from sleep or occur during a particular stage of sleep. Two troubling parasomnias, nightmares and night terrors, have been well described in the sleep laboratory. Nightmares are long, disturbing dreams with a visual quality to the images; they awaken the sleeper. When they occur in the sleep laboratory, they arise from REMS. The occurrence of frequent nightmares has been associated with higher rates of certain forms of psychopathology, but the mechanisms of this linkage are unknown. Night terrors, which typically involve screaming, sleep walking, and the appearance of extreme fright, arise during stage 4 of NREMS. Massive autonomic arousal and poor recall of the episodes are characteristic of night terrors. They commonly begin in the preadolescent period and typically diminish in frequency or disappear within a few years. The mechanisms that cause nightmares and night terrors are poorly understood.

One often-discussed issue is whether the content of normal dreams or nightmares has a special significance in terms of the psychological make-up of individuals. The classic explanation of Sigmund Freud was that dreams reflect hidden psychological conflicts that can only be expressed in disguised fashion during sleep. Current neurophysiologists cite the marked brain stem influence on REMS (dream sleep) in animal models, and they argue that the content of dreams is determined by activation of sensory and motor centers in the brain. Whether the universal mechanisms underlying REMS physiology activate specific memories to produce psychologically meaningful dreams remains a challenging question at the interface of sleep research and psychiatry.

A newly described parasomnia is reminiscent of REMS minus atonia in cats with pontine lesions that eliminate the usual paralysis of REMS. Some adults, approximately 50% of whom have no detectable neurological abnormality in wakefulness, have lived for years with a peculiar sleep disorder in which they have incurred head and other injuries. At various times during the night, some of these individuals get out of bed and dive straight into a radiator or other object or assume a firing position with an imaginary rifle. If awakened, they may state that they were being chased or were firing at enemies. Often such patients must be tied to their beds at night to prevent injury. Careful evaluation in the sleep laboratory reveals that they exhibit the bizarre behaviors during REMS. Hence, the disorder has been dubbed *REMS behavior disorder,* and its existence was suggested by the work with REMS without atonia in cats.

Selected Psychiatric Disorders

Sleep is commonly disturbed in a variety of psychiatric conditions including depression and post-traumatic stress disorder. We have seen that NREMS, REMS, and waking have very different electrophysiological properties. REMS involves a change in the extent of activity in cholinergic, noradrenergic, and serotonergic neurons relative to NREMS or wakefulness. The states of sleep result from the recruitment of populations of neurons at diverse sites rather than the mere turning on and off of a discrete center within the brain. The concept of increased cholinergic activity in REMS compared to NREMS coupled with a relative decline in noradrenergic and serotonergic activity in NREMS has parallels in contemporary theory of mood disorders.

Major depression (see Chapter 17) is a common psychiatric illness characterized by depressed mood, appetite disturbance, difficulties with concentration and memory, suicidal thinking, excessive guilt, and nighttime or early morning awakening. In contrast to a normal sleep cycle, REMS in patients with major depression often occurs early (i.e., within the first 90 min of sleep). Rapid eye movements themselves may be more frequent, especially during the first REMS episode. These changes have been thought to be relatively specific to depression, although shortened REMS onset times have sometimes been reported in schizophrenia.

The increased "pressure" to enter REMS during major depression has been postulated to reflect enhanced cholinergic activity within the CNS. It has also been argued that depression reflects a deficiency in noradrenergic or serotonergic activity. As noted earlier, REMS in cats can be induced by cholinergic agents, and serotonergic and noradrenergic activity declines in REMS. If depressed individuals had enhanced cholinergic activity, this might provide a "push" into REMS with lower noradrenergic activity removing inhibition of REMS. Interestingly, cholinergic agents have been found to reduce the time to enter REMS in individuals susceptible to depression. Furthermore, medications that improve depression are commonly believed to enhance the activity of serotonergic and noradrenergic neurons (see Chapter 17), and these medications all suppress REMS. REMS and mood thus may share some regulatory mechanisms. While it is too simplistic to describe either REMS or depression as the outcome of a "balance" between cholinergic and other influences, the concept of shared regulatory mechanisms remains useful for guiding research and conceptualizing some aspects of mood disorders.

The theme of hypervigilance is prominent in one psychiatric disorder, *post-traumatic stress disorder,* in which individuals previously exposed to a life-threatening event such as combat, natural disaster, or rape have marked intrusions of thoughts of the event into consciousness, sometimes beginning years after the incident. These individuals report being "on the lookout" or experiencing dramatic nighttime dreams or daytime flashbacks that are visual replicas of the original event. The strongly visual nature of these frightening dreams is reminiscent of the vividly pictorial aspects of the classic nightmare arising from REMS. The disturbance may stem from a dysregulation of the mechanisms underlying REMS. Thus, preliminary work suggested that Vietnam War veterans suffering from the disorder also have a disturbance of REMS. When these veterans were examined in the sleep laboratory, it was found that the percentage of sleep time devoted to REMS was increased, more rapid eye movements were observed, the time of onset of REMS was more variable, and phasic leg movements in REMS were unusually prominent. Thus, patients displayed evidence of a disturbed regulation of REMS. REMS is itself a state in which the brain functions in an alerting mode. Waking flashbacks, consisting of visual images of the traumatic event, may involve the inappropriate activation of alerting mechanisms of REMS and consequent dreaming during waking.

SUMMARY

The concept of sleep as a homogeneous state has been transformed by over 30 years of research in human and animal sleep laboratories. The recognition of NREMS and REMS as distinct varieties of sleep has produced an exponential growth in our understanding of the neural mechanisms underlying sleep. This knowledge has fostered hypotheses about how the sleep/wake cycle is organized and regulated in the context of more sophisticated description and treatment of a variety of human disorders. The concepts of sleep as a time of altered homeostatic control and REMS as a paradoxical state involving activation of alerting and orienting mechanisms suggest novel approaches to clinical research. Although the hypotheses require refinement, the application of basic science to clinical sleep studies continues vigorously.

BIBLIOGRAPHY

Original Articles

Aserinsky E, Kleitman N. Regularly occurring periods of eye motility, and concomitant phenomena, during sleep. *Science* 1953;118:273–274.

Aston-Jones G, Bloom FE. Activity of norepinephrine-containing locus coeruleus neurons in behaving rats anticipates fluctuations in the sleep-waking cycle. *J Neurosci* 1981;1:876–886.

Dement WC, Kleitman N. Cyclic variations in EEG during sleep and their relation to eye movements, body motility, and dreaming. *Electroencephalogr Clin Neurophysiol* 1957;9:673–690.

Hobson JA, McCarley RW. The brain as a dream state generator: an activation–synthesis hypothesis of the dream process. *Am J Psychiatry* 1977;134:1335–1348.

Jouvet M. Recherches sur les structures nerveuses et les mécanismes responsables des différentes phases du sommeil physiologique. *Arch Ital Biol* 1962; 100:125–206.

McGinty DJ, Harper RM. Dorsal raphe neurons: depression of firing during sleep in cats. *Brain Res* 1976;101:569–575.

Morrison AR, Bowker RM. The biological significance of PGO spikes in the sleeping cat. *Acta Neurobiol Exp (Warsz)* 1975;35:821–840.

Ross RJ, Ball WA, Sullivan KA, Caroff SN. Sleep disturbance as the hallmark of posttraumatic stress disorder. *Am J Psychiatry* 1989;146:697–707.

Steriade M, Pare D, Parent A, Smith Y. Projections of cholinergic and non-cholinergic neurons of the brainstem core to relay and associational thalamic nuclei in the cat and macaque monkey. *Neuroscience* 1988; 25:47–67.

Books and Reviews

Hartmann E. *The nightmare: the psychology and biology of terrifying dreams.* New York: Basic Books; 1984.

Kryger MH, Roth T, Dement WC. *Principles and practice of sleep medicine.* Philadelphia: WB Saunders; 1989.

Morrison AR. Brain-stem regulation of behavior during sleep and wakefulness. In: Sprague JM, Epstein AN, eds. *Progress in psychobiology and physiological psychology.* Vol. 8. New York: Academic Press; 1979: 91–131.

Parmeggiani PL, Morrison AR. Alterations in autonomic function during sleep. In: Loewy AD, Spyer KM, eds. *Central regulation of autonomic functions.* Oxford: Oxford University Press; 1990:367–386.

Steriade M, McCarley RW. *Brainstem control of wakefulness and sleep.* New York: Plenum Press; 1990.

11

Biological Rhythms

Gary E. Pickard and Patricia J. Sollars

Since the present moment is both an end and a beginning of time, though not of the same time, but the end of what has passed and the beginning of the future, just as a circle has its convexity and its concavity in the same thing in some way, so is time always at a beginning and at an end; and because of this, time is thought to be always distinct. For it is not of the same thing that the moment is both a beginning and an end, since if it were, it would be two opposites simultaneously and in the same respect. And time will certainly not come to an end, for there is always a beginning of it.

Aristotle,
Physics trans. by Hippocrates G. Apostle (Indiana University Press, 1969, p. 86)

- Circadian rhythms are characterized by three major properties: entrainment, free-running rhythms, and temperature compensation.

- Circadian pacemakers function as biological clocks.

- The direction and amplitude of light-induced shifts are phase-dependent.

- The phase-shifting effects of light are mediated by the retina.

- The hypothalamic suprachiasmatic nucleus (SCN) is an important component of the circadian system.

- The retinohypothalamic tract is a nonvisual retinal pathway.

- The suprachiasmatic nucleus is a circadian oscillator.

- Splitting of the circadian rhythm of wheel-running activity requires at least two circadian oscillators.

- Spontaneous internal desynchronization of human circadian rhythms sometimes occurs.

- SCN-lesioned rats entrain to restricted feeding schedules.

- SCN homografts restore circadian rhythms to arrhythmic hosts.

- SCN heterografts determine clock autonomy.

- The pineal gland is an important component of the circadian system.

- Sleep disturbances are associated with depression.

- Phototherapy can be an effective treatment for seasonal affective disorder.

■ Chapter Overview

This chapter describes how the examination of many diverse organisms, from plants to insects to humans, gradually led to the conclusion that endogenous circadian oscillations are a pervasive property of biological organization and that they function as biological clocks. The neural basis of the generation of circadian rhythms is presented next, followed by a discussion of the role of the pineal gland and melatonin in circadian rhythms. The chapter concludes with a section on the human circadian system, its role in some psychiatric illnesses, and a description of noninvasive phototherapeutic techniques used for seasonal depression that have been developed as a direct result of animal research.

Rhythmic processes in animals and plants exhibit a wide range of periodicities, from milliseconds to years per cycle. In fact, biological rhythmicity is so commonplace in nature that for centuries such rhythms were assumed to represent merely a passive consequence of a periodic environment. It is now recognized that circadian rhythms (Latin *circa* = about; *dies* = day) are fundamental endogenous adaptations made by eukaryotic organisms in response to the relentless cycle of day and night. The suggestion that daily rhythms are endogenous was first presented in 1729, when the French astronomer Jean Jacques d'Ortous de Mairan described the persistence of leaf movements in plants placed in total darkness. Unfortunately, the significance of de Mairan's findings—that daily rhythms are not a passive response to the environment—remained unappreciated for two centuries.

It was while watching bees search for marmalade on his breakfast table in the Swiss Alps in the summer of 1910 that the psychiatrist August Forel noticed the insects returning at the same time each day whether or not food was present. This led Forel to suggest that bees might possess a *Zeitgedächtnis*—a memory for time. In the 1920s von Frisch

and Beling, while studying the behavior of individual bees in the laboratory, more carefully examined their capacity to measure the passage of time. Sugar water was presented to bees at the same time of day for several days; when it was not offered, the bees continued to arrive at the testing station on time. These investigators then showed that the daily timekeeping system was endogenous by repeating their experiments in a salt mine, removed from environmental time cues.

The suggestion that humans also possessed an internal timing mechanism came with the advent of rapid travel across multiple time zones. In 1931, when Wiley Post flew eastward around the world in $8\frac{1}{2}$ days, he discovered the relevance of his internal clock when he recognized that his flying abilities were adversely affected by the rapid time zone displacement. His sleep was disrupted, his attention span and alertness were diminished, and he had a general feeling of uneasiness; in short, he was the first person to experience jet lag. Post's physiology was unable to keep up with him as he traversed the globe in 208 hr because his biological clock could not adjust quickly enough to the new local times.

PROPERTIES OF CIRCADIAN RHYTHMS

Circadian rhythms are characterized by three major properties. During the 1950s,

Biological Bases of Brain Function and Disease, edited by Alan Frazer, Perry B. Molinoff, and Andrew Winokur. Raven Press, Ltd., New York © 1994.

Pittendrigh and his colleagues began to develop the theoretical framework necessary to understand the properties of endogenous circadian systems. Their work determined that circadian rhythms are manifestations of *circadian pacemakers,* which are self-sustained biological oscillators. Circadian pacemakers are characterized by three major properties: (1) *entrainment* (their synchronization to environmental cycles); (2) *free-running rhythmicity* (their continued oscillation under constant conditions); and (3) *temperature compensation* (the stability of period length under changes in ambient temperature).

Entrainment

The most powerful environmental agent underlying entrainment of the endogenous circadian pacemaker is the light/dark cycle, although other elements such as food availability and temperature variation may also serve to synchronize some organisms to the external milieu. In addition, social interactions may play an important role in the entrainment of humans as well as other animals for which communication is a significant component of the behavioral repertoire. Under the entrained condition (e.g., while living under a light/dark cycle), the physiological and behavioral organization of an organism establishes a regular phase relation to the external environment (Fig. 1). Furthermore, when internal synchrony is maintained among an individual's various systems (i.e., endocrine, nervous, immune, etc.) while entrained, its capacity to function in the external environment is enhanced. The problems associated with jet lag, for example, illustrate the consequence of desynchronization among different circadian rhythms resulting from disparate rates of re-entrainment among the body's systems.

Free-Running Rhythms

In the absence of an environmental cycle, circadian pacemakers free-run (Fig. 1) and

express their endogenous, genetically determined period, which is only approximately equal to 24 hr. The period of circadian rhythms is species-typical, with the period expressed by individuals of each species generally being narrowly distributed around the group mean, e.g., *Mus musculus* (house mice) $\approx$ 23.6 hr; *Mesocricetus auratus* (golden hamsters) $\approx$ 24.1 hr; *Homo sapiens* (humans) $\approx$ 25 hr. The variety of circadian periods expressed under constant conditions has provided the most compelling evidence of the endogenous nature of circadian rhythmicity. It is difficult to imagine that unrecognized geophysical cues could be responsible for generating such a broad range of circadian periods. Despite the unlikelihood of this possibility, experiments have been performed specifically to discredit the suggestion that unknown temporal cues produced by the earth's rotation are responsible for generating circadian rhythms. In 1962, Hamner and his colleagues demonstrated that circadian rhythms persist in a number of diverse organisms even when they are placed on a turntable rotating counter to the earth's rotation at the South Pole. Indeed, the putative participation of geophysical effects in the generation of circadian rhythms has recently been completely eliminated by the observation of the continued expression of a free-running circadian rhythm of vegetative spore formation in the bread mold *Neurospora crassa* maintained for 7 days in constant darkness on the space shuttle Columbia while it orbited the earth every 90 min.

Temperature Compensation

Temperature compensation of circadian pacemakers (i.e., the conservation of circadian period observed over rather wide temperature ranges) has been described in a number of cold-blooded organisms. Most biochemical processes double their rate of reaction with every 10°C increase in temperature; however, free-running circadian rhythms change very little with such changes in am-

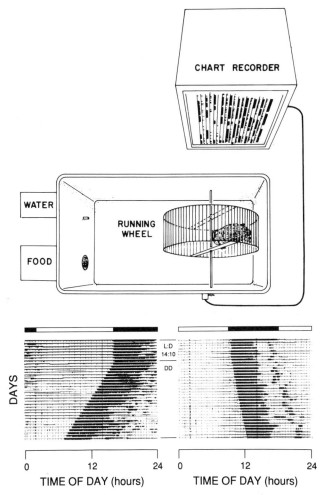

FIG. 1. Method of recording rodent wheel-running activity. Each activity wheel rotation results in a microswitch closure that produces a deflection of a pen on a multichannel chart recorder. The continuous records for each channel are cut into sections representing 24-hr intervals and are presented with successive days arranged vertically. The wheel-running activity records of a mouse (left) and a hamster (right) are presented to illustrate (1) entrainment to a light/dark cycle of 14 hr light/10 hr darkness (first 7 days) followed by (2) a free-running circadian rhythm upon release into constant darkness (DD). Period in DD is approximately 23.6 and 24.1 hr for mouse and hamster, respectively.

bient temperature. *This stability of circadian period is taken by most investigators to reflect the functional significance of the circadian system as a biological clock.* Indeed, a biological clock would not keep very accurate time if it sped up and slowed down as the ambient temperature rose and fell. Although temperature compensation is clearly most meaningful for cold-blooded organisms, it might also be valuable for hibernating mammals such as

ground squirrels. Neural components of the ground squirrel circadian system are among the most metabolically active components of the brain while animals are in deep torpor with a core body temperature as low as 2°C.

Circadian Pacemakers as Biological Clocks

It is by their self-sustaining oscillatory nature and their capacity to be entrained by the environmental light/dark cycle that circadian pacemakers provide proper phasing of physiological processes with the external world. In so doing, circadian pacemakers in effect recognize local time and therefore can be said to function as biological clocks. It is believed that these clock-like functions bestow on an organism the significant adaptive advantage of being able to predict or anticipate environmental factors on a daily basis and to foresee seasonal changes as well. For example, it would clearly be advantageous for the nocturnally foraging rodent to return to its burrow in anticipation of dawn rather than to wait for the morning sunrise and the awakening of diurnal predators before seeking safety.

CIRCADIAN RHYTHMS SHIFTED BY BRIEF LIGHT PULSES

The direction and amplitude of light-induced shifts are phase-dependent. The formal processes underlying photic entrainment of circadian rhythms have been extensively examined by looking at the effects of brief light pulses (15 to 60 min in duration) administered to rodents maintained in constant darkness. One of the species used most frequently in these experiments is the golden hamster because of the precision it displays in the circadian rhythm of wheel-running activity (Fig. 1). The onset of wheel-running activity is used as a phase indicator and is arbitrarily defined as circadian time (CT) 12. Light pulses cause shifts in the phase of the circadian activity rhythm, with both the direction and the amplitude of the shift dependent on the point in the cycle (*phase*) at which the light pulse is presented (Fig. 2A). Phase-dependent shifts of the endogenous free-running oscillator are described by a *phase-response curve* (PRC) (Fig. 2B).

The general form of the light-induced PRC is very consistent among mammals whether diurnal or nocturnal. The PRC is characterized by three regions: (1) a period coincident with the subjective day, where light is ineffec-

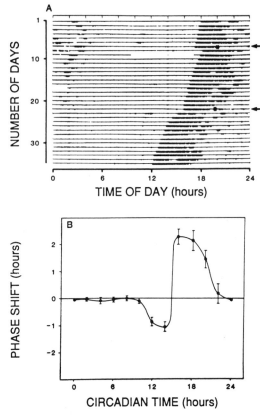

FIG. 2. Effect of brief light pulses on the circadian rhythm of wheel-running activity of the hamster. **A**: Wheel-running activity record of a hamster free-running in constant darkness illustrating the effect of exposure to 15 min of light on the days indicated by arrows and at the times indicated by asterisks. The first light pulse produced a phase delay and the second light pulse produced a phase advance in the onset of wheel-running activity. **B**: A phase–response curve illustrating the effect of 60-min light pulses presented at various times relative to the hamster's circadian time. Onset of wheel running is defined as circadian time (CT) 12. Phase advances are plotted as positive and phase delays as negative. Each point represents the mean and standard deviation of six animals. Modified from Takahashi JS, Zatz M. *Science* 1982;217:1104.

tive in producing phase shifts (CT 0–CT 10); (2) a region early in the subjective night where light pulses produce phase delays (CT 10–CT 14); and (3) a zone late in the subjective night where light affects phase advances (CT 16–CT 24) (Fig. 2B). Since the endogenous circadian system is photosensitive early or late in the subjective night (i.e., at dusk and at dawn), light encountered around those times of day serves to adjust (or shift) the internal oscillator in order to maintain its appropriate temporal relation to the environmental day/night cycle. Thus, in the hamster, with an endogenous period of 24.1 hr, the endogenous clock must phase-advance approximately 6 min each day in order to maintain stable entrainment with a 24-hr environmental cycle, whereas a mouse, with an endogenous period of 23.6 hr, must phase-delay its circadian system 24 min each day to remain stably entrained. In the former case, it is the light encountered at dawn that is the effective entraining signal, and in the latter case light perceived at dusk is the phase-setting cue. The limits of entrainment to light/dark cycles are determined by the maximal amount of phase shift an individual can affect in a single day.

The phase-shifting effects of light are mediated by the retina. Mammals, including humans, rely solely on their eyes for photic entrainment; the circadian pacemaker of a blinded mammal free-runs regardless of the lighting conditions. This is evident in the sleep/wake record of a blind graduate student who sought medical help for his chronic insomnia and daytime sleepiness (Fig. 3). While living in the hospital under instruction to sleep only when he felt sleepy, he displayed a free-running sleep/wake cycle with a 24.8-hr period. When released from the hospital, his sleep again became fragmented and he napped repeatedly during work hours. It can be seen in the lower half of Fig. 3 that these naps are an extrapolation of his free-running 24.8-hr sleep/wake rhythm as he tried to maintain a 24-hr schedule. In this instance, social cues that might have stood in the stead of photic cues were apparently not a sufficiently potent *zeitgeber* (entraining agent) to entrain his circadian system.

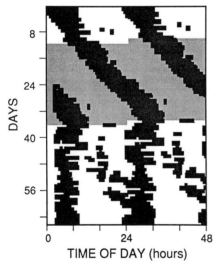

FIG. 3. Sleep/wake pattern of a blind subject. Time spent asleep is depicted by the dark-shaded areas. Successive days are presented top to bottom and the data are double-plotted over a 48-hr time interval to facilitate visualization of the circadian rhythm. First 12 days are at home with the use of an alarm clock. Stippled interval represents an ad-lib sleep/wake, work, and meal schedule while in the hospital. On day 37 the subject returned home and attempted to readjust to a 24-hr day but his fragmented sleep maintains the phase and period of his free-running rhythm clearly expressed during the previous hospital stay. Modified from Miles LEM, Raynal DM, Wilson MA. *Science* 1977;198:421.

THE NEURAL BASIS OF CIRCADIAN RHYTHMS

The hypothalamic suprachiasmatic nucleus (SCN) is an important component of the circadian system. The search for the neural locus of mammalian circadian rhythmicity began with the work of the psychiatrist Curt Richter, who placed lesions in various regions of the rat brain and observed their effects on eating, drinking, and locomotor activity rhythms. Lesions placed in the ventromedial anterior hypothalamus abolished the observed rhythms, but Richter provided no further detail. Other investigators lesioned various components of the visual system based on the strategy that photic information reaches the circadian system via visual projections from the retina. However, ablation of all known visual projections in the primary and accessory optic pathways had no effect on circadian behavior unless the optic nerves were severed, which resulted in blindness and free-running circadian rhythms.

In 1972, a previously unidentified retinal projection to the hypothalamus, the *retinohypothalamic tract* (RHT), was described by two laboratories working independently, using a newly developed autoradiographic tract tracing procedure. Hendrickson and her coworkers and Moore and Lenn injected a mixture of radioactive amino acids into the vitreous humor of the eyes of mammals from a number of different species, and subsequently visualized labeled retinal synaptic terminals on a tightly packed cluster of small neurons in the hypothalamus situated immediately dorsal to the optic chiasm, the *suprachiasmatic nucleus* (SCN). Then, to determine whether disruption of this newly identified retinal projection to the hypothalamus would eliminate entrainment, the SCN was lesioned. However, in addition to disrupting entrainment, SCN ablation abolished circadian rhythmicity as illustrated in the disruption of the circadian pattern of wheel-running activity depicted in Fig. 4. The initial SCN lesion studies provided the catalyst for the ongoing investigation of the role of the SCN in the generation of circadian rhythms and of the role of the RHT in mediating entrainment.

Improvements in techniques for the tracing of neuroanatomic pathways in the central nervous system have made it possible to examine retinal projections to the hypothalamus in a wide variety of species in all vertebrate classes. Figure 5 is an example of this projection demonstrated by *horseradish peroxidase* (HRP) histochemistry. The HRP enzyme was injected into the vitreous humor of one eye and allowed to be transported to the retinal terminals where it was detected histochemically (see Chapter 1). It is believed that the RHT has been highly conserved through evolution and is a common feature of the optic system of all vertebrates.

The retinohypothalamic tract is a nonvisual retinal pathway. Many of the features of the organization of the RHT serve to empha-

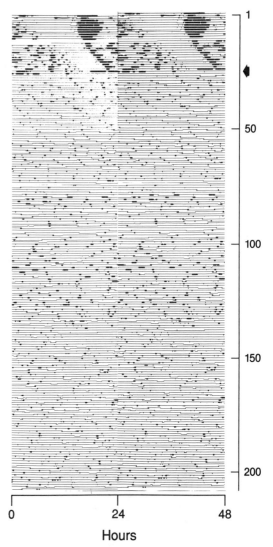

FIG. 4. Wheel-running activity record (double-plotted) of a suprachiasmatic nucleus (SCN)-lesioned hamster maintained in constant dim red light throughout. On the day indicated by the arrow, a small lesion that completely destroyed the suprachiasmatic nuclei was made in the anterior hypothalamus. The circadian rhythm of wheel-running activity became disrupted following the lesion and remained noncircadian for the remainder of the experiment (approximately 185 days).

size the nonvisual nature of this retinal projection. In the absence of all visual projections except the RHT, an animal is rendered behaviorally blind (i.e., unable to make simple visual discriminations). However, this same

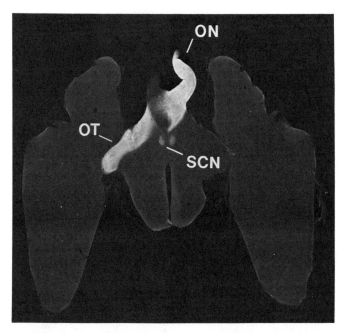

FIG. 5. Photomicrograph of a hamster brain section illustrating the retinohypothalamic tract. Five microliters of a horseradish peroxidase (HRP) solution was injected into the vitreous humor of the right eye and 24 hr later the HRP was demonstrated histochemically. As seen in this brain section prepared in the horizontal plane, the right optic nerve (ON) is heavily labeled. After crossing in the optic chiasm, the labeled nerve continues as the optic tract (OT). On either side of the midline, immediately caudal to the optic chiasm, is the retinal terminal field over each SCN. Rostral is at the top of the photomicrograph.

animal is able to entrain to the light/dark cycle via the RHT, which is both sufficient and necessary for entrainment. The retinal ganglion cells that give rise to the RHT are very few in number (less than 1% of the total ganglion cell population of the retina) and are distributed somewhat randomly across the entire retinal surface. These cells have a very simple morphology, with only a few sparsely branching, long dendrites (Fig. 6) and a large receptive field, suggesting a high degree of convergence of input from retinal photoreceptors. Moreover, these cells do not exhibit the center-surround receptive field organization (two circular, concentric zones that are antagonistic) typical of most ganglion cells. The firing rate of these ganglion cells changes directly as ambient illumination intensity increases, and the cells are commonly referred to as luminosity detectors. It can be concluded that these cells are well suited for their role of conveying information to the circadian system regarding the phase of the environmental light/dark cycle.

The suprachiasmatic nucleus is a circadian oscillator. In the 20 years since the original studies demonstrating that SCN ablation rendered rats' drinking and locomotor activity arrhythmic, a large body of indirect evidence has accumulated in support of the hypothesis that the mammalian SCN is crucially involved in the generation of circadian rhythms in a broad range of behavioral and physiological phenomena. This evidence has been obtained primarily from lesion studies conducted in several different species, including primates. These studies have demonstrated that bilateral destruction of the SCN abolishes circadian rhythms in many behavioral and physiological parameters including eating, drinking, wheel-running activity, sleep, temperature, pineal *N*-acetyltransferase, adrenal corticosterone, and estrous cyclicity. Taken together, lesion stud-

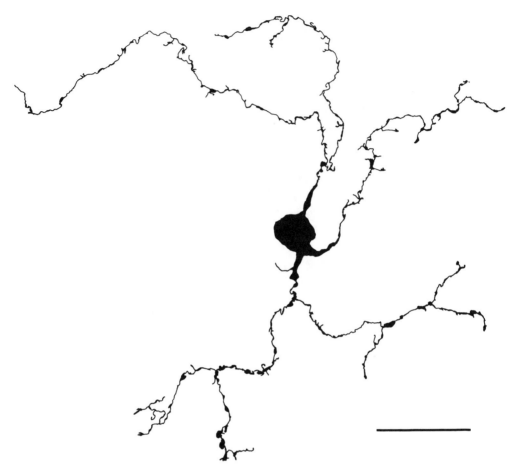

FIG. 6. Retinal ganglion cell afferent to the suprachiasmatic nucleus (SCN) of the hamster. To identify the population of retinal ganglion cells that project to the SCN, the SCN was injected with retrograde tracers that were transported to the retina. The uncomplicated morphology of the dendrites of this cell is typical of the ganglion cells that project to the SCN. Calibration bar = 50 μm.

ies support the idea that the SCN functions as a circadian oscillator. However, all lesion studies suffer from interpretive ambiguities, and SCN ablation studies in particular cannot differentiate between the possibilities that (1) destruction of the SCN region is directly responsible for the loss of circadian behavior or (2) destruction of the SCN region merely lesions a nodal point through which other structures in the brain may regulate circadian behavior.

More direct evidence supporting the role of the SCN as a central circadian oscillator has been obtained from studies that showed a circadian rhythm of metabolic activity in the SCN of several species including monkeys, cats, mice, rats, and hamsters. Further, the electrophysiological studies of Inouye and Kawamura provided some of the most compelling evidence of the SCN's oscillatory nature. These investigators demonstrated the persistence of a circadian rhythm of in vivo multiunit electrical activity in the SCN after it had been surgically separated from the surrounding hypothalamus. Although circadian rhythms of neuronal firing patterns were observed in numerous other brain sites in the intact animal, these vanished without exception when their connections to the SCN were severed. In addition, other investigators have shown that electrical stimulation of the rodent SCN can alter the phase of the circadian rhythm of wheel-running activity and that the phase shift is dependent on the time of stimulation. Finally, oscillations in neural activity and peptide secretion have been revealed in SCN hypothalamic slice preparations maintained in vitro, although typically these preparations do not remain viable long enough to establish whether the oscillations are fully self-sustained.

THE CIRCADIAN SYSTEM AND MULTIPLE CIRCADIAN OSCILLATORS

The above-mentioned studies leave no doubt that the SCN is a circadian oscillator; however, they do not eliminate the possibility that the SCN is simply one component in a complex multioscillatory system that functions as the circadian pacemaker (the pacemaker is defined as that which is responsible for determining species-typical circadian behavior). The lines of evidence that appear to support such a multioscillatory pacemaking system are (1) the phenomenon of splitting, which occurs in several species of mammals housed in conditions of constant environmental lighting; (2) the spontaneous internal desynchronization of certain circadian rhythms in humans; and (3) observations of a food-entrainable oscillator that is evident in animals with complete ablation of the SCN.

Splitting of the circadian rhythm of wheel-running activity requires at least two circadian oscillators. One of the strongest indications that multiple oscillators underlie the organization of circadian behavior is provided by the phenomenon of *splitting.* When splitting occurs, the circadian rhythm of wheel-running activity dissociates or splits into two distinct bouts of activity. At the onset of splitting (which occurs in the hamster after several weeks in constant light), the two activity components free-run with different circadian periods for several days until they stabilize approximately 180° out of phase

(Fig. 7). The attainment of the stabilized antiphase relationship between activity bouts is also accompanied by a change in period of the split activity rhythm (Fig. 7). On the basis of the splitting phenomenon it has been suggested that the circadian pacemaker is composed of at least two coupled circadian oscillators since it is difficult to envisage a system consisting of a single circadian oscillator that can express two different circadian periods concurrently.

The simplest explanation of splitting suggests that the two coupled oscillators requisite for this phenomenon may simply be represented by the bilaterally symmetrical SCN. Indeed, each SCN is anatomically connected to its contralateral counterpart and splitting may merely be the result of the physiological uncoupling of the paired SCNs. Evidence consistent with the suggestion that the two SCNs represent a coupled circadian oscilla-

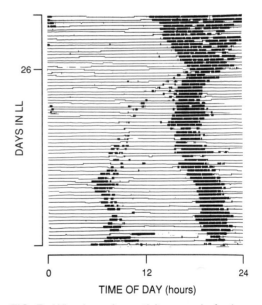

FIG. 7. Wheel-running activity record of a hamster illustrating the "splitting" phenomenon. After 26 days under constant light (LL) conditions, the single bout of wheel-running activity dissociates or "splits" into two bouts of activity that initially free-run with different periods until they stabilize in an antiphase relationship. Modified from Ellis GB, McKlveen RE, Turek FW. *Am J Physiol* 1982;242:R44.

tory system is provided by unilateral SCN ablation studies. Animals demonstrating normal (nonsplit) circadian behavior continue to express circadian rhythms after unilateral SCN ablation, although usually with a reduction in period. This observation indicates that a single SCN can function as a circadian oscillator. Furthermore, unilateral SCN destruction abolishes split activity rhythms and results in the establishment of a single circadian rhythm of activity with a period usually different from both the split and presplit rhythms (Fig. 8). In addition, the metabolic activity of the two SCNs has been shown to be bilaterally asymmetrical in hamsters expressing split activity rhythms. These data suggest that coupling between the bilaterally paired SCNs is an important component of the organization of the circadian pacemaker

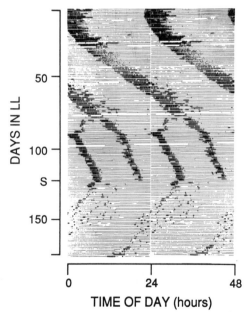

FIG. 8. Wheel-running activity record of a hamster demonstrating the abolition of splitting following unilateral suprachiasmatic nucleus (SCN) destruction. After approximately 75 days under constant light (LL) conditions, wheel-running activity splits. The S indicates the day of surgery when the animal received a unilateral SCN lesion that resulted in the abolition of the split condition and the induction of a single circadian rhythm with a very short period. Modified from Pickard GE, Turek FW. *Science* 1982;215:1119.

in mammals. Bilaterally symmetrical circadian oscillators have also been demonstrated in the circadian systems of invertebrates such as the sea hare, *Aplysia californica,* in which the two eyes contain loosely coupled circadian oscillators, and the cockroach, in which the two optic lobes serve that function.

Spontaneous internal desynchronization of human circadian rhythms sometimes occurs. The second indication of the presence of a multioscillator system in mammals comes from the examination of the circadian rhythms of humans maintained in temporal isolation. The German physician Jürgen Aschoff pioneered the study of human circadian rhythms in the 1960s by having volunteers live in isolation in an underground bunker for several weeks. Under these conditions the subjects' circadian system free-ran and usually expressed a period of about 25 hr. On occasion, however, it was reported that the subjects' circadian rhythms spontaneously desynchronized. It seemed that the rhythm of body temperature continued to oscillate with a period of about 25 hr whereas the sleep/wake rhythm lengthened to a period of about 32 hr, and the two rhythms usually free-ran with independent periods until the termination of the experiment.

In these experiments, subjects were requested to organize their days by avoiding naps and delimiting subjective days by a major wake episode followed by a major sleep episode; initiation and termination of sleep were signaled by the pressing of a button. However, some subjects could not avoid napping and pressed another button to indicate the beginning and end of each nap. Naps were not considered sleep and were not included in the original analysis of the sleep/wake cycle data. However, subject-defined "naps" were sometimes 8 hr in duration. Recent reanalysis of the original data from over 150 cases of spontaneous internal desynchronization by Zulley and coworkers indicates that when naps are included as sleep, the sleep/wake cycle remains in synchrony with core body temperature. That the subjects discriminated between two groups of long sleep episodes, calling one a nap and the other major sleep, may indicate that their "psychological day" had become dissociated from their "physiological day" rather than an internal desynchronization between physiological components. Under this analysis it is no longer necessary to posit a multioscillatory system in humans.

SCN-lesioned rats entrain to restricted feeding schedules. The third line of evidence in support of a multioscillatory circadian system is provided by the observation that rats with complete bilateral destruction of the SCN are able to anticipate a limited daily phase of food availability. The food-entrainable oscillator is apparent as a pronounced increase in activity that anticipates the daily time of restricted food availability and that free runs for several cycles before damping out when *ad libitum* feeding conditions are renewed. The data indicate the existence of a circadian system that is entrainable to limited food access and is both anatomically and functionally distinct from the light-entrainable SCN. However, this phenomenon has been demonstrated only in the rat, and the anatomic locus of this extra-SCN circadian system is unknown.

NEURAL TRANSPLANTATION AND THE SCN AS CIRCADIAN PACEMAKER

SCN homografts restore circadian rhythms to arrhythmic hosts. Neural transplantation procedures have become a powerful tool for evaluating the functional role of brain structures and recently have been used to address the autonomy of the SCN as the circadian pacemaker in rodents. Several laboratories have been successful in restoring circadian rhythmicity to arrhythmic animals by the technique of *homograft transplantation* (i.e., transplantation between donors and hosts of the same species). Embryonic hypothalamic tissue containing the SCN is implanted in the third ventricle of rats or hamsters rendered arrhythmic by SCN lesioning, and within weeks of the implantation surgery circadian

rhythmicity is recovered. These findings are consistent with previous work implicating the SCN as the circadian pacemaker in rodents. However, these experiments cannot discern whether the implanted SCN tissue alone is responsible for generating the restored rhythm or whether it establishes functional connections with another circadian oscillator (or oscillators) outside the SCN, forming a coupled pacemaker system responsible for generating circadian behavior.

SCN heterografts determine clock autonomy. To determine whether the donor tissue alone is responsible for restoring circadian rhythmicity to SCN-lesioned hosts, *heterograft transplantation* (between donors and hosts of different species) has been conducted. Since the period of the circadian rhythm of activity is species-typical, the period of the restored rhythm in heterograft experiments can be used to determine whether the donor, the host, or an interaction between donor and host is responsible for the restored circadian behavior. Therefore, the demonstration that mouse SCN implanted in arrhythmic SCN-lesioned hamsters establishes circadian activity with a mouse-typical period (Fig. 9) suggests that the SCN determines this species-typical characteristic of circadian rhythmicity and thus acts as an autonomous circadian pacemaker in the mouse. However, rat SCN implanted in SCN-lesioned hamsters restores circadian rhythmicity with a period significantly shorter than that of an intact rat (Fig. 10). It appears, therefore, that the SCN alone is not sufficient to determine the rat's species-typical circadian period and that it is not the autonomous circadian pacemaker in the rat circadian system. Rather, in this species, it seems that the SCN is one component of a multioscillator pacemaking system, an interpretation consistent with the evidence for an extra-SCN food-entrainable circadian oscillator in the rat.

Species differences in the organization of the circadian system are not limited to mammals and are well documented among non-mammalian vertebrates. Circadian oscilla-

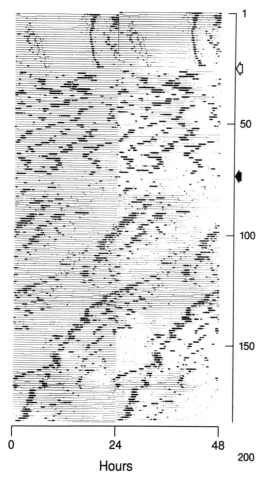

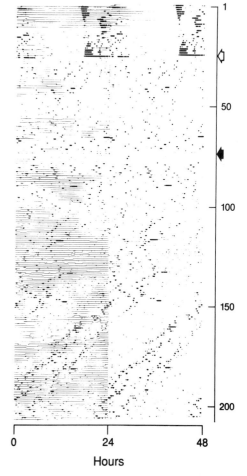

abolishes circadian activity rhythms. A similar procedure in several other species of birds and lizards merely induces a change in the period of the free-running circadian activity rhythm, while pinealectomy has no effect at all on the circadian locomotor rhythm in the desert iguana (*Dipsosaurus dorsalis*). Thus it is clear that the organization of the circadian system in many species (mammals and non-

FIG. 9. Hamster wheel-running activity record (double-plotted). Animal was maintained in constant dim red light. On the day indicated by the upper arrow, the suprachiasmatic nucleus (SCN) was lesioned and the circadian rhythm of wheel running disrupted. On the day indicated by the lower arrow, fetal mouse hypothalamic tissue containing the SCN was implanted in the lesion site. Soon after the transplantation surgery the circadian rhythm of wheel running was restored with a mouse-typical period.

FIG. 10. Hamster wheel-running activity record (double-plotted). On the day indicated by the upper arrow, the suprachiasmatic nucleus (SCN) was lesioned, resulting in the disruption of the circadian rhythm of wheel running. On the day indicated by the lower arrow, fetal rat hypothalamic tissue containing the SCN was implanted in the lesion site. The restoration of circadian activity is clearly evident although the period of the activity rhythm is not rat-typical.

tors of lizards and birds are located in several different loci including the hypothalamus, the eyes, and the pineal gland. The importance of each of these sites in regulating circadian activity rhythms varies considerably among species. For example, removal of the pineal gland in several species of passerine birds and in the lizard *Anolis carolinensis* mammals) is quite distinct and may range from a single, autonomous circadian pacemaker in the SCN to a hierarchically organized, multioscillatory system in which the position of the individual component oscillators in the hierarchy varies among species. Indeed, as Winfree speculated, the ubiquity of circadian systems in the biological world suggests that natural selection may have favored those individuals whose internal dynamics matched the planet's daily rotation regardless of the precise mechanism that may have evolved to do so.

PINEAL GLAND

The pineal gland is an important component of the circadian system. The pineal gland of almost all vertebrates rhythmically produces the hormone melatonin and releases it into the circulation (the armadillo being one notable exception). Circulating se-

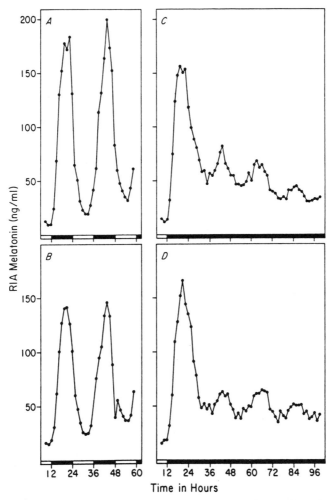

FIG. 11. Comparison of the rhythms of melatonin release from chick pineals maintained in vitro. The light treatments are indicated at the bottom of each panel. **A** and **B** are two individual pineals from a 60-hr LD 12:12 experiment. **C** and **D** are two individual pineals from a 96-hr experiment in constant conditions (dim red light). From Takahashi JS, Hamm HE, Menaker M. *Proc Natl Acad Sci USA* 1980;77:2319.

rotonin (see Chapter 6) is rapidly converted to melatonin in the pineal by a two-step process that results in high nighttime levels and low daytime levels. In nonmammalian vertebrates such as birds and lizards, the pineal is not dependent on neural connections from the brain and remains both rhythmic and photosensitive in vitro (Fig. 11). Rhythmic melatonin secretion from isolated pineals and from dispersed pineal cell cultures can persist for several cycles in constant darkness, thereby establishing the endogenous nature of the circadian rhythm in the pineal. The photosensitive nature of nonmammalian pineals is indicated by the entrainment of melatonin secretion from pineals maintained in vitro under light/dark cycles. In addition, light administered to the pineal either in vivo or in vitro during the dark phase of the light/dark cycle, when melatonin levels are high, induces a very rapid drop in melatonin production.

In contrast, the SCN in mammals, including humans, is responsible for maintaining circadian rhythmicity in the secretion of pineal melatonin. Disruption of the neural pathway from the SCN to the pineal anywhere along its multisynaptic route abolishes the circadian rhythm of melatonin secretion; the mammalian pineal is therefore a passive oscillator driven by the SCN (Fig. 12).

Melatonin is secreted during the dark portion of the day/night cycle, and consequently the length of the night is reflected by the duration of melatonin secretion; as day length changes with the seasons, so does the duration of nocturnal melatonin secretion. Many animals have developed mechanisms whereby the duration of elevated melatonin levels in the circulation serves as a signal for the modulation of several hypothalamic neuroendocrine systems (see Chapter 9). For example, in the autumn, when day length falls below a critical threshold (12.5 hr light per day for the golden hamster), the lengthening pulse of melatonin secretion effects a shutdown of the reproductive system by reducing the secretion of luteinizing hormone–releasing hormone (LHRH) from the hypo-

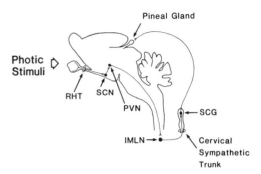

FIG. 12. Summary of the neural circuit controlling the circadian rhythm of pineal melatonin release. Photic signals are transmitted from the retina to the suprachiasmatic nucleus (SCN) by the retinohypothalamic tract (RHT). Efferent fibers exiting the SCN dorsocaudally innervate the hypothalamic paraventricular nucleus (PVN), which projects monosynaptically to sympathetic preganglionic neurons in the intermediolateral nucleus (IMLN) of the spinal cord; preganglionic fibers enter the cervical sympathetic trunk and synapse on postganglionic neurons in the superior cervical ganglion (SCG). Postganglionic fibers from SCG neurons exit the SCG via the internal carotid nerve and innervate the pineal gland. Disruption of any component of this circuit beginning with the SCN abolishes the circadian rhythm of pineal melatonin secretion. From Pickard GE, Turek FW. *J Comp Physiol* A 1985; 156:803.

thalamus. Thus, by monitoring the circadian rhythm of melatonin secretion, mammals can predict or anticipate the changing seasons and turn off their reproductive systems before the onset of winter when conditions become less than optimal for the survival of their young.

RELATION OF THE HUMAN CIRCADIAN SYSTEM TO MENTAL DISORDERS

The acute ill effects suffered from flying across multiple time zones and the adverse physiological and mental effects associated with shift work schedules (in which 15% to 25% of the work force in Western industrial countries is engaged) can be attributed to alterations in the phase of the endogenous circadian system. This results in a transient internal temporal dissociation or a lack of synchronization among various bodily rhythms. The causal connection between the circadian system and mental disorders is, however, much harder to demonstrate, despite the fact that rhythmicity has long been thought related to psychiatric illnesses.

Sleep disturbances are associated with depression. The relationship between depression and alterations in sleep has been known for centuries and is well documented: disturbances in the duration (total sleep time), timing (latency to first REM, or rapid eye movement, sleep), and continuity of sleep (increased wakefulness) are among the most common symptoms in depression (see Chapter 17). In addition, sleep deprivation can induce short-lived remission of depression. Chronobiological considerations have increasingly been applied both to theories of normal sleep physiology (see Chapter 10) and to hypotheses about the pathophysiology of depression.

One hypothesis that has been proposed to account for the relationship between sleep and depression suggests an abnormal phase relationship between two circadian oscillators, one controlling REM sleep and body temperature and the other controlling the sleep/wake cycle. The body temperature rhythm is suggested to be advanced relative to sleep in depressives (phase advance hypothesis). The clinical evidence available is not entirely consistent with this hypothesis and there now appears to be no need to propose that different circadian oscillators regulate body temperature and sleep in humans (see above).

Borbély has offered another hypothesis concerning the relationship between sleep and depression based on the assumption that two separate processes underlie normal sleep regulation. One process is determined by sleep and waking (process S), whereas the other is controlled by a circadian oscillator (process C), independent of the sleep/wake cycle. The model suggests that sleep propensity is determined by a combination of both processes. Process S is hypothesized to be a factor reflecting increased propensity to sleep as duration of prior wakefulness increases; process C reflects the circadian propensity to sleep at various times around the clock.

Some investigators have suggested that process S is deficient or accumulates slowly in the depressed state. This hypothesis does not require multiple circadian oscillators controlling different functions and is consistent with a large body of data. For example, it is well known that sleep and sleep propensity are not determined exclusively by prior waking time. A clear demonstration of this is found in the example of a man who stayed awake for 11 days and then slept only 14 hr. Moreover, a circadian rhythm in sleep propensity is well documented; in temporal isolation, major sleep episodes occur around the minimum of core body temperature (the circadian rhythm of core body temperature is used as a phase indicator). The circadian system may therefore play an indirect role in depression although there is still much to be learned about the relationship between sleep, circadian rhythms, and depression.

Phototherapy can be an effective treatment for seasonal affective disorder. A form of cyclic depression that recurs annually during the winter was recognized several years ago. Winter depression, or *seasonal affective disorder* (SAD), is characterized by lethargy, sleep disturbances, carbohydrate craving, weight gain, and clinical depression. *Phototherapy* (treatment with bright light) has been shown to be a dramatic, noninvasive therapeutic treatment for SAD patients.

Interest in the application of phototherapy to patients with SAD was stimulated by the discovery of Lewy and coworkers in 1980 that nocturnal melatonin secretion in humans could be suppressed by bright light but not by ordinary room light. When it was later realized that only bright light had antidepressant effects on SAD patients, it was hypothesized that phototherapy exerted its antidepressant effects by altering melatonin secretion. Since bright light also changes the timing of the onset of melatonin secretion in humans, as it does in animals, it has been suggested that SAD is a result of an abnormality of the circadian system.

If the circadian system plays a primary role in SAD, the timing of light application would be an important aspect of the mechanism of phototherapy (i.e., the antidepressant effects of light treatment should be phase-dependent). However, the available evidence indicates that SAD patients respond equally well to light presented in the morning and evening. It would seem apparent that current simple models fail to adequately explain either the pathophysiology of SAD or the mechanism of action of phototherapy. The influence of the changing seasons on human affect and the mechanisms by which phototherapy can offset these seasonal changes await further understanding.

SUMMARY

Biological rhythms in the 24-hr range are a fundamental property of nature. Considerable progress has been made in identifying the components of the circadian system in mammals. The suprachiasmatic nucleus of the hypothalamus is a vital component of the circadian system and functions as an autonomous circadian pacemaker in at least some animals. The SCN pacemaker is entrained to the environmental day/night cycle via direct projections from the retina. This pathway is both necessary and sufficient to synchronize the endogenous circadian system to the external day/night cycle.

Resetting the phase of the circadian system can produce a constellation of effects described as "jet lag." In addition, symptoms similar to jet lag are experienced by shift workers. While the role of the circadian system in affective disorders remains to be established, the application of phototherapy for seasonal affective disorder offers an indica-tion that rational manipulations of the circadian system may have beneficial therapeutic effects.

BIBLIOGRAPHY

Original Articles

Daan S, Beersma DGM, Borbély AA. Timing of human sleep: recovery process gated by a circadian pacemaker. *Am J Physiol* 1984;246:R161–R178.

Inouye S-IT, Kawamura H. Persistence of circadian rhythmicity in a mammalian hypothalamic "island" containing the suprachiasmatic nucleus. *Proc Natl Acad Sci USA* 1979;76:5962–5966.

Lewy AJ, Wehr TA, Goodwin FK, Newsome DA, Markey SP. Light suppresses melatonin secretion in humans. *Science* 1980;210:1267–1269.

Pickard GE, Turek FW. Splitting of the circadian rhythm of activity is abolished by unilateral lesions of the suprachiasmatic nuclei. *Science* 1982;215:1119–1121.

Pittendrigh CS. Circadian rhythms and the circadian organization of living systems. *Cold Spring Harbor Symp Quant Biol* 1960;25:159–184.

Stephan FK, Zucker I. Circadian rhythms in drinking behavior and locomotor activity are eliminated by hypothalamic lesions. *Proc Natl Acad Sci USA* 1972;69:1583–1585.

Zulley J, Campbell SS. Napping behavior during "spontaneous internal desynchronization": sleep remains in synchrony with body temperature. *Human Neurobiol* 1985;4:123–126.

Books and Reviews

Kupfer DJ, Monk TH, Barchas JD, eds. *Biological rhythms and mental disorders.* New York: Guilford Press; 1988.

Rosenwasser AM. Behavioral neurobiology of circadian pacemakers: a comparative perspective. *Progr Psychobiol Physiol Psychol* 1988;13:155–226.

Rusak B, Zucker I. Neural regulation of circadian rhythms. *Physiol Rev* 1979;59:449–526.

Takahashi JS, Zatz M. Regulation of circadian rhythmicity. *Science* 1982;217:1104–1111.

Turek FW. Circadian neural rhythms in mammals. *Annu Rev Physiol* 1985;47:49–64.

Winfree AT. *The timing of biological clocks.* New York: WH Freeman (Scientific American Library); 1987.

12

Learning and Memory
Behavioral Studies

Thomas W. Abrams

The path of the inborn reflex [“unconditioned reflex”] is already completed at birth; but the path of the signalizing reflex [“acquired reflex” or “conditioned reflex”] has still to be completed in the higher nervous centres.

There should be no theoretical objection to the hypothesis of the formation of new physiological paths and new connections within the cerebral hemispheres. Since the especial function of the central nervous system is to establish most complicated and delicate correspondences between the organism and its environment we may not unnaturally expect to find there . . . a highly developed connector system superimposed on a conductor system. . . . Conditioned reflexes are phenomena of common and widespread occurrence: their establishment is an integral function in everyday life. We recognize them in ourselves and in other people or animals under such names as 'education,' 'habits,' and 'training;' and all of these are really nothing more than the results of an establishment of new nervous connections during the post-natal existence of the organism.

I. P. Pavlov,
*Conditioned Reflexes: An Investigation of the Physiological Activity
of the Cerebral Cortex,* 1927
Trans. by G. V. Anrep, ed. (New York: Dover Publications, Inc., 1960, pp. 25–26)

- Learning can be considered as the process by which an animal's behavior is altered as a result of experience.

- There are three recognized forms of nonassociative learning: habituation, sensitization, and dishabituation.

- Habituation is the waning of responses to individual stimuli.

- Sensitization is an enhanced response following preexposure to a particular stimulus.

- Dishabituation is the restoration of a habituated response to one stimulus as a result of the presentation of a second novel stimulus.

- Associative learning is learning about relationships between stimuli.

- In classical conditioning, two stimuli are presented in a specific temporal relationship during training so that one stimulus, the conditioned stimulus (CS), provides some information about the occurrence of the second stimulus, the unconditioned stimulus (US or UCS).

- Instrumental conditioning occurs when the presentation of a stimulus depends on the performance of a particular behavior by the subject.

- Higher order features of classical conditioning are not restricted to higher animals.

- There are two principal schools of thought about how memory is presented in the brain using, respectively, cellular or diffuse models.

- Neural changes may be distributed throughout an entire neuron or restricted to a specific synapse.

- Identification of the cellular locus of plastic changes is an important challenge.

This chapter gives a brief introduction to the study of learning and provides a behavioral context for the material in Chapter 13, which considers biophysical and biochemical mechanisms of neural plasticity (i.e., alteration of neuronal properties) during learning. Because progress in understanding cellular mechanisms of learning has occurred in the context of studies of very simple forms of learning, this chapter focuses on simple forms of nonassociative and associative learning. The last section of the chapter discusses the general types of neural mechanisms that are theoretically likely to contribute to learning.

Learning about events or stimuli in the world enables individual organisms to adapt their behavioral responses to changing environmental circumstances. Mechanisms that allow behavioral adaptation within an animal's lifetime are so fundamentally important for success that they appeared early in evolution and are present in virtually all species with central nervous systems. *Learning can be considered as the process by which an animal's behavioral response is altered as a result of experience.* In general, in experimental studies of learning, an animal is provided with a controlled experience, and its behavior is assessed at a later time; if its behavior at the assessment time is altered as a function of the experience during training, then learning may have occurred. In order to determine whether behavior at the assessment time is altered as a function of the particular experience during training, it is necessary to compare the behavior of control groups of animals that are treated differently during the training period but are tested under identical circumstances at the assessment time. Obviously, the careful design of control group treatments is critical for conclusions about the nature of learning.

Biological Bases of Brain Function and Disease, edited by Alan Frazer, Perry B. Molinoff, and Andrew Winokur. Raven Press, Ltd., New York © 1994.

SIMPLE FORMS OF LEARNING

Three Forms of Nonassociative Learning: Habituation, Sensitization, and Dishabituation

Habituation

Nonassociative changes in behavioral response occur as the result of the presentation of a single stimulus and can be considered the most elementary forms of learning. In one class of nonassociative behavioral plasticity, the repeated presentation of a particular stimulus during the training period results in a decreased response to the same stimulus at the assessment time. For example, the startle response produced by a sound is reduced if an animal has received repeated prior presentations of the sound. *Such waning of responses to individual stimuli is termed* habituation. If the stimulus presentation is terminated, the habituated response gradually recovers (Fig. 1A). Habituation shows stimulus specificity. When responses to one particular stimulus decline substantially after this stimulus is presented repeatedly, responses to another stimulus that differs only slightly in intensity or location may show much less reduction.

Despite showing stimulus specificity, habituation is not considered by some psycholo-

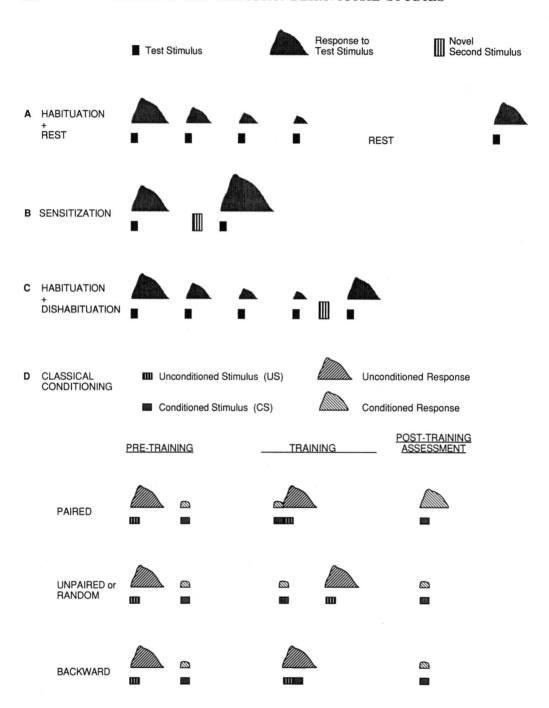

gists to represent true learning. However, from a mechanistic point of view, a decline in responsiveness, even if it occurs at a peripheral locus in sensory neurons, need not be fundamentally different from decreases in responsiveness of a central neuron or central synapse; in some cases, the underlying mechanisms could be identical.

It should be noted that while most studies of habituation are designed to present only a single stimulus, some authors have emphasized that the presentation of the habituating stimulus occurs in some particular experimental context or setting. An animal may actually be learning about a relationship between the stimulus and the context. Habituation effects have been found to be reduced if the animal is tested in a second setting. Thus, even habituation may involve the formation of associations.

Sensitization

Preexposure to a particular stimulus can also result in an effect opposite to that of habituation, namely, enhancement of subsequent responses. Such enhancement is termed sensitization. There are two types of sensitization, depending on whether the test stimulus is identical to or distinct from the sensitizing stimulus. Presentation of one stimulus may in some cases result in an enhancement of the response when the same stimulus is presented subsequently. For example, the mobbing response of some birds to a predator is transiently increased in birds that were recently exposed to the predator. Alternatively, presentation of an independent stimulus may produce an augmentation of the response to the test stimulus (Fig. 1B). Many protective reflex responses to relatively innocuous test stimuli are enhanced after the presentation of a more threatening or stronger stimulus. Sensitization generally shows less stimulus specificity than habituation, increasing the animal's responsiveness to a variety of stimuli.

Dishabituation

Dishabituation is the restoration of a habituated response to one stimulus as a result of the presentation of a second novel stimulus. It is similar to sensitization except that the response to the test stimulus is first decremented by repeated presentations of this stimulus prior to the presentation of another novel stimulus (Fig. 1C). Dishabituation could represent an elimination of habituation (reversal of the habituation process) or it could simply represent sensitization in an instance where the response to the test stimulus has been previously depressed. Even if dishabituation involves a second mechanism that reverses habituation, stimuli that produce dishabituation could simultaneously trigger sensitization; thus, the enhancement of a decremented response could be the result of two processes.

FIG. 1. Simple forms of nonassociative and associative learning. **A**: Habituation and recovery. When a test stimulus is delivered repeatedly, the animal's response to the stimulus declines gradually. After habituation, the response recovers to the initial control level if there is a rest period without stimulation. **B**: Sensitization. The response to a test stimulus is enhanced when tested following the presentation of a second novel or strong stimulus. **C**: Dishabituation. After habituation, the response to a test stimulus recovers, at least partially, following the presentation of a second novel or strong stimulus. **D**: Classical conditioning. Before training, the unconditioned stimulus (US) elicits the unconditioned response, while the conditioned stimulus (CS) elicits either no response or a different response. After CS-US pairing during training, in which the CS is repeatedly presented shortly before the US, the animal's response to the CS is altered. Note that the conditioned response to the CS during the post-training assessment period is not identical to the response to the US; in fact, the two responses may be quite different. The change in the response to the CS is associative as it requires the appropriate pairing of the CS and US. If the two stimuli are presented unpaired or in a random temporal relationship, the response to the CS is either not altered or is changed differently than with CS-US pairing. Backward pairing, in most paradigms, does not result in the same associative change as forward pairing.

Associative Learning: Learning About Relationships

Associative learning is learning about relationships between stimuli. The two most widely studied forms of associative learning are classical, or Pavlovian, conditioning and instrumental, or operant, conditioning. In classical conditioning, an animal learns about relationships between stimuli. In instrumental conditioning, an animal learns about relationships between its behavior and a stimulus. Of the various forms of associative learning, classical conditioning seems to offer the greatest promise for analysis of underlying neural mechanisms and is most extensively studied by neuroscientists at present. In addition, some neurobiological investigations of learning utilize instrumental tasks, such as spatial learning paradigms, which are discussed later in this chapter.

Classical Conditioning

In classical conditioning, two stimuli are presented in a specific temporal relationship during training so that one stimulus, the conditioned stimulus (CS), provides some information about the occurrence of the second stimulus, the unconditioned stimulus (US or UCS). Later, the animal is presented with the CS alone to determine whether its response to the CS has changed (Fig. 1D). In most traditional classical conditioning paradigms, prior to training, the CS has relatively little biological significance whereas the US is a biologically important stimulus that produces an unconditioned response (UR or UCR). During training, the CS is presented immediately prior to the US. The animal comes to know that the CS predicts the occurrence of the US and responds appropriately; thus, after training, when the CS is presented alone, it elicits a conditioned response that it did not elicit before. The Russian physiologist Ivan Pavlov, in his earliest conditioning experiments on dogs, used a "neutral stimulus," the sound of a metronome, as a CS, and food, which evoked an innate salivation reflex, as a US. After the metronome had been paired several times with the food, the sound alone was able to elicit salivation. Thus the dog learned that the metronome predicted the arrival of food.

Although the learned response to the CS, the conditioned response, often resembles the unconditioned response to the US, this is not always the case. For example, in conditioned suppression paradigms, a tone is paired with shock during training. When presented alone after training, the tone now results in a cessation of activity; in contrast, the shock alone results in a large increase in activity. One might interpret such a response in conditioned suppression to indicate that after the tone the animal is anticipating the shock, waiting immobile in a state of "fear."

Instrumental Conditioning

Instrumental conditioning occurs when the presentation of a stimulus depends on the performance of a particular behavior by the subject. In instrumental conditioning, the presentation of a stimulus depends on the performance of a particular behavior by the animal. This contrasts with classical conditioning in which the presentation of the CS and US occur independently of the animal's behavior. For example, in some instrumental conditioning paradigms, the appropriate response by an animal can result in delivery of food or avoidance of shock. Such stimuli act as rewards or reinforcers of a behavioral response. During the training period, the animal learns the relationship between its response and a reinforcer; as a result of this training, the probability of a response is altered when measured at the assessment time.

The Nature of What Is Learned During Classical Conditioning

During the 60 years since the time of Pavlov, studies of classical conditioning have revealed it to be a far richer and more complex form of learning than once was appreciated.

If one is to attempt to analyze the neural mechanisms underlying conditioning, it is important to understand in more depth what animals learn about relationships during conditioning. Indeed, it is a serious challenge for a cellular analysis of conditioning to account for the various features of conditioning described below.

1. Conditioning depends on how informative the CS is about occurrence of the US— contiguity is not sufficient. Pavlov originally found that the CS should begin before and overlap temporally with the US for effective conditioning to occur. Thus, temporal contiguity was believed to be critical for an animal to learn to associate the CS with the US. Numerous studies have now demonstrated that it is not contiguity, but contingency, or how well the CS predicts US occurrence, that determines whether conditioning will result. Two experimental examples powerfully illustrate this feature of conditioning:

a. *Unannounced USs degrade learning.* The American psychologist Robert Rescorla analyzed the effects of extra unpaired USs on learning. He used a conditioned suppression paradigm in which a tone, the CS, by being paired with a shock, the US, comes to elicit a cessation of behavior, a conditioned "fear" response; rats anticipating shock remain immobile. Rescorla demonstrated that even when the number of shocks paired with tones remained constant, learning decreased with increasing numbers of extra shocks not preceded by CSs. Thus learning is proportional to how well the CS predicts the occurrence of the US. In an analogous manner, preexposure to the US before CS-US pairing begins greatly reduces the conditioning produced by pairing. The unannounced US makes the CS a poorer signal of the US occurrence.

b. *Kamin blocking effect.* Using a compound CS consisting of two simultaneous stimuli, Leon Kamin demonstrated blocking of conditioning to the second CS when

one of the CSs had previously signaled the US. In Kamin's protocol, a noise was paired with a shock in phase I of training. Then, in phase II, the noise was delivered together with a light prior to the shock. Rats showed no behavioral suppression to the light alone. In contrast, control rats that were conditioned to the compound CS, without prior training with noise paired with shock, showed a conditioned fear response to either the sound or the light alone. Thus, for animals that had received prior noise-shock training and for which the noise effectively predicted the shock, the light provided no additional information and could not effectively serve as a CS.

2. Pairing is usually effective only if the CS and US occur together within a particular temporal window and in the appropriate sequence. With each particular conditioning paradigm there is a narrow range of interstimulus intervals for effective CS-US pairing. In most forms of classical conditioning, CS onset must precede US onset if the animal is to learn the predictive relationship. Thus in many paradigms, simultaneous or backward pairing of the two stimuli is relatively ineffective despite the fact that there is temporal contiguity (Fig. 2). Backward pairing sometimes results in conditioned inhibition—a reduction in the probability that the conditioned response will be elicited by the CS; because with backward pairing, the CS precedes relatively long periods without a US, it comes to signal US-free periods for the animal. This sequence requirement for effective CS-US pairing is consistent with the concept that learning depends on how informative the CS is. One of the most puzzling aspects of the interstimulus interval function from a mechanistic point of view is that the optimal interval for effective pairing may shift if the interval between pairing trials is altered. Thus, the window for effective pairing appears to be relative rather than absolute.

3. Conditioning may involve learning relationships between two "neutral" stimuli that

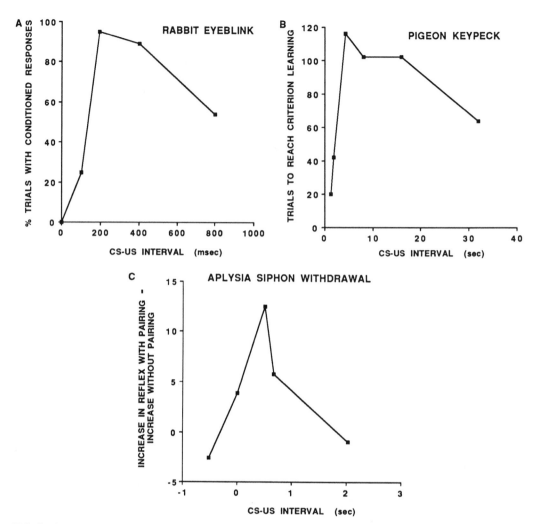

FIG. 2. Dependence of associative learning on interstimulus interval for three classical conditioning paradigms. **A**: Interstimulus interval function for conditioning of rabbit eye blink in which tone (CS) is paired with puff to the eye (US). **B**: Interstimulus interval function for conditioning of pigeon keypeck in which illumination of a key (CS) is paired with food (US). **C**: Interstimulus interval function for conditioning of *Aplysia* siphon withdrawal in which a weak siphon touch (CS) is paired with a tail shock (US). In each graph, the ordinate represents some measure of the relative amount of associative learning as a function of the interval between the CS and US. Notice that both simultaneous onset of CS and US and backward presentations of the two stimuli (US onset preceding CS onset) produce relatively poor associative learning. Notice too that the optimum interval for CS-US pairing varies substantially with the paradigm used. From Rescorla RA. Behavioral studies of Pavlovian conditioning. *Ann Rev Neurosci* 1988;11:329-352 and Abrams TW, Kandel ER. Is contiguity detection in classical conditioning a system or a cellular property? Learning in *Aplysia* suggests a possible molecular site. *Trends Neurosci* 1988;11:128-135.

initially lack biological significance. Conditioning has been achieved with two initially neutral CSs using two-phase conditioning paradigms, in both second-order conditioning and sensory preconditioning. In second-order conditioning, during phase I of training, CS_1 is paired with the US. During phase II, CS_2 is paired with CS_1, which now effectively functions as a US. When tested subsequently, CS_2 evokes the same conditioned response that CS_1 produced after being paired with the US in phase I. In sensory preconditioning, the reciprocal pairing sequence is utilized. In phase I, two neutral CSs are paired with one another. In phase II, CS_1 is paired with the US. When tested during the assessment period, CS_2 is able to elicit the same conditioned response as CS_1, indicating that the animal has learned a relationship between the two CSs in phase I.

Higher order features of classical conditioning are not restricted to higher animals. Although many of the special features that characterize classical conditioning in vertebrates suggest relatively sophisticated cognitive processing of information, many of these same higher order features of classical conditioning have also been observed in invertebrates with simple nervous systems. For example, Christie Sahley and Alan Gelperin found that food avoidance conditioning in the garden slug *Limax* shows a number of higher order features seen in vertebrates. Pairing of carrot or potato odor with contact with a bitter-tasting quinidine solution resulted in these garden slugs avoiding the paired odor. *Limax* showed Kamin blocking, very similar to that seen in rats: after slugs were trained with carrot odor paired with quinidine, they failed to learn to avoid potato odor when potato odor and carrot odor were presented simultaneously paired with quinidine in the second phase of training. *Limax* also showed reduced conditioning if they were preexposed to the US, quinidine, before being trained with carrot odor paired with quinidine. Thus, as in vertebrates, the magnitude of associative learning was dependent on how well the CS predicted the occurrence of the US.

The marine snail *Aplysia californica* has been used extensively to study simple forms of nonassociative and associative learning. In classical conditioning of the defensive withdrawal reflex of *Aplysia,* presentation of unannounced USs block conditioning. Moreover, for the snails to learn the relationship between the CS and the US, the two must be paired in a precise temporal manner. The US must follow the CS within a brief time window of approximately 1 sec (Fig. 2C). Interestingly, as in many vertebrate conditioning paradigms, there is a sequence requirement that the CS begin first. Backward pairing, even with substantial temporal overlap, results in no associative learning; moreover, simultaneous presentation of the two stimuli is much less effective than if there is a 0.5-sec delay before US onset. Thus, even in these simple marine snails, learning about relations between the CS and US depends on how informative the CS is.

GENERAL ASPECTS OF THE NEURAL BASIS OF LEARNING

Cellular vs. Diffuse Models of How Information Is Stored in the Mammalian Brain

There are two principal schools of thought about how memory is presented in the brain using, respectively, cellular or diffuse models. For much of this century there have been two schools of thought concerning how memories are represented in the brain. One school originated with the speculations of early neuroanatomists at the end of the nineteenth century. Lugaro, Tanzi, and Ramon y Cajal, after observing morphological changes in synaptic structures during embryonic development, hypothesized that learning could result from similar alterations in synaptic connections between neurons. An alternative point of view was advocated by neuroscientists such as Karl Lashley and E. Roy John, who believed that information responsible for learned behaviors is represented diffusely throughout the cortex. The original arguments for diffuse memory storage came from ablation experiments such as those of Lashley in which relatively large areas of cortex were removed. No single ablation eliminated all of a particular memory. Lashley believed that there was no relationship between memory impairment and the location of a lesion;

he found that the deficit was simply proportional to the amount of cortex removed, suggesting that all of the cortex was equivalent or "equipotential." In his influential review article "In Search of the Engram," Lashley concluded that there was no localized engram, or memory trace, to be found and that "well-defined conditioned reflex paths" (neural pathways) did not underlie learned behaviors. He stated that "It is not possible to demonstrate the isolated localization of a memory trace anywhere within the nervous system. The engram is represented throughout" either a substantial region of the cortex or the entire cortex.

A more recent proponent of the diffuse memory perspective has been E. Roy John. Based on the earlier lesion studies and on findings from relatively crude electrophysiology, John argued that learning does not result from the "establishment or facilitation" of a specific series of synaptic connections. He was strongly impressed by the observation that responses of individual cortical neurons to sensory stimuli are commonly variable and that many cortical neurons are "nonspecific" in that they are broadly tuned (i.e., they are excitable by a range of stimuli). In contrast, John found that population responses (or field potentials), recorded from substantial amounts of neural tissue, correlated well with sensory stimuli and with learning. John believed that these field potentials were emergent phenomena unrelated to individual neurons or individual synapses. Instead, he proposed that field potentials represent electrical activity that is somehow synchronized throughout the brain. He argued that learning is based on "the establishment of temporal patterns of ensemble activity, rather than the elaboration of new pathways or connections." Clearly, John's position is the antithesis of the view that learning results from changes in neuronal or synaptic properties.

Both Lashley and John came to logical, though extreme conclusions from their experimental results. Based on the results of extensive neurobiological studies since the time of Lashley, there are now alternative views of how information is represented in the mammalian brain; diffuse memory storage need not be invoked to explain the results of Lashley and John. In particular, two aspects of the functional organization of the mammalian brain are relevant to an understanding of their findings.

1. Multiple representations of information. Many types of information are processed in parallel in multiple areas of the cortex. This does not imply, however, that all information is represented in a diffuse manner everywhere in the brain. Rather, there are specific regions in which particular types of information are represented. For instance, there are at least 15 maps of visual space in different regions of the cortex, though the precise type of visual information in each region may vary. Moreover, within a given region, different subareas or different populations of neurons may code different types of information. For example, in area 17 of the visual cortex, different sites respond to different regions of the visual field; within a given area, neurons differ in their preferences for stimulus orientation or direction of movement. Similarly, in the somatosensory system, different parts of the body are mapped onto different locations of the postcentral gyrus in cortex. Like visual maps, these somatosensory maps are highly specific, such that even different regions of a single digit are mapped to slightly different sites within the cortex; for example, adjacent phalanges are represented by groups of neurons approximately 400 μm apart. Thus, although a given type of sensory or motor information is represented in multiple regions of cortex, these representations are often quite specific.

2. Populations of neurons code information or behaviors. According to our current understanding of cortical organization, single cortical neurons do not represent complex stimuli or produce movements or behaviors. Rather, populations of active neurons represent events and determine behavior. Moreover, in many areas of the cortex and other areas of the brain, neurons have broadly tuned responses in that they can be activated by a range of stimuli. However, the fact that neurons are coarsely tuned does not mean that they are nonspecific as John believed. Instead, the profile of neuronal activity within a population differs dramatically depending on the stimulus or movement represented. Computer models reveal that large populations of neurons with broadly tuned responses can represent information very efficiently and produce very accurate behavioral responses. The strategy of having complex information represented in a distributed fashion by substantial populations of neurons makes the output of the nervous system relatively consistent and accurate, and insensitive to variability or jitter in the activity of individual neurons.

These two features of cortical neural organization—multiple representations in different regions and coarse tuning of many cortical neurons—were misunderstood by Lashley and John. Their conclusion that information and memories are represented diffusely in some form that is independent of individual neurons or synapses is undoubtedly incorrect. A more widely accepted model today is that information is represented by large populations of neurons and vast numbers of synapses. *Changes in behavior as a result of experience are probably a consequence of changes in the properties of substantial numbers of individual neurons and very large numbers of synapses: this phenomenon is termed* neural plasticity.

Interestingly, Wolff Singer and Charles Gray recently found that cortical visual neurons responding to a single object tend to fire in oscillatory patterns that are transiently synchronized. This transient synchronization of oscillations may temporarily link together large arrays of neurons involved in processing related information. This observation that oscillatory firing may be synchronized across cortical areas does not mean that the response properties of individual neurons are nonspecific; rather, it simply means that complex information is processed by large arrays of neurons acting in concert.

Classes of Neural Plasticity

Neural changes may be distributed throughout an entire neuron or restricted to a specific synapse. A substantial variety of neural changes may contribute to the behavioral changes produced by experience (Fig. 3). In the case of a cell-wide change, the plasticity could influence excitability, synaptic interactions, or both. Changes that affect synaptic transmission could be localized to either the pre- or the postsynaptic cell (Fig. 3). Obviously, multiple plastic mechanisms could occur in various combinations. For example, a high-frequency burst of action potentials in a presynaptic neuron could, in principle, result in (1) an enhancement of transmitter release from this neuron, (2) an increase in postsynaptic sensitivity to transmitter, and (3) an increase in postsynaptic excitability—all at the same time. From a conceptual point of view, alteration of a synapse is a more appealing candidate for a neural mechanism of learning than a change in excitability. While a change in excitability influences a neuron's response to all synaptic inputs, a change in synaptic transmission, whether it is due to a pre- or a postsynaptic modification, has the possibility of being localized to a single synapse. Such plasticity at selected synaptic connections could mediate highly specific types of learning.

The neuronal activity responsible for triggering an alteration in a neural pathway might occur either within the pathway that undergoes the change or within a modulatory pathway that causes neurons in a second pathway to undergo the modification. These two alternatives are termed *homosynaptic* and *heterosynaptic plasticity,* respectively. Modification of a pathway by activity in the pathway itself could occur simply as a consequence of spike activity, perhaps because of the accumulation of Ca^{++} entering through voltage-sensitive Ca^{++} channels; such Ca^{++} elevation could influence either excitability

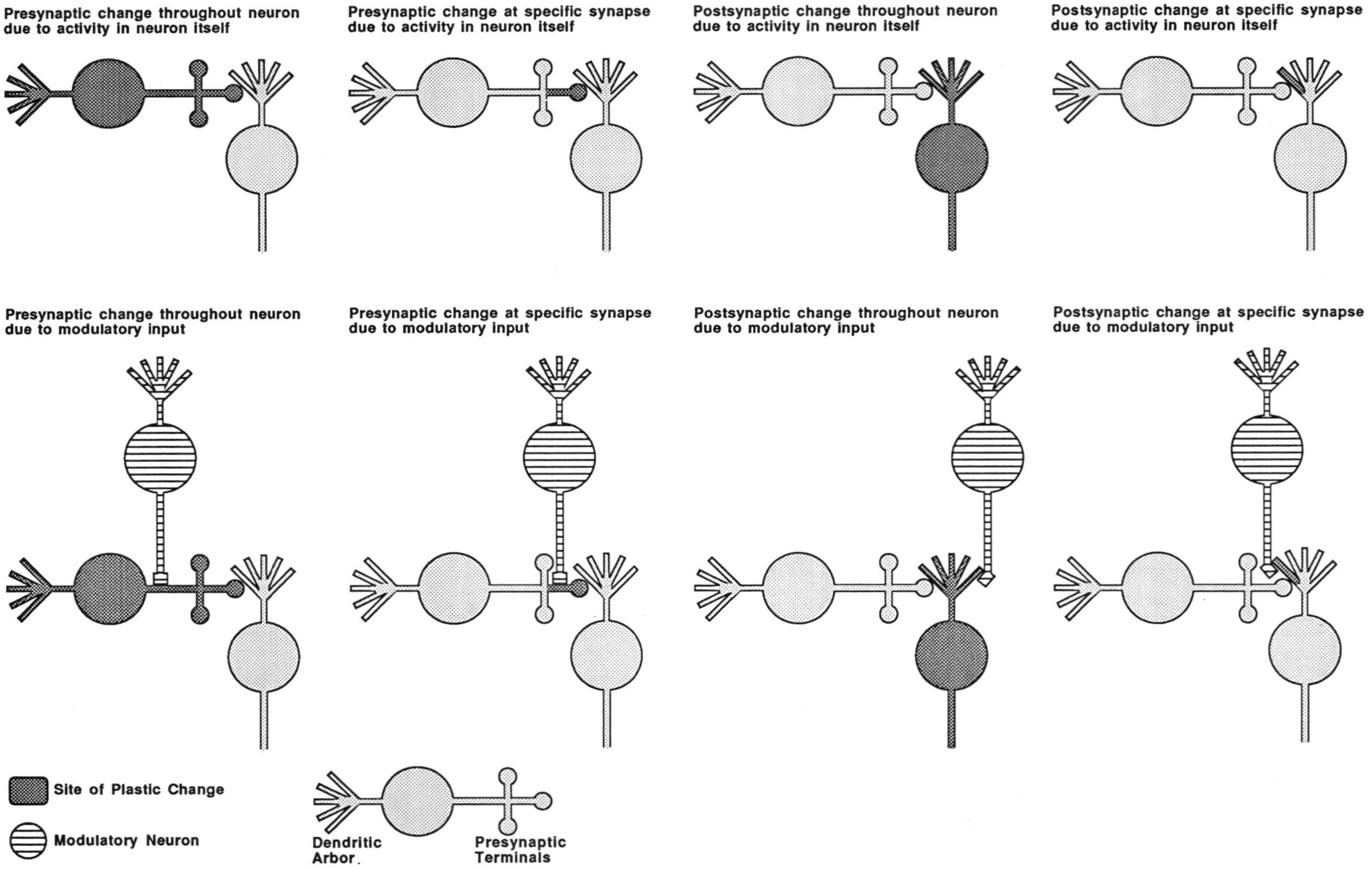

Presynaptic change throughout neuron due to activity in neuron itself

Presynaptic change at specific synapse due to activity in neuron itself

Postsynaptic change throughout neuron due to activity in neuron itself

Postsynaptic change at specific synapse due to activity in neuron itself

Presynaptic change throughout neuron due to modulatory input

Presynaptic change at specific synapse due to modulatory input

Postsynaptic change throughout neuron due to modulatory input

Postsynaptic change at specific synapse due to modulatory input

Dendritic Arbor

Presynaptic Terminals

Site of Plastic Change

Modulatory Neuron

or transmitter release. Alternatively, a synaptic change could be a consequence of the activation of the synapse, such as through the depletion of the releasable pool of transmitter or the desensitization of postsynaptic receptors. A third alternative is that the release of transmitter at synapses within a pathway may activate modulatory receptors as well as conventional receptors. (While conventional receptors produce very transient excitatory or inhibitory currents, modulatory receptors alter neuronal function over longer time periods.) Situations in which the same synapses that produce conventional rapid synaptic potentials also initiate modulatory changes may actually be quite common since many classes of neurons are now known to release both conventional and modulatory transmitters at their synapses; however, there are also known instances where single neurotransmitters activate both conventional excitatory receptors and modulatory receptors at single synapses.

Identification of Neurotransmitters Involved in Learning

It is an important challenge for neurobiologists seeking to understand neural plasticity during learning to specifically identify the cellular locus of changes that occur and to discriminate which neurons are responsible for triggering these changes. The analysis of modulatory factors that initiate neural plasticity is frequently approached with a combination of pharmacological and behavioral techniques. Studies that use a receptor antagonist or that deplete stores of a monoamine neurotransmitter have led to the "identification" of a number of neurotransmitters with central roles in learning. However, it is essential to distinguish permissive effects of a mod-

ulatory transmitter from signaling functions in which a modulatory neurotransmitter acts to initiate plasticity in a neural pathway during learning. In the former case, a modulatory neurotransmitter may be essential for maintaining a neural circuit in an appropriate state so that it is capable of undergoing plastic changes, even though this transmitter may not have a critical signaling function for initiating plasticity during learning. To decide whether a neurotransmitter actually plays a central role during a given instance of neural plasticity, one must first identify which neurons are responsible for initiating the changes.

SUMMARY

The chapter has reviewed simple forms of learning including habituation, sensitization, classical conditioning, and instrumental conditioning. It was emphasized that during conditioning, the animal learns substantially more about the relationship between two paired stimuli than simply temporal contiguity. The chapter then discussed how learned information may be represented in the nervous system. Early models proposed that information is represented in a distributed manner within the central nervous system. More modern views indicate that complex information is indeed processed by large constellations of neurons. Nevertheless, it is clear that these representations depend upon the activity and properties of individual neurons. In principle, there is a wide variety of cellular changes in neurons that may contribute to learning; such changes may be initiated either homosynaptically or heterosynaptically and may be either cell-wide or synapse specific. The following chapter discusses

FIG. 3. Classes of neural plasticity that could contribute to behavioral changes during learning. *Top row:* Plastic changes that result from activity in the pre- and/or postsynaptic neurons themselves. *Bottom row:* Plastic changes that result from input from a modulatory cell. Changes can be localized to either the pre- or postsynaptic neuron, and the changes may be relatively widespread throughout the cell or restricted to a given synapse. For cell-wide changes or for specific postsynaptic changes, either excitability (i.e., initiation of action potentials) or synaptic transmission could be altered. Regions of neuron undergoing plastic change are shown as darker.

some of the specific cellular changes that have been identified during simple forms of learning.

BIBLIOGRAPHY

Original Articles

Sahley C, Rudy JW, Gelperin A. An analysis of associative learning in a terrestrial mollusc. I. Higher-order conditioning, blocking and a transient US pre-exposure effect. *J Comp Physiol* 1981;144:1–8.

Books and Reviews

Hearst E. Fundamentals of learning and conditioning. In: Atkinson RC, Hernstein RJ, Lindzey G, Luce RD, eds. *Steven's handbook of experimental psychology.* 2nd Ed. Vol. 2: *Learning and Cognition.* New York: Wiley; 1988:3–109.

Pavlov IP. *Conditioned reflexes: an investigation of the physiological activity of the cerebral cortex.* Translated and edited by GV Amrep. London: Oxford University Press; 1927.

Rescorla RA. Pavlovian conditioning: it's not what you think it is. *Am Psychologist* 1988;43:151–160.

Squire LR. *Memory and brain.* New York: Oxford University Press; 1987.

13

Learning and Memory
Cellular Studies in Simple Neural Systems

Thomas W. Abrams

The extension, the growth, and the multiplication of the appendages of the neuron do not stop at birth; they continue and nothing is more striking than the difference between the length and the number of the cellular ramifications, of the second and third order, in a newborn and an adult man.

The new cellular extensions do not grow at random; they have to orient themselves according to major neural currents or according to intracellular associations which are the object of repeated action of will. . . .

The ability of the neurons to grow in an adult and their power to create new associations can explain learning and the fact that man can change his ideological systems. Our hypothesis can even explain the conservation of very old memories such as memories from youth in an old man and in an amnesiac or in a mental patient, because the association pathways that have existed for a long time and have been exercised for many years are probably very powerful and were formed at the time when the plasticity of the neuron was at its maximum.

S. Ramón y Cajal,
Histologie du système nerveux (Madrid: Instituto Ramón y Cajal, 1955 ed., pp. 888–890)

▶ Key Concepts ───────────────────────────────

- Neural changes during behavioral plasticity can occur in parallel at multiple neural loci.

- Plasticity in the siphon sensory neuron-to-motor neuron synapse is due to presynaptic changes.

- During sensitization, strong noxious stimuli excite several populations of modulatory interneurons that release at least three or four facilitatory transmitters which act presynaptically to enhance synaptic transmission from the siphon sensory neurons.

- Multiple facilitatory processes in the siphon sensory neurons contribute in parallel to strengthening of the gill and siphon withdrawal reflex during dishabituation and sensitization.

- During sensitization, alterations occur at other neural loci in addition to the sensory neuron-to-motor neuron synapses.

- During long-term sensitization there is a reduction in a K^+ current in sensory neurons, as in short-term sensitization.

- Presynaptic release sites show a change in morphology with long-term learning.

- Protein synthesis is required in a critical time window during and/or shortly after training.

- Cyclic AMP can trigger long-term presynaptic facilitation of sensory neuron-to-motor neuron connections.

- Long-term sensitization is accompanied by persistent activation of the cAMP-dependent protein kinase.

- Long-term potentiation (LTP) has many features that make it a strong candidate for a mechanism of associative learning.

- Hippocampal place cells code for the animal's location in space.

- The response properties of hippocampal place cells must arise through learning.

- LTP is consistent with Hebb's proposal: presynaptic activity must occur coincident with postsynaptic depolarization.

- LTP is triggered by a postsynaptic signal, a rise in intracellular Ca^{++}.

- The NMDA receptor-gated channel allows a transient Ca^{++} rise when activated in an associative manner.

- In the postsynaptic neuron both kinases and proteases may be involved in the induction of LTP cascade.

- If postsynaptic processes are required for initiating LTP, a retrograde messenger must initiate presynaptic enhancement of transmitter release.

- Protein synthesis is required for induction of the late phase of LTP.

■ Chapter Overview ────────────────────────────

This chapter considers three examples of experimental systems in which a cellular approach has been taken. The first system discussed, a flexion reflex in vertebrates mediated by a relatively simple spinal circuit of neurons, was perhaps the earliest preparation in which mechanisms underlying behavioral plasticity were analyzed. Although relatively little is understood about the cellular basis of this form of plasticity, this model illustrates some important issues at the behavioral level, as well as some central problems facing cellular analysis. The second system that is described is the invertebrate marine mollusc *Aplysia californica*, which has been used for the study of the neural basis of learning and behavioral plasticity. The nervous system of this snail is very useful for electrophysiological studies because it contains relatively few neurons. The final system that is considered is a long-lasting form of synaptic strengthening in the hippocampus, termed long-term potentiation (LTP). Since LTP has associative features, it would seem to be a reasonable candidate mechanism for learning.

Ever since the first neuroanatomists examined the fine structure of synaptic regions of the central nervous system, neurobiologists have been intrigued by the possibility that alterations in synaptic connections between neurons could occur as a result of experience. The study of anatomical, cellular, and molecular bases of synaptic changes that underlie behavioral changes during learning remains one of the most exciting and challenging areas of neurobiology today.

Neurobiologists attempting to characterize the neural loci that undergo changes during learning and the neural pathways that are responsible for triggering these changes have found it necessary either to investigate very simple forms of learning in vertebrates, which may be mediated by relatively simple neural circuits, or to study relatively primitive forms of learning in invertebrates with simple nervous systems. During the past decade or two, substantial progress has been made in understanding some of the cellular mechanisms responsible for neural plasticity in these simple systems.

Biological Bases of Brain Function and Disease, edited by Alan Frazer, Perry B. Molinoff, and Andrew Winokur. Raven Press, Ltd., New York © 1994.

PLASTICITY IN A SPINAL FLEXION REFLEX

In 1898, the great British physiologist Charles Sherington first described plasticity in the reflex of a spinal cat (an animal with a transected spinal cord). With repeated stimuli, the flexion response habituated; with rest, it recovered. The American physiologist C. Ladd Prosser subsequently showed that after habituation of the flexion response in the spinal animal, it was possible to cause the flexion response to recover (to dishabituate) with a pinch to the paw. Thus, when neurobiologists later sought to study nonassociative plasticity at the cellular level, they looked for simple reflexes that exhibited plasticity. Alden Spencer, Richard Thompson, and their colleagues carried out a detailed analysis of plasticity in the flexion reflex in cats whose spinal cords had been sectioned at the thoracic level. When flexion of the hindleg was elicited by weak electrical stimuli to the skin, the response decremented dramatically if the skin stimulus was presented at 10-sec intervals; with longer intervals of 30 sec or more, there was little or no decrement (Fig. 1A). After the flexion response had habituated, a

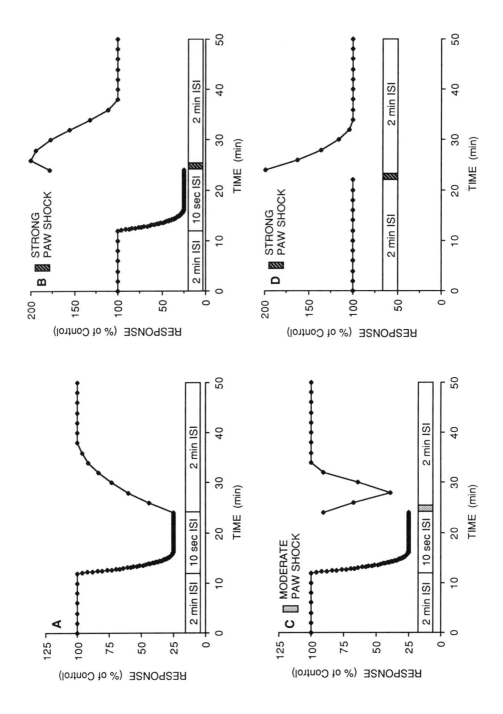

strong stimulus, such as a pinch or shock to the paw, resulted in substantial recovery of the decremented response (i.e., the response dishabituated) (Fig. 1B).

What is the relationship between cellular mechanisms underlying dishabituation and sensitization? It seemed possible that this recovery of the habituated flexion reflex by a strong stimulus could represent the reversal of the process responsible for the decrement, restoring the reflex to its nondecremented state. To better understand the nature of dishabituation, Spencer and Thompson compared the enhancement of the response with strong and weak dishabituating stimuli. Several observations suggested that dishabituation did not simply reflect an elimination of habituation. With strong paw shocks, the response was augmented to a level greater than the initial control level (Fig. 1B). Moreover, with weaker paw shocks, the response increased, but only transiently, even though it was tested at relatively long interstimulus intervals (Fig. 1C). The reflex then recovered slowly, indicating that some of the initial response decrement remained after the dishabituation had decayed. These results suggested that the response enhancement represented an additional facilitatory process. Consistent with this possibility, it was found that a paw pinch could enhance subsequent flexion responses even when the response had not been previously decremented (Fig. 1D). Thus, paw shock produced sensitization of the flexion reflex. The enhancement of a habituated response might simply represent sensitization overlaid on habituation. Stated differently, the enhancement of a habituated response (dishabituation) and the enhancement of a nonhabituated response (sensitization) may result from identical mechanisms. Spencer and colleagues were unable to explore the relationship between dishabituation and sensitization at a cellular level; this issue will be reexamined below in the discussion of cellular studies on a simpler reflex circuit in an invertebrate.

Changes in the Neural Circuit for the Reflex

Spencer and Thompson then attempted to identify the changes occurring in the neural circuit for the flexion reflex in the cat during habituation, dishabituation, and sensitization. They recorded intracellularly from leg motor neurons and observed changes in the amplitude of excitatory postsynaptic potentials (EPSPs) produced in the motor neurons by stimulation of sensory neuron axons lo-

---

FIG. 1. Plasticity in the flexion reflex. The flexion reflex in a cat with the spinal cord transected anteriorly was elicited by giving a very weak electrical stimulus to the lower surface of the paw. The response measured was the contraction of the tibial muscle. **A:** Habituation of flexion response. When a weak skin stimulus is given at a 10-sec interstimulus interval (ISI), the response amplitude rapidly decrements. When the ISI is increased to the longer 2-min interval used originally, the response recovers. **B:** Dishabituation of the habituated flexion response. After the flexion response is habituated by repeated presentation of the weak paw stimulus at a 10-sec ISI, a strong paw shock is delivered; the shock results in enhancement of the response amplitude above the original control level. The response is then tested at a long interval that does not produce habituation; the enhanced response gradually decays to its initial control level. **C:** Dishabituation of the habituated flexion response following a moderate paw shock. Notice, in contrast to B, that following the moderate shock the flexion response does not recover to control levels. Notice, too, that after the dishabituating stimulus, the dishabituation wears off, although the response is tested at a nonhabituating ISI, revealing that some amount of habituation remains; this residual habituation then decays gradually. **D:** Sensitization of the flexion response. Presentation of a strong paw shock results in a transient enhancement of the nondecremented flexion response. These hypothetical results are adapted from the results of Spencer WA, Thompson RF, Neilson DR Jr. Response decrement of the flexion reflex in the acute spinal cat and transient restoration by strong stimuli. *J Neurophysiol.* 1966;29:221–239.

cated in a peripheral nerve from the leg. These changes in EPSP amplitude paralleled the behavioral changes that occurred in the flexion reflex. With long interstimulus intervals there was no decrement of the EPSP, while with short interstimulus intervals (e.g., 1 sec) there was a rapid decline in EPSP amplitude. Finally, as in the habituation of the flexion response, a decremented synaptic response could be restored in either of two ways —by increasing the interval between stimuli or by stimulating a second peripheral nerve with a brief, high-frequency train of stimuli (e.g., 100 stimuli/sec for 4 sec). These changes in the EPSP recorded in leg motor neurons occurred independently of changes in muscle properties or in the responsiveness of sensory neurons to cutaneous stimuli. Thus, these central changes are likely to be responsible for the changes in the reflex during habituation, during recovery with rest, or during dishabituation with a strong second stimulus such as a paw pinch.

Input from sensory neurons excited by peripheral nerve stimulation reaches motor neurons via two routes. Sensory neurons make direct excitatory monosynaptic connections with motor neurons. In addition, sensory neuron stimulation results in indirect polysynaptic potentials produced by interneurons that synapse onto motor neurons; these interneurons are themselves excited by activation of the sensory neurons either through direct connections or through other interneurons. When Spencer, Thompson, and Neilson used peripheral nerve stimuli that produced primarily monosynaptic EPSPs in motor neurons, they observed that these synaptic connections were not altered. Thus, the changes responsible for the depression and recovery of the synaptic input to motor neurons must occur within interneurons or at interneuron-to-motor neuron synapses. Although some efforts were subsequently made to examine plasticity in interneurons, the fact that the principal changes of interest were taking place in more complex portions of the neural circuit made further analysis of this system difficult.

Neural changes during behavioral plasticity can occur in parallel at multiple neural loci. Spencer and Thompson addressed an important additional issue: whether the decrement in the EPSP was due to a decline in excitatory connections or to an increase in inhibitory modulation of the reflex circuit. In the spinal cord, there is direct inhibitory synaptic input to motor neurons; sensory neurons and interneurons also receive inhibitory input. To explore the possible contribution of changes in inhibition to the decrease in the polysynaptic excitatory input from sensory neurons, Spencer and his colleagues blocked the major class of inhibitory synapses in the spinal cord, which use the transmitter γ-aminobutyric acid (GABA). Two antagonists of GABAergic synapses, strychnine and picrotoxin, had no effect on depression of polysynaptic EPSPs produced by repeated stimulation of sensory neurons. This suggested that depression involved a decrease in excitation within the circuit for the reflex rather than an increase in inhibition. MacDonald and Pearson reexamined the role of inhibition in habituation of the flexion response, both in rats with intact central nervous systems and in spinal animals. As Spencer and colleagues had observed in the case of the polysynaptic EPSP, MacDonald and Pearson found that in animals with spinal transection decrement of the flexion response was unaffected by antagonists of GABAergic inhibitory synapses. However, they observed that intact rats showed greater habituation of the flexion reflex; moreover, this decrement of the flexion response was substantially reduced by GABA antagonists. Thus, in intact animals, two processes contribute to behavioral habituation of the flexion reflex: (1) there is a decrement in the polysynaptic EPSP within the spinal cord and (2) there is an increase in inhibitory modulation of the circuit for the flexion response; this inhibition involves input from supraspinal pathways. This observation that learning can utilize parallel changes at multiple neural loci has now been made in a number of neurobiological studies of behavioral plasticity.

These studies of the vertebrate flexion reflex yielded some preliminary, though indirect, insights into the types of neural changes that might contribute to behavioral plasticity. However, the complexity of the neural circuitry involved combined with the fact that most of the changes occurred within interneurons that were difficult to identify and study directly made a direct cellular analysis impractical. To investigate the cellular basis of learning, it is advantageous to be able to directly record from neurons that are involved in the behaviors being studied and that exhibit plasticity. This has been an important criterion for neurobiologists who have looked for simple model systems in which to analyze cellular mechanisms of learning.

LEARNING IN THE MARINE SNAIL *APLYSIA*

A simpler system used by the American neuroscientist Eric Kandel and his colleagues to study the neural basis of learning is the marine mollusc *Aplysia californica.* This snail's nervous system has relatively few neurons, many of which have large pigmented cell bodies and are unique and reidentifiable from animal to animal. Thus, it is possible to identify individual neurons and synapses that have specific roles in producing a behavior and to return to these same identified cells in different animals or following a training procedure that results in behavioral modification. The behavioral response studied in many analyses of behavioral plasticity in *Aplysia* is the defensive withdrawal reflex.

Plasticity in the Defensive Withdrawal Reflex of *Aplysia*

Aplysia has an external respiratory organ, the gill, located dorsally. The gill is partially covered by a sheet of skin called the mantle, which ends posteriorly in a siphon through which water bathing the gill is pumped out when the gill contracts (Fig. 2). The mantle and gill are enclosed by two laterally located flaps of skin, the parapodia, which meet at the dorsal midline when closed. When the siphon is extended, it projects out through the parapodia. In response to either weak tactile stimulation of the siphon or mantle or stronger stimuli elsewhere on the body, the animal withdraws the gill and siphon within the protective folds of the parapodia. Kandel and his colleagues found that this simple protective withdrawal reflex undergoes several forms of plasticity: habituation, dishabituation, and sensitization. Repeated presentations of a weak tactile stimulus to the siphon result in rapid decrement of the withdrawal response. Stroking the skin or shocking the body wall produces sensitization of the nonhabituated response or recovery of the habituated response. These changes in the reflex are very similar to changes in simple vertebrate flexion reflexes described earlier in this chapter.

Vincent Castellucci and his colleagues have been able to identify many of the sensory neurons responsible for responding to tactile stimulation of the siphon as well as the motor neurons that produce gill and siphon retraction. The sensory neurons, motor neurons, and interneurons that mediate the defensive withdrawal reflex are located within a single ganglion, the abdominal ganglion. Several clusters of small mechanosensory neurons on the ventral surface of the left hemiganglion project out the siphon nerve and innervate the siphon skin. Approximately 14 known motor neurons innervate the siphon and approximately six known motor neurons project to the gill. A substantial part (approximately 25% to 50%) of the excitatory synaptic input to the gill and siphon motor neurons in response to tactile stimuli comes directly from sensory neurons, monosynaptically. In addition, polysynaptic excitatory input comes indirectly via interneurons that receive excitatory synapses from the sensory neurons and in turn make excitatory connections with gill and siphon motor neurons. For two decades, there has been a major effort by a number of laboratories to analyze the changes in the monosynaptic sensory

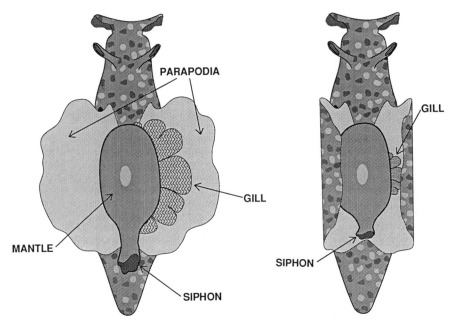

FIG. 2. *Aplysia* defensive withdrawal reflex. The mantle overlies the respiratory organ, the gill. Posteriorly, the mantle ends in a siphon. The mantle and gill are located between two protective flaps, the parapodia. A tactile stimulus to the siphon, the mantle, or elsewhere on the body surface, including the tail, if sufficiently strong, results in the withdrawal of the siphon and gill within the protective parapodia.

neuron-to-motor neuron connection that contribute to the behavioral changes. Indeed, synaptic changes have been identified that parallel various forms of behavioral plasticity in the defensive withdrawal reflex. As the withdrawal reflex decrements with repeated stimulation of the siphon, so does the amplitude of the monosynaptic EPSP decline with repeated activation of the sensory neuron. As the habituated behavioral response is augmented after a strong noxious stimulus or a rest period, so does the monosynaptic connection increase in amplitude with dishabituating stimuli or rest. As the nonhabituated withdrawal reflex is enhanced after a strong sensitizing stimulus, so is the sensory neuron-to-motor neuron synapse strengthened by facilitatory transmitter that is released by sensitizing stimuli (Fig. 3).

Presynaptic Plasticity: Inferences from a Quantal Analysis

Plasticity in the siphon sensory neuron-to-motor neuron synapse is due to presynaptic changes. To distinguish whether the changes responsible for alterations in synaptic transmission during synaptic depression and synaptic facilitation take place presynaptically or postsynaptically, Castellucci and Kandel carried out a quantal analysis of the synaptic plasticity at this synapse. In studies at the neuromuscular junction under low-release conditions (achieved with low-Ca^{++}, high-Mg^{++} saline), Jose del Castillo and Bernard Katz had originally demonstrated in 1954 that the synaptic potentials produced by stimulation of the presynaptic motor neuron fluctuate in amplitude in a quantal manner. Thus individual synaptic events can be analyzed to be multiples of unitary potentials. One evoked potential is composed of one to five unitary potentials, the number varying statistically. A unitary potential, or quantum, is assumed to represent the release of a single synaptic vesicle. With some stimuli, no synaptic potential is detectable, indicating that no vesicles are released. On average, the amplitude of a synaptic potential is equal to the mean number of unitary potentials or quanta per

NON-DEPRESSED   **DEPRESSED**

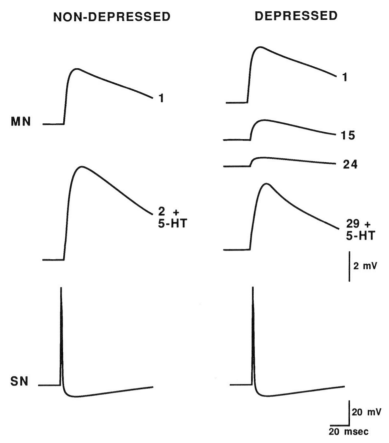

FIG. 3. Facilitation of sensory neuron to motor neuron synapse in *Aplysia*. The facilitatory transmitter serotonin (5-hydroxytryptamine; 5-HT) is normally released by modulatory interneurons during dishabituating or sensitizing stimuli. In this experiment, bath application of 5-HT was substituted for natural noxious stimuli that excite these facilitatory interneurons. The sensory neuron was caused to fire action potentials with intracellular current stimuli at 30-sec intervals. A single action potential in the presynaptic sensory neuron is shown below; two or three synaptic responses in the motor neuron are shown above, with stimulus number indicated at the right. **Left:** facilitation of nondepressed synapse; after the first stimulus, 5-HT was applied. **Right:** depression of synapse with repeated activation and subsequent facilitation; after 5-HT was washed out, this same synapse showed gradually increasing depression; application of 5-HT prior to the 29th stimulus resulted in reversal of synaptic depression and facilitation above the initial amplitude (compare EPSP 29 and EPSP 1).

EPSP times the amplitude of an individual unitary potential:

$$V_{EPSP} = ma$$

where m is the mean number of quanta released per presynaptic action potential and a is the average amplitude of the response to a single vesicle (the quantal response); m equals the number of releasable vesicles (N) times the probability (p) that an individual vesicle will be released by a single action potential. By carrying out a statistical analysis of synaptic transmission under low-release conditions, one can estimate m and a as did del Castillo and Katz. Such a quantal analysis can be a powerful approach for determining whether a change in synaptic transmission is due to a pre- or postsynaptic alteration. The average amplitude of a quantum, or unitary potential, is dependent on both presynaptic and postsynaptic factors: the amount of transmitter per vesicle, the receptor density at the synapse, and the postsynaptic cell's resting conductance. (The postsynaptic resting conductance influences the postsynaptic potential for a given synaptic current according to Ohm's law:

$$V_{EPSP} = I_{EPSP}/g_{neuron}$$

or

$$V_{EPSP} = I_{EPSP} \times R_{neuron}$$

where I_{EPSP} is the synaptic current and g_{neuron} is the resting neuronal conductance, equal to the reciprocal of the resting neuronal resistance R_{neuron}.) In contrast, the mean number of quanta released per action potential is solely dependent on presynaptic factors—Ca^{++} influx and the release process itself. Analyzing the sensory neuron-to-motor neuron synaptic connection under low-release conditions in 1976, Castellucci and Kandel found that during the synaptic depression that results from repeated activation of the siphon sensory neuron, the mean number of quanta released declined in parallel with the amplitude of the EPSP, while the quantal amplitude remained unchanged. Similarly,

during synaptic facilitation produced by a train of stimuli applied to a peripheral nerve that contains sensory neuron axons (a substitute for a strong tactile stimulus), mean number of quanta released increased while the amplitude of the unitary EPSP remained constant (Fig. 4). Thus, in this system, both synaptic depression and synaptic facilitation result from presynaptic changes in the siphon sensory neurons. The changes in transmitter release from these siphon mechanosensory neurons are an important contributor to experience-dependent changes in the defensive gill and siphon withdrawal reflex.

Mechanisms Underlying Depression of Synaptic Transmission from Sensory Neurons

At least two types of changes in the presynaptic terminals of the sensory neurons contribute to the decrease in transmitter release with repeated activation of the sensory neu-

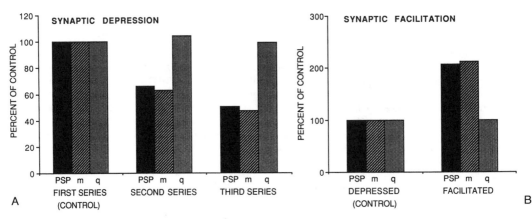

FIG. 4. Quantal analysis of synaptic depression and synaptic facilitation at sensory neuron–to–motor neuron synapses. A quantal analysis of *Aplysia* siphon sensory neuron–to–motor neuron synapses was conducted on synapses in control, depressed, and facilitated states. EPSP amplitude is the size of the mean postsynaptic potential; a is the mean amplitude of an individual quantum; m is the mean quantal content (or mean number of quanta per EPSP). **A:** Quantal analysis during synaptic depression. Each series consisted of PSPs produced by five action potentials in the sensory neuron stimulated at 10-sec intervals. **B:** Quantal analysis during synaptic facilitation. After the sensory neuron had been stimulated repeatedly at 10-sec intervals, a train of stimuli were given to a nerve leading to the abdominal ganglion to produce facilitation of the depressed synapse. In each case, the mean quantal content changes in parallel with the EPSP amplitude, while the quantal amplitude remains unchanged, suggesting that at these synapses the changes underlying both synaptic depression and synaptic facilitation occur presynaptically. Data adapted from Castellucci V, Kandel ER. Presynaptic facilitation as a mechanism for behavioral sensitization in *Aplysia*. *Science* 1976;194:1176–1178.

ron synapses. One change that can be measured relatively directly is a depression in Ca^{++} current with repeated depolarization of the sensory neuron. Some types of Ca^{++} channels inactivate fairly rapidly with prolonged depolarization of the membrane in a manner analogous to inactivation of Na^+ channels, except more slowly. In *Aplysia*, such Ca^{++} channel inactivation contributes to reduced transmission with repeated activity in sensory neurons. A second type of change makes a substantial contribution to the reduction in transmitter release but is difficult to characterize directly. Evidence for this second change comes from studies that found that in depressed synapses, even with prolonged depolarization of the presynaptic sensory neurons, which should allow substantial Ca^{++} influx, transmitter release remained minimal. Thus, it appears that with synaptic depression some aspect of the release process itself becomes inactivated (e.g., the pool of releasable vesicles coupled to release sites in presynaptic active zones may become depleted). Through ultrastructural analysis of serial sections of *Aplysia* ganglia in which a single sensory neuron had been injected with a visualizable marker and then stimulated repetitively for many minutes to depress its synaptic connections, Craig Bailey indeed found that the number of vesicles within 30 nm of the vesicle release sites (or active zones) was decreased twofold. In contrast to the sensory neuron synapses, most neuronal synapses do not show such substantial synaptic depression; the depression of transmitter release that occurs specifically in these siphon mechanosensory neurons may have evolved as a mechanism for behavioral habituation.

Mechanisms Underlying Presynaptic Facilitation of Synaptic Transmission from Siphon Sensory Neurons

Modulatory Neurotransmitters

During sensitization, strong noxious stimuli excite several populations of modulatory interneurons that release at least three or four facilitatory transmitters which act presynaptically to enhance synaptic transmission from the siphon sensory neurons. Perhaps the most important of these modulatory transmitters is serotonin (5-hydroxytryptamine, 5-HT; see Chapter 6), since depletion of 5-HT greatly reduces facilitation of sensory neuron-to-motor neuron synapses produced by sensitizing stimuli as demonstrated by David Glanzman and his colleagues. Two peptide transmitters, the small cardioactive peptides SCP_A and SCP_B, also produce facilitation of these synapses. The SCPs are products of a single gene and are probably coreleased by SCP-containing modulatory neurons that project to the abdominal ganglion. The relative contribution of this peptidergic input is not known. Finally, a small cluster of facilitator interneurons in the abdominal ganglion use a transmitter that is yet unidentified. 5-HT and both SCPs act to stimulate adenylyl cyclase in the sensory neurons, producing a rise in intracellular levels of the second messenger cAMP (see Chapter 4).

Multiple K^+ Currents Are Modulated by Facilitatory Transmitters and cAMP

Marc Klein, Joseph Camardo, Steven Siegelbaum, and Eric Kandel demonstrated that increased cAMP-dependent protein phosphorylation closes a particular K^+ channel called the S-K^+ channel (Fig. 5). In addition, as shown by Douglas Baxter and John Byrne and by Bruce Goldsmith and Thomas Abrams, at least one other K^+ current, a transient, steeply voltage-dependent K^+ current, is modulated by facilitatory transmitter and 5-HT. Since outward current flowing through K^+ channels is responsible for the repolarization of the membrane during the action potential, this reduction in K^+ current broadens the action potential in the sensory neurons. Klein and Kandel proposed that prolongation of the sensory neuron action potential could be a presynaptic mechanism for facilitating synaptic transmission from

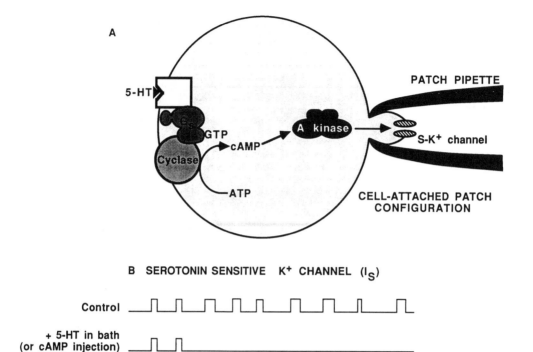

FIG. 5. 5-HT acts via the intracellular messenger cAMP to close the S-K$^+$ channel. **A:** Single-channel recording configuration. A fire-polished patch pipette is used to record currents through a single S-K$^+$ channel in *Aplysia* sensory neurons in the cell-attached patch configuration. Once an S-K$^+$ channel is identified, channel activity can be recorded under control conditions or after the application of serotonin to the bath. Alternatively, cAMP can be injected into the cell body of the sensory neuron. **B:** Outward currents through single S-K$^+$ channels under control conditions and in the presence of 5-HT. Outward single-channel currents can be recorded at depolarized transmembrane potentials (V_m) as the channel flips briefly from the closed state to the open state. After the application of 5-HT, the channel shifts to a steady closed state. The fact that 5-HT applied outside the pipette can influence an ion channel in the pipette implies that an intermediary intracellular messenger must couple the 5-HT receptor to the K$^+$ channel. Consistent with this, injections of cAMP into the sensory neuron produce similar closing of S-K$^+$ channels.

the sensory neurons; with a longer action potential, there is more time for Ca^{++} influx and thus more transmitter release with each action potential. Because Ca^{++} channels open relatively slowly compared with Na$^+$ channels, even a small increase in the duration of the action potential could have a relatively large effect on transmitter release. For example, a 20% broadening of the action potential can increase the EPSP amplitude by 46%.

A Second Facilitatory Process That Contributes to Reversal of Synaptic Depression and Enhancement of the Habituated Reflex

Binyamin Höchner, Klein, and Kandel found that in synapses that had been substantially depressed due to repeated activation of the sensory neuron, prolongation of the sensory neuron action potential was relatively ineffective in facilitating the sensory neuron-to-motor neuron synapse. Nevertheless, application of 5-HT could effectively facilitate these depressed synapses, suggesting that 5-HT initiates a second facilitatory process causing a restoration of the synapse to its undepressed state. Perhaps this second facilitatory process involves an increase in the rate of translocation of synaptic vesicles into the releasable pool of vesicles located adjacent to release sites, as suggested by Kevin Gingrich and Byrne. Alternatively, this reversal of synaptic depression may involve modulation of some aspect of the release process itself that has been inactivated by repeated action potentials in the sensory neuron. There is evidence that cAMP-dependent phosphorylation can trigger this second facilitatory process as well as the reduction in K^+ current, though other intracellular messenger systems, such as protein kinase C, may also be involved (Fig. 6).

Multiple facilitatory processes in the siphon sensory neurons contribute in parallel to strengthening of the gill and siphon withdrawal reflex during dishabituation and sensitization. Given these results, one would expect that after habituation of the defensive withdrawal reflex, when synapses from the si-phon sensory neurons have become depressed, modulation of K^+ current and prolongation of the presynaptic action potential should be relatively ineffective in producing facilitation and restoring the reflex response. However, once facilitatory transmitters such as 5-HT have initiated the process responsible for reversing synaptic depression, the spike broadening produced by cAMP would further enhance release of transmitter. Thus, both processes contribute in parallel to dishabituation of the gill and siphon withdrawal reflex. Both processes may also contribute to facilitation of sensory neuron synapses that have not been intentionally depressed by the experimenter; however, in nondepressed synapses, the process involving modulation of the release process or vesicle mobilization makes a relatively smaller contribution to facilitation. It is likely that all sensory neurons, even in nonhabituated animals, have had some recent activity, and thus their vesicle release capacity may be at a less than maximal state.

During sensitization, alterations occur at other neural loci in addition to the sensory neuron-to-motor neuron synapses. Various other sites within the neural circuit for the defensive withdrawal reflex were recently ex-

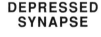

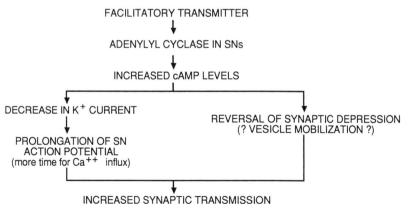

FIG. 6. Flow diagram of the cellular mechanism underlying presynaptic facilitation in the siphon sensory neurons of *Aplysia*. Two parallel processes contribute to facilitation.

amined by William Frost and colleagues in an effort to identify additional plastic changes that contribute to enhancement of the defensive withdrawal reflex during behavioral sensitization. As described above, the siphon sensory neurons make excitatory synaptic connections with a number of interneurons as well as with motor neurons. One group of these interneurons consists of the three L30 neurons, which inhibit excitatory interneurons in the neural circuit for the withdrawal reflex. A sensitizing stimulus or application of 5-HT causes a reduction in the strength of the inhibitory synaptic connections from L30 neurons to these excitatory interneurons. This decrease in the normal inhibition of the withdrawal reflex appears to result from presynaptic inhibition of synaptic transmission from the L30 cells. A second group of interneurons, the L29 cells, receive excitatory input from the siphon sensory neurons and make both fast excitatory synaptic connections with motor neurons and slow facilitatory connections with sensory neurons. When the L29 neurons are strongly excited by noxious stimuli, they undergo a frequency-dependent potentiation of their synaptic connections with motor neurons. Following sensitizing stimuli, there is a decrease in synaptic transmission from interneurons that inhibit the withdrawal reflex and an increase in synaptic transmission from excitatory interneurons within the circuit for the reflex. Recent studies by Louis-Eric Trudeau and Castellucci and by Thomas Carew and his colleagues suggests that a reduction in inhibition contributes importantly to the enhancement of the reflex during sensitization. Thus, even within the simple nervous system of *Aplysia,* behavioral plasticity results from parallel plastic changes at multiple neural loci.

Conditioning of the Defensive Withdrawal Reflex

In addition to being modulated through nonassociative forms of learning, the defensive withdrawal reflex can be classically conditioned using a paradigm developed by Carew, Edgar Walters, and Kandel. A very light touch to the siphon, which elicits a brief, small gill and siphon withdrawal, serves as the CS; a moderate tail shock, which elicits a strong defensive withdrawal response, serves as the US. If during training this weak siphon stimulus is paired with the tail shock, then after a series of pairing trials the response to that same weak CS is markedly enhanced, both in its amplitude and in its duration. It is as if the animal learns that the siphon touch predicts the occurrence of the tail shock, and alters its response to the CS. Since the noxious US is of modest intensity and brief duration, it produces little sensitization if delivered by itself. Similarly, if the CS and US are both presented during training in a random or unpaired relationship, there is little or no enhancement of the reflex response to the siphon touch. Thus, the learning is associative. As described earlier, conditioning requires that the CS and US be paired in a precise temporal manner: the onset of the US must occur within about 1 sec of the onset of the CS, and the CS must begin before the US (see Chapter 12, Fig. 2C).

Activity-Dependent Facilitation

The analysis of cellular changes contributing to conditioning was influenced by the earlier studies on nonassociative plasticity in the defensive withdrawal reflex which had specified the neural circuit for the reflex and characterized changes that contribute to a similar reflex enhancement during sensitization. It seemed likely that the aversive US strengthens the input from the CS sensory neurons during conditioning by activating the same facilitatory interneurons that enhance synaptic transmission from these sensory neurons during sensitization. However, classical conditioning selectively increases the withdrawal response only when the siphon sensory neurons have been excited by the CS just prior to the delivery of the tail shock US. In 1983, Bob Hawkins, Abrams, Carew, and Kandel identified an associative form of synaptic plasticity, activity-dependent facilitation in siphon sensory neurons, that could account for this pairing specificity in the conditioning of the reflex. At the same time, Walters and Byrne demonstrated the existence of activity-dependent facilitation in a second group of *Aplysia* mechanosensory neurons. In activity-dependent facilitation, the response of sensory neurons to facilitatory input is enhanced if they fire action potentials immediately before the facilitatory input arrives. Activity-dependent facilitation in the siphon sensory neurons was first demonstrated using a training paradigm very similar to that used in the behavioral conditioning experiments: instead of stimulating the siphon with a light touch, siphon sensory neurons were activated with intracellular current pulses; instead of measuring the duration of the siphon withdrawal response, the amplitude of monosynaptic EPSPs from sensory neurons was measured in siphon motor neurons. After a series of pairing trials, EPSPs from sensory neurons that have had their activity paired with the US show substantially more facilitation than EPSPs from sensory neurons whose activity was not paired. Such activity-dependent enhancement of presynaptic facilitation occurs during training when the CS, which excites the siphon sensory neurons, is paired with the US, which produces the facilitatory input. Since the siphon sensory neurons are the pathway for the afferent input to the reflex from the CS, any modulation of their synapses must affect the strength of the reflex; thus, this associative facilitation of their synaptic connections is an important contributor to the associative changes produced by conditioning.

Activity-dependent facilitation in *Aplysia* mechanosensory neurons resembles the regular form of presynaptic facilitation that occurs in these neurons in the absence of paired activity, except that recent spike activity in the sensory neurons enhances the facilitation process. Initial characterizations of the changes accompanying activity-dependent facilitation demonstrated that, like regular facilitation in these cells, this associative form of facilitation involves a prolongation of the presynaptic action potential and a reduction

in outward current. However, sensory neurons whose spike activity was paired with tail shock showed a greater reduction in outward K^+ current and a greater broadening of the action potential than did sensory neurons whose activity was specifically unpaired with tail shock. Thus, activity-dependent facilitation may use the same cAMP-dependent mechanism as regular facilitation in the sensory neurons, but in an enhanced form. Indeed, the elevation in cAMP levels in response to the facilitatory transmitter 5-HT is greater when spike activity or membrane depolarization is paired with application of 5-HT (Fig. 7). Thus, it appears that inputs from the CS and the US converge within the sensory neurons and interact to produce an associative facilitation of synapses within the CS pathway.

Which component of the action potential interacts with the biochemical cascade to increase the facilitation response? During an action potential, Ca^{++} influx occurs through voltage-sensitive Ca^{++} channels, and intracellular Ca^{++} levels rise transiently beneath the membrane. These Ca^{++} transients are responsible for eliciting vesicle exocytosis, but Ca^{++} elevations can also modulate other cellular processes. In the siphon sensory neurons, Ca^{++} influx is necessary for activity-dependent enhancement of the facilitation response. When Ca^{++} influx was eliminated during the paired action potentials in the sensory neurons during training, the paired activity no longer enhanced the facilitation response—even though Na^+ influx, K^+ efflux, and membrane depolarization still occurred. This suggested the possibility that Ca^{++} influx may enhance the stimulation of cAMP synthesis by facilitatory transmitter (Fig. 10).

The Ca^{++}/Calmodulin-Sensitive Adenylyl Cyclase Provides a Molecular Site of Convergence for the Signals From the CS and US

The analysis of activity-dependent facilitation suggested that within the nervous system

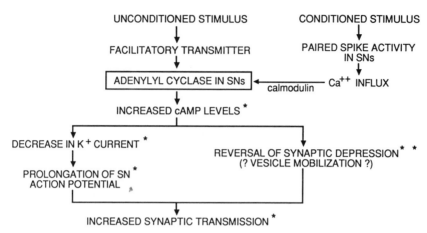

FIG. 7. Flow diagram of enhancement of presynaptic facilitation in *Aplysia* sensory neurons by paired activity in the sensory neurons. *, Enhanced by paired spike activity; **, presumably enhanced by paired spike activity.

of *Aplysia,* the CS and US were represented by two signals: the CS results in Ca^{++} influx in the sensory neurons of the CS pathway, while the US results in release of facilitatory transmitter. Where do these two signals from the CS and US converge and interact? The evidence that cAMP synthesis is enhanced by paired spike activity suggested that Ca^{++} may potentiate the activation of adenylyl cyclase by facilitatory transmitter. Thus, adenylyl cyclase may serve as a molecular site of convergence for the inputs from the CS and the US.

In mammalian brain, adenylyl cyclase is stimulated by Ca^{++} via the Ca^{++}-binding protein calmodulin. Similarly, adenylyl cyclase in the central nervous system of *Aplysia* is stimulated by Ca^{++} via calmodulin. The level of Ca^{++} needed to stimulate the enzyme is approximately 1 to 5 μM, which is above basal levels in *Aplysia* neurons but within the range of free Ca^{++} that is reached during trains of action potentials. Moreover, the same adenylyl cyclase catalytic unit that interacts with calmodulin in a Ca^{++}-dependent manner is also stimulated by the stimulatory G protein G_S, which couples the receptor to the catalytic unit of the cyclase (Fig. 8) (see Chapter 4). Thus, the Ca^{++}/calmodulin-dependent cyclase is dually regulated by Ca^{++} and by stimulatory transmitters that activate G_S. Under appropriate assay conditions,

Ca^{++}/calmodulin enhances the activation of the cyclase by facilitatory transmitter. In particular, Yoram Yovell and Abrams obtained evidence suggesting that Ca^{++}/calmodulin binding to adenylyl cyclase may accelerate

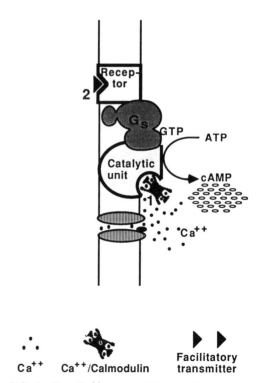

FIG. 8. The Ca^{++}/calmodulin-sensitive adenylyl cyclase is dually regulated.

the activation of the enzyme by transmitter and G_s. When exposure to facilitatory transmitter is brief, optimal activation of the cyclase requires the temporal pairing of Ca^{++} and transmitter. Moreover, the cyclase appears to display a sequence preference analogous to that shown by the behavioral conditioning (see Chapter 12, Fig. 2): just as the CS must precede the US, Ca^{++}, the cellular representation of the CS, must precede 5-HT, the cellular representation of the US, for optimal activation of the cyclase.

Long-Term Plasticity in the Defensive Withdrawal Reflex of *Aplysia*

If the stimuli that produce short-term habituation or sensitization of the gill and siphon withdrawal reflex are repeated for an hour, for a few hours, or for a few days, the animals demonstrate a long-term change in the withdrawal reflex. Thus, training with repeated weak stimuli to the siphon that is continued over 4 days results in long-term habituation that can last more than 3 weeks. Similarly, if repeated sensitizing stimuli, such as shocks to the body wall, are given over a few hours, animals show enhancement of the withdrawal response when they are tested 24 hr later. If the training is continued for several days, the animals show long-term sensitization that persists for more than 2 weeks. During long-term habituation, the synaptic connections between siphon sensory neurons and gill and siphon motor neurons show long-term depression. During long-term sensitization, these same monosynaptic connections from siphon sensory neurons show long-term enhancement. In addition, there is a decrease in the number of detectable synaptic connections between siphon sensory neurons and motor neurons during long-term habituation and an increase in the incidence of detectable connections during long-term sensitization. Thus, monosynaptic connections that undergo transient changes during short-term behavioral plasticity also undergo persistent changes that contribute to long-term behavioral plasticity.

It should be noted that *long-term* and *short-term* are relative terms that do not necessarily refer to two discrete forms of learning. Processes underlying very short-term behavioral plasticity and very long-term learning are likely to be different; however, there may be a series of mechanisms of plasticity that overlap temporally and underlie learning lasting from minutes to years.

Cellular mechanisms underlying long-term sensitization of the gill and siphon withdrawal reflex include the following:

1. During long-term sensitization there is a reduction in a K^+ current in sensory neurons, as in short-term sensitization. Scholz and Byrne found that during long-term synaptic facilitation, there is a reduction in the same $S-K^+$ current that is decreased via cAMP-dependent phosphorylation during short-term presynaptic facilitation in the sensory neurons. This suggests that elevated cAMP-dependent phosphorylation may also contribute to long-term synaptic plasticity in this system.

2. Presynaptic release sites show a change in morphology with long-term learning. Craig Bailey and Mary Chen compared the presynaptic arbors of the siphon sensory neurons in control animals and animals that had received 4 days of sensitization training with four shocks per day. The active zones (or vesicle release sites) of sensory neurons were larger and more numerous in long-term sensitized animals, and there was a nearly two-fold increase in the number of vesicles associated with active zones. Furthermore, sensory neurons in long-term sensitized animals had more than twice as many varicosities—the presynaptic swellings along the length of fine neuronal branches at which release occurs in *Aplysia* neuropil (the region of invertebrate ganglia where neuronal processes interdigitate, forming synapses) (Fig. 9). Conversely, in long-term habituated animals, reductions were observed in incidence of active zones, active zone area, density of vesicles near release sites, and numbers of varicosities. These changes in the synaptic re-

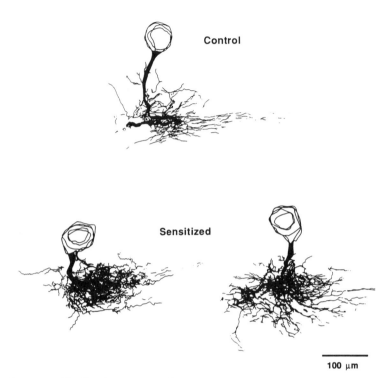

Control

Sensitized

100 μm

FIG. 9. Long-term sensitization is accompanied by a proliferation of sensory neurons' presynaptic processes within the ganglion. Adapted from Bailey CH, Chen M. Long-term sensitization in *Aplysia* increases the number of presynaptic contacts onto the identified gill motor neuron L7. *Proc Natl Acad Sci USA* 1988;85:9356–9359.

lease sites and the numbers of vesicles in the releasable pool would be expected to produce large increases and decreases in synaptic transmission from siphon sensory neurons in long-term sensitized and long-term habituated animals, respectively.

3. Protein synthesis is required in a critical time window during and/or shortly after training. A series of 5-min applications of 5-HT to sensory neurons and motor neurons in coculture over 2 hr resulted in a 70% increase in the amplitude of the monosynaptic EPSP measured 24 hr later. Treating the neurons with an inhibitor of either mRNA synthesis (actinomycin D or α-amanitin) or protein synthesis (anisomycin or emetine) completely blocked the long-term facilitation by serotonin without affecting short-term facilitation. Because the protein synthesis inhibition produced by anisomycin was rapidly re-

versible, it was possible to define the precise time period in which protein synthesis is necessary. Inhibition of protein synthesis was only effective in blocking long-term synaptic facilitation when the inhibition occurred during and for 1 or 2 hr after the exposure to 5-HT. Inhibiting mRNA or protein synthesis at later times did not interfere with long-term facilitation, even when the inhibitors were applied for as long as 22 hr beginning shortly after the termination of the exposure to 5-HT. This suggests that it is not necessary to have RNA transcription and protein translation continue for an extended period to produce a strengthening of synaptic connections. Instead, regulatory proteins may have their expression altered during and immediately after "training" with 5-HT; these regulatory proteins may in turn influence processes that are responsible for an increase in synaptic strength 24 hr later.

By labeling newly synthesized proteins with [^{35}S]methionine or [^{3}H]leucine, it is possible to detect changes in protein synthesis in sensory neurons that have received prolonged exposure to 5-HT. It has been possible to identify two groups of proteins that are transiently increased in their synthesis during two periods within several hours after extended exposure to 5-HT. The earliest detectable increase occurs within 30 min after the onset of extended exposure to 5-HT; one can speculate that the proteins showing an early increase in expression are regulatory proteins that trigger the later delayed changes in protein synthesis that have been observed.

4. Cyclic AMP can trigger long-term presynaptic facilitation of sensory neuron–to–motor neuron connections. To see whether cAMP-dependent phosphorylation can induce long-term facilitatory changes in sensory neurons, Scholz and Byrne, and Samuel Schacher and his colleagues injected cAMP into the cells or exposed them to cell permeant cAMP analogs. Twenty-four hours later, sensory neurons showed a reduction in K$^+$ current, and sensory neuron–to–motor neuron synapses were facilitated. Leonard Cleary, Fidelma Nazif, and Byrne found that cAMP injections also trigger an increase in branch points and varicosities in the sensory neuron. In addition, cAMP analogs induce the same changes in protein synthesis as does 5-HT. This suggested that repeated or persistent elevations in cAMP levels may initiate long-term synaptic facilitation in sensory neurons by causing changes in gene expression. Genes that are switched on by cAMP are activated by a nearby cAMP-responsive element (CRE). When the cAMP-dependent protein kinase is activated, one of the substrate proteins that it phosphorylates is a transcription regulator (the CRE-binding protein or CREB protein), which when phosphorylated can bind to and activate the CRE. By injecting synthetic DNA with the CRE sequence that binds the CREB protein, Pramod Dash, Hochner, and Kandel were able to block long-term facilitation of synaptic transmission from sensory neurons.

5. Long-term sensitization is accompanied by persistent activation of the cAMP-dependent protein kinase. The cAMP-dependent protein kinase holoenzyme consists of a tetramer of two regulatory and two catalytic subunits. When the two catalytic subunits of the kinase are bound to the two regulatory subunits, the active site of each catalytic unit is blocked. When intracellular cAMP levels rise, cAMP binds to each regulatory unit and the holoenzyme dissociates, freeing the catalytic units to phosphorylate substrate proteins. When cAMP levels fall, the regulatory subunits no longer have cAMP bound and are able to reassociate with the catalytic subunits, which terminates their phosphorylating activity. The American neurochemist James Schwartz and his colleagues found that in long-term sensitized animals the number of regulatory subunits of the cAMP-dependent kinase was reduced by approximately 25% whereas the number of catalytic units was not altered. Such a reduction in regulatory units would be expected to result in persistent activation of the catalytic subunits even after cAMP levels declined when sensitization training had ended. This reduction in the number of regulatory subunits appears to require protein synthesis, as do long-term sensitization and long-term facilitation of sensory neuron synapses. Perhaps new proteins expressed increase proteolytic degradation of the regulatory subunits. The regulatory subunits are also more susceptible to degradation when the holoenzyme tetramer is dissociated (i.e., when cAMP binds). This suggests that degradation would be enhanced when changes in gene expression that promote proteolysis are induced by initial facilitatory input and when subsequent facilitatory input triggers additional transient rises in cAMP, making the regulatory subunits particularly vulnerable to proteolysis. Such a mechanism involving repeated exposures to facilitatory transmitter could underlie the requirement for repeated training trials for initiation of long-term sensitization and long-term learning in general.

ROLE OF THE HIPPOCAMPUS IN LEARNING IN MAMMALS

In the several decades since Spencer and his colleagues carried out their studies on plasticity in the flexion reflex, numerous attempts have been made to identify the neural circuits involved in simple forms of learning in vertebrates. In some instances it has been possible to specify the neural loci that play critical roles in learning. For example, Richard Thompson and his colleagues demonstrated that associative changes in the cerebellum play a critical role in conditioning of the rabbit eye blink. Nevertheless, as yet little is known about the cellular processes underlying the neural changes that contribute to learning. In 1973, Timothy Bliss and Terje Lømo, studying the mammalian hippocampus, discovered a new type of neural plasticity known as *long-term synaptic potentiation.* Although it has not been directly demonstrated to be involved in any behavior, *long-term potentiation has many features that make it a strong candidate for a mechanism of associative learning.* During recent years, there has been substantial progress in analyzing the biophysical and biochemical events that trigger long-term potentiation. Hippocampal plasticity is discussed in the remainder of this chapter.

The hippocampus was strongly implicated in learning and memory in a seminal clinical study of a neurology patient, H.M., who was treated for severe epilepsy by bilateral removal of much of the hippocampus, the amygdala, and the parahippocampal gyrus. Because of this surgical treatment, H.M. became amnesic and was able to remember new events for only very brief periods. In other mammals, including primates and rodents, experimental lesions of the hippocampus and parahippocampal gyrus have been shown to affect learning. In rodents, the hippocampus appears to play an important role in learning spatial information. For instance, lesions of the hippocampus interfere with learning to navigate in various types of mazes.

Hippocampal Place Cells

Hippocampal place cells code for the animal's location in space. Physiologists recording from the hippocampus of freely moving rats have found that a large percentage of pyramidal cells in three regions of the hippocampus, CA1, CA3, and the dentate gyrus, are selectively activated when the animal is in a particular area of its environment. Different individual pyramidal neurons represent different regions of the rat's environment. These cells, termed *place cells,* are strikingly different from most other neurons that are excited by external stimuli in that no single sensory modality and no particular stimulus is required to activate these neurons. Rather, these cells are excited by the constellation of cues that could inform an animal as to its location in space; any single cue can be eliminated and the place cell will still respond appropriately in its preferred location. Furthermore, if animals are placed in a familiar environment and the lights are turned off, place cells fire in the same location in which they normally would respond as the animal runs around in the dark. Thus, even in the absence of visual or other spatial cues, place cells maintain their preferences for specific locations. In a commonly used test, a rat is provided food at one particular point in a simple, four-arm maze. After it has become familiar with the maze, the animal is placed in the maze in the dark. On trials in which the rat orients correctly and moves to the normally rewarded location, place cells fire maximally in the same locations as in the light. On trials in which the animal is confused and seeks the food in another location, place cells have their optimal locations shifted in a manner that corresponds to the animal's orientation error.

The response properties of hippocampal place cells must arise through learning. The response properties of place cells imply that each rat has a map of the entire area in which it is allowed to run. Such a map must be generated through learning. More specifically, both the recognition of the constellation of cues that signal a particular location and the knowledge of spatial relationships among locations that allows place cells to respond appropriately as an animal moves in the absence of cues (i.e., in the dark) must arise as a result of experience. The observation that place cells develop their properties through experience is consistent with the hypothesis that the hippocampus is involved in spatial learning.

Long-Term Potentiation in the Hippocampus

Bliss and Lømo developed a protocol that induced a long-lasting form of synaptic strengthening in the hippocampus, which they called long-term potentiation, or LTP. Within the hippocampus, four sets of synapses are capable of undergoing LTP: the synapses from the incoming perforant path axons to the dentate granule cells in the dentate gyrus (or fascia dentata), the synapses from the dentate granule cell axons (called mossy fibers) to the CA3 pyramidal cells, the synapses from fimbrial neurons to the CA3 pyramidal cells, and the synapses from the CA3 pyramidal cell axons (called the Schaeffer collaterals and commissurals) to the CA1 pyramidal cells. In LTP, a brief, high-frequency stimulation of the presynaptic neurons (e.g., 125 stimuli in 0.5 sec or 200 stimuli in 10 sec) results in a strengthening of the synaptic connection that persists for an extended period—at least days or weeks in the intact animal (Fig. 10B). In addition to being long–lasting and very rapidly induced, LTP would seem to be a reasonable candidate mechanism for learning in that it has associative features.

LTP as an Associative Form of Synaptic Plasticity

When a group of presynaptic neurons in the hippocampus is excited by a weak extracellular stimulus that can activate only axons in a limited region, high-frequency stimulation of this small population results in a brief increase in these neurons' synaptic connections with postsynaptic pyramidal cells. Such an enhancement of synaptic connections lasting minutes after high-frequency stimulation is termed post-tetanic potentiation (a tetanus is a high-frequency train of stimuli) and occurs at synapses in many neural systems. In contrast, a similar but stronger intensity train of stimuli, which brings a larger population of presynaptic axons to threshold, results in a long-term synaptic enhancement that persists without noticeable decline after post-tetanic potentiation has decayed (i.e., strong stimulus levels are effective in inducing LTP). Why does this long-term synaptic potentiation require the activation of a large population of presynaptic neurons?

An understanding of the associative nature of hippocampal LTP came from studies by Tom Brown and colleagues and by Bengt Gustafsson and Holger Wigstrom in which they explored what conditions would effectively produce long-term enhancement of the synaptic inputs from small populations of presynaptic cells. Because axons making synaptic connections with a given postsynaptic pyramidal cell arrive from different neighboring regions, it is possible to stimulate independently nonoverlapping populations of presynaptic neurons. As explained above, high-frequency stimulation of one small population of axons results in transient post-tetanic potentiation, but not long-term potentiation, of these synaptic inputs (Fig. 10C). High-frequency stimulation of a separate large population of presynaptic neurons has little effect on the synaptic connections from the small population, although the synaptic connections from the large population undergo long-term potentiation. However, LTP of the synaptic inputs from the small population of neurons results if stimulation of the small population of axons occurs simultaneously with high-frequency stimulation of the large population of presynaptic axons (Fig. 10C). This paired stimulation is reminiscent of the pairing of neural inputs that would be expected to occur in many forms of classical conditioning: prior to training, one

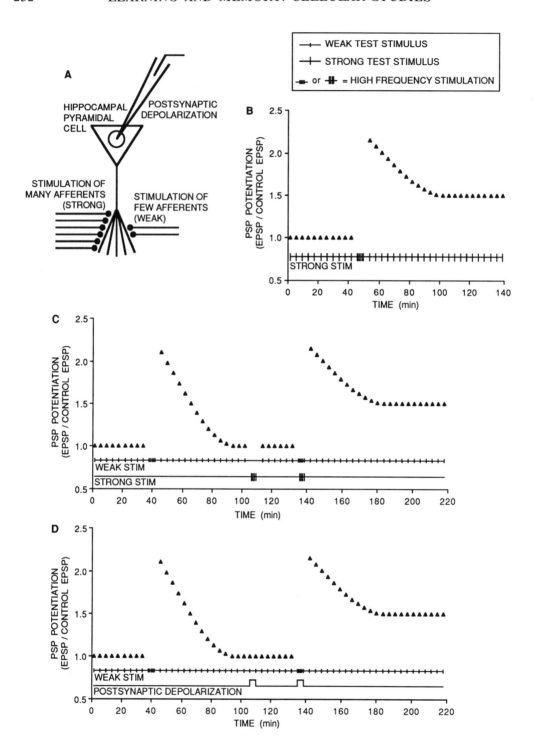

input activated by the US effectively excites postsynaptic neurons while a second input activated by the CS is too weak to strongly excite postsynaptic cells; with stimulus pairing, the synaptic input from the CS is strengthened, so that it is now sufficient to trigger postsynaptic activity and a behavioral response.

LTP is consistent with Hebb's proposal: presynaptic activity must occur coincident with postsynaptic depolarization. How does stimulation of a large population of presynaptic axons that is temporally paired with activity in a small population of presynaptic axons cause long-term enhancement of the synaptic connections from this small population? The two groups of axons could interact in two possible ways. On the one hand, the large population could somehow directly modulate the small group of presynaptic neurons. Alternatively, by powerfully exciting the postsynaptic neuron, stimulation of the large population of presynaptic axons could alter the interaction between the small population of presynaptic neurons and the post-

synaptic cell. One way a mechanism involving powerful postsynaptic excitation could work would be if induction of LTP required the pairing of presynaptic activity and postsynaptic depolarization. By altering the membrane potential of a postsynaptic pyramidal cell with intracellular current injection during high-frequency presynaptic stimulation, Gustafsson and Wigstrom, Robert Malinow and John Miller and Brown and his colleagues demonstrated that postsynaptic depolarization is indeed required for induction of LTP. Thus, hyperpolarizing the postsynaptic neuron during high-frequency stimulation of a large population of presynaptic axons effectively blocks induction of LTP. Reciprocally, the synaptic connections from a small population of presynaptic neurons undergo long-term potentiation if activation of these cells is paired with injection of depolarizing current into the postsynaptic cell (Fig. 10D).

A similar requirement for paired pre- and postsynaptic activity in initiation of persistent modification of synaptic strength was

FIG. 10. Various experimental treatments capable of inducing long-term potentiation (LTP) of synaptic connections in hippocampus. **A:** Experimental configuration. Synaptic responses recorded intracellularly in a postsynaptic pyramidal cell in the CA1 region of hippocampus. Two separate populations of presynaptic axons (or afferents) from CA3 pyramidal cells can be activated with different-strength stimuli: a weak stimulus that activates a small number of axons and a strong stimulus at a second location that activates a nonoverlapping, large number of axons. The postsynaptic cell potential can also be changed by injecting current intracellularly. The two different-strength stimuli at the two locations are indicated by short and long vertical lines. **B:** A high-frequency train of stimuli that excites the large population of presynaptic axons produces LTP of the synaptic inputs from this population. EPSP potentiation represents the relative amplitude of the EPSP from the population of presynaptic axons stimulated during the individual test stimuli. Note that an early, transient post-tetanic potentiation decays, leaving a persistent potentiation (i.e., LTP) of these synaptic connections. **C:** Pairing high-frequency stimulation of a large population of axons with high-frequency stimulation of a small population of presynaptic axons produces LTP of the synaptic inputs from the small population. Individual test stimuli are given to excite the small population of presynaptic axons (upper line). A high-frequency stimulus that excites this small population of axons produces only transient post-tetanic potentiation but no LTP. A high-frequency train of stimuli that excites the large population of axons (lower line) produces no enhancement of the synaptic connections from the small population of presynaptic axons. When two trains of stimuli are given that simultaneously excite the small and large populations of axons, the synaptic connections from the small population of axons undergo LTP that is evident after the decay of post-tetanic potentiation. **D:** Pairing postsynaptic depolarization with high-frequency stimulation of a small population of presynaptic axons produces LTP of these synaptic inputs. While a high-frequency train of stimuli that excites the small population of presynaptic axons alone produces postsynaptic potentiation of their synaptic inputs, and depolarization of the postsynaptic cell has no effect on these synaptic inputs, when postsynaptic depolarization is paired with high-frequency presynaptic stimulation, the input from this small population of presynaptic axons is strengthened in a long-term manner.

first proposed by the Canadian psychologist D. O. Hebb in 1949 in a theoretical discussion:

> When an axon of cell A is near enough to excite a cell B and repeatedly or persistently takes part in firing it, some growth process or metabolic change takes place in one or both cells such that A's efficiency, as one of the cells firing B, is increased. The most obvious and I believe much the most probable suggestion concerning the way in which one cell could become more capable of firing another is that synaptic knobs develop and increase the area of contact between the afferent axon and efferent soma . . . [and] dendrites.

Thus, LTP operates according to Hebb's postulate, although in LTP it is postsynaptic depolarization rather than firing of postsynaptic action potentials that is critical.

Mechanisms of LTP Induction

LTP is triggered by a postsynaptic signal, a rise in intracellular Ca^{++}. The cellular mechanisms underlying LTP have been most extensively analyzed in the CA1 region of the hippocampus. At the synapses between CA3 pyramidal cell axons and CA1 pyramidal cells, the critical initial signal in induction of LTP is influx of Ca^{++} into the postsynaptic pyramidal cell. The essential role of Ca^{++} was first suggested by experiments of Gary Lynch and his colleagues in which LTP was effectively blocked by injection of the Ca^{++} chelator EGTA into the postsynaptic pyramidal cell. More recently, Roger Nicoll and Robert Zucker and their colleagues showed that experimentally induced transient elevations in postsynaptic intracellular Ca^{++} in the postsynaptic neuron trigger persistent enhancement of synaptic inputs.

The NMDA receptor–gated channel allows a transient Ca^{++} rise when activated in an associative manner. Glutamate is believed to be the principal neurotransmitter at these synapses. These pyramidal cells have multiple types of glutamate receptors, identified by their preferred agonists, including *N*-methyl-D-aspartate (NMDA) receptors, quisqualate/α-amino-3-hydroxy-5-methyl-4-isoxazole-

propionic acid (AMPA) receptors, and kainate receptors (see Chapter 7). The primary route for Ca^{++} influx into postsynaptic CA1 pyramidal cells is through the NMDA receptor channel rather than through voltage-sensitive Ca^{++} channels activated by depolarization. In CA1 pyramidal cells, the NMDA receptor does not play a major role in normal excitatory synaptic transmission; the depolarizing current during the normal EPSP is carried primarily through channels gated by quisqualate/AMPA receptors. In contrast, the NMDA receptor is centrally involved in the induction of LTP. The NMDA receptor channel shows unusual properties in that it requires two events to be effectively opened. First, it requires the binding of glutamate, which causes the channel to undergo a conformational change into the open state. However, under normal conditions, Mg^{++} ions, held in place by the negative charges on the inside of the postsynaptic membrane, block the pore of the channel. Only when the postsynaptic pyramidal cell spine undergoes a large depolarization is the Mg^{++} blockade relieved. Thus, Ca^{++} influx through the NMDA receptor–gated channel requires the temporal coincidence of (1) glutamate binding and (2) postsynaptic depolarization. The NMDA receptor's requirement for postsynaptic depolarization paired with the release of glutamate from an individual presynaptic terminal can explain the associative nature of LTP. A strong synaptic input that effectively depolarizes the postsynaptic pyramidal cell paired with the simultaneous activation of individual presynaptic neurons effectively triggers Ca^{++} influx through the NMDA receptor and long-term enhancement of the synaptic connections from these active presynaptic neurons.

There are interesting parallels between the associative activation of the NMDA receptor channel during LTP and the associative activation of the Ca^{++}/calmodulin-sensitive adenylyl cyclase in *Aplysia* during activity-dependent facilitation. In each case, two signals converge in an associative manner and interact not at the level of neural circuits but at the level of single molecules. In each case, a change in a critical second messenger results when these two signals converge at a single molecular site. In the case of LTP the molecule is a membrane-bound receptor, whereas in the case of activity-dependent facilitation the associative molecule is a membrane-bound enzyme. Figure 11 compares the associative activation of these two molecules.

In the postsynaptic neuron both protein kinases and proteases may be involved in the induction of LTP cascade. How does the Ca^{++} transient in the postsynaptic spine trigger LTP? At least three enzymes have been suggested as playing essential roles in the initiation of LTP. The earliest molecular hypothesis for LTP was proposed in 1984 by Gary Lynch and Michel Baudry, who suggested that a specific Ca^{++}-activated protease, calpain, cleaved cytoskeletal elements so as to unmask or allow insertion of additional glutamate receptors in the postsynaptic membrane. Consistent with this hypothesis, leupeptin, a tripeptide inhibitor of calpain, interfered with both LTP and some forms of learning. More recently, two protein kinases have been demonstrated to be essential for the induction of LTP. Injection of a specific peptide inhibitor of either Ca^{++}/calmodulin-dependent kinase II or protein kinase C into the postsynaptic pyramidal cell effectively blocks LTP. The observation that inhibiting either kinase prevents induction of LTP suggests that perhaps the two protein kinases are activated in a serial fashion as part of the cascade for initiating LTP. Interestingly, Ca^{++}/calmodulin-dependent kinase type II is found at extremely high densities in the postsynaptic regions of the spines, leading to the proposal that this enzyme may play an important role in the regulation of synaptic transmission. Recent experiments of Thomas O'Dell, Kandel, and Seth Grant have implicated another protein kinase, a tyrosine kinase, in induction of LTP.

Contribution of Presynaptic vs. Postsynaptic Changes to LTP

Either of two classes of mechanisms could underlie LTP. First, there could be increased transmitter release from each presynaptic neuron; such enhanced release could occur from the original number of release sites or from an expanded number of release sites. Second, there could be increased response to neurotransmitter in the postsynaptic spine. A variety of evidence supports both a presynaptic and a postsynaptic locus for the change that underlies the increased strength of synaptic connections. Consistent with a postsynaptic contribution, when specific agonists were applied experimentally, the postsynaptic sensitivity to a quisqualate/AMPA agonist was observed to increase during LTP. This would suggest that there may be alterations in the quisqualate/AMPA class of receptors. On the other hand, one series of studies has shown that release of [^{3}H]glutamate that accompanies stimulation of presynaptic axons is increased in parallel with LTP. Recently, Charles Stevens and Richard Tsien and their colleagues carried out quantal analyses of the synaptic connections between CA3 neurons and CA1 neurons before and after induction of LTP. Their data support this possibility of a presynaptic change; in parallel with an increase in EPSP amplitude, the number of quanta released per stimulus was found to increase without a change in the size of individual quanta. As discussed earlier, a change in mean number of quanta per synaptic potential clearly indicates a change in the presynaptic release process. A number of morphological changes in synaptic ultrastructure have been reported including an increase in the number of synaptic contacts.

If postsynaptic processes are required for initiating LTP, a retrograde messenger must initiate presynaptic enhancement of transmitter release. One attractive group of candidates for such a retrograde signal is the family of messenger molecules that are derived from arachidonic acid. Arachidonic acid is cleaved from membrane phospholipids by the enzyme phospholipase A_2. As in the case of other intracellular messenger systems, the enzyme that initiates the cascade is activated by receptors via one of the class of GTP-binding proteins (G proteins). Arachidonic acid and its metabolites are unusual regulatory messen-

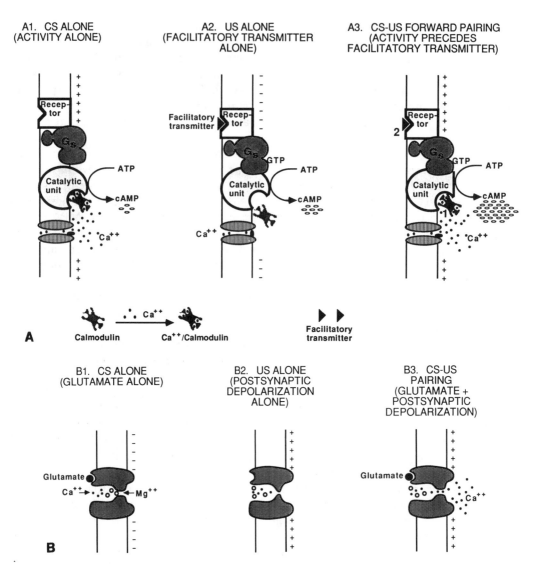

FIG. 11. Summary of molecular hypotheses for associative synaptic plasticity in *Aplysia* sensory neurons and mammalian hippocampal neurons. In both models, associative activation of a membrane-bound protein gates activation of an intracellular messenger that triggers synaptic modification. **A:** Stimulus convergence at the adenylyl cyclase may underlie activity-dependent facilitation in *Aplysia* sensory neurons. A1, Presentation of the conditioned stimulus alone results in activity in the siphon sensory neurons; this depolarization, in turn, causes Ca^{++} influx into these cells. The elevation in Ca^{++} acts via calmodulin to increase cyclase activity, resulting in a small rise in cAMP, the second messenger that triggers synaptic facilitation. A2, Presentation of the unconditioned stimulus alone results in release of facilitatory transmitter and moderate stimulation of cyclase activity, causing a modest amount of presynaptic facilitation and modest strengthening of the defensive withdrawal reflex. A3, Paired presentation in which sensory neuron activity immediately precedes facilitatory transmitter results in dual activation of the adenylyl cyclase and enhanced synthesis of cAMP, causing enhanced presynaptic facilitation and more effective strengthening of the withdrawal reflex. **B:** Stimulus convergence at the NMDA-type glutamate receptor channel may underlie associative long-term potentiation in the CA1 region of the hippocampus. B1, Activity of a small number of presynaptic neurons (equivalent to a CS) results in release of glutamate from their presynaptic terminals. Glutamate binds to the NMDA-type glutamate receptor, causing its channel to open; however, the permeability of the channel remains low because Mg^{++} ions are held in the pore by the negative potential on the inside the membrane. Thus, there is no influx of Ca^{++}. B2, A large number of additional synaptic

ger molecules in that they are lipid-permeable and can therefore act both intracellularly and intercellularly, influencing neighboring cells. However, recently substantial evidence has accumulated that another cell-permeant second-messenger, nitric oxide, may serve as the retrograde signal. Nitric oxide (NO) was first identified as a second messenger in studies of the peripheral vascular system where it was identified as endothelium-derived relaxing factor. Recently, Schuman and Madison, as well as O'Dell and his colleagues, found that inhibitors of NO synthase, the enzyme that inhibits NO, block induction of LTP. Moreover, both studies observed that extracellular application of hemoglobin, a cell-impermeant protein that binds NO, interferes with induction of LTP. This effect of hemoglobin may be interpreted as indicating that the NO signal must pass through the extracellular compartment before it acts on its target. This blockade by an extracellular inhibitor is consistent with the model that NO acts as a retrograde signal between adjacent cells. Interestingly, Small, O'Dell, Kandel, and Hawkins have found that application of NO to hippocampal slices can induce persistent potentiation of synaptic connections, but only if the NO is paired with activation of the presynaptic neurons. Thus, it may be that if NO is released from the postsynaptic neurons during LTP, this retrograde messenger selectively enhances synaptic transmission from those presynaptic axons that are active. Such an activity-dependent response to an extracellular modulatory signal is formally quite similar to the gating of presynaptic facilitation in *Aplysia* sensory neurons by activity that is paired with facilitatory transmitter. The role of NO as a retrograde messenger is integrated with other aspects of the current hypothesis concerning LTP in Fig. 12.

Protein synthesis is required for induction of the late phase of LTP. Inhibitors of protein synthesis are able to completely block the induction of the late phase of LTP, lasting beyond 1–2 hours. This suggests that in the hippocampus, as in *Aplysia* sensory neurons, long-term synaptic plasticity requires protein synthesis.

Link Between LTP and Spatial Learning

As discussed at the outset of the discussion of hippocampal LTP, because of its rapid induction, stable persistence, and associative nature, this form of synaptic plasticity has seemed hypothetically an attractive candidate for a cellular mechanism of learning. Although in rodents the hippocampus plays a critical role in spatial learning and hippocampal pyramidal cells have response properties to multimodal sensory cues that enable these neurons to code the spatial position of the animals in an environment, there has been limited evidence linking LTP to spatial learning. Until recently, the suggestion that LTP contributes to spatial learning was based primarily on the observation that administration of NMDA receptor antagonists to the CNS of intact behaving animals resulted in impairment of spatial learning in rats. However, blockade of NMDA receptors is likely to have effects in addition to interfering with induction of LTP. Recently, two studies used recombinant DNA techniques including homologous recombination for insertion of mutant genes into embryonic stem cells to create mutant strains of mice lacking one of two protein kinases previously shown to be

---

inputs to the postsynaptic neuron (equivalent to a US alone) results in effective postsynaptic depolarization which relieves the Mg^{++} blockade; however, because the channel has not been opened by transmitter, there is also no Ca^{++} influx. B3, Release of glutamate from a single presynaptic neuron paired with postsynaptic depolarization (equivalent to CS-US pairing) results in channel opening in the absence of a Mg^{++} blockade, so that Ca^{++} influx can occur. Influx of Ca^{++} into the postsynaptic neuron acts as the intracellular signal that triggers long-term potentiation of the synapse. From Abrams TW, Kandel ER. Is contiguity detection in classical conditioning a system or a cellular property? Learning in *Aplysia* suggests a possible molecular site. *Trends Neurosci* 1988;11:128–135.

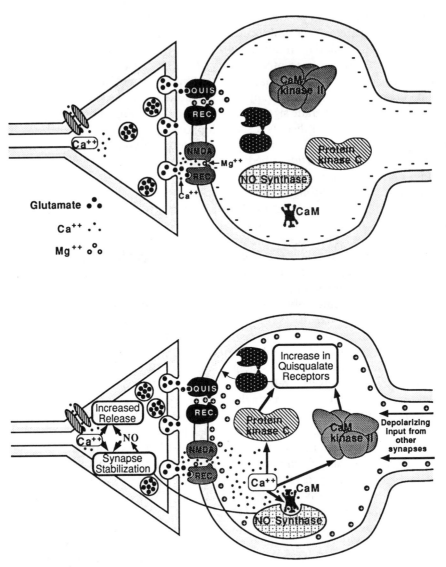

FIG. 12. Model for induction of long-term potentiation in the hippocampus. Coincidence of presynaptic activity with postsynaptic depolarization allows the NMDA-type glutamate receptor to trigger synaptic enhancement. **Top:** Glutamate release from presynaptic terminal in the absence of additional depolarizing input to the postsynaptic spine. Although glutamate binds to the postsynaptic receptor, the NMDA channel remains blocked by Mg^{++} ions. **Bottom:** Glutamate release paired with other depolarizing inputs. Postsynaptic inputs depolarize the spine, which relieves the Mg^{++} blockade, allowing Ca^{++} influx when glutamate is bound to the NMDA receptor. Postsynaptic Ca^{++} triggers synaptic enhancement, perhaps by stimulating two Ca^{++}-sensitive protein kinases (CaM kinase II or protein kinase C); these Ca^{++}-sensitive enzymes somehow result in an increase in sensitivity to glutamate in the postsynaptic cell that occurs through modulation of quisqualate AMPA/(QUIS) receptors (shown here as insertion of new quisqualate receptors). Ca^{++} is also shown activating nitric oxide (NO) synthase, via CaM. NO synthase synthesizes NO, which, because it is cell-permeant, can diffuse to the presynaptic cell. This retrograde signal may then act to increase transmitter release from presynaptic terminals. The action of NO on the presynaptic terminals is shown as dependent on Ca^{++} influx that results from presynaptic activity.

necessary for induction of LTP. Alcino Silva and colleagues and Seth Grant and colleagues found that two mouse strains that were mutant in either Ca^{++}/calmodulin-dependent kinase II or Fyn tyrosine kinase did not show LTP. Both mutant strains are impaired in spatial learning tasks with complex arrays of cues. Interestingly, the mice deficient in Ca^{++}/calmodulin-dependent kinase II are capable of simpler associative learning tasks, where associations with arrays of spatial cues are not necessary. Based on similarity in the requirements for specific protein kinases, these recent results would suggest that LTP may be fundamentally involved in spatial learning, although not in some other forms of associative learning.

SUMMARY

This chapter has reviewed several simple neural systems in which neurobiologists have attempted to characterize cellular mechanisms of plasticity contributing to behavioral changes that occur during learning. Through a number of cellular studies, it has been possible to gain insights into the nature of mechanisms that contribute to neural plasticity during learning.

For example, we know that existing synaptic connections are altered during learning. In the instances analyzed, learning is accompanied by modification of existing synaptic connections rather than growth of neurons to targets in novel regions of the nervous system with which they would not otherwise connect. This does not mean, on the level of some individual neurons, that new synaptic connections may not form (or that existing connections may not be eliminated). In other words, during this process of synaptic modification, some potential target neurons may receive synapses from individual presynaptic cells which already had projected to the appropriate region but which had not previously connected with these target cells; alternatively, some existing synaptic connections may be completely retracted.

It has been frequently observed that plasticity during learning is triggered by second-messenger systems. Second messengers, including cAMP, diacylglycerol, and Ca^{++}, commonly produce their effects by activating protein kinases; in turn, kinases can modulate proteins involved in various cellular processes or regulate gene expression. Alternatively, some second messengers such as Ca^{++} or arachidonic acid metabolites may interact directly with enzymes or ion channels.

It has been established that short-term learning involves covalent modification of existing proteins. Similarly, existing proteins may be modified in long-term learning. Such modifications include phosphorylation, proteolytic cleavage, and possibly methylation.

Long-term learning often involves changes in gene expression. Recent studies in *Aplysia* suggest that some of the genes whose transcription is altered are regulatory; these genes in turn influence synthesis of other proteins. Also, in long-term learning there may be changes in the morphology of synaptic connections. Active zone release sites may be altered in size or structure, and specialized postsynaptic regions, such as dendritic spines, may be changed in shape. Fine branches of pre- or postsynaptic neurons may be altered to permit an increase or decrease in the incidence or strength of synaptic connections.

The existing proteins altered during either short-term or long-term learning may include ion channels, proteins involved in transmitter release, and receptors.

It can be stated that although some systems have been studied extensively, at present there is no instance of learning in which underlying cellular mechanisms are completely understood. Clearly, much work has yet to be done in this important and exciting field.

BIBLIOGRAPHY

Original Articles

Chang F-LF, Greenough WT. Transient and enduring morphological correlates of synaptic activity and efficacy change in the rat hippocampal slice. *Brain Res* 1984;309:35–46.

Davies SN, Lester RA, Reymann KG, Collingridge GL. Temporally distinct pre- and post-synaptic mechanisms maintain long-term potentiation. *Nature* 1989;338:500–503.

Eskin A, Garcia KS, Byrne JH. Information storage in the nervous system of *Aplysia:* specific proteins affected by serotonin and cAMP. *Proc Natl Acad Sci USA* 1989;86:2458–2462.

Frost WN, Clark GA, Kandel ER. Parallel processing of short-term memory for sensitization in *Aplysia. J Neurobiol* 1988;19:297–334.

Hochner B, Klein M, Schacher S, Kandel ER. Additional component in the cellular mechanism of presynaptic facilitation contributes to behavioral dishabituation in *Aplysia. Proc Natl Acad Sci USA* 1986;83:8794–8798.

Kauer JA, Malenka RC, Nicoll RA. A persistent postsynaptic modification mediates long-term potentiation in the hippocampus. *Neuron* 1988;1:911–917.

Klein M, Shapiro E, Kandel ER. Synaptic plasticity and the modulation of the Ca^{2+} current. *J Exp Biol* 1980;89:117–157.

Lynch MA, Errington ML, Bliss TVP. Long-term potentiation of synaptic transmission in the dentate gyrus: increased release of [14C]glutamate without increase in receptor binding. *Neurosci Lett* 1985;62:123–129.

Malenka RC, Kauer JA, Zucker RS, Nicoll RA. Postsynaptic calcium is sufficient for potentiation of hippocampal synaptic transmission. *Science* 1988;242:81–84.

Montarolo PG, Goelet P, Castellucci VF, Morgan J, Kandel ER, Schacher S. A critical period for macromolecular synthesis in long-term heterosynaptic facilitation in *Aplysia. Science* 1986;234:1249–1254.

Nowak L, Bregestovski P, Ascher P, Herbet A, Prochiantz A. Magnesium gates glutamate-activated channels in mouse central neurones. *Nature* 1984;307:462–465.

Schacher S, Castellucci VF, Kandel ER. cAMP evokes long-term facilitation in *Aplysia* sensory neurons that requires new protein synthesis. *Science* 1988;240:1667–1669.

Scholz KP, Byrne JH. Intracellular injection of cAMP induces a long-term reduction of neuronal K^+ currents. *Science* 1988;240:1664–1666.

Siegelbaum SA, Camardo JS, Kandel ER. Serotonin and cyclic AMP close single K^+ channels in *Aplysia* sensory neurons. *Nature* 1982;299:413–417.

Thompson RF. The neural basis of basic associative learning of discrete behavioral responses. *Trends Neurosci* 1988;11:152–155.

Williams JH, Errington ML, Lynch MA, Bliss TVP. Arachidonic acid induces a long-term activity-dependent enhancement of synaptic transmission in the hippocampus. *Nature* 1989;341:739–742.

Books and Reviews

Abrams TW. Activity-dependent presynaptic facilitation: an associative mechanism in *Aplysia. Cell Mol Neurobiol* 1985;5:123–145.

Abrams TW, Kandel ER. Is contiguity detection in classical conditioning a system or a cellular property? Learning in *Aplysia* suggests a possible molecular site. *Trends Neurosci* 1988;11:128–135.

Agranoff BW. Learning and memory. In: Siegel GJ, Agranoff BW, Albers RW, Molinoff PB, eds. *Basic neurochemistry*, 5th ed. New York: Raven Press; 1994 (in press).

Bailey CH, Chen M. Structural plasticity at identified synapses during long-term memory in *Aplysia. J Neurobiol* 1989;20:356–372.

Gustafsson B, Wigström H. Physiological mechanisms underlying long-term potentiation. *Trends Neurosci* 1988;11:156–162.

O'Keefe J. A review of hippocampal place cells. *Progr Neurobiol* 1979;13:419–439.

Squire LR. *Memory and brain.* New York: Oxford University Press; 1987.

14

Animal Behavioral Approaches

William D. Essman and Irwin Lucki

Paleontologists had been digging up bones for so long that they had forgotten how little information could be gleaned from a skeleton. Bones might tell you something about the gross appearance of an animal, its height and weight. They might tell you something about how the muscles attached, and therefore something about the crude behavior of the animal during life. They might give you clues to the few diseases that affected bone. But a skeleton was a poor thing, really, from which to try and deduce the total behavior of an organism.

Michael Crichton,
Jurassic Park (New York: Ballantine Books, 1990, p. 394)

- A variety of behavioral pharmacological procedures are used to assess the relevance of animal models to specific clinical behavioral dysfunctions.

- The criteria for behavioral experiments include both pharmacological and behavioral components.

- Selectivity means that a model must be able to differentiate between drugs that are effective in treating a particular human disorder and those that are not.

- The potency of a drug is measured by determining the dose of the drug that produces a functional effect, such as a behavioral or biochemical action.

- For some clinical disorders there are demonstrable interactions between drugs. These interactions may range from antagonism (attenuation of one drug's effects by administration of another) to synergism (a greater than additive effect of two compounds administered simultaneously).

- An animal test of a drug relies on the test being relevant to the clinical disorder.

- Validity in behavioral pharmacology describes the relationship between the results from a behavioral experiment and the clinical observations of the disorder it models.

- There are three levels of validity: predictive, face, and construct.

- Animal self-administration studies play a crucial role in understanding human substance abuse.

- Elicited behavior generally refers to observable behaviors produced by a drug.

- Drug discrimination experiments are designed to characterize the subjective effects of drugs in animals.

- Drug signatures in operant paradigms are determinations of the effects of drugs on patterns of responding engendered by different operant schedules.

- Two of the most important characteristics of a drug are its selectivity and its efficacy.

- Site of action is another critical aspect of neuropharmacological investigation.

- Depending on the drug, repeated administration may lead to tolerance on the one hand or supersensitivity on the other.

■ Chapter Overview ────────────────────────────

This chapter focuses on studies that use behavioral pharmacological methods to identify drugs that could be useful in alleviating patient suffering and to investigate the behavioral, neurochemical, and neuroanatomic mechanisms through which the psychotherapeutic compounds act. First the chapter describes how the relevance of a particular animal study to a human disorder is assessed in terms of behavioral criteria and validity. Then it describes two broad types of animal behavioral pharmacology experiments that strive to attain different goals in examining the behavioral properties of drugs: those evaluating clinical efficacy and those demonstrating neurobiological mechanisms mediating the effects of known drugs or drugs of abuse. Also discussed is a third broad category involving characterization of the neurobiological substrates of psychoactive drug action. Finally, the chapter discusses some of the advantages behavioral studies present that are critical to the understanding of the biological bases of behavior.

The field of behavioral pharmacology uses concepts and techniques derived from both pharmacology and psychology to study the interactions between drugs and behavior. Some behavioral pharmacology studies investigate the behavioral or psychological processes that are altered by administration of a drug. For example, such studies may determine what doses of drugs alter locomotor activity, lever-pressing behavior, feeding, sexual behavior, and aggression. Other behavioral pharmacology studies are more concerned with discovering the neurobiological substrates that mediate particular behavioral effects. The integration of behavioral or psychological with neurobiological research approaches provides a basis for the systematic study of the actions of drugs that are pertinent to their clinical effects in humans.

Historically, behavioral pharmacology emerged during the decade of the 1950s from the need to study drugs with specific behavioral effects that could successfully treat certain psychiatric disorders. For example, the introduction of chlorpromazine in the 1950s provided psychiatrists with a drug that selectively reduced patients' psychotic symptoms. Even though chlorpromazine had effects in the clinic, there was at that time no clear explanation of its behavioral or neurochemical effects. Behavioral techniques became one of the important research tools for the investigation of chlorpromazine and the psychotherapeutic drugs that followed. This legacy is evident today in behavioral pharmacology studies concerned with the treatment of medical diseases and disorders with strong behavioral symptoms. Currently, areas of intense behavioral investigations include psychiatric disorders (e.g., schizophrenia, depression, anxiety), diseases with neurological manifestations (e.g., Parkinson's disease, Alzheimer's disease), management of pain (e.g., postoperative pain, chronic pain), and disorders of drug use (e.g., alcoholism, drug abuse). In each of these instances, the principal complaint of the patients involves a psychological or behavioral dysfunction that impairs normal functioning in everyday life.

Animal behavior experiments provide an important basis for addressing questions as to the clinical relevance of the pharmacological effects of drugs. For example, one of the most important properties of drugs is their ability to activate or block receptors. These effects are often termed *functional properties* of

Biological Bases of Brain Function and Disease, edited by Alan Frazer, Perry B. Molinoff, and Andrew Winokur. Raven Press, Ltd., New York © 1994.

drugs. Behavioral experiments provide functional evidence for the mechanisms of action of established therapeutic compounds by providing measures of drug effects, sometimes called response endpoints, that are related to the clinical effects of drugs in humans. Behavioral studies also provide a basis for investigating the mechanisms of action of novel therapeutic compounds by comparing their properties to known clinically effective drugs. Chemists are now capable of creating compounds with more targeted neurochemical effects, such as agonists or antagonists at specific neurotransmitter or neuropeptide receptors. However, it is not always clear as to which diseases these compounds are best suited to treat. Behavioral studies can provide evidence that specific neurochemical tools may be developed as effective medicines. Compounds with neurochemical effects that are targeted at a specific disease process and that lack serious side effects or effects on other neurochemical systems can be identified using behavioral studies. Since clinical trials are the most expensive aspect of drug discovery (see Chapter 17), it is important that every effort be exerted to identify the compounds most likely to produce therapeutic effects without serious side effects before the compounds are nominated for evaluation in humans. Significant behavioral side effects, such as abuse potential, behavioral sedation, neurological abnormalities, or psychotomimetic or anxiogenic subjective effects, may limit the medicinal utility of the most efficacious drug. Animal behavior experiments can indicate which compounds might be effective for various disorders, which may be likely to produce impairing behavioral side effects, and how new therapeutics might compare to currently prescribed drugs.

ASSESSMENT OF THE CRITERIA FOR AND VALIDITY OF BEHAVIORAL EXPERIMENTS

A variety of behavioral pharmacological procedures are used to assess the relevance of animal models to specific clinical behavioral dysfunctions. Animal behavior is often studied in psychopharmacology with the purpose of discovering assays that parallel human disorders as closely as possible. Such experimental paradigms are called *animal models.* The behaviors of animals under different experimental conditions are studied to simulate behavioral or psychological processes in the laboratory that are thought to be important to the clinical syndromes shown by human patients. Psychiatric disorders are generally diagnosed on the basis of reports of subjective mood or thought disturbances and the appearance of associated somatic symptoms. Furthermore, the effects of drugs on the behavioral model may be interpreted as operating on the modeled subjective states, such as altering anxiety or depression. These factors make it tempting to construct animal models based on anthropomorphic representations of human psychological processes. However, this practice can be misleading. Human observers can never exactly characterize the internal psychological processes of infrahuman species. It is also impossible to "diagnose" a rat or monkey as having depression or schizophrenia, for example, because the internal mood or thought disturbances that are a critical part of the human diagnostic criteria cannot be modeled in animals. Behavioral descriptions of psychiatric patients that do not rely on internal states, such as disturbances of motor activity, reinforcement mechanisms, feeding behavior, or sensory-motor function, will provide the most valuable information concerning objective psychological processes that can be modeled in animals. The current trend to include more overt, rather than subjective, behavioral characteristics of patients in psychiatric diagnostic criteria will improve the design of animal models directed at specific clinical disorders.

Five General Criteria for Behavioral Experiments

The criteria for behavioral experiments include both pharmacological and behavioral components. The first step in determining whether an animal model will provide a useful tool for studying a human psychiatric dysfunction involves assessing the model in terms of the characteristics it shares with the human syndrome. These characteristics represent similarities between human and animal behaviors and their responses to drug administration that are important to elucidating the behavioral and neurochemical mechanisms underlying psychiatric disorders. As such, they constitute a set of standards with which the animal paradigms are evaluated. A successful model is often called an animal *screen,* since it may be used to screen new drugs for potential clinical efficacy. In practice, an animal behavioral assay does not have to fulfill all of these criteria to be useful. However, the more criteria the paradigm meets, the more useful it will be in screening new drugs.

Selectivity

Selectivity means that a model must be able to differentiate between drugs that are effective in treating a particular human disorder and those that are not. Useful behavioral tests must demonstrate selectivity. Therefore, the most important criterion for a behavioral test is that it show positive effects for known clinically efficacious drugs (called *criterion drugs*) and negative effects for compounds known to be ineffective for treating the disorder being modeled. This means that an assay must minimize both *false positives* and *false negatives.* False positives represent compounds that show activity in a particular test but have no demonstrable clinical efficacy. False negatives represent compounds with known therapeutic activity that do not produce the desired effects in the behavioral paradigm. The model has the greatest probability of screening only those compounds likely to be of clinical use if both of these conditions are met.

Potency Relationships

The potency *of a drug is measured by determining the dose of the drug that produces a* *functional effect, such as a behavioral or biochemical action.* The potency criterion is necessitated by the fact that drugs produce more than just one effect. A behavioral assay must show relative potencies among criterion drugs that match their clinical potencies to ensure that the assay measures the actions of the compounds responsible for their therapeutic effects rather than side effects of the drugs. For example, the relative potencies of antipsychotics in an animal model should match their potencies in providing relief from psychotic symptoms and not their potencies in producing motor impairment, a side effect of some typical antipsychotics. Potencies of drugs to produce a common behavioral effect in animals can be compared with either their clinical effects or their side effects in humans. If the relative potencies among drugs in a behavioral experiment do not match their clinical therapeutic potencies, then it is possible that the behavioral test is measuring a common side effect of the drugs. It is important that drug effects on animal models be based on their primary therapeutic effects rather than their side effects to ensure that the models are identifying compounds with true therapeutic potential.

Temporal Characteristics

The temporal characteristics criterion reflects the observation that the behavioral effects of drugs may change with their chronic administration. For example, patients do not generally display improvement immediately after the first drug treatment in disorders such as schizophrenia and depression but require continued treatment for weeks before the drug's therapeutic effects emerge. Therefore, a behavioral test that purports to act as an animal model of these disorders should show at least some temporal delay in the effects it displays. Alternatively, certain side effects of drugs, such as the sedation that accompanies anxiolytic benzodiazepine therapy, may demonstrate *tolerance* in that the side effects are decreased with continued benzodiazepine administration whereas the therapeutic effects of the benzodiazepines continue. Therefore, a model of anxiolytic behavioral effects should not demonstrate tolerance following chronic drug administration. This would match the time course of the anxiolytic actions of benzodiazepines in clinical practice. As with the criterion for appropriate potency relationships, the ability to demonstrate similar temporal characteristics between clinical effects and results from a behavioral assay provides evidence that both are measures of the same drug actions.

Drug Interactions

For some clinical disorders there are demonstrable interactions between drugs. These interactions may range from antagonism *(attenuation of one drug's effects by administration of another) to* synergism *(a greater than additive effect of two compounds administered simultaneously).* Again, behavioral assays should show interactions comparable to any observed in clinical practice to ensure that the behavioral test is measuring the therapeutic functions of the drug.

Theoretical/Psychological Relevance

An animal test of a drug relies on the test being relevant to the clinical disorder. The relevance criterion is perhaps the hardest to satisfy. This criterion demands that an animal test rely on some behavioral or psychological process of theoretical importance to the disorder. For example, if the clinical syndrome presents with a significant component of fear or anxiety, the behavioral test should also measure a similar element of "fear" (as opera-

tionally defined in the assay). Of all the criteria, this is perhaps the most difficult to meet, because it relies on aspects of clinical syndromes that are not well defined.

As stated above, animal behavioral tests rely on the measurement of overt behavioral responses. In contrast, human clinical syndromes such as depression often rely on subjective verbal reports of dysfunctions of internal mood states. It is truly difficult to establish whether the overt responses of animals are due to the identical internal states reported by psychiatric patients. Correspondingly, it has not yet been determined whether behavioral processes assessed by certain animal models are also demonstrated as behavioral dysfunctions by human patients. In addition, the different psychological variables that are responsible for a clinical disorder are not generally completely understood or identified. However, it is thought that animal behavior research can contribute information about the psychopathology of psychiatric diseases by examining the behavioral processes that are altered by psychotherapeutic drugs.

Levels of Validity

Validity *in behavioral pharmacology describes the relationship between the results from a behavioral experiment and the clinical observations of the disorder it models.* Once a particular animal test has been analyzed for its ability to meet these criteria, it may be evaluated accordingly. *There are three levels of validity: predictive, face, and construct* (see Table 1). As indicated in the table, the three levels of validity are hierarchical in nature. Higher levels of validity indicate progressively greater congruence between an animal

TABLE 1. *Validity of behavioral models of drug action*

Level of validity[a]	Necessary criteria
I. Predictive validity	Selectivity, potency relationships
II. Face validity	Temporal characteristics, drug interactions (in addition to criteria for predictive validity)
III. Construct validity	Theoretical relevance (in addition to criteria for predictive and face validity)

[a] Each level of validity is indicated with the criteria necessary to reach that level. In addition, models at one level should have met the criteria for the preceding level.

model and its relevant human disorder. The section below describes how the ability of a behavioral paradigm to meet the specific criteria of selectivity, potency relationships, temporal characteristics, drug interactions, and theoretical relevance is used to assign the assay a level of predictive, face, or construct validity.

Predictive Validity

The predictive validity of a model is evaluated on the basis of its ability to accurately differentiate between drugs that are clinically efficacious in the human disorder being modeled and those that are not. A model at this level of validity has met the criteria of selectivity (i.e., it has a minimum of false positives and false negatives) and potency relationships (i.e., it gives appropriate results concerning the relative potencies between compounds). Although models at this level of validity can be useful for identifying new clinically effective compounds, their principal utility is usually limited to identifying compounds with pharmacological mechanisms similar to those of known therapeutic drugs. New therapeutic compounds with novel pharmacological mechanisms of action sometimes fail to produce appropriate effects in these models. When this happens, assessments of predictive validity must be readjusted to incorporate a new class of therapeutic drug. For example, some animal behavior tests for antipsychotic drug action have relied on the ability of neuroleptics to produce motor impairments, e.g., catalepsy or psychomotor retardation. Clozapine, a neuroleptic that produces neurochemical effects different from those of typical neuroleptics, was not identified as a clinically efficacious drug in these standard behavioral procedures. The efficacy of clozapine in the treatment of human schizophrenic patients called into question the utility of these behavioral assays for screening new antipsychotics. New behavioral screens for antipsychotic drugs will have to be developed that include clozapine as an active compound.

Face Validity

The face validity of an animal experiment is evaluated on the basis of behavioral and pharmacological qualities that can be demonstrated to be similar to those of the human disorder it models. For some investigators, one aspect of face validity is the morphological similarity between the animal behavior and the dysfunctional human behavior (e.g., motor impairments in models of Parkinson's disease or abnormal oral behaviors in models of tardive dyskinesia). Other aspects of face validity concern the temporal properties of drug administration and appropriate drug interactions. A model meeting these criteria can be assumed to measure some function of therapeutic drugs that is important in the human psychiatric disorder. For example, a delayed onset of action in a model of antidepressant drug action indicates that the pharmacological effects measured by the behavioral assay are similar to those mediating the therapeutic effects of drugs in depressed human patients, since antidepressant drugs appear to have such a delayed onset of clinical effects.

Construct Validity

The construct validity of a model is assessed by determining a direct theoretical relationship to the human disorder being modeled. The goal of such a model is to develop an assay in which the clinical syndrome and the behavior measured in the animal test rely on similar psychological or behavioral processes (e.g., anxiety, reinforcement mechanisms, despair, etc.). Such an animal study represents the closest approximation possible to the actual human psychiatric disorder. The behaviors in the assay and in the disorders must be homologous rather than analogous. *Homologous* behaviors have the same psychological and neurophysiological origins. *Analogous* behaviors look similar, at least on superficial inspection, but occur through different mechanisms. As indicated above, the criterion of theoretical or psychological relevance is the most difficult to meet. Construct validity is correspondingly difficult to attain. However, the conceptions of animal models of psychiatric disorders at this level are important for their implications regarding the etiology of psychiatric illnesses. If an assay can unequivocally meet the criteria for construct validity, then it provides a model that should identify behavioral, neurochemical, and anatomical factors most relevant to a particular clinical dysfunction.

Examples of Behavioral Models

The selection of an animal model with a particular level of validity depends on the goals of the experiment. If the model is to be used to identify new psychotherapeutic compounds from a series of chemicals that affect a particular neurotransmitter, a level of predictive validity may be all that is necessary. On the other hand, if a researcher is investigating the neurochemical mechanisms that mediate a human disorder, a model with face or construct validity would be more appropriate. With the variety of assays currently available, behavioral pharmacologists are generally able to tailor studies to their particular needs.

Two animal models provide concrete examples of how behavioral criteria and validity assessments are applied to actual behavioral screens. The first model is used to screen antidepressant drugs and represents the level of predictive validity. The second model is used to evaluate the abuse potential of new compounds and demonstrates the properties of construct validity. Each model is successful in achieving the goals of its own level of validity and therefore each is a useful tool in behavioral pharmacology.

Antidepressant Drugs—Predictive Validity

The assay to be described measures the effects of antidepressant drugs on the behavior of rats responding in an operant experimental chamber under a differential reinforcement of low rates (DRL) 72-sec schedule, which was developed by Seiden and coworkers. In this procedure, animals are placed in experimental chambers that contain a response lever and mechanism for presenting the subjects with either food or water. After first training the animals to press the response lever for food, the animals are placed in a test situation in which they are reinforced only if they withhold their response for at least 72 sec. This means that subjects are reinforced for incorporating long pauses into their lever-pressing behavior. If the subject waits for at least 72 sec before making a response, it is given a food pellet. A response made prior to the 72-sec interval does not produce food, but instead resets a clock that measures the interval back to 72 sec. Normal subjects are only moderately successful in obtaining reinforcement under this schedule; they generally receive few reinforcers during the test. A special effect of antidepressant drugs is to change this behavior so as to increase the number of reinforcers the animals receive during the session. This occurs when the subjects treated with antidepressants are more effective in withholding their responses for the entire 72-sec interval.

Figure 1 shows the effects of several tricyclic antidepressant drugs (see Chapter 17) on the rates of responding and reinforcement in rats responding on the DRL 72-sec schedule. Each of these drugs significantly increases the number of reinforcements the animals receive and decreases their overall rates of responding. The antidepressants do not produce a general disruption of behavior. Instead, responses appear to be withheld more effectively after treatment with antidepressants so that more responses are placed near to or beyond the 72-sec criterion.

The characterization of the DRL 72-sec procedure as possessing predictive validity is based on the following experimental results. First, this test passes the criterion of selectivity. Increases in reinforcement rate in this procedure are produced by most clinically effective antidepressants, including tricyclic

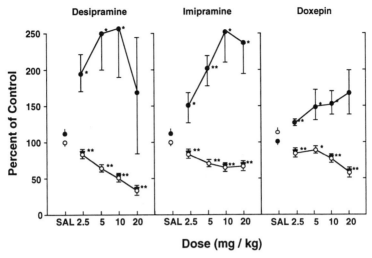

FIG. 1. Effects of tricyclic antidepressants on response rate (open circles) and reinforcement rate (closed circles) in rats responding under a differential reinforcement of low rates 72-sec schedule. Percentage of control rates (responses or reinforcement) is indicated on the ordinate and dose of drug in mg/kg on the abscissa. All three tricyclic antidepressants produced a significant decrease in response rate and increase in reinforcement rate. $*p < .05$; $**p < .01$. Reprinted from O'Donnell JM, Seiden LS. Differential-reinforcement-of-low-rate 72-second schedule: Selective effects of antidepressant drugs. *J. Pharmacol. Exp. Ther.* 1983;224:80–88.

antidepressants such as desipramine and imipramine, monoamine oxidase inhibitors (MAOIs) such as phenelzine and iproniazid, and novel "second-generation" antidepressants such as mianserin and trazodone (see Chapter 17). Also, compounds from several pharmacological classes other than antidepressants have proven ineffective in increasing rates of reinforcement (see Table 2), suggesting that the detection of false positives is minimal using this behavioral response. There are only a few false negatives, such as nomifensine, a compound with stimulant as well as antidepressant properties. The stimulant properties of nomifensine might account for its failure to demonstrate antidepressant-like effects in this model, since stimulant compounds are known to produce increases in response rates on DRL schedules.

Second, the DRL 72-sec procedure appears to pass the relative potency criterion. This criterion is difficult to assess with many antidepressant drugs because their clinical potencies are similar. However, some potency comparisons can be made. Tranylcypromine, an antidepressant that is an inhibi-

tor of monoamine oxidase and one of the more potent antidepressants (see Chapter 17), is more than four times as potent as the atypical antidepressant trazodone in this assay. The clinical potencies of these compounds are different by 6- to 10-fold, with tranylcypromine being more potent than trazodone. As observed in medical treatment, most of the other compounds appear to be of approximately equal potency.

The DRL 72-sec behavioral assay clearly exhibits predictive validity by meeting the selectivity and relative potency criteria. However, this procedure cannot be said to possess either face or construct validity. As stated above, demonstration of appropriate temporal characteristics and drug interactions endow face validity on an assay. No reliable drug interactions are known that either attenuate or potentiate all known antidepressant treatments, so the DRL 72-sec procedure does not have the burden of meeting this criterion. The same cannot be said of the necessity of appropriate temporal characteristics. The DRL 72-sec assay demonstrates immediate effects of antidepressants. As mentioned

TABLE 2. *Characterization of the DRL 72-sec behavioral assay: a model of antidepressant drug action*[a]

Drug and class	Activity
Antidepressants	
Desipramine	+
Imipramine	+
Nortryptyline	+
Amitryptyline	+
Doxepin	+
Tranylcypromine	+
Iproniazid	+
Phenelzine	+
Mianserin	+
Trazodone	+
Zimelidine	+
Neuroleptics	
Chlorpromazine	−
Haloperidol	−
Pimozide	−
Clozapine	−
Antihistamines	
Diphenhydramine	−
Anxiolytics	
Ethanol	−
Chlordiazepoxide	−
Pentobarbital	−
Stimulants	
Amphetamine	−
Nomifensine	−
Bupropion	−

Adapted from Seiden and O'Donnell, 1985.

[a] Examples of drugs from different pharmacological classes and their activity in the DRL 72-sec test. +, Active in the test; −, inactive in the test.

previously, a period of chronic drug administration is considered necessary to produce amelioration of depressive symptoms. In one study, chronic administration of the antidepressant imipramine increased its efficacy in the DRL 72-sec procedure. While this is consistent with the temporal criterion, similar studies with other antidepressants have not yet been conducted. Since most antidepressants have only been shown to produce effects on DRL responding following acute treatment, face validity has not been demonstrated. In addition to failing the criteria for construct validity by lacking face validity, the DRL 72-sec procedure also fails the special criterion for construct validity because it demonstrates no apparent psychological relationship to depression.

Drugs of Abuse—Construct Validity

Animal self-administration studies play a crucial role in understanding human substance abuse. The second example concerns self-administration experiments that are used to model substance abuse. This type of assay demonstrates predictive, face, and construct validity. In these studies, drug is administered to animals by intravenous, oral, or other route, contingent on the performance of a specified response, generally a bar press. Animals rapidly learn to respond in order to receive certain drugs. Compounds are said to function as positive reinforcers if they support responding in one of two conditions: (1) if they function as reinforcers in naive animals (i.e., the promotion or increase of new behaviors); or (2) if they sustain responding in animals trained to self-administer a different drug (i.e., the maintenance of responding in what is known as a substitution test).

Compounds that are positive in drug self-administration experiments usually produce drug-seeking behavior or addiction in humans. Figure 2 shows results from two experiments examining the self-administration of two drugs of abuse, heroin and morphine. The typical pattern of the dose–effect function for drug reinforcement is clear; responding increases as the dose is increased from a low, inactive dose until some maximum is reached. At higher doses, responding decreases, possibly due to toxic or incapacitating drug effects. The maximum level of responding produced by a drug is the critical measure of drug self-administration experiments. If the animals respond at levels significantly above those maintained by saline, the drug functions as a positive reinforcer.

Self-administration experiments meet all of the criteria for predictive validity. First, the assays show high selectivity. All compounds that are commonly abused by humans will also support self-administration; opioids, stimulants, sedative-hypnotics, some antihistamines, alcohol, dissociative anesthetics, and, under certain conditions, benzodiazepines, will all cause animals to continue to

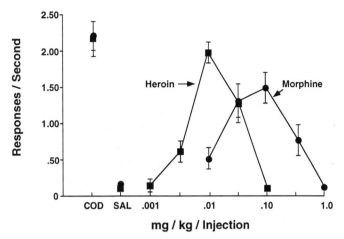

FIG. 2. Self-administration of heroin and morphine in rhesus monkeys trained to self-administer codeine (IV). Points over COD indicate control levels of codeine self-administration prior to the heroin or morphine substitution tests. Points over SAL indicate control levels of saline self-administration prior to the same tests. Response rates (in responses/sec) are indicated on the ordinate and doses of heroin or morphine (in mg/kg/injection) are indicated on the abscissa. Both heroin and morphine supported levels of self-administration similar to those with the training drug codeine, with heroin being approximately one order of magnitude more potent than morphine. Redrawn from Young AM, Swain HH, Woods JH. Comparison of opioid agonists in maintaining responding and in suppressing morphine withdrawal in rhesus monkeys. *Psychopharmacology* 1981;74:329–335.

respond in order to receive them. Hallucinogens present a special case because they are not self-administered in animal experiments. Their atypical pattern of use in humans (i.e., sporadic abuse over a limited time and failure to develop strong drug-seeking behavior) may explain why animal experiments do not detect them as they do other established classes of drugs of abuse. This atypical pattern may be important for understanding the abuse of this class. In addition, self-administration experiments also demonstrate appropriate potency relationships for abused compounds. For example, the opiates heroin, morphine, and codeine support self-administration with the rank order of potency heroin > morphine > codeine. This is the same potency relationship these compounds show in human opiate abusers. A similar potency relationship holds for the stimulants amphetamine and cocaine, with amphetamine being more potent in both humans and animals. With the satisfaction of both the selectivity and relative potency criteria, it is clear that these procedures possess good predictive validity.

Self-administration experiments also meet the additional criteria necessary for face validity. The temporal characteristics of drug-taking behavior in animals have been studied by allowing the animals constant access to a drug for an extended period, sometimes several weeks or more. Under these conditions, animals follow temporal patterns of self-administration that match those of human addicts. The clearest example of these effects may be found in the alcohol self-administration literature. Monkeys that are allowed constant access to alcohol engage in extended periods of self-administration, or "binges," followed by periods of abstinence, in which the animals might even go into a state of withdrawal. This pattern resembles that seen in many human alcoholics. Similar comparisons are difficult for other abused substances that are not as readily available as alcohol in human society. Nevertheless, the results obtained have tended to support the idea that animals and humans show similar patterns of drug intake over time. The next criterion involves drug interactions. Again, self-administration experiments in animals generally demonstrate interactions similar to those in human drug abuse. For example, opioid antagonists such as naloxone block the effects of opiates such as heroin in humans (see Chapter 20) and also increase the doses of opiate agonists such as heroin necessary to maintain self-administration in animals. The evidence suggests that self-administration experiments meet the criterion of appropriate drug interactions.

The criterion of theoretical relevance for self-administration assays is met by these procedures and determines the basis of their claim of construct validity. There is a growing acceptance of the idea that drugs are abused initially by humans because they produce reinforcing interoceptive stimuli, or positive subjective effects (see Chapter 20). This is precisely the operational definition of the function drugs perform in self-administration experiments in animals. In other words, the properties of drugs that lead to their abuse by humans are the same properties that are measured in drug self-administration procedures. The behavioral significance of these procedures for the human disorder it models is therefore one of the most compelling in the behavioral pharmacology literature. Based on a simple functional relationship, the theoretical relevance of self-administration to human drug abuse is met, and therefore the construct validity for the animal model is established. Animal experiments have been crucial in developing this theoretical advance in the understanding of human substance abuse. Indeed, researchers have recently begun to study human drug abuse under laboratory conditions using procedures originally developed for the study of animal self-administration.

NEUROPHARMACOLOGY OF PSYCHOTHERAPEUTIC COMPOUNDS

Another broad category of behavioral experiments involves characterization of the neurobiological substrates of psychoactive drug action. The use of animal behavior experiments to study drug action is one of the best ways to determine the effects of drugs that are likely to be relevant to their clinical actions. Alterations in neurobiological functioning are thought by many investigators to underlie both the behavioral effects of drugs in animals and their therapeutic effects in human psychiatric patients. A suggestion derived from this perspective is that human psychiatric patients may have some identifiable abnormality in a neurotransmitter or in a neurophysiological or neuroanatomic system that is specific to their disorder. The abnormal system may therefore serve as the ultimate target of drug intervention. This may occur through a direct effect of the drug on the neurobiological system, called a primary effect of the drug. Alternatively, the drug may produce effects on a secondary system that corrects or alleviates the behavioral symptoms of the disorder. This occurs when the drug's primary effect is on a neurotransmitter that interacts with the abnormal system. Behavioral experiments are well suited for the study of both the primary and secondary effects of drugs on behavior, since they are conducted in live animals with intact nervous systems that demonstrate interactions between neurobiological systems. Some animal behavior models may reproduce the primary neurochemical or behavioral disturbances that are present in human disorders. Other animal behaviors may be better at detecting drugs that alleviate symptoms of behavioral disorders.

The next section describes several types of behavioral assays used to investigate the neurobiological mechanisms of action of drugs. The section following that discussion examines several areas of research that use these behavioral techniques to characterize different aspects of the neurobiology of psychotherapeutic drugs. Taken together these sections provide a feeling for the types of investigations carried out to determine the neurobiological basis of drug action.

Behavioral Experiments in Neuropharmacology

Three types of behavioral paradigms that have been used to address questions of the neuropharmacological or neurobiological bases for the effects of drugs are *elicited behaviors, drug discrimination,* and *drug signatures.* Each type of experiment utilizes the ability of drugs to alter the behavior of organisms in a way that depends on the precise functional properties of the compounds in the central nervous system.

Elicited Behaviors

Elicited behavior generally refers to observable behaviors produced by a drug. While all effects of drugs in behavioral pharmacology can be considered elicited, or caused by the compounds in some sense, the term "elicited behavior" generally refers to the functional effects of these drugs on unconditioned behavior. Drugs can elicit behaviors that animals would not normally exhibit under the environmental and historical circumstances characterizing the experimental paradigm. Table 3 lists behaviors that are elicited by drugs that stimulate different subtypes of serotonin and dopamine receptors. Agonists selective for these different neurotransmitter receptors each produce a distinct behavioral response. The behaviors elicited by these ago-

nists may be either exaggerations or attenuations of normal behaviors, such as locomotion, grooming, head shaking, sniffing, or rearing, or may involve the adoption of highly abnormal postures or movements that are virtually absent from the normal repertoire of the subject, such as the serotonin syndrome. Elicited behaviors are known to be caused by the stimulation of certain neurotransmitter receptors because different agonists at the same receptor produce similar behavioral effects and antagonists at that receptor block the effects of agonists. Dopamine antagonists also elicit a specific behavioral response, i.e., the production of catalepsy, which has been used to quantify the behavioral actions of these drugs. Because the specific behaviors elicited by these agonists and antagonists are directly related to their pharmacological actions, they provide convenient response end points for investigations of a functional response produced by stimulation of a particular neurotransmitter receptor.

Drug Discrimination

Drug discrimination experiments are designed to characterize the subjective effects of drugs in animals. Most if not all psychoactive compounds produce changes in subjective states, often referred to as *interoceptive stimuli.* These stimuli can be readily identi-

TABLE 3. *Directly observable behaviors elicited by serotonergic and dopaminergic drugs*[a]

Drug class	Behavior
Serotonin	
5-HT$_{1A}$ agonists	Serotonin syndrome (reciprocal forepaw treading, hindlimb abduction, lateral head weaving, tremor, rigidity, Straub tail)
5-HT$_{1B}$ agonists	Increased locomotor activity
5-HT$_{1C}$ agonists	Decreased locomotor activity
5-HT$_2$ agonists	Head shakes
Dopamine	
Antagonists	Catalepsy; inhibition of dopamine agonist–induced behaviors
D$_1$ agonists	Grooming; enhanced mouth movements
D$_2$ agonists	Reduced/enhanced locomotion (depending on dose); sniffing; rearing; yawning; emesis

Adapted from Clark and White, 1987; Glennon and Lucki, 1988; and Sandberg et al., 1988.

[a] Examples of behaviors that have been connected to activation or blockade of selected receptors for serotonin and dopamine.

fied and differentiated from one another by experienced human drug users. For example, human addicts can reliably report whether they have been given heroin, cocaine, or a barbiturate. Drug discrimination procedures are methods by which a researcher can query a nonhuman subject about the identity of a particular drug based on the interoceptive stimuli it produces in the animal. In the standard drug discrimination paradigm, the presence or absence of the drug stimulus is used as a cue to enable an animal to select an appropriate response to acquire some reward, such as food or water, or to avoid some aversive stimulus, such as a mild electric shock. This is usually accomplished using an operant apparatus, in which responses on one lever deliver reinforcement in the presence of the drug stimulus and responses on a second lever only produce reinforcement in the absence of the drug. In well-trained subjects, drugs that share similar stimulus properties with the training drug, i.e., produce similar subjective effects, will produce responding on the drug-appropriate lever. Drugs that produce different interoceptive stimuli reliably produce responses on the lever associated with the nondrug state.

A second drug discrimination method uses the drug-induced stimulus as a conditioned stimulus (CS) in a classically conditioned taste aversion paradigm called a *discriminated taste aversion* (DTA). In these procedures, a drug (or nondrug) stimulus is paired with an injection of some noxious substance, such as lithium chloride, after the subject has consumed a substance with a novel taste, such as water flavored with saccharin. The nondrug (or drug) state is paired with administration of some innocuous substance, such as physiological saline, following consumption of the same flavored substance. Under these conditions, animals will consume less of the novel flavor in the presence of the stimulus paired with the noxious injection than in the presence of the stimulus paired with the harmless injection. The drug therefore acts as a "cue," indicating whether fluid consumption will or will not be followed by a period of discomfort.

Figure 3 shows the results of such an experiment conducted with the drug 8-hydroxy-2-(di-*n*-propylamino)tetralin (8-OH-DPAT), an agonist at the serotonin$_{1A}$ (5-HT$_{1A}$) receptor. After training, increasing doses of 8-OH-DPAT cause a progressive decrease in the amount of saccharin consumed when saccharin has been paired with lithium chloride in the presence of 8-OH-DPAT. As in the operant discrimination task, drugs that share stimulus properties with the training drug induce a similar pattern of behavior in the DTA paradigm (e.g., a reduction of intake of the flavored substance) if the training drug has been paired with a noxious injection. Figure 3 demonstrates such a generalization for the 5-HT$_{1A}$ receptor agonists buspirone and ipsapirone. These compounds produce a decrease in saccharin consumption similar to the decrease with the training drug 8-OH-DPAT in the conditioned subjects. In contrast, the 5-HT$_{1B/1C}$ receptor agonists trifluoromethylphenylpiperazine (TFMPP) and *meta*-chlorophenylpiperazine (m-CPP) did not produce a selective decrease in saccharin consumption in the 8-OH-DPAT-trained rats. These results indicate that the stimulus properties of 8-OH-DPAT are mediated by the 5-HT$_{1A}$ receptor and demonstrate how drug discrimination techniques can provide a pharmacological characterization of the stimulus properties of drugs.

Drug Signatures

Drug signatures *in operant paradigms are determinations of the effects of drugs on patterns of responding engendered by different operant schedules.* As suggested in the drug discrimination section, operant behavior (generally bar pressing in an operant chamber) has been extensively used to examine the properties of drugs. Many of these investigations have determined the effects of psychoactive compounds on the behavior produced by various schedules of reinforcement. A schedule of reinforcement describes what an animal has to do to obtain reinforcement and when that reinforcement will occur based on the animal's behavior. In practice,

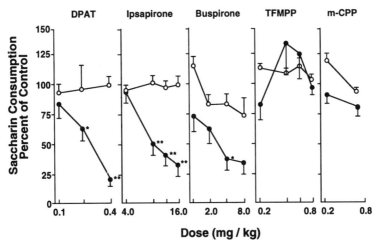

FIG. 3. Changes in saccharin consumption during generalization test trials in rats trained to discriminate the 5-HT$_{1A}$ agonist 8-OH-DPAT from saline and in unconditioned controls in a discriminated taste aversion drug discrimination procedure. In this procedure, administration of 8-OH-DPAT was followed by administration of LiCl following drug training sessions; saline training sessions were followed by saline administration. Percentage of control saccharin consumption is indicated on the ordinate and dose of drug in mg/kg is indicated on the abscissa. The 5-HT$_{1A}$ agonists 8-OH-DPAT, ipsapirone, and buspirone all decreased saccharin intake in the conditioned animals (closed circles) at doses that did not decrease consumption in the unconditioned control animals (open circles). The 5-HT$_{1B/1C}$ agonists TFMPP and m-CPP did not decrease saccharin intake selectively in these animals. *$p < .05$; **$p < .01$ Reprinted from Lucki I. Rapid discrimination of the stimulus properties of 5-hydroxytryptamine agonists using conditioned taste aversion. *J Pharmacol Exp Therapeut* 1988;247:1120–1127.

the schedule of reinforcement determines that a reinforcer, such as a food pellet or a positively reinforcing drug, or a punisher, such as an electric shock or an aversive drug, will be delivered to an animal when it presses a lever a specified number of times or after a specified period of time. The DRL schedule described in the section on drug screening is one such schedule, whereas experiments that determine the reinforcing properties of drugs use schedules of drug administration to assess whether particular drugs are likely to possess significant abuse potential, i.e., whether they can serve as reinforcers. Most comprehensive introductory psychology textbooks provide an explanation of the basic schedules used in behavioral pharmacology. Several classes of psychoactive drugs produce reliable changes in behavior under certain schedules of reinforcement that may be related to their mechanism of action. For example, many psychoactive compounds produce rate-

dependent effects (increases in response rates under schedules that produce low rates of responding and decreases in response rates under schedules that engender high rates of responding). Other actions of drugs on operant behavior can be restricted to particular pharmacological or therapeutic classes. Hallucinogens produce increases in pausing after reinforcement on schedules that require a particular number of responses to attain reinforcement (fixed ratio, or FR, schedules). Neuroleptics produce decreases in responding to avoid electric shock at doses that do not interfere with responding to escape electric shock. Drugs of abuse maintain responding leading to their administration (see section on drugs of abuse above). Benzodiazepines increase behavior maintained under schedules involving punishment at doses that do not affect unpunished behavior (see below). Compounds that share effects in one of these specific operant paradigms are likely to produce at least some similar neuropharmacological actions.

Types of Neuropharmacological Investigation

Several kinds of experimental questions are asked by behavioral pharmacologists concerning the neuropharmacology of psychotherapeutic agents. Each of these types of experiment provides part of the information necessary to understand how a drug acts, where it acts, and how its actions may be altered by previous histories of drug administration in the animals used in the experiments. The results from the various experiments can then be brought together to form a composite picture of the neuropharmacological processes likely to mediate various aspects of human abnormal behavior. This section will describe three of these broad areas of research and provide examples of specific experiments from the types of procedures outlined above that have been used to address each question.

Pharmacological Classification

Two of the most important characteristics of a drug are its selectivity *and its* efficacy. *Selectivity* refers to the relative potency of drugs for actions at receptors, and for a specific drug reflects those receptors or neurotransmitter systems at which the drug acts most potently. *Efficacy* refers to whether a drug acts as an agonist (stimulates the receptor) or an antagonist (binds to the receptor without producing stimulatory effects). A *pharmacological* classification of a compound is therefore intended to provide information about the receptors mediating the effects of a compound and whether the drug is acting as an agonist or an antagonist. A *behavioral* pharmacological classification is concerned with the same issues; however, the principal focus of behavioral experimentation is to determine which neurotransmitter receptor system(s) mediate(s) the behavioral effects of the drug. This is an important point that is sometimes overlooked. Animal behav-

ior experiments provide information on the functional properties of drugs that are related to the neurotransmitter receptors on which the drugs act. These experiments may therefore be used to arrive at a pharmacological classification of drugs as they affect the behavior of animals. An example of a drug signature paradigm that provides pharmacological information concerning therapeutic agents is the conflict procedure in rats and monkeys. In a conflict study, subjects are trained to respond for food in an operant paradigm with two different components. In one component, animals are rewarded with food under some schedule of reinforcement (e.g., after a variable number of responses, called a variable ratio, or VR, schedule). In the conflict component (generally indicated with some novel stimulus not present in the first component, e.g., a light or tone that is present only in the second component), subjects are also rewarded with food; however, responses in this component are also punished, generally by electric shock. In well-trained subjects, responding is primarily confined to the nonpunished periods. Few if any responses occur in the conflict period. Benzodiazepines such as diazepam (Valium), which are antianxiety drugs (see Chapter 19), selectively increase responses in this conflict component without altering responses in the unpunished period. This effect is shown in Fig. 4 for the benzodiazepine chlordiazepoxide (CDP; Librium). As the dose of CDP is increased, the number of punished responses increases. This effect of CDP occurs at doses that have no rate-increasing effects on unpunished responding (Fig. 4).

Several lines of evidence indicate that this procedure can be used to provide a pharmacological characterization of benzodiazepines (see Chapter 19). Other benzodiazepine agonists are also active in the conflict procedure. Their rank order of potency in increasing punished responding agrees closely with the potency of their clinical effects, which are thought to occur selectively through the benzodiazepine receptor. As would be expected for a benzodiazepine receptor-mediated effect, benzodiazepine antagonists such as flu-

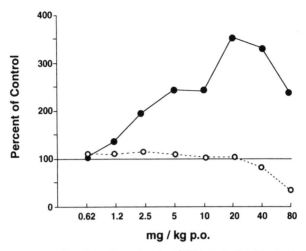

FIG. 4. Dose–response curve for chlordiazepoxide (CDP) on behavior controlled by two different schedules of reinforcement: punished fixed ratio (closed circles) and unpunished variable interval (open circles). Percentage of control response rates is indicated on the ordinate and dose of CDP in mg/kg (PO, or orally administered) is indicated on the abscissa. CDP increased response rates of punished behavior at doses that had no effect on unpunished behavior (2.5–20.0 mg/kg). Reprinted from Sepinwall J, Cook L. Behavioral pharmacology of antianxiety drugs. In: Iversen L, Iversen S, Snyder S, eds. *Handbook of psychopharmacology.* Vol. 13: *Biology of mood and antianxiety drugs.* New York: Plenum Press; 1978:345–393.

mazenil attenuate the effects of benzodiazepine agonists in the conflict procedure. Pharmacological selectivity is further suggested by the fact that compounds from other pharmacological classes do not cause such selective increases in punished responding. Even other clinically efficacious nonbenzodiazepine anxiolytics such as buspirone (see Chapter 19) are weakly active or inactive in conflict paradigms in rats and monkeys. These results suggest that the actions of benzodiazepines in the conflict procedure are produced through the benzodiazepine receptor.

It is important to note that this procedure may be used only to provide a *pharmacological* classification if it is conducted in rats or monkeys. In pigeons, the atypical anxiolytic buspirone is also active in conflict paradigms. Pigeons therefore appear to provide a *therapeutic* classification of anxiolytics.

Localization of Function

Site of action is another critical aspect of neuropharmacological investigation. Behavioral experiments may also be directed at determining the particular neurobiological substrates mediating the behavioral effects of drugs. In these investigations, researchers attempt to ascertain the brain region or nucleus on which a compound acts to produce a selected behavioral effect. This may be accomplished in two ways. First, electrolytic or chemical lesions of discrete brain regions may be made and the effects of these lesions on the behavioral actions of drugs determined. If a lesion of a particular area alters the effect of a drug, this suggests that the site either contains the receptors through which the drug acts to produce that behavior or is involved in the neural circuit that mediates the behavior. Second, the drug may be injected directly into a particular brain region. If the local injection of low doses of the drug produces the desired behavioral action, the selected locus is implicated in that action of the drug. The region cannot be said to mediate all the effects of the drug; different behavioral effects may have different anatomic loci. If the behavior under investigation is not observed, the specific brain region may not be involved in the behavior under study. At times the effects of drugs may require simultaneous stimulation of several brain regions at once. By localizing particular behavioral actions to discrete regions in the brain, new therapeutic approaches to a particular disorder may be indicated by known interactions between neurotransmitter systems in those loci.

An example that illustrates the direct-injection approach may be found in the localization of the discriminative stimulus properties of cocaine. In these experiments, rats were trained to discriminate cocaine from saline in a standard two-lever operant paradigm described above. Following training, these subjects were implanted with cannulae directed at selected brain nuclei known to bind cocaine. Cocaine was then administered directly to these discrete regions and the animals were allowed to select levers in the operant chamber as in a standard discrimination test. After injection of cocaine into the nucleus accumbens, rats responded on the cocaine-appropriate lever, indicating that the drug produced an effect in this area that mimicked its stimulus properties when administered peripherally. Injection of cocaine into other brain regions resulted primarily in saline-appropriate responding. These observations suggest that the ability of cocaine to produce its interoceptive stimuli is mediated within a particular brain area, the nucleus accumbens.

Effects of Pharmacological History on Drug Actions

Depending on the drug, repeated administration may lead to tolerance on the one hand or supersensitivity on the other. Pharmacological history can affect both behavioral and clinical responses to drugs. The repeated administration of many psychoactive compounds leads to selective alterations in the behavioral effects of drugs. For example, the repeated administration of morphine leads to a reduction of the analgesia produced by this drug or by certain other opiates. Such a reduction in the effect of a drug is called *tolerance.* Tolerance to a drug is characterized by both a reduction in the effect produced by a

given dose of drug and an increase in the dose of drug necessary to produce a particular level of effect. Both of these characteristics are true for tolerance to the analgesia produced by morphine; the analgesia produced by a given dose of morphine is decreased by chronic administration, and a larger dose of morphine is needed to produce pain relief after repeated administration of the drug. A different response to repeated drug administration is observed for certain drugs. Chronic administration of amphetamine, a drug that releases endogenous dopamine and therefore acts as an indirect dopamine agonist, leads to an increase in some of its behavioral effects. This kind of increase, known as *supersensitivity,* is characterized by an increase in the effect produced by a given dose of drug, or a reduction in the dose of drug necessary to produce a particular level of effect. Supersensitivity can be seen in both the locomotor-stimulating effects of relatively low doses of amphetamine and the potential for higher doses of this drug to induce stereotypy (see Table 3). This is indicated by the fact that the doses of amphetamine necessary to produce locomotion are reduced by prior administration of amphetamine. Also, doses of amphetamine that previously had only induced locomotion may elicit stereotyped behaviors after prior amphetamine administration.

Demonstrations of tolerance or supersensitivity are valuable in themselves and may be useful in understanding certain aspects of the clinical use of drugs. However, behavioral experiments may also be used to determine the alterations in specific neuropharmacological systems likely to underlie instances of tolerance or supersensitivity. By utilizing behavioral responses associated with particular neurotransmitter systems, researchers can investigate how chronic administration of therapeutic drugs, similar to that often necessary in the treatment of psychiatric disorders such as depression or schizophrenia, changes the functional properties of those neurotransmitter systems.

Serotonin (5-hydroxytryptamine; 5-HT) is a neurotransmitter with several different receptor subtypes that mediate its effects in the central nervous system (see Chapter 6). Drugs that are selective for certain of these subtypes elicit behaviors that can be clearly differentiated from each other (see Table 3). For example, agonists selective for the 5-HT_{1A} subtype of receptor induce behaviors in rats that are known collectively as the serotonin syndrome. This syndrome includes abduction or spreading of the hindlimbs, reciprocal forepaw treading, head weaving, rigidity, tremor, and flat body posture. In contrast, agonists selective for the 5-HT_2 receptor produce a rapid axial rotation of the head about the longitudinal axis known as the head shake but do not elicit the serotonin syndrome. Chronic administration of clinically effective antidepressant drugs from a variety of classes—tricyclics, monoamine oxidase inhibitors (MAOIs), and atypicals—have been reported to selectively reduce the ability of 5-HT_2 receptor agonists to induce the head shake response. In contrast, chronic administration of MAOIs, but not other classes of antidepressant drugs, reduces the ability of agonists at the 5-HT_{1A} receptor to elicit the serotonin syndrome. These results suggest that chronic antidepressant treatments alter the function of 5-HT systems in a discrete manner rather than producing a general modification of serotonergic activity. These selective changes in responsiveness to certain serotonergic agonists may mimic alterations in response to endogenous serotonin that are important to the clinical effect of antidepressant drugs.

The examples in this section demonstrate how behavioral methods can be used to address basic scientific questions about the neuropharmacology of drugs. No single behavioral method is specific to a given neuropharmacological question. Any of the paradigms could theoretically be used to provide valid information in each research classification.

SUMMARY

This chapter provides a framework for the description of different uses of behavioral techniques in neuropharmacology. In drug-screening procedures, behavioral paradigms are assessed according to how well they meet five criteria: selectivity, potency relationships, temporal characteristics, drug interactions, and theoretical or psychological relevance. The criteria met by a particular assay determines the type of validity ascribed to it: predictive, face, or construct. These levels of validity are used to determine the value of the model as a drug screen. In neuropharmacological investigations, researchers may use elicited behaviors, drug discrimination techniques, and drug profiles in operant paradigms to address questions concerning the pharmacological properties, neuroanatomic locus, and historical factors that mediate drug actions.

There are distinct advantages to the behavioral assessment of drug actions. Investigations of the behavioral effects of drugs provide a clear functional relevance to a particular measure of drug effect. This is not true of every method that employs isolated organs or cell systems to determine drug effects. It is often difficult to relate what is happening in a test tube to what is occurring neurochemically in a psychiatric patient. Behavioral techniques have the advantage of providing a measure of drug action that is obviously of behavioral and psychological relevance. There are also distinct neurochemical advantages to working in whole animals. The metabolic and physiological processes that can be assumed to affect drug actions or to alter the identity of the actual chemical that enters the central nervous system and alters brain function are intact in behaving animals and thus more closely mimic the clinical condition. Finally, drug effects on whole animals reflect the actions of a drug on all relevant pharmacological systems and may provide information on ways in which these systems interact to produce their effects that are not discernible from isolated systems. Behavioral methods provide a complement to other physiologically based techniques, yielding information that aids interpretation of more biochemically oriented investigations, just as biochemical studies yield insights that shape behavioral experiments.

BIBLIOGRAPHY

Original Articles

Lucki I. Rapid discrimination of the stimulus properties of 5-hydroxytryptamine agonists using conditioned taste aversion. *J Pharmacol Exp Therapeut* 1988; 247:1120–1127.

McGuire PS, Seiden LS. The effects of tricyclic antidepressants on performance under a differential-reinforcement-of-low-rates schedule in rats. *J Pharmacol Exp Therapeut* 1980;214:635–641.

Tyre NC, Iversen SD, Green AR. The effects of benzodiazepines and serotonergic manipulations on punished responding. *Neuropharmacology* 1979;18:689–695.

Wood DM, Emmett-Oglesby MW. Mediation in the nucleus accumbens of the discriminative stimulus produced by cocaine. *Pharmacol Biochem Behav* 1989;33:453–457.

Young AM, Swain SD, Woods JH. Comparison of opioid agonists in maintaining responding and in suppressing morphine withdrawal in rhesus monkeys. *Psychopharmacology* 1981;74:329–335.

Books and Reviews

Barry H III. Classification of drugs according to their discriminable effects in rats. *Fed Proc* 1974;33: 1814–1824.

Clark D, White FJ. D1 dopamine receptor: the search for a function. A critical evaluation of the D1/D2 dopamine receptor classification and its functional implications. *Synapse* 1987;1:347–388.

Frazer A, Offord SJ, Lucki I. Regulation of serotonin receptors and responsiveness in the brain. In: Sanders-Bush E, ed. *The serotonin receptors.* New York: Humana Press, 1988:319–362.

Glennon RA, Lucki I. Behavioral models of serotonin receptor activation. In: Sanders-Bush E, ed. *The serotonin receptors.* New York: Humana Press; 1988: 253–293.

Sanberg PR, Bunsey MD, Giordano M, Norman AB. The catalepsy test: its ups and downs. *Behav Neurosci* 1988;102:748–759.

Seiden LS, O'Donnell JM. Effects of antidepressant drugs on DRL behavior. In: Seiden LS, Balster RL, eds. *Behavioral pharmacology: the current status.* New York: Alan R Liss, 1984:323–338.

Sepinwall J, Cook L. Behavioral pharmacology of antianxiety drugs. In: Iversen LL, Iversen SD, Snyder SH, eds. *Handbook of psychopharmacology.* Vol. 13. *Biology of mood and antianxiety drugs.* New York: Plenum Press; 1978:345–393.

Woods JH. Behavioral pharmacology of drug self-administration. In: Lipton, MA, DiMascio A, Killam KF, eds. *Psychopharmacology: A generation of progress.* New York: Raven Press; 1978:595–607.

15

Methods for the Study of Brain–Behavior Relationships

Ruben C. Gur and Raquel E. Gur

This is a gift that I have, simple, simple; a foolish extravagant spirit, full of forms, shapes, objects, ideas, apprehensions, motions, revolutions; these are begot in the ventricles of memory, nourished in the womb of pia matter, and delivered upon the mellowing of occasion.

William Shakespeare,
Love's Labour's Lost, (Holofernes to Nathaniel and Dull)

- Broca's approach to the study of the brain—referred to as the "lesion method"—has been applied successfully and is the source of much information on brain-behavior relationships.

- During the 1960s, an array of techniques for studying brain-behavior relationships, particularly the role of hemispheric specialization, was developed by cognitive psychologists.

- More recently, anatomic and functional neuroimaging have begun to provide important information about brain-behavior relationships.

- The neuropsychological assessment method provides quantitative behavioral data.

- Because most current neuropsychological assessment batteries do not measure affect and emotional functioning, our understanding of the neural underpinnings of human emotion is very rudimentary.

- Neuroanatomic methods can image brain anatomy in living subjects.

- Neurophysiological methods provide information about dynamic features of brain activity.

- Isotopic techniques for imaging neurophysiology make use of the fact that active neurons have a metabolic need for oxygen and glucose. Furthermore, rates of cerebral blood flow change in response to this need.

- Positron emission tomography (PET) provides in vivo measures of biochemical and physiological processes with three-dimensional resolution.

- Behavioral dimensions studied with neuroimaging can help to identify neural networks.

- The challenge is to integrate behavioral theories on regional brain function with anatomic and physiological neuroimaging data.

■ Chapter Overview ─────────────────────────────

This chapter reviews the recent history of the study of brain–behavior relationships in humans and describes some of the prevailing classical methods for examining how brain regions regulate aspects of behavior. This is followed by a description of the new techniques for neuropsychological assessment and neuroimaging, which can be combined to provide powerful and rigorous tools for advancing our understanding of brain–behavior relationships. Some of the results of these applications are described. The chapter also discusses the integration of neuropsychological and neuroimaging methods to yield more definitive answers to age-old mind–brain questions than would be possible with the fragmented use of individual techniques.

Understanding how the brain regulates behavior, ranging from sensory perceptions and motor responses to abstract reasoning, memory, and emotion, has always been an intriguing challenge. Philosophers and scientists have presented different views on how mental activity relates to brain processes, and several puzzles were identified. For example, the French philosopher René Descartes wondered how a unitary consciousness could emanate from a brain that consists of two hemispheres connected only by fibers. He resolved this by suggesting that the seat of the "soul" is in the pineal gland, which is not divided in two.

Obviously, to achieve an understanding of the neural substrates of behavior, which is arguably the most complex aspect of our existence as living organisms, a rather refined comprehension of brain organization including mechanisms of action needed to be established. This has proved to be a foreboding task, and only recently have the necessary techniques been developed to make us optimistic that major breakthroughs are at hand. But investigators have not been waiting idly for such methods to emerge, and important insights have already been achieved with classical techniques.

Biological Bases of Brain Function and Disease, edited by Alan Frazer, Perry B. Molinoff, and Andrew Winokur. Raven Press, Ltd., New York © 1994.

EVOLUTION OF THIS FIELD OF STUDY

The beginnings of the study of brain–behavior relationships were less than glorious. Having only the external measurements of the shape of the skull to provide data on brain structure, early investigators attempted to relate variations in skull conformation to mental "faculties." This endeavor, termed *phrenology,* rapidly led to proliferation of theories without any reasonable evidence, and the field was shunned by reputable scientists. The whole idea that aspects of behavior could be "localized" to specific brain regions was challenged and considered nonsensical.

Broca's approach to the study of the brain —referred to as the "lesion method"—has been applied successfully and is still the source of much information on brain–behavior relationships. Naturally occurring and man-made lesions provided much early information on brain–behavior relationships. However, toward the end of the nineteenth century, evidence began to accumulate that different brain regions might be specialized for regulating complex behavior such as speech. Pioneering studies by Bouillaud and Dax were largely ignored, but in the 1860s two case reports by the French neurosurgeon Paul Broca captured the imagination of a new generation of investigators. Broca decided to examine speech localization by studying the brains of patients who had impaired speech without loss of their general intellectual abilities. He reasoned that speech is an important human faculty, and if it cannot be localized, there is little hope for localizing others. The first patient he described had a limited vocabulary but was able to use it to communicate effectively. For example, he could only say the words for the first three digits, but he used the first two properly and said "3" for any number larger than 2. In the latter case he used his fingers to indicate the precise number he intended. Postmortem examination of this patient's brain showed a lesion in the third frontal "convolution" of the left hemisphere. A second patient with similar symptoms also had a left hemispheric lesion, leading Broca to propose that language functions are localized in the left hemisphere.

Broca's German contemporary Carl Wernicke showed later that left hemispheric lesions more posterior to "Broca's area" are associated with normal verbal fluency but impaired comprehension of verbal material. Such patients, unlike the "Broca-type" aphasics who have impoverished speech, talk fluently and with adequate vocabulary. However, they fail to comprehend the content of verbal messages communicated to them. At about this time, the British neurologist Hughlings-Jackson showed other associations between location of lesions and behavioral deficits, and his work demonstrated an important role of the right hemisphere in spatial processing. Thus patients with right hemispheric lesions do not lose their ability to speak or their verbal comprehension. They do, however, have difficulties in learning spatial layouts and recognizing faces, and they may have additional spatial difficulties.

This pioneering work became an intensively studied area with eminent investigators piecing together data from brain-damaged patients to construct and test theories on brain regulation of behavior. Some of the most influential among this century's investigators are the Russian neuropsychologist A. R. Luria at Moscow University and the Ameri-

can neurologist Norman Geschwind from Harvard. The lesion method has been enhanced and extended by studies on the behavioral effects of brain surgery, such as corpus callosotomy and temporal lobectomy for the treatment of intractable epilepsy. The American neuropsychologists Roger Sperry, Jerre Levy, Michael Gazzaniga, and their colleagues at Caltech proposed several important principles for the organization of consciousness based on examination of patients after callosal disconnection surgery (known as commissurotomy when the anterior commissures are also disconnected, or corpus callosotomy when only the callosum is cut; see Chapter 22). This work contributed to arguably one of the most baffling yet fundamental principles of brain organization: *laterality.* Complementing findings on the effects of unilateral brain damage, these studies showed dramatically, in the same individuals, that the two hemispheres have a rather profound asymmetry in cognitive processing. For example, when such patients are asked to hold a paper clip in their right hand they can state verbally that they are holding a paper clip. However, when the paper clip is placed in the left hand, which sends sensory input to their separated right hemisphere, they are unable to say what they are holding. It is possible to demonstrate that their right hemisphere "knows" the answer but is unable to talk. This can be done, for example, by asking patients to identify by palpation the object they have just palpated.

During the 1960s, an array of techniques for studying brain–behavior relationships, particularly the role of hemispheric specialization, was developed by cognitive psychologists. The methods of the cognitive psychologists capitalize on the notion that transfer across the corpus callosum (the body of nerve fibers connecting the two hemispheres) results in some loss of information. Stimuli are presented very briefly in one visual field, and speed and accuracy of its processing are related to side of stimulation. The brief presentation is necessary because it requires approximately 120 msec for a subject to foveate (i.e., focus vision to an off-center target). Such studies have shown, for example, that verbal material is processed more accurately when presented to the right visual field (hence being initially perceived by the left hemisphere). By contrast, spatial stimuli (such as dots that have to be localized, faces, orientation of lines) are processed more accurately when presented to the left visual field. These effects are very pronounced in patients who have undergone callosum sectioning for treatment of intractable epileptic seizures, where right visual field presentation of linguistic material is easily recognized and restated by the patient but when the same material is presented to the left visual field the patient cannot repeat the words (see Fig. 1). In normal subjects, the effects are not nearly as dramatic but can still be demonstrated.

Similarly, in the auditory modalities, words presented to the right ear are perceived more accurately than left-ear presentations of the same words or syllables. Lateralized effects are also found in the haptic (touch) and olfactory modalities. Other psychological methods for studying hemispheric specializa-tion include recording the direction of motor orientation (e.g., lateral eye movements) during problem solving, evaluation of chimeric stimuli such as faces, and examination of the relationship between sensory and motor indices of asymmetry such as handedness and sighting dominance. These methods have been used to examine hemispheric asymmetries in several behavioral dimensions related both to cognition and to affect. For example, such methods helped to demonstrate right hemispheric superiority for perception and expression of negative emotions.

Beginning in the middle of this century, work by Arthur Benton and his colleagues at the University of Iowa and Harold Goodglass and Edith Kaplan at Boston University has incorporated psychological testing into the study of patients with brain lesions; these studies have helped to further refine the hypotheses and test them more rigorously using quantitative analyses. For example, instead of having to rely on a clinical judgment that a patient seems not to understand sentences with the ease one would expect from someone of his or her level of education, standard

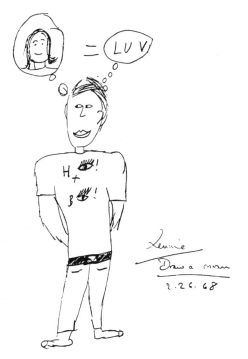

FIG. 1. Drawing by a young commissurotomy patient who was instructed to draw a man. Note how he has spontaneously drawn the picture of a woman's face as connected to the right hemisphere and a nonsense syllable (LUV), which is pronounced as the word *love,* coming from the left hemisphere. Thus, the face and feelings associated with it are on the right, the words are on the left. From Levy J. Cerebral asymmetries as manifested in split-brain man. In Kinsbourne M, Smith LW, eds. *Hemispheric disconnection and cerebral function.* Springfield IL: Charles C Thomas; 1974.

tests of sentence comprehension have been developed that can be scored in a uniform fashion across laboratories so that performance can be compared to that of normal subjects with comparable levels of age and education. The sensitivity of behavioral measures used for correlation with brain parameters has been improved with the introduction of techniques for quantifying functions such as abstract thinking, speech fluency and comprehension, memory, attention, sensory perception, and motor activity. These measures are obtained by psychological tests, and the linkage between the behavioral measures and regional brain function is referred to as *neuropsychological assessment,* which is described in the next section.

The methodology of neuropsychological assessment has enabled researchers to develop rather elaborate hypotheses on brain–behavior relationships based on lesion effects. These hypotheses have become incorporated into the neurological workup. Relationships were found between behavior and several brain dimensions. In general, the anterior parts of the brain are more involved in the outflow or "expressive" behavior, whereas the posterior parts regulate sensory perception, computation, understanding of material, and generally "receptive" processing. Thus, the back of one's brain "perceives," "evaluates," and "thinks," while the front plans and acts. The laterality effects we discussed suggest that left hemispheric regions are superior for language analysis and speech production whereas the right hemisphere serves spatial abilities. Other evidence suggests hemispheric asymmetry for emotional processing, although it is generally believed that subcortical regions play the more prominent role in emotional regulation. Possibly, subcortical brain regions provide regulation of drive states (hunger, thirst) and establishment of emotional input into fundamental learning processes, whereas in cortical areas more refined processing takes place including complex reasoning and synthesis. For example, Ross and Mesulam reported loss of emotional prosody, or speech intonation, with right hemispheric lesions homotopic (same area, on the other side) to Broca's region; others reported loss of the sense of humor and emotional control with lateralized cortical lesions.

More recently, anatomic and functional neuroimaging have begun to provide important information about brain–behavior relationships. The advent of methods for imaging of regional brain anatomy using x-ray computed tomography (CT) or magnetic resonance imaging (MRI) has expedited the progress of lesion–behavior research because the investigator is no longer required to wait for postmortem data to localize the lesion. This not only improves the rate at which knowledge can be accumulated but also makes interpretations more accurate since behavior is measured at the same time that lesion data are available. Pathological findings, on the other hand, have to be related to behavioral data collected much earlier; in the meanwhile, there might have been changes in the lesion. An example of how behavior can be linked to brain regions by the lesion method combined with anatomic neuroimaging is illustrated in Fig. 2.

FIG. 2. X-ray computed tomography (**A**) and corresponding templates (**B**) of a 34-year-old woman obtained a few hours after she developed left hemiplegia and severe left visuospatial neglect. She appeared unaware of her defects, specifically denying that there was anything wrong with her left limb (anosognosia). Note that most of the territory of the right middle cerebral artery is occupied by an area of decreased density. This includes cortex and white matter in the frontal, temporal, and parietal lobes, as well as the insula and the region of the basal ganglia. The lesion spares the thalamus. The ventricular system is deviated to the left, a typical sign of edema. At this stage, it is not possible to discriminate the infarcted areas from the areas of edema. From Damasio H, Damasio AR. *Lesion analysis in neuropsychology.* New York: Oxford University Press; 1989.

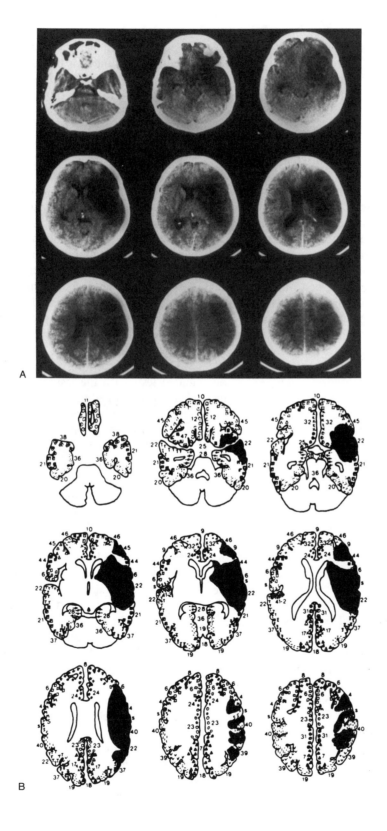

Although anatomic neuroimaging is a vast step forward, it is limited in that it provides data on brain structure only. Regional brain activity is reduced not only in the area of the lesion but also in functionally connected areas, and this is not observable with neuroanatomic imaging. As indicated by electroencephalography (EEG), a method for measuring the rate of electric discharge in neural tissue, abnormal activity can be the source of severe behavioral manifestations such as epileptic seizures (see Chapter 22), sometimes without any abnormalities detectable by anatomic neuroimaging methods. Furthermore, EEG can show changes in activity induced by performance of tasks and this too will not show up on anatomic neuroimaging. The study of the relationship between task performance and regional brain activation has tremendous potential for helping us to understand brain regulation of behavior, since the investigator no longer depends on finding patients with specific location and type of lesion in order to search for behavioral correlates. Instead, task conditions can be controlled experimentally, in normal subjects, to document effects of stimuli on regional brain activity. This has required the availability of a relative newcomer in the array of methods, loosely termed *functional neuroimaging.*

This wholly new technology has its roots in the early work of Seymour Kety and Carl Schmidt in the Department of Pharmacology at the University of Pennsylvania in the 1940s but did not attain wide applicability and some maturity until the 1980s. These methods are termed functional neuroimaging because regional brain physiological activity is measured in vivo (i.e., in the intact organism). The applications of this methodology to the study of brain–behavior relationships are increasing rapidly, and several important processes have been investigated.

NEUROPSYCHOLOGICAL ASSESSMENT

The neuropsychological assessment method provides quantitative behavioral data. Neuro-psychological testing has evolved as a means of obtaining reliable psychometric measures of behavioral functions that have been linked to brain systems and processes. Thus, tests of verbal fluency can help quantify the extent of speech (aphasic) deficits associated with anterior left hemispheric lesions (Broca-type aphasia); tests of verbal comprehension can help assess deficits of posterior left hemispheric lesions; and spatial-constructional tests can help determine whether spatial deficits attributable to posterior lesions of the right hemisphere (as suggested by Hughlings-Jackson) are present. The psychometric tests add the aspect of standardization and quantitation, which are invaluable components of systematic clinical assessment and research. In this way, clinical impressions can be buttressed by more objective data that show how a patient, or a group of patients, performs relative to a normative sample.

The power of joining psychometrically validated tests with the lesion method is most clearly exemplified in the work of clinical investigators such as Benton, Goodglass, Kaplan, and Reitan. Their studies, and those of numerous others who followed their lead, show systematic and reliable relationships between deficits on behavioral measures and regional brain dysfunction. The result is that we now have a rather solid body of knowledge demonstrating correlations between the presence and location of lesions and impairment in major behavioral dimensions. Based on this evidence, an experienced neuropsychologist can make an informed prediction of the location and severity of brain lesions after inspecting the pattern of neuropsychological test scores, and, conversely, if the location of lesions is known, the neuropsychologist can help identify those aspects of disturbed behavioral functioning attributable to the lesion. Some of the more salient findings linking deficits to brain regions are summarized in Table 1.

Because most current neuropsychological assessment batteries do not measure affect and emotional functioning, our understanding of the neural underpinnings of human

TABLE 1. *Deficits in behavioral dimensions and corresponding areas of brain damage associated with these deficits*

Behavioral deficit	Impaired brain region
Abstraction, mental flexibility	Frontal lobe
Speech fluency	Frontotemporal, left
Comprehension	Temporoparietal, left
Prosody (intonation)	Frontotemporal, right
Memory	
Verbal	Temporal and frontal, left
Figural/facial	Temporal and frontal, right
Motor	Precentral sulcus, contralateral
Sensory	Postcentral sulcus, contralateral
Attention/neglect	Parietal, frontal, right
Spatial processing	Temporoparietal, right
Face recognition	Parietal, right
Calculation (arithmetic)	Temporoparietal, left
Emotional expression	Frontotemporal, right

emotion is very rudimentary. William James, a founder of modern psychology, emphasized the need to study the three facets of human behavior that he described as *cognition* (computational activity), *conation* (related to will, motivation, need states), and *affect* (emotion). However, while psychologists have made impressive progress in studying cognition, affect has been somewhat neglected in neuropsychology. Nonetheless, some initial work is encouraging. Consistent with the notion of cortical involvement in emotional processing, evidence has been obtained for greater right hemispheric involvement in emotional tasks. For example, emotions are expressed more intensely on the left side of a face (Fig. 3) and perceived more accurately when presented to the left visual field.

It also appears that the cortical representation of emotion parallels that for cognition in that receptive and expressive aspects are processed in posterior and anterior regions, respectively. Affective disturbances have been consistently documented in patients following destructive as well as irritative (such as in epilepsy) brain lesions. For example, outbursts of uncontrollable laughter or crying may occur following destructive lesions, and laughter as well as crying has been observed during ictus (a seizure) in patients with focal epilepsy (see Chapter 22). However, more work is needed to develop standard neuropsychological assessment procedures for quanti-

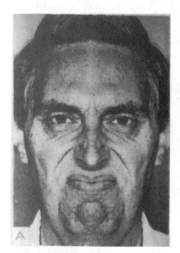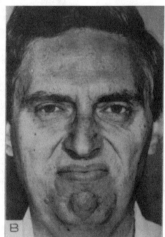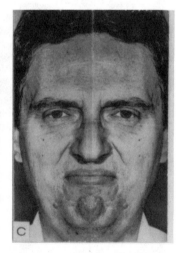

FIG. 3. An example of (**A**) left-side composite, (**B**) original, and (**C**) right-side composite of the same face. The face is expressing disgust. Note that the left-side composite (A) expresses the emotion more intensely than the right-side composite (C). The photograph of the original face was obtained courtesy of P. Ekman (*Pictures of facial affect,* Consulting Psychologists Press, Palo Alto, CA, 1976), and printed with permission of the poser.

fying emotional processing so that it can be linked to regional brain function. Once this is accomplished, tests of emotional processing can be incorporated into neuropsychological test batteries. This will be particularly important for application of neuropsychological assessment in patients with psychiatric illnesses.

NEUROIMAGING METHODS

Neuroanatomic methods can image brain anatomy in living subjects. The two major techniques currently available are CT and MRI. MRI has virtually replaced CT since it can display brain structures and many lesions with exquisite detail (Fig. 4). MRI is an imaging method based on the nuclear energy levels of hydrogen atoms. These levels can be split in the presence of a large external magnetic field, and their imaging is based on the water content of the tissue. These methods can be used for establishing links between brain regions and behavior. If a lesion is detected with CT or MRI, then we can infer

that at least some of the patient's behavioral deficits, documented clinically or by neuropsychological testing, have been caused by destruction of brain tissue, and hence this region is implicated in regulating the impaired behavior. A danger is that it might be concluded that a brain region is exclusively involved in regulating the impaired behavioral function when in fact it may only be a component of a larger neural "network" that regulates the behavior.

Neurophysiological methods provide information about dynamic features of brain activity. Behavior is affected not only by the anatomic integrity of the neural tissue but by the level, distribution, and dynamic features of neural activity. The capacity of brain regions to become active in response to task demands is likely to be of particular importance for establishing brain–behavior relations. In clinical populations, behavioral deficits can be more extensive than those attributable to the death of neurons in regions showing anatomic destruction on CT. They can be caused by brain cells that are not dead but are either insufficiently active or too active. Some grave

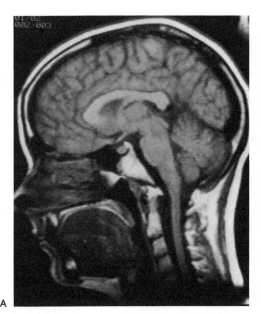
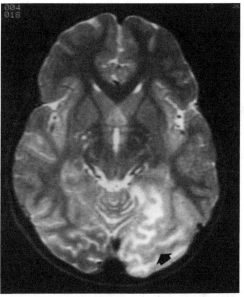

FIG. 4. MRI: **(A)** A sagittal view of a normal brain. **(B)** An axial view of a cerebral infarct. Individuals with lesions in this area usually have difficulty in understanding language.

forms of brain dysfunction are caused by abnormalities in regional brain physiological activity in the absence of anatomic destruction. For example, epilepsy has severe behavioral manifestations and there is evidence for interictal (i.e., between-seizures) chronic deficits in cognitive and emotional functioning. Several techniques for physiological neuroimaging demonstrate abnormalities corresponding to an epileptogenic focus, yet CT or MRI scans are frequently uninformative or even normal.

Of the several physiological techniques that merit inclusion in the neuroimaging family, the oldest is EEG and the associated methods for recording of evoked potentials (EP). However, standardized methods for generating topographic displays of regional EEG/EP measures have only recently been developed. BEAM (brain electric activity mapping) is an acronym that has been widely used (although it is a trade name and there are other systems that utilize a similar principle) for methods to display quantified EEG/EP parameters in gray or color-scaled topographic displays of brain activity (Fig. 5).

Isotopic techniques for imaging neurophysiology make use of the fact that active neurons have a metabolic need for oxygen and glucose. Furthermore, rates of cerebral blood flow (CBF) change in response to this need. Therefore, it could be hypothesized that when individuals perform cognitive tasks their brain metabolism rates increase. If this can be established, then measures of such rates obtained during the performance of cognitive tasks can help generate experimental data to delineate brain regions necessary for regulating specific cognitive processes. Such measures can also help identify regions of abnormal physiological activation associated with behavioral deficits. As indicated above, the isotopic techniques for measuring cerebral metabolism and blood flow can be traced to the pioneering method of Kety and Schmidt for measuring whole-brain metabolism and blood flow. Their technique uses intracarotid injection of nitrous oxide, and measurement of arteriovenous differences in the concentration of nitrous oxide yields accurate and reproducible data on brain metabolism and blood flow. The main drawbacks of this method for neurobehavioral research are (1) it provides only whole-brain, not regional, values and (2) it is invasive and risky.

Safe regional determinations of CBF were first made possible by the introduction of the xenon-133 clearance techniques for measuring regional CBF (rCBF). As in the nitrous oxide method, differences between input and output of tracers are used to calculate rates of tissue activation. The highly diffusible xenon-133 gas can be administered, in trace amounts, mixed in air or in saline (physiological salt solution). Its concentration in brain regions is measurable by scintillation detectors. The rate of clearance of xenon-133 permits accurate quantitation of rCBF in the fast-clearing gray matter compartment as well as calculation of mean flow (gray and white matter). Initial applications, using carotid injections, were invasive and only measured one hemisphere at a time. In 1975 Walter Obrist and colleagues at Duke University reported the xenon-133 inhalation technique and presented models for quantifying rCBF with this noninvasive procedure. The technique permits simultaneous measurements from both hemispheres, and the number of brain regions that can be measured depends on the number of detectors. Initial studies were performed with up to 16 detectors, 8 over each hemisphere, but commercial systems with 32 detectors are now available and recently a system was introduced that enables the placement of up to 254 detectors. The main limitation of the technique is that it is optimal for measuring rCBF on the brain surface near the skull and thus is limited to the study of cortical brain regions.

Positron emission tomography (PET) provides in vivo measures of biochemical and physiological processes with three-dimensional resolution. PET is used with radionuclides that decay through the emission of positrons (the antiparticles of electrons). The radionuclides are usually given intravenously and are taken up by tissue. Through the emission of a positron, the radionuclides get rid of their energy and undergo the process of annihilation when the positron interacts with an electron. The two photons emitted from each annihilation event travel in opposite directions, and the energy generated is measured by an array of detectors. Detection of annihilation in two opposite detectors at the identical time indicates the presence of the isotope in the volume separating the detectors. Using computed tomography principles, these coincidental counts generate images reflecting the regional rate of radionuclide uptake. Depending on the radionuclide used, various physiological parameters can be measured and imaged including, at present, oxygen and glucose metabolism, blood flow, and density and affinity of certain neurotransmitter receptors. Several commercial instruments are now available for such measurements, but this is an expensive technology. The PET device itself can be purchased for about $1 million (for the cheapest system), but the short half-life of the isotope requires the availability of a dedicated particle accelerator (cyclotron), at a cost of perhaps $2–3 million. In addition, a team of physicists, radiochemists, nuclear medicine experts, and technologists is needed to operate the system. The images obtained with current generation PET scanners are very detailed. To relate this physiological information to anatomic regions of interest, an atlas of brain anatomy is required. Such computerized "atlas" databases have been established with digitized images of sliced brains. Multiple brain "slices" can be obtained with PET (Fig. 6).

Another important application of PET is for assessment of the density and affinity of receptors for neurotransmitters. Ligands have already been developed for imaging D_2 dopamine receptors, and ligands for other receptors are currently being developed and investigated. PET thus has the potential to provide the important link between anatomy and physiological activity that is mediated by excitatory and inhibitory effects of neuro-

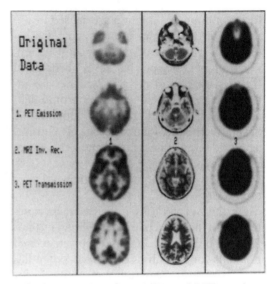

FIG. 6. Raw data from MRI and PET used as input for merging. MRI data were acquired at 4.2-mm intervals with a slice thickness of 4.0 mm using an inversion recovery pulse sequence (TE = 30 msec, TI = 300 msec, RT = 1276 msec). Transmission and emission PET data were also acquired, although only the emission data are shown in this image set. Note the alignment of sections in terms of scaling, angle, and level. From Mazziotta JC, et al. Region of interest issures: the relationship between structure and function in the brain. *J Cereb Blood Flow Metab* 1991;11:A51–A56.

transmitters. The investigation of this poorly understood link is crucial.

Another technique more recently introduced for three-dimensional imaging is single-photon emission computed tomography (SPECT). This technique uses photon-emitting radionuclides that, unlike positron emitters, do not require the availability of a dedicated cyclotron. However, at present the reliability of the quantitation with available radionuclides that can be safely administered is still very problematic, and much work is required to make SPECT applicable in systematic neurobehavioral research. SPECT can also be used for studying neurotransmitters, and ligands for imaging both D_1 and D_2 dopamine receptors have been described.

Behavioral dimensions studied with neuro-

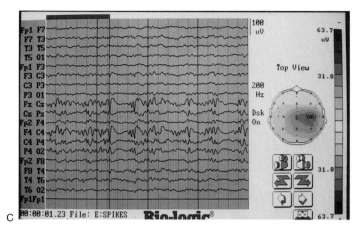

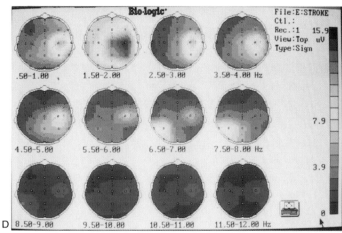

Fig. 5. (*Continued.*) Examples of topographic displays of electrophysiological data. **C:** In another example of a voltage map, the map displays the maxima of a spike obtained from an epileptic that is indicated by the red cursor on the continuous EEG display. **D:** This display is of an EEG that has been subjected to frequency analysis; the 12 integrated spectral bands are plotted topographically. In a patient with a right cerebrovascular accident (CVA), the low-frequency range of activity (first three maps) is concentrated over the right hemisphere.

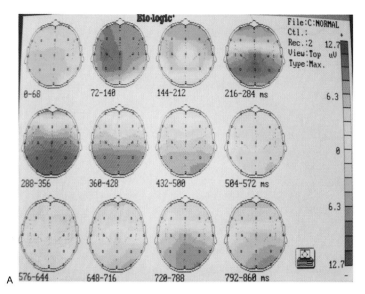

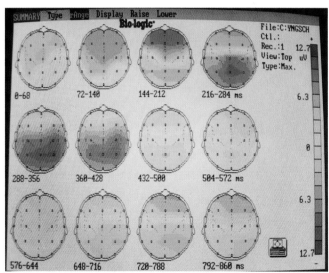

FIG. 5. Examples of topographic displays of electrophysiological data. **A:** Integrated voltages of evoked responses for 12 latency windows following stimulus onset are mapped. In this case, averaged evoked response amplitudes to a rare stimulus (oddball P300 paradigm) from a normal subject are shown. Note the posterior maxima in the 288- to 356-msec latency window. **B:** Data similar to (A) but obtained from a schizophrenic patient. Note the overall decreased amplitude when compared with the normal subject, as well as the right-sided skew of the positive potential, especially at the 288- to 356-msec latency window.

(continued on reverse)

imaging can help to identify neural networks. Mental activity, as a product of the activity of brain regions, has metabolic costs. The regional distribution of activity is determined by neurotransmitter systems operating on neural networks, with regional specificity. To understand how the brain regulates behavior it would help to investigate this entire chain. Neuroimaging, although still in its infancy, can contribute to our understanding of behavioral regulation. Described below are some of the findings that may illustrate the potential of neuroimaging for studying the neural basis of behavior.

NEUROANATOMY AND BEHAVIOR

Several studies have examined the relationship between cognitive dimensions and neuroanatomic data. For example, left hemispheric superiority in language processing has been related to CT evidence that language-related structures are larger on the left, and some studies have correlated performance of cognitive tasks with CT measures of atrophy. Relationships have been suggested between the extent and location of anatomic lesions and the severity and pattern of behavioral deficits. For example, large anterior lesions in the left hemisphere are usually associated with greater deficits in speech output than smaller lesions in these areas.

There is much need for better normative data on control subjects and more precise quantitation of the CT and MRI results. The most widely used technique for obtaining the neuroanatomic measures is to trace brain regions on the image and calculate their area using planimetry. A more rigorous method would be to apply segmentation algorithms (i.e., methods for computerized classification of image elements, or voxels, into tissue type such as brain vs. cerebral spinal fluid (CSF) or gray vs. white matter) with established reliability and validity. Volumetric measures of brain tissue using such algorithms are likely to be more sensitive to relatively subtle differences that can be associated with normal vari-

ability. For example, using a segmentation algorithm of MRI obtained in normal subjects, a linear decrease in brain volume and increase in CSF volume were associated with aging. The effect was more pronounced in men than women (Fig. 7).

NEUROPHYSIOLOGY AND BEHAVIOR

The physiological neuroimaging techniques measuring blood flow and glucose or oxygen metabolism are more suitable than the neuroanatomic methods for dynamic studies of brain–behavior relationships. These techniques can be expected to give measures that are influenced not only by basal variability (among normal subjects and between patients and controls), but also by environmental stimuli that can lead to changes in regional brain activity. This sensitivity of the physiological measures to environmental demands can be utilized to design experimental procedures in which the environmental factors are rigorously controlled so as to test hypotheses on brain–behavior relationships. Thus, subjects can be studied both at resting baseline states and while performing behavioral tasks.

With regard to the influence of stimuli, the techniques are sensitive to changes in brain activity produced by sensory stimulation and show specific effects on blood flow or metabolism for visual, auditory, and somatosensory modalities. For example, visual stimuli increase activity in occipital regions, whereas auditory stimulation produces increases of activity in temporal auditory cortex. Several studies have also examined the effects of cognitive tasks, consistently reporting increased metabolic activity during cognition compared to resting baseline. Regional specificity to task demands has also been documented. For example, in an early experiment we wanted to test statistically whether there was greater physiological activation in regions that serve specific cognitive functions. A sam-

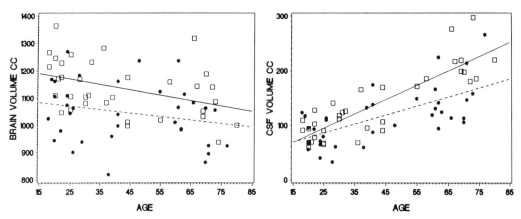

FIG. 7. Scatterplots and regression lines showing the relationship between age and brain volume (**left**) and age and cerebrospinal fluid (CSF) volume (**right**). Values for men are represented by squares and a solid regression line; values for women are represented by circles and a dashed regression line. Note that the effect is more pronounced in men than in women. From Gur RC, et al. Gender differences in age effect on brain atrophy measured by magnetic resonance imaging. *Proc Natl Acad Sci USA* 1991;88:2845–2849.

ple of normal right-handed young men was studied, and measurements of rCBF were performed with the xenon-133 inhalation technique at rest and during the performance of verbal (analogy problems) and spatial (gestalt-completion) tasks.

The verbal task was chosen because of evidence that performance of this task involves predominantly left hemispheric processing. By contrast, performance on the gestalt-completion task is impaired with right hemispheric damage. Both tasks reliably increased CBF across regions. The increase was hemispherically asymmetrical only for the verbal task, which produced greater increases in left hemispheric rCBF. For the spatial task, the increase was bilaterally symmetrical when the entire sample was examined. However, subjects who had greater increases in right hemispheric rCBF performed better than subjects who had the reverse asymmetry of CBF change from baseline. In a subsequent experiment, the same verbal task and a different spatial task (line orientation) were administered to a sample of right- and left-handed males and females. Gender and handedness are dimensions of individual differences that have been shown to influence the direction and degree of hemispheric cognitive specialization. In this second study of

rCBF (Fig. 8), females had higher rCBF and left handers differed from right handers in the pattern of hemispheric activation. Right handers replicated the greater left hemispheric increases of rCBF for the verbal task and showed greater right hemispheric increases with the spatial task. Left handers did not show this pattern. These results indicated that rCBF measured with the xenon-133 technique is sensitive not only to the effects of cognitive effort on regional brain activity but to individual differences affecting the direction and degree of hemispheric specialization for cognitive function.

Subsequent studies with rCBF and PET have confirmed and extended these findings. In most cases, the results confirmed hypotheses that had been generated from earlier observations. But, as often happens when new technology is applied, some of the results were unforeseen. For example, a PET study with the same verbal analogy and spatial line orientation tasks described above showed asymmetrical effects in the expected temporo-parietal regions that had been implicated by clinical observations of brain damage. However, a less established hypothesis proposed in 1972 by the British neuropsychologist Colwyn Trevarthen was also supported by the data. Trevarthen suggested that neural

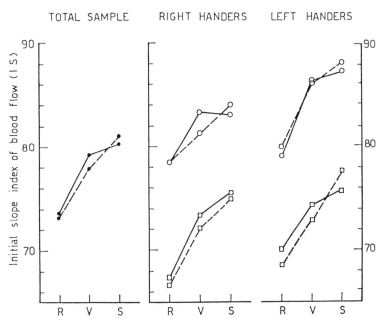

FIG. 8. Initial slope (IS) index of blood flow to the left (———) and right (– – –) hemispheres for the total sample (●) and for right- and left-handed females (○) and right- and left-handed males (□) during performance of resting (R), verbal (V), and spatial tasks (S). As can be seen, cerebral blood flow increased in both hemispheres for both tasks, but the increase is slightly greater in the left for the verbal and in the right for the spatial task. This is clearer for right handers than for left handers. From Gur RC, et al. Sex and handedness differences in cerebral blood flow during rest and cognitive activity. *Science* 1982;217:659–6611. Copyright 1982 by the AAAS.

activation of lateralized cognitive processes could "spill over" to motor brain regions and produce orientation to the contralateral hemispace. Thus, when people have verbal thoughts, they will orient themselves to the right, and when they have spatial cognitions, they will orient themselves to the left. This hypothesis received some confirmation in studies examining the effects of verbal and spatial tasks on the direction of conjugate lateral eye movements while individuals were reflecting on the answers to test items. The PET study showed that the effects of the tasks on rCBF were asymmetrical not only in the temporoparietal regions but also in regions controlling the orientation response (Fig. 9). This cognitive-motor network may explain, for example, cognitive deficits that have been found in patients suffering from movement disorders such as Parkinson's disease.

Another behavior that received additional neurophysiological examination by the new

techniques is anxiety. A behavioral "law," traced to the results of an animal study by Yerkes and Dodson in 1908, posits a curvilinear, "inverted-U" relationship between anxiety and performance. Performance is not very good when anxiety is extremely low, since the attentional and arousal components required for optimal performance are missing. At extremely high anxiety, however, performance also deteriorates. The brain mechanisms responsible for this phenomenon could not be studied without the availability of neuroimaging techniques. Initial findings with PET and the xenon-133 technique showed that this inverted-U relationship between anxiety and performance is paralleled by changes in cortical metabolism and blood flow. The subjects with low and high anxiety (who performed poorly) also had lower cortical CBF than the subjects with medium anxiety (who performed better). This suggests a neural mechanism that reduces cortical activ-

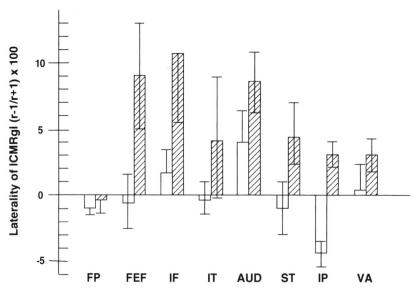

FIG. 9. Laterality scores of glucose metabolism for seven regions of interest in subjects receiving the verbal task (empty bars) and the spatial task (crosshatched). FP, frontal pole; FEF, frontal eye field; IF, inferior frontal; IT, inferior temporal; AUD, auditory cortex; ST, superior temporal; IP, inferior parietal; VA, visual association. From Gur RC, et al. A cognitive–motor network demonstrated by positron emission tomography. *Neuropsychologia* 1983;21:601–606.

ity in high anxiety, perhaps reflecting a shift toward activation of subcortical regions which are more important in fight-or-flight situations.

Other PET and xenon-133 studies have examined regional brain involvement in attention. These studies helped to establish, for example, the existence of a network of brain regions that animal neuroanatomic studies have implicated in attentional processing. In humans, these regions show greater right hemispheric activation. Further elaboration of attentional processes in relation to regional brain activity was elegantly carried out in a series of studies using PET measures of CBF by the American neuropsychologist Michael Posner, the neurologist Marcus Raichle, and their colleagues at Washington University in St. Louis.

Physiological studies examining regional brain abnormalities in neuropsychiatric populations have usually used resting conditions. However, clearer results may be obtained in these populations by the use of activation procedures. Since the behavioral abnormalities occur in response to environmental trig-

gers, regional abnormalities in brain activity may be undetected at rest but become apparent in the pattern of changes in activity produced by task activation. This was documented in a sample of patients with unilateral cerebral infarcts. Few studies have examined both resting and activated conditions in psychiatric populations (see Chapter 18). Such studies could improve diagnostic accuracy and might help identify patterns of abnormal activation in specific forms of psychopathology. A potentially productive strategy would be to identify regional abnormalities in brain anatomy and physiological activity associated with focal and nonfocal brain disease and to relate the abnormal pattern to behavioral impairment.

INTEGRATING BEHAVIORAL AND NEUROIMAGING DATA

The challenge is to integrate behavioral theories on regional brain function with anatomic and physiological neuroimaging data. In addition to the anatomic information on the integrity of brain regions, such as is now available from x-ray CT and MRI scans, the PET and xenon-133 techniques provide information on regional brain physiological activity, and topographic EEG techniques complement our armamentarium of data on regional brain function with information on electric activity. Imaging technology provides means for integrating such multifaceted data in a comprehensible manner, but theory is needed to guide our understanding of how the activity of the brain is related to behavior.

In the process of formulating theories on brain regulation of behavior, the pattern of test performance is used to link regional brain involvement with specific behaviors. The pattern of deficits is used in clinical practice to implicate brain regions putatively affected by a disease. The process of testing neurobehavioral theories can be helped by quantification of theoretical statements concerning regional brain involvement in the regulation of specific behaviors. We have proposed an algorithm that applies such a quantification to standard neuropsychological test scores. The algorithm yields a value for each brain region, which reflects expectations that the region is neurally compromised given the pattern of scores. These regional values can be examined statistically to test the behavioral hypotheses against clinical data and other neuroimaging data. They can also be presented topographically using standard procedures for translating numbers into a gray scale or a color scale. This facilitates comprehension of the spatial distribution of implicated regions. Initial testing of the algorithm in clinical cases and populations was encouraging. There was consistency between the behavioral images and the location of the lesion in patients with unilateral cerebral infarcts (Fig. 10).

The topographic displays showed correspondence with clinical and CT data and were congruent with the clinical interpretation of the neuropsychological data. Note that in both cases the behavioral image suggested that regions considerably larger than the CT lesion were behaviorally "hypofunctional," including a contralaterally homotopic region. This was not detected by the

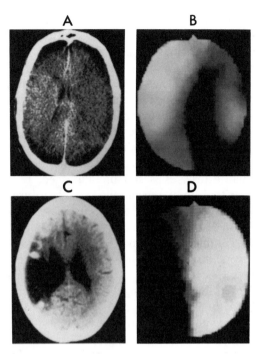

FIG. 10. CT scans and corresponding behavioral images of two patients with cerebral infarcts, one in the right hemisphere (**A** and **B** for CT and behavioral image, respectively) and one in the left (**C** and **D**). The CT scans were reversed so that the left hemisphere is to the viewer's left. From Gur RC, et al. Behavioral imaging: a procedure for analysis and display of neuropsychological test scores. I. Construction of algorithm and initial clinical evaluation. *Neuropsychiatry Neuropsychol Behav Neurol* 1988;1:53–60.

clinical evaluation and may reflect inadequacy in the spatial resolution of the behavioral images. However, it could also be a true behavioral manifestation of remote physiological effects of focal lesions. Comparison of the behavioral images with PET and CT scans should make it possible to evaluate which behavioral effects are accompanied by remote physiological suppressions.

DIRECTIONS FOR FUTURE RESEARCH AND LONG-TERM POTENTIAL OF NEUROIMAGING TECHNIQUES

The impact of neuroimaging technology is only beginning to surface. Some techniques are still in the process of evolving toward optimal resolution and standard scanning procedures. Normative data are lacking, and only embryonic steps have been taken to identify neural networks regulating human behavior. Although several brain diseases can already be reliably detected by neuroimaging (e.g., stroke, Alzheimer's disease, epilepsy), the diagnostic utility of the techniques for the vast majority of neurological and for all psychiatric diseases is still unestablished. It is clear that no one technique is likely to provide all the answers. Each has its relative advantages and limitations and yields data that are complementary but overlapping in part. Several immediate steps are necessary to harness this technology in the service of improved theoretical insight on normal brain–behavior functions and diagnosis and treatment of psychopathology.

One of the first steps would be the application of these techniques to patients with destructive brain lesions, such as those produced by stroke, head trauma, or brain tumors, to help in determining the extent and topographic distribution of anatomic brain damage and abnormal (suppressed or abnormally increased) metabolic activation. In addition to abnormalities of baseline physiological activity, behavioral deficits can stem from failure of brain regions to become activated in response to task demands. Neurobehavioral probes, which are standard behavioral activation procedures combined with neuroimaging studies of regional brain physiological activity, will become a useful tool for hypothesis testing as well as for diagnosis and evaluation of treatment effects.

Another step would be to combine the ability of PET to image the distribution of neurotransmitters with its measurements of topographic distribution of metabolism to understand how neurotransmitter systems regulate behavior. It would be revealing, for instance, to compare Parkinson's disease with Alzheimer's disease (see Chapter 23). Dopamine deficiency seems responsible for the symptoms of the former, and some evidence suggests the involvement of cholinergic pathways in the latter. Neuroimaging of

neurotransmitter receptor density as well as the distribution of physiological activity in these populations can be compared to that of schizophrenia, where there is evidence for increased dopamine availability. Such studies can progress in a complementary fashion in brain diseases with specific pathology in comparison to disorders of behavior where the brain pathology is unclear, and the metabolic studies could help identify regional brain involvement. For example, studies of reading disability and other learning disabilities could help test hypotheses on regional brain dysfunction that underlie these disorders.

But looking at pathology and deficit is only one side of the coin. Normal individuals vary considerably in behavior and abilities, and studying the relationship between this variability and regional brain physiology could shed light on the neural underpinnings of this variability. For example, exceptionally talented individuals in the sciences, arts, and humanities could be evaluated. Again, this should be done at rest and during neurobehavioral probe procedures. How does the regional brain activity of a mathematician differ from that of an architect? Which brain regions does a mathematician activate when using calculus? Which brain regions does a lawyer activate when preparing or presenting a case? Could we train individuals to activate appropriate brain regions and thereby enhance their abilities? The new technology permits us to begin to address such questions.

Thus far the cognitive dimension of behavior has received the greatest attention, particularly in the examination of verbal and spatial tasks in relation to hemispheric activation. But emotion and conative or motivational factors could also be studied with the techniques. The studies on anxiety, attention, and affect described above can be refined and extended to other dimensions (such as additional emotions), and new dimensions can be explored (such as pleasure–pain). Studies of populations representing a range of normal and abnormal behaviors could be informative in understanding regional brain involvement in the regulation of behavior and of considerable relevance to the diagnosis and treatment of dysfunction. The key could be to integrate data from both anatomic and physiological methods.

SUMMARY

Methods for investigating brain-behavior relationships in humans, initially restricted to lesion studies, have been enriched by standardized neuropsychological assessment batteries and, more recently, the application of neuroimaging. The chapter presented the evolution, advantages, and limitations of these sources of information. This combined methodology, even in its present state, is uniquely equipped to help us understand normal variability in brain function, as well as the regulation of behavior in pathological states, because it is suitable for rigorous experimentation. This is embodied in the application of neurobehavioral probes to physiological neuroimaging studies. Such an integrated approach holds much promise for elucidating aspects of the neurobiology of behavior.

BIBLIOGRAPHY

Original Articles

Gur RC, Gur RE, Rosen AD, Warach S, Alavi A, Greenberg J, Reivich M. A cognitive-motor network demonstrated by positron emission tomography. *Neuropsychologia* 1983;21:601–606.

Ross ED, Mesulam M-M. Dominant language functions of the right hemisphere? Prosody and emotional gesturing. *Arch Neurol* 1979;36:144–148.

Sackeim HA, Greenberg MS, Weiman AL, Gur RC, Hungerbuhler JP, Geschwind N. Hemispheric asymmetry in the expression of positive and negative emotions. Neurologic evidence. *Arch Neurol* 1982;39: 210–218.

Books and Reviews

Benton AL, Hamsher K, Varney N, Spreen O. *Contributions to neuropsychological assessment:* a clinical manual. New York: Oxford University Press; 1983.

Damasio H, Damasio AR. *Lesion analysis in neuropsychology.* New York: Oxford University Press; 1989.

Geschwind N. Disconnexion syndromes in animals and man. *Brain* 1965;88:237–294, 585–644.

Goodglass H, Kaplan E. *The assessment of aphasia and related disorders.* 2nd Ed. Philadelphia: Lea & Febiger; 1983.

Gur RC, Gur RE. The impact of neuroimaging on human neuropsychology. In: Weingartner HJ, Lister RG, eds. *Perspectives on cognitive neuroscience.* New York: Oxford University Press; 1991:417–435.

Lezak MD. *Neuropsychological assessment.* 2nd Ed. New York: Oxford University Press; 1983.

Luria AR. *Higher cortical functions in man.* 2nd Ed. New York: Plenum Publications; 1980.

McKenna P, Warrington E. The analytical approach to neuropsychological assessment. In: Grant I, Adams KM, eds. *Neuropsychological assessment of neuropsychiatric disorders.* New York: Oxford University Press; 1986:31–47.

Mesulam M-M, ed. *Principles of behavioral neurology.* Philadelphia: FA Davis; 1985.

Reivich M, Gur R, Alavi A. Positron emission tomography studies of sensory stimuli, cognitive processes and anxiety. *Human Neurobiol* 1983;2:25–33.

16

Genetic Approaches to Mental Illness

R. Arlen Price

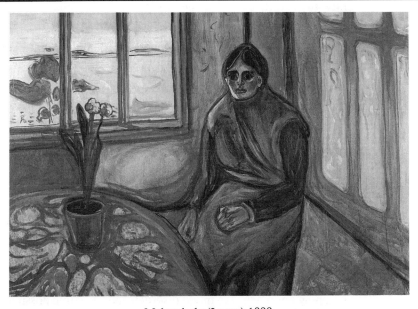

Melancholy (Laura) 1899

The light and the colors penetrated my soul and my body, in which my sick blood flowed. Melancholy . . . I ran out to escape this eerie creature.

Edvard Munch

The paintings of the Norwegian artist Edvard Munch often focused on strong human emotions. In this particular painting, Munch is said to have examined his connection with his sister's illness through his own "sick blood." Munch apparently suffered from many of the same symptoms of anxiety and depression that affected his sister, and later was himself hospitalized for a time. It is common for mental illness to run in families, and shared genes, referred to by Munch as "sick blood," appear to be a large part of the reason.

- There appear to be at least three broad classes of heritable mental disorders. In descending order of their population prevalence they are mood disorders, including depression and mania; anxiety disorders, including panic, phobic, and obsessive-compulsive disorders; and psychotic disorders, especially schizophrenia.

- Studies aimed at detecting and characterizing genetic influences on behavior present special problems.

- Psychiatric illnesses are by far the most common of all classes of human diseases.

- Explicit phenotype definitions are essential to any clinical, biological, epidemiological, or genetic study.

- Case-control family studies compare familial and population rates of illness.

- Currently, twin studies provide the most common means of testing for genetic involvement.

- The greater concordance for mood disorders of identical twins over fraternal twins suggests genetic involvement.

- Adoption studies provide the best means of separating genetic and environmental effects, but restricted access to adoption records makes such studies difficult to carry out, particularly in the United States.

- Mendel's observations of inheritance were remarkable for their insight and experimental nature.

- There appears to be no simple mode of inheritance for any of the mood disorders.

- At present there is no one mechanism to explain the biological basis of any mood disorder.

- The genes causing cystic fibrosis and Duchenne's muscular dystrophy were found using the gene mapping approach.

- Gene mapping approaches to mood disorders have become possible only within the last few years.

- A shift of emphasis away from global explanations for mental illness may reduce the etiological complexity of these disorders.

- There is hope that we can soon understand the genetic bases of mood disorders well enough to predict who is vulnerable and effectively prevent or treat disease by focusing only on those individuals.

This chapter focuses on the common genetic strategies that have been applied to mental illnesses and on one of the most common and well-researched forms of mental illness—the mood disorders. Topics discussed include the epidemiological significance of mental illness in our country, phenotype definition, familial aggregation, genetic involvement and mode of inheritance, gene mapping approaches, complex inheritance of mental illnesses, and the constructive use of genetic heterogeneity. The chapter concludes with a consideration of future approaches and the potential of genetic counseling and prevention to help individuals and families.

For centuries, perhaps millennia, common folk wisdom has held that mental illness runs in families. Implicit theories of cause have ranged from environmental ones (e.g., reaction to extreme loss) to supernatural ones (e.g., enchantment or witchcraft). However, a recurring belief has been that tendencies to become mentally ill are "in the blood" or, to borrow an Old Order Amish expression, "Siss im blut." That is, many people have the impression that mental illnesses are inherited genetically. Modern scientific investigations have confirmed some of these common-sensical notions about the causes of mental illness. Virtually all mental disorders do run in families, and most appear to be influenced substantially by genes. The emerging picture from recent research is that mental illness is made up of a collection of genetically distinct but clinically overlapping disorders. Complex causal mechanisms probably determine the distinctive forms of these disorders as well as their interrelationships.

There appear to be at least three broad classes of heritable mental disorders. In descending order of their population prevalence they are mood disorders, *including depression and mania;* anxiety disorders, *including panic, phobic, and obsessive-compulsive disorders; and* psychotic disorders, *especially* schizophrenia. The strategies for understanding all these psychiatric disorders are the same, and much of what we know about them genetically is similar.

GENETIC STRATEGIES FOR CLINICAL RESEARCH

Studies aimed at detecting and characterizing genetic influences on behavior present special problems. Table 1 presents a series of steps that should be followed when undertaking genetic research on newly defined disorders or disorders whose definitions are evolving. Although most mood disorders fall into the latter category, some, e.g., late luteal phase dysphoric disorder (premenstrual syndrome; PMS) and rapid cycling bipolar disorder, fall into the former category as disorders only recently recognized by the scientific community. All of the points outlined in Table 1 are important and will be considered separately, and most represent topics that recur in genetic research on mental illness. Reliable *phenotype definition* (where phenotype refers to an observable trait) according to standard criteria is essential to any genetic study. It is important to establish *familial aggregation* (that the trait runs in families) before undertaking more extensive genetic studies. Unless a mental illness is more common in family members of a person with the illness than in the general population, it is unlikely that genes significantly influence risk for the illness. Histories

Biological Bases of Brain Function and Disease, edited by Alan Frazer, Perry B. Molinoff, and Andrew Winokur. Raven Press, Ltd., New York © 1994.

TABLE 1. *Genetic strategies in clinical research: steps in identifying individual genes causing mental illness*

Step	Strategy
1. Phenotype definition	Diagnostic criteria and standardized assessment
2. Familial aggregation	Epidemiological studies of familial and population risks
3. Genetic involvement	Genetic and nongenetic causes of familial aggregation: twin and adoption studies
4. Mode of inheritance	Multigene, a few genes, single gene, or major gene Associations and interactions
5. Heterogeneity	Define homogeneous subgroups
6. Specific mechanisms	Biological studies of candidate genes Gene mapping

obtained from clinical interviews may strongly suggest a familial pattern of illness but are more often inconclusive because such interviews lack sufficient structure and sensitivity to detect all illnesses of relatives. Case-control family studies (e.g., a comparison of families of mentally ill and physically ill patients) are an alternative that can clearly establish familial aggregation. Since illnesses may cluster in families because of shared living conditions as well as genes, it will be important to examine twins and adoptees to assess the presence and extent of *genetic involvement* as opposed to the influence of family environment. Family studies are also necessary to detect the specific *mode of inheritance* (e.g., multigene or single gene). Family studies also should focus on questions of biological and genetic subtyping by examining the relationship of familial risk to clinical features, biological markers, and comorbid conditions (i.e., other, co-occurring disorders). Such studies will be useful in identifying markers for *heterogeneity,* i.e., clinical features that signify distinct genetic illnesses. Once genetic influence has been established and major gene involvement has been suggested it will be appropriate to pursue molecular genetic and gene mapping studies to determine *specific mechanisms.* At that point, genetic linkage and association studies can provide bridges between family studies of clinical phenotypes and molecular studies of genes at the level of DNA. Studies of biological markers may suggest candidate genes that play primary causal roles in each type of mental illness. Each of these major points will be considered in turn.

SIGNIFICANCE

Psychiatric illnesses are by far the most common of all classes of human diseases. At any given time in the United States, more than one person in ten (10.9%) is mentally ill. The illnesses include mood, anxiety, and psychotic disorders, but of these the mood disorders are the most common (about 7% of the total population). The implications are staggering: at least 25 million Americans are now suffering from some form of mental illness, and about 17 million of those have a severe mood disorder.

PHENOTYPE DEFINITION

Explicit phenotype definitions are essential to any clinical, biological, epidemiological, or genetic study. Although the prominent clinical features of mood disorders are described elsewhere in this volume (see Chapter 17), some features are reviewed here because genetic studies are strongly influenced by phenotype definitions. In particular, clinical and genetic trait definitions are not always the same. It is important in beginning any genetic study to think carefully about trait definitions, especially boundaries between distinct disorders and areas of overlap in which two or more disorders cannot be distinguished.

A phenotype is an observed trait, like height, eye color, or mood. A genotype is the genetic makeup of an individual, often expressed with respect to a particular gene or genes. The strength of the relationship between phenotype and genotype is embodied in the concept of heritability. Literally, it is the correlation between the two. For example, an additive quantitative trait such as stature will have a high correlation between the number of growth-promoting genes a person carries and the person's height. The correlation will be lower for recessive genes and the trait phenotype because individuals with one gene copy cannot be distinguished from those with none.

For many years rigorous definitions of mental illnesses were lacking. For example, the development and acceptance of standardized criteria for bipolar disorder and major depressive disorder and the utilization of standardized assessment instruments have made it possible to generalize findings from disparate studies. These diagnostic criteria are the result of extensive discussions among psychiatrists, psychologists, and epidemiologists. In the United States, the most commonly used diagnostic criteria are catalogued in the *Diagnostic and Statistical Manual of Mental Disorders* (DSM) of the American Psychiatric Association, which is currently in its third edition (DSM-III-R), and the *International Classification of Diseases* (ICD) of the World Health Organization (WHO), now in its ninth edition (ICD-9). Several standardized semistructured interview procedures have been devised to provide the information necessary for making DSM-III-R and ICD-9 diagnoses, including some that may be administered by nonclinicians. The diagnostic criteria are constantly changing and so must be kept in mind in interpreting the results from different studies. Often, for example, differences in diagnostic criteria may explain differences in results among studies.

One source of confusion in describing mood disorders is that some psychiatric terms are a part of common language and experience. When depressed, people usually feel sad. When manic, people usually feel speeded up. What distinguishes a well individual's response to a particularly bad or good day from that of an individual with a mood disorder are its severity, duration, and distinct qualities that suggest a disruption of normal biological processes and needs, like sleeping, eating, and sex. Severity and duration of the mood states are judged relative to everyday experience and to common reactions to important life experiences that occur more rarely (e.g., death of a loved one or news of an important success). Specific symptoms (e.g., sleep and appetite disturbances) can indicate that the mood state is severe enough to have a biological cause. Most useful in genetic studies are outward manifestations of the mood disorder (the phenotype) that are closely related to an underlying genetic cause (the individual's genotype).

Often the boundaries between different types of mood disorder are difficult to establish. People who become manic almost always also become depressed, either just after the manic period or on a completely different occasion. Thus, manics are usually called *bipolar*. People who only become depressed are said to have major depressive disorder and are often called *unipolar*. People with chronic but somewhat less severe depressed mood that lasts for years are said to have *dysthymia*. Obviously, clinical conditions that are vaguely defined are unlikely to have clearly evident genetic mechanisms.

A more detailed presentation of clinical aspects of mood disorders can be found in Chapter 17.

FAMILIAL AGGREGATION

Case-control family studies compare familial and population rates of illness. Before constructing elaborate genetic hypotheses it is essential to establish that familial aggregation exists. This requirement is particularly important for mental disorders with a high population base rate. For example, if a disorder is very common (say, indigestion), most families will have at least one member who is "affected"—even though the disease is not genetic.

For phenotypes that can be measured quantitatively (e.g., height, weight, or IQ), familial aggregation may be described by standard correlation methods. For qualitative phenotypes (e.g., presence or absence of a mood disorder), aggregation is described by concordances (identity of phenotypes in two relatives) or by conditional probabilities (risk for illness in relatives, given that one individual, the proband or index case, is ill). These familial risk estimates are meaningful only when compared with the risk in the general population, often estimated by the risk to relatives of normal controls.

The genotype is constant during an individual's lifetime (with the exception of some somatic cell mutations), even though some genes may not have observable effects until certain periods in life. Thus, it is the lifetime risk for mood disorders that is most relevant to genetic studies. The lifetime risk or morbid risk is the chance that any particular individual will develop a mood disorder at some time during his or her life. It is calculated from the ratio of the number of individuals who are affected to the number who are at risk in a specified population.

Mood disorders may begin at any time during an individual's life, but most often the first onset is between the ages of 15 and 55. Thus, a well person at age 60 is unlikely to develop a mood disorder, with the possible exception of depression associated with dementia. A well child at age 5, however, has lived through little if any of the interval during which he or she will be at risk for developing a mood disorder. Thus, a well state at age 5 gives little information about an underlying state of vulnerability to illness during a lifetime, say, by the time a child reaches age 60. Because of variable age of onset, estimates of risk for mood disorders are usually adjusted for age so as to reflect the cumulative risk for individuals over their whole lifetimes.

As estimated from results of nationwide community surveys, the age-adjusted lifetime population risks for bipolar mania and unipolar depression are about 1% and 6%, respectively, with equal rates of bipolar disorder in men and women and a 2:1 female-to-male ratio for unipolar depression. Another 3% of the population, mostly women, suffer from a chronic but somewhat less severe form of depression known as dysthymia.

National surveys have also identified families of patients with mood disorders (index cases) and families of well individuals (normal controls). This approach, called the case-control family study, compares familial and general population rates of illness. In first-degree relatives (parents, siblings, and children) of unipolar depressed patients, the risk of depression is about 28%, whereas the risk of bipolar disorder is the same as the population risk, about 1%. In first-degree relatives of manic-depressive patients, there is a 4% risk of bipolar disorder and a 23% risk of unipolar depression. Taken together, the familial risk is about the same in the two types of mood disorders, but mania appears to be limited to families of manics. The fact that both types of mood disorders are found in bipolar individuals and their relatives suggests a continuity between these extreme mood states, but the fact that there is no increased risk of mania in the families of depressed patients suggests the possibility that unipolar depression is etiologically distinct from bipolar manic depression (Table 2).

The concept of relative risk compares rates of illness among family members to rates in the general population. On the one hand, familial risk figures indicate that more than two thirds of first-degree relatives of individuals with major mood disorders will not have a serious illness themselves. It is encouraging

TABLE 2. *Familial and population risk for mood disorders (%)*

Index case	Bipolar illness	Unipolar depression
Normal	1	6
Unipolar	1	28
Bipolar	4	23

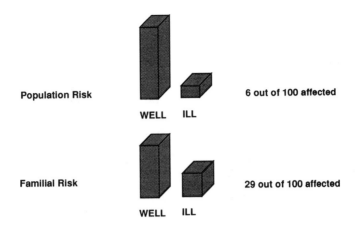

Relative Risk: 29 to 6 (Approximately 5 to 1)

FIG. 1. More than one person in 20 will develop a major mood disorder at some time during his or her lifetime. If a parent or sibling has already had a major illness, the risk increases to between 1 in 4 and 1 in 3. Although the majority of relatives will never develop a mood disorder themselves, the relative risk—the proportional increase in risk due to having an ill family member—is about 4:1; that is, someone with an ill family member is about four times as likely to become ill as someone with family members who are all well.

news that most relatives should be well or at least will not have a severe mood disorder. On the other hand, the familial risk of more than 1 in 4 (27% to 29%) is quite high, particularly when understood as relative risk, about 4:1 (27–29% vs. 7%). Therefore, having a close relative with a major mood disorder increases one's own risk about fourfold over that of someone who has no ill first-degree relatives (Fig. 1).

GENETIC INVOLVEMENT

Currently, twin studies provide the most common means of testing for genetic involvement (Fig. 2). Because twins account for slightly more than 1% of all live births (approximately 1 in every 83 births), twinning is sufficiently common to provide the necessary samples for genetic investigations. Twin births may be divided roughly equally into three types: identical (single-egg) twins, same-sex fraternal (two-egg) twins, and opposite-sex fraternal (two-egg) twins. Fraternal twinning (analogous to human litter or clutch size) is at least to some degree genetic.

The greater similarity of identical twins, who share all genes, as compared to fraternal twins, who share on average only half, suggests genetic influence.

However, such studies may be hampered by genetic and environmental entanglements. For instance, the two types of twins may have unequal environmental similarity (e.g., more similar names, diet, dress, activities, and expectations of identical twins), different procedures may be used for case identification (e.g., more similar identical twin pairs coming to attention), and there may be different degrees of diagnostic bias (e.g., a clinician basing the diagnosis of one twin in part on information about the identical twin). Obviously, potential differences such as these complicate the interpretation of some twin studies.

Probably the most comprehensive twin study of mood disorders was conducted in Sweden. This study found that the concordance rates (proportion of pairs in which both twins were ill) for bipolar disorder were higher in identical (.62) than in fraternal (.08) twins. Concordance rates were even higher when depressed cotwins of bipolars were con-

Identical Twinning

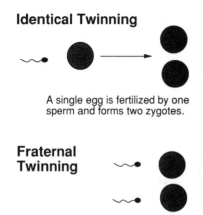

A single egg is fertilized by one sperm and forms two zygotes.

Fraternal Twinning

Two eggs are fertilized by two sperm and form two zygotes.

FIG. 2. Identical twins, also called monozygotic, arise when a single egg is fertilized by one sperm and the zygote splits to form two separate fetuses. The two resulting individuals have identical genetic material in all their cells, although their phenotypes may differ because of random differences in development processes, X-chromosome inactivation in women, or exposure to different environments, including intrauterine competition. Fraternal twins, also called dizygotic, are formed from two separate eggs and two separate sperm. They are genetically related as are normal siblings, sharing on average half their genes. Under this "natural experiment," genetic effects are inferred if the identical twins have more similar phenotypes than fraternal twins. Critics point out that this method may overestimate genetic influence if environments of identical twins are substantially more similar than those of fraternal twins. Large differences in degree of similarity of identical twins and other genetic relatives may also arise whenever multiple genes are required for disease expression, a pattern that has been noted for mood disorders and schizophrenia.

sidered concordant (.80). The concordance rates for unipolar depression were also higher for identical (.43) than for fraternal (.18) twins, but including bipolar–unipolar twin pairs as concordant did not change the concordance rates appreciably. Although there is some variability among other twin studies, the overall message is fairly consistent. *The greater concordance for mood disorders of identical twins over fraternal twins suggests genetic involvement.* On the other hand, the fact that concordance is far less than perfect

(1.00) demonstrates that genetic determinism is not everything. The twin studies also confirm that bipolar disorder tends to "breed true" in particular families and suggests that bipolar illness may be more highly familial (at least in identical twins) and, possibly, more strongly influenced by some genetic process than is unipolar depression. The very high concordance of identical twins, who share all genes, relative to fraternal twins and other family members, who have segregated genes, suggests that genetic interaction (variability in gene expression due to "background" genotype at several genetic loci) may be important in mental illnesses.

Adoption studies provide the best means of separating genetic and environmental effects, but restricted access to adoption records makes such studies difficult to carry out, particularly in the United States (Fig. 3). Of the five adoption studies that have been completed, most were small, and the evidence from these studies has been mixed. Two studies supported genetic influence in that risk to separated biological relatives (an index of shared genotype) was higher than risk to adoptive relatives who had lived together (an index of shared environment). Two studies were weakly positive but statistically equivocal. The one study that was clearly negative included "neurotic" depression (e.g., dysthymia), which may be a mild and nongenetic mood complaint. Thus, although the evidence from adoption studies is scant, the results are consistent with those from twin studies. The familial aggregation of mood disorders appears to be accounted for in part by the shared genetic vulnerability of biological relatives.

MODE OF INHERITANCE

Mendel's observations of inheritance were remarkable for their insight and experimental nature. More than 90 years before the structure of the genetic material (DNA) was understood, the principles by which genes are transmitted across generations and some of

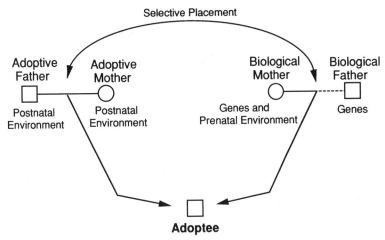

Adoptee

FIG. 3. The logic of the adoption method is portrayed in this figure. An adult adoptee had been separated from his biological parents at birth and raised by unrelated adoptive parents. The adoption study design works best in the absence of selective placement, the matching of characteristics of his biological and adoptive relatives. Any resemblance of the adoptee to his biological parents will be due to transmitted genes and exposure to the intrauterine environment provided by the biological mother. The biological father is connected to the diagram by a dashed line because information is often difficult to obtain about the fathers of children given up for adoption. In the absence of selective placement, any resemblance of the adoptee to his adoptive parents should be due to his exposure to shared postnatal environment.

the ways in which genotypes may be related to observed phenotypes were first described by Gregor Mendel. Mendel was an Augustinian monk living in Brunn, Moravia (now part of Czechoslovakia) who experimented with plants in the monastery garden. Mendel was the first to describe the genetic material as discrete elements inherited separately from both parents. In addition, he described a mechanism for recessive inheritance, which requires two gene copies for the phenotype to be expressed, and dominant inheritance, which requires only one gene copy (Fig. 4). Although more complicated forms of single-gene expression and multigene traits have been described, Mendel's laws still hold for many human genetic diseases, especially the relatively rare ones, such as phenylketonuria, cystic fibrosis, neurofibromatosis, and Duchenne's muscular dystrophy. For common diseases, including but not limited to psychiatric illnesses, multiple gene involvement is probably the rule.

There appears to be no simple mode of inheritance for any of the mood dis- *orders.* Some studies suggest that when the onset of illness occurs early in life, genetic and possibly major gene inheritance (a single gene with relatively large effects) may be somewhat more likely for both major depressive disorder and bipolar disorder than are *multifactorial* inheritance (multiple genetic and environmental causes).

In a few bipolar families, such as in the Old Order Amish living in eastern Pennsylvania, the large number of affected relatives in two or more generations suggests a dominantly expressed major gene (only a single gene copy being necessary for disease development). However, this mode of inheritance is not certain. For example, in relatively inbred population isolates such as the Old Order Amish, a frequently occurring recessive gene (requiring two gene copies) may appear dominant because the recessive disease is transmitted through the mating of *homozygous* (two-gene) affected individuals with common *heterozygous* (one-gene) carriers. In such families, about half the children would carry two gene copies and become ill. A gene can be-

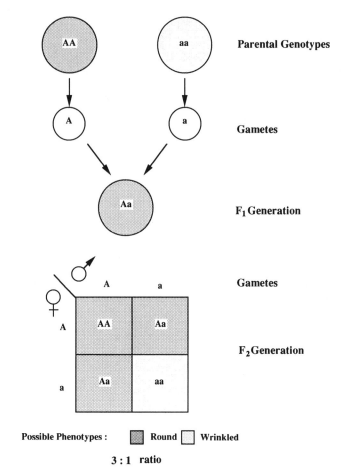

FIG. 4. Mendel's law of segregation. Discrete genetic elements called genes occur as identical pairs in homozygous individuals with the "true breeding" phenotypes, shaded and white. The genes separate (or segregate) to form gametes, which then combine to form a "hybrid" heterozygote that expresses the phenotype of only one of the parents, the shaded type. Combining the gametes through random mating of the hybrids results in one quarter true breeding individuals of each parental type and one half hybrids. Although the concept of dominance must have been known at least implicitly to animal and plant breeders for several millennia, Mendel was the first to formalize the concept into the 3:1 expected ratio of parental phenotypes in the offspring (F_2) of matings between hybrid individuals (F_1). In this example, the shaded phenotype is said to be dominant to white, which is said to be recessive.

come this common in an isolated group either by its initial presence in a small founding population (in this case some 31 families) or because of the random loss of some normal (not mutated) genes during meiosis in the small population (called *genetic drift*).

In some other non-Amish families, the lack of father-to-son transmission suggests an X-linked gene. However, if the X-linked hypothesis were true, then yet another sex-influenced mechanism would be necessary in other families to account for the even sex ratio for mania in the population.

Patterns of inheritance may be further complicated by genetic interactions at different gene loci (epistasis), gene–environment interactions, nongenetic forms of disease, and cross-assortative mating (e.g., marriage of a woman with unipolar depressive illness to a man with bipolar disorder), which can bring two or more different predisposing genes into the same family. To make matters still more complicated, individual families carrying common disease genes may assume virtually any pattern of single-gene inheritance by chance alone, even though multiple genetic loci are involved.

BIOLOGICAL MECHANISMS

At present there is no one mechanism to explain the biological basis of any mood disorder. Biological hypotheses are potentially important in genetic studies because they suggest mechanisms that can be confirmed or disconfirmed. This approach involves the identification of specific genetic mechanisms once the biological defect has been identified. Phenylketonuria, a recessively inherited metabolic disorder that can lead to mental retardation, provides a model for this genetic approach. It was known that this disease was due to an inability to metabolize the amino acid phenylalanine. That knowledge prompted work that led to the isolation of the gene for phenylalanine hydroxylase. Genes from affected individuals could be shown to have been inactivated through mutation.

There are either many or few biological clues to the genetic causes of mood disorders —depending on how one chooses to look at the data. Associations have been reported between mood disturbances and several neurotransmitter systems, including levels of neurotransmitters themselves, receptors, enzymes involved in synthesis and metabolism, precursors, metabolites, and the activity of their second-messenger systems. Associations have also been reported with somatic illnesses and endocrine function, especially hypothyroidism. The most intriguing clues have come from the identification of drugs that are effective in treatment. The effectiveness of lithium, monoamine oxidase inhibitors, and tricyclic antidepressants suggests that the availability of neurotransmitters at nerve terminals could provide a mechanism for mood disorders. It has even been hoped that the mechanism might be as simple as having too little of a neurotransmitter such as serotonin. Through clinical association studies, most biological mechanisms that are at all plausible have received at least some empirical support. Unfortunately, few consistent associations have been found. Thus, although some of these hypotheses may prove to be true in some cases, no single mechanism has yet been found that will consistently explain the biological basis of even a small subset of mood disorders. Thus, at present there are no biological phenotypes that may safely be substituted for clinical phenotypes in genetic studies. It is humbling to acknowledge that we have so much to learn.

GENE MAPPING

The genes causing cystic fibrosis and Duchenne's muscular dystrophy were found using the gene mapping approach. In the gene mapping approach to determining genetic mechanisms, an attempt is made to find a gene, generally through genetic linkage studies, when the biological defect is unknown. Two genes are linked if they are located close together (a maximum of 50 million DNA base pairs apart, but usually much closer) on the same chromosome (Fig. 5). Linkage is detected by the association of genotypes at two gene loci either in families, in the general population, or in both (Fig. 6 and Table 3). The genes responsible for cystic fibrosis and Duchenne's muscular dystrophy were identified through their association with known genetic markers (e.g., genes with known locations). The markers can be selected merely for systematic coverage of the genome or can be "candidate genes" suggested because of biological associations with the illness. This approach is being applied in a number of studies of mood disorders.

In the past the limiting factor in gene mapping approaches to mood disorders was our inability to define specific human genotypes that could be used as genetic markers. Until a little over 15 years ago there were few genetic

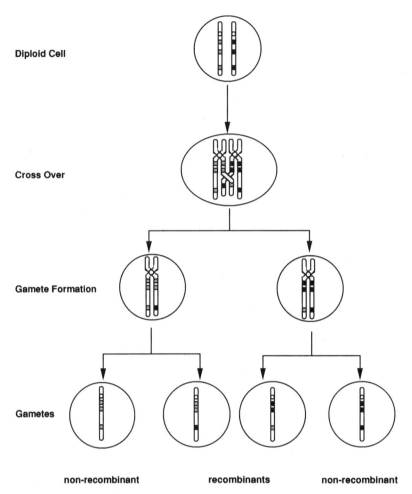

FIG. 5. Mendel pointed out that genes that determine different phenotypes usually segregate (divide and pass into gametes) independently, even though we now know there are perhaps 50,000–100,000 genes that are placed on only 23 pairs of chromosomes. Genes that lie on the same chromosome are usually passed on independently because of the process of genetic recombination; genetic material is exchanged between the parental chromosomes through physical crossovers that occur early in meiosis. The only exception to this rule is for genes that are physically very close to each other, within about 50 million DNA base pairs. Such deviations from independent assortment of genes into gametes provides a means of identifying the location of disease genes through their association with known genetic markers.

markers that could be used as reference points. Various proteins found in blood and saliva provided only about 50 such markers scattered over the 22 pairs of nonsex chromosomes (autosomes) and the sex chromosomes (X and Y).

Since the development of molecular cloning methods in the 1970s, there has been an exponential rise in the number of genetic markers that can be used in genotyping, in- cluding cloned genes, complementary DNAs synthesized from known polypeptide se- quences, and "anonymous" DNA fragments (segments of DNA isolated at random and without any known function). In general, genotyping for these markers depends on in- dividual differences in DNA sequence identi- fied as restriction fragment length polymor- phisms (RFLPs) (Fig. 7). RFLPs are inherited variations in DNA sequences that result in

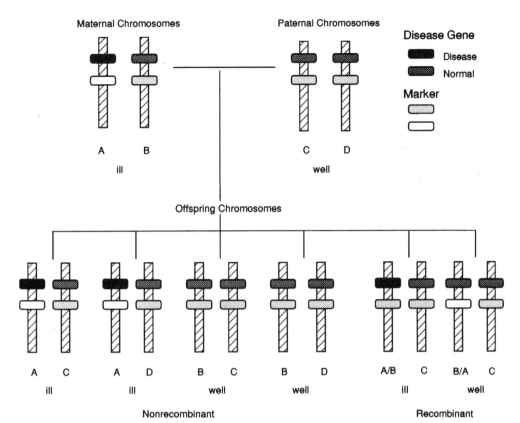

FIG. 6. Linkage between disease gene and marker. A mother carries one copy of a disease gene (black) that is located near a marker with known genotype (white). The mother's homologous chromosome carries a normal gene at the disease locus (dark shading) and a different marker genotype (light shading). The father is homozygous for both the normal "disease" gene and the lightly shaded marker genotype. The disease gene represented in black always appears with the marker genotype represented by white unless there has been a physical crossover. If the disease gene and marker are on different chromosomes or far apart (beyond 50×10^6 bp) on the same chromosome, then recombinants and nonrecombinants will occur with equal frequency. If the disease gene and marker are physically close together, then nonrecombinants will predominate. If the "marker" and the disease gene happened to be the same, then no recombinants would ever be observed. It is through these types of disease/marker associations that many genetic diseases have been located. Modeled in part after White and Lalouel, *Sci Am* 1988;258:40–48.

DNA fragments of different lengths when digested with site-specific enzymes known as restriction endonucleases. Now such markers number in the thousands. More important, several hundred markers are roughly evenly spaced over the whole genome, i.e., one or more known markers every few million base pairs of DNA sequence. Even newer sequence-based polymorphisms, e.g., individual variations in short sequence repeats (SSR) identi-

TABLE 3. *Requirements for gene mapping studies of mood disorders*

Requirement	Methodological approach
1. Prior clinical hypotheses	E.g., disease definitions
2. Clinical/biological homogeneity	Family subsets defined by childhood onset, comorbid disease associations, or biological markers
3. Model free quantitative methods	E.g., those using only affected family members
4. Need for replication	Nonreplication alone not evidence for genetic heterogeneity

A: Variation in Restriction Site

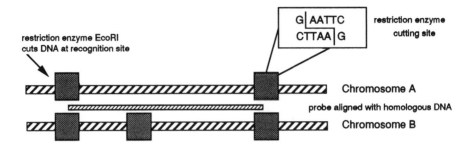

B: Variation in Repeated Sequences

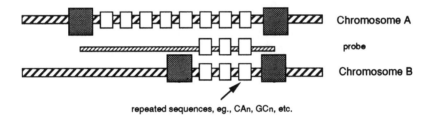

C: Identification of RFLP's

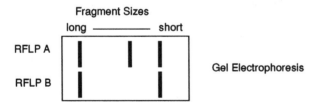

FIG. 7. Restriction fragment length polymorphisms (RFLPs) consist of inherited individual differences in DNA sequences that result when total genomic DNA is digested with a DNA sequence–specific restriction enzyme. Here the enzyme *Eco*RI recognizes the palindromic sequence GAATTC (for the bases guanine, adenine, thymine, and cytosine) and cuts each DNA strand between the G and A. **A:** All individuals have *Eco*RI sites flanking the region identified by a radioactively labeled probe with a homologous DNA sequence. However, individuals differ in having the central site. **B:** All individuals have the same flanking restriction sites but differ in the length of the intervening sequence due to the presence of varying numbers of tandemly repeated sequences. Some markers, called microsatellites, are sufficiently variable (e.g., in CAn, GCn, etc.) that polymorphisms may be identified by amplifying the specific region using the polymerase chain reaction (PCR). The differences or polymorphisms are identified by separating the resulting fragments according to size by gel electrophoresis. **C:** The polymorphisms described in A and B as they might appear on a gel, with RFLP A giving three bands and RFLP B giving two. Modeled in part after White and Lalouel, *Sci Am* 1988;258:40–48.

fied through the use of the polymerase chain reaction (PCR), now make many markers accessible to investigators without the necessity of maintaining separate clones. It is remarkable that only 7 years after the feasibility of constructing a human gene map was suggested in 1980, the first provisional map consisting of approximately 400 markers spanning roughly 95% of the human genome was completed.

Much work is now under way to achieve a high-resolution (about 1 million base pair marker separation) human gene map. As a part of the cooperative Human Genome Project, efforts have also been focused on developing a physical map of contiguous DNA segments and eventually determining the sequence of all 3×10^9 base pairs in the human genome. The goal set for the genome project is that it be completed by the year 2005. Regardless of whether the entire project is finished at that time, the increase in the amount of genetic information available within the next 10 to 15 years will be staggering. The subsequent availability of sequence information on all 50,000 to 100,000 human genes and their various regulatory sequences will revolutionize clinical and scientific work on human disease. During a time of extraordinarily rapid change truth may sound like hyperbole. The fact is that within the next few years all clinical and scientific practice in psychiatry will be fundamentally changed by genetic research.

MAPPING GENES FOR MOOD DISORDERS

Gene mapping approaches to mood disorders have become possible only within the last few years. These are exciting but also troubling times for clinical research on complex human diseases such as the mood disorders. The technology of molecular biology is appealing to researchers of mood disorders because the approach offers an allure of certainty to murky areas in which diseases are understood only in terms of their phenomenology, treatment is restricted to management of symptoms, and effective prevention is largely unknown. Genetics, particularly linkage and association studies, provides a means of bridging the gap between the clinical level (the observed phenotype) and the molecular level (the genetic cause) (Fig. 8). There has been a great deal of excitement about the potential of such studies and euphoria over initial results. But, after the first few years, failed studies and other apparently successful ones that have defied replication have produced something close to clinical depression in some researchers!

Linkage of bipolar disorder to an X chromosome marker (color blindness) was first reported more than 20 years ago. Other investigators in different parts of the world (e.g., Israel and Belgium) have been able to replicate these findings. However, only a few of the families that appear to have an X-linked pattern (e.g., have no father-son transmission) show a linkage between mood disorder and X-linked markers. Furthermore, some investigators who have examined many such families have been frustrated by finding no linkage to X markers. Finally, different researchers have reported linkages to RFLPs associated with two markers located on the distal long arm of the X chromosome (Blood Clotting Factor 9 and glucose-6-phosphate-dehydrogenase, G6PD), which are themselves unlinked!

About 10 years ago, there was another period of excitement over a report of linkage of bipolar disorder to the human major histocompatibility complex (MHC) system located in the middle short arm of chromosome 6. However, no other investigators have been able to present a convincing replication, and new data from the original investigators do not support the original finding.

Probably the most excitement generated by a linkage finding resulted from a report of linkage of bipolar disorder to RFLPs identified by genetic markers located on the distal short arm of chromosome 11. Some of the reasons for excitement appeared to be sound: the linkage was found in a population isolate having limited genetic variability and rela-

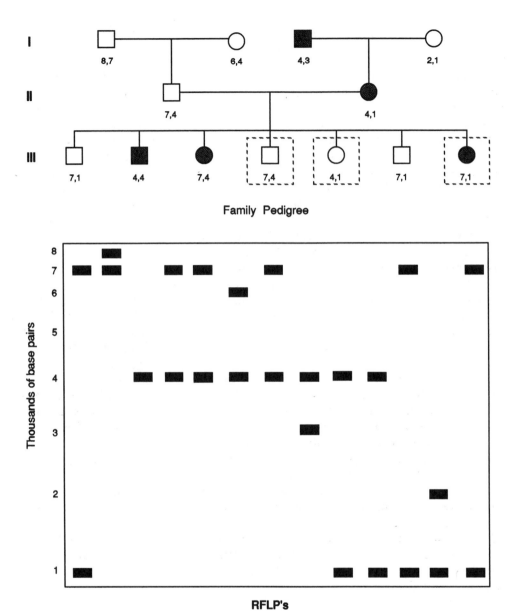

FIG. 8. Segregation of a disease phenotype with a genetic marker in a three-generation family. The dominantly expressed disease gene originates in the pedigree from the maternal grandfather in generation I, who has marker genotype 4,3. He passes on the disease gene along with the 4,000-bp (4-kb) marker polymorphism identified by gel electrophoresis. The mother in generation II passes on the disease and the 4-kb fragment to two of her children in generation III. The three generation III individuals outlined by the dashed line represent inconsistency in disease–marker associations that are commonly observed in complex diseases in general and in psychiatric disorders in particular. In one case (individual 4,1), the 4-kb polymorphism was inherited from the unaffected father in generation II, demonstrating that the marker is associated with but not completely linked to the disease in the population. Thus, the unaffected individual with marker genotype 4,1 presumably inherited the normal gene from the mother along with the 1-kb polymorphism. The affected offspring with marker genotype 7,1 could have been due to a recombination event that placed the disease with the 1-kb polymorphism of the mother; the disease could have arisen because of the presence of another gene or could be due to nongenetic causes. The unaffected offspring with genotype 7,4 could be accounted for by a recombination event in the mother placing the normal gene with the 4-kb polymorphism or could be a case of reduced gene penetrance, a well phenotype in a gene carrier. For mental illnesses reduced penetrance appears to be common and could be due to the offspring's genotype at other genetic loci (genetic interaction or epistasis) or to differences in environmental exposures.

tively few confounding factors such as alcoholism and drug abuse to complicate the mood disorder phenotype. However, the excitement appears to have been exaggerated by an unwarranted mystique associated with this first report of an apparent connection between mental illness and "DNA" as opposed to older types of genetic markers (apparently, even modern day scientists are susceptible to superstition!). As with the X and MHC linkages, several groups failed to replicate the original chromosome 11 report with other family data. Based on new data from the original population, the finding was withdrawn a little less than 4 years later.

OTHER PSYCHIATRIC ILLNESSES

Virtually all common forms of mental illness, including schizophrenia, anxiety disorders, and substance abuse disorders, run in families. Over the years, most of these illnesses have been examined in twin studies and a few in adoption studies. All appear to be influenced, at least in part, by genes, some substantially so. Schizophrenia, panic disorder, and alcoholism have received the most study. In addition to indicating genetic influence, studies of these disorders provide similar stories of frustrated searches for the causative genes. For example, specific candidate genes or gene locations have been proposed, disconfirmed, and withdrawn for schizophrenia, alcoholism, and panic disorder within the last few years.

COMPLEX INHERITANCE OF MENTAL ILLNESSES

The reasons for these initial difficulties in identifying genes for mood disorders and other forms of mental illness are understandable. Modern genetic approaches have worked only with relatively rare diseases that involve simple dichotomies (well vs. ill) and for which the mode of inheritance is well known (e.g., dominantly inherited, such as Huntington's disease). The mental disorders, on the other hand, are not simple clinically, biologically, or genetically.

Multiple possible disease boundaries separate disorders of mood from other psychiatric disorders. Standard phenotype definitions based on the clinical phenomenology have made it possible to understand the epidemiology of mood disorders (e.g., the estimation of population base rates). However, it seems unlikely that distinct genetic diseases can be found by focusing on clinical or biological phenomena that are common to all mood disorders. Clearly, other approaches are needed.

CONSTRUCTIVE USE OF GENETIC HETEROGENEITY

A shift of emphasis away from global explanations for mental illness may reduce the etiological complexity of these disorders. The understanding of the genetic basis of other complex, nonpsychiatric disorders has progressed in a very different way: by splitting common conditions like breast cancer or diabetes into subsets based on some clinical or biological characteristic shared by some but not all individuals afflicted with the disease. Using this approach, gene locations have recently been identified for early-onset familial breast cancer and for a non-insulin-dependent childhood form of diabetes (maturity onset diabetes of the young; MODY). The study of these complex disorders may provide a useful analogy for the mood disorders. For example, continuity of symptoms across all ill individuals in the areas of early breast tumors and glucose intolerance, respectively, helped researchers understand the epidemiology of breast cancer and diabetes (e.g., base rates for breast cancer and diabetes). However, clues about the genetic basis of these diseases were discovered only by focusing on individual patient differences that breed true in families.

It is possible that several etiologically distinct illnesses produce similar mood disturbances. High familial risk for bipolar and recurrent unipolar depression, particularly with early onset, suggests that there are genetic subforms of affective illness. Again, such a shift of emphasis away from global explanations (e.g., a single gene for all mood disorders) is an important step in reducing the etiological complexity of these disorders to manageable proportions, but many difficulties lie ahead.

THE FUTURE

Various methodological approaches will be important in the coming years. In an area where phenotype definitions are sometimes arbitrary, it is essential that disease boundaries be defined prior to the undertaking of genetic association and mapping studies. At least initially, it appears safest to take a "splitting" rather than a "lumping" approach to mental disease classification. Splitting will help us to identify homogeneous biological and genetic disease subtypes from among the mixed group of mentally ill people. Age of onset and biological associations may provide the clues for defining genetically meaningful subsets. Once a disease gene has been identified, it may be possible to lump some clinical subtypes together by studying the range of clinical expression in carriers of the same disease gene. Linkage methods that use only pairs of severely affected relatives require larger sample sizes than some other sampling designs. However, these "affected family member" approaches have the distinct advantage of being "model-free" in that they do not require assumptions about mode of inheritance. The mode(s) of inheritance of mood disorders are unknown (e.g., whether a phenotype results from dominant or recessive gene expression). However, such information on gene expression is irrelevant if only "ill" phenotypes are selected. Finally, failures to replicate results, like those reported in the recent psychiatric literature, may not be taken as an indication of genetic heterogeneity. Replication always has been essential in all areas of science, and genetic

mapping of psychiatric illnesses is no exception.

COUNSELING AND PREVENTION

The prospect of genetic counseling and the prevention of psychiatric illness may bring both hope and foreboding. *There is hope that we can soon understand the genetic bases of mood disorders well enough to predict who is vulnerable and effectively prevent or treat disease by focusing only on those individuals.* The acquisition of any new knowledge or power is always accompanied by a sense of uneasiness until enough experience has been amassed to ensure its proper utilization. Ideally, approaches will be found that minimize human suffering without limiting human diversity or individual acceptance. At present, geneticists have little of immediate tangible value to offer to families—only impersonal relative risk figures (e.g., those in Table 2 and Fig. 1). In the future, the new tools of genetics should allow us to offer much more in the way of information, prevention, and clinical care.

SUMMARY

Mental illnesses are made up of genetically distinct but clinically overlapping disorders. Genetic mechanisms probably determine the distinctive form of these disorders as well as their interrelationships. The three major classes of heritable mental disorders are: mood disorders (depression and mania), anxiety disorders (panic, phobic, and obsessive-compulsive), and psychotic disorders (schizophrenia). Genetic approaches to mental illness usually require the establishment of reliable phenotype definitions, familial aggregation, genetic involvement, mode of inheritance, biological associations, markers for genetic heterogeneity, and gene identification through gene mapping or biological studies.

Some reliability in phenotype definitions for mental illnesses has been achieved in recent years, and most mental illnesses have been found to aggregate in families. However, there are no consistent biological associations, and no specific genes have been identified for mental illness. Genes are likely to be identified in the near future through molecular genetic and gene mapping studies. The identification of the genes should improve our ability to predict, treat, and at times even prevent the occurrence of mental illness.

BIBLIOGRAPHY

Original Articles

Andreasen NC, Rice J, Endicott J, Coryell W, Grove WM, Reich T. Familial rates of affective disorder. *Arch Gen Psychiatry* 1987;44:461–469.

Botstein D, White RL, Skolnick M, Davis RW. Construction of a genetic linkage map in man using restriction fragment length polymorphisms. *Am J Hum Genet* 1980;32:314–331.

Kelsoe JR, Ginns EI, Egeland JA, Gerhard DS, Goldstein AM, Bale SJ, et al. Re-evaluation of the linkage relationship between chromosome 11p loci and the gene for bipolar affective disorder in the Old Order Amish. *Nature* 1989;342:238–243.

McGuffin P, Sargeant M, Hetti G, Tidmarsh S, Whatley S, Marchbanks RM. Exclusion of a schizophrenia susceptibility gene from the chromosome 5q11–q13 region: new data and a reanalysis of previous reports. *Am J Hum Genet* 1990;47:524–535.

Regier DA, Boyd JH, Burke JD Jr, Rae DS, Meyers JK, Kramer M, et al. One-month prevalence of mental disorders in the United States. *Arch Gen Psychiatry* 1988;45:977–986.

Weissman MM, Leaf PJ, Tischler GL, Blazer DG, Karno M, Bruce ML, et al. Affective disorders in five United States communities. *Psychol Med* 1988;18:141–153.

Books and Reviews

Gottesman IL II. *Schizophrenia: the epigenetic puzzle.* Cambridge, UK: Cambridge University Press; 1982.

Plomin R, DeFries J, McClearn G. *Behavioral genetics: a primer.* 2nd Ed. San Francisco: WH Freeman; 1989.

Suzuki K. Molecular genetic approaches to inherited neurological degenerative disorders. In: Siegel GJ, Agranoff BW, Alpers RW, Molinoff PB, eds. *Basic neurochemistry,* 5th ed. New York: Raven Press; 1994 (in press).

Tsuaung MT, Faraone SV. *The genetics of mood disorders.* Baltimore: Johns Hopkins University Press; 1990.

Watson JD, Gilman M, Witkowski J, Zoller M. *Recombinant DNA.* 2nd Ed. Second Edition), San Francisco: WH Freeman; 1990.

White R, Lalouel J-M. Chromosome mapping with DNA markers. *Sci Am* 1988;258:40–48.

17

Mood Disorders

Mark S. Bauer and Alan Frazer

All his life he suffered spells of depression, sinking into the brooding depths of melancholia, an emotional state which, though little understood, resembles the passing sadness of the normal man as a malignancy resembles a canker sore.

William Manchester,
The Last Lion, Winston Spencer Churchill, Vol. I: *Visions of Glory*
(New York: Little, Brown and Company, 1989, p. 23)

- Mood disorders are distinct from normal variations in mood.

- Phenomenology provides the cornerstone for the classification of mood disorders.

- In bipolar disorder, persons with depression also experience episodes of mania or hypomania.

- Dysthymia and cyclothymia are less severe forms of mood disorder.

- Mood disorders are common and tend to recur.

- Mood disorders are serious illnesses.

- New drug development is a time-consuming and highly regulated process.

- Three classes of antidepressant drugs are currently marketed: tricyclic antidepressants (TCAs), monamine oxidase inhibitors (MAOIs), and second-generation or atypical antidepressants.

- Antidepressants most probably act by affecting central noradrenergic and/or serotonergic neurotransmission.

- The mainstay of treatment for acute manic or hypomanic episodes is lithium.

- Substantial interest has arisen in the use of certain anticonvulsants in bipolar disorder.

- Two sets of models have been used in the attempt to understand the mechanisms that underlie mood disorders: the psychological model and the biomedical model.

The first sections of this chapter summarize what is known about mood disorders from a descriptive, or phenomenological, vantage point. The latter sections review psychopharmacological treatments of these disorders. The chapter concludes with a discussion of conceptual issues pertaining to the mood disorders.

The recognition of certain moods, or feeling states, as distinctly abnormal is as old as recorded history. The cause of such nonnormal moods has been variously ascribed to spiritual, moral, cultural, and biological factors. Two eras have had a particular influence on our current views of mood disorders: the late nineteenth century and the 1950–1960s. The late nineteenth century saw the development of systematic observation of persons with disordered feelings and behavior, focusing on the characteristics and course of their pathology. These descriptive methods constitute the core of our current approach to mood disorders. They also laid the groundwork for the seminal observations in the 1950–1960s that certain chemical compounds could normalize mood and behavior in depressed and manic individuals.

Among the most important psychiatric researchers in the nineteenth century were Sigmund Freud and the German psychiatrist Emil Kraepelin. Freud, though better known for his development of psychoanalytic theory and technique for the treatment of the neuroses, wrote one of the early landmark works in the classification of mood disorders. In *Mourning and Melancholia* Freud clearly differentiated depression from grieving. Although sadness was a prominent feature of both depression and mourning, the former was characterized by a pervasive loss of self-esteem, whereas in the latter a sense of loss of something outside the self was central. Freud

emphasized the distinctly different quality of depressed mood in melancholia.

Kraepelin studied patients with severe, recurrent, debilitating psychiatric illnesses. At this time scientific psychiatry was in its infancy and little had been done even to describe the clinical features of such patients beyond labeling them insane. Kraepelin's major contribution was to separate such severely ill patients on the basis of progression of the illness (natural history). He showed that patients with mood disorders, which he grouped together as "manic-depressive insanity," did much better in the long run than patients with schizophrenia, which he called "dementia praecox" to emphasize its early onset (praecox) and the inevitable global decline in function (dementia). Thus Freud and Kraepelin provided two core observations that have remained valid up to the present day: (1) mood disorders are characterized by a distinct, nonnormal subjective experience, and (2) psychiatric illnesses, including mood disorders, run their course in a specific manner and in this way are similar to "medical" illnesses.

In the 1950s, several clinical scientists made the remarkable observation that depressed persons treated with drugs affecting brain monoamines improved in mood. In addition, disparate symptoms including changes in mood, appetite, sleep, ability to concentrate, and general energy level improved concurrently. It was proposed that such varied symptoms form a distinct syndrome and that this syndrome was due to abnormalities of brain monoamine systems.

The study of mood disorders has progressed parallel with that of other medical ill-

Biological Bases of Brain Function and Disease, edited by Alan Frazer, Perry B. Molinoff, and Andrew Winokur. Raven Press, Ltd., New York © 1994.

nesses: the delineation of the syndromes proceeds by the gathering of clinical observations, description of the natural history of the illness, and response to treatment. Though the study of behavioral pathology is admittedly more complex than the study of pathology in isolated organ systems, and though the knowledge base for mood disorders and other psychiatric syndromes lags behind that for other biomedical fields, the data summarized below suggest that the mysteries of the neural basis of mood disorders will continue to yield to careful clinical and laboratory research.

DIAGNOSIS

Mood disorders are distinct from normal variations in mood. The classification of mood disorders is best conceptualized in terms of episodes and disorders. *Episodes* denote discrete periods of time of altered function. Usually episodes are time-limited, i.e.,

they have a definitive onset and termination. Onset may be abrupt and clear or slow and insidious. Some episodes do not clearly resolve but rather go on to become chronic conditions. Nevertheless, once an affective, or mood, episode is identified (e.g., depression, mania, hypomania), the person is considered to have, or have had, a mood disorder. The pattern and type of episodes over time determine the *type of disorder.* There are four main mood disorders. Major depressive disorder (single episode or recurrent) and bipolar disorder are sometimes called "major" mood, or affective, disorders. Dysthymia and cyclothymia are sometimes called "minor" disorders (Fig. 1).

Phenomenology provides the cornerstone for the classification of mood disorders. In its psychiatric usage, phenomenology refers to the study of how patients act and feel. Observations of patients by clinicians (signs) and reports of the patients' subjective experience (symptoms) provide the core data for de-

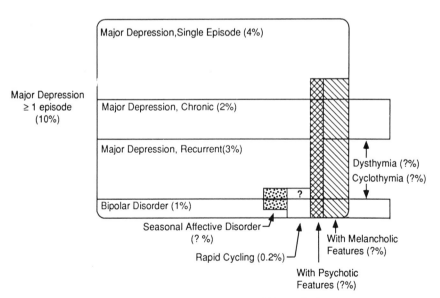

FIG. 1. Distribution of mood disorders in the population. While all of us have been sad or "blue" at times, a significant proportion (1 in 10) will have an episode of major depression. Of those, 40% will have no further episodes, but 50% will go on to a chronic or recurrent course. Another 10% (1% of the total population) will develop manic or hypomanic episodes and be diagnosed with bipolar disorder. Each category of mood disorder may have several subtypes as indicated.

scriptive psychiatry. This approach to psychiatric diagnosis was not widely accepted, at least not in the United States, until the 1970s. Prior to that time, many theoretic schemata, biological and psychological in origin, provided competing approaches to psychiatric illnesses including mood disorders.

The move toward codified description as the cornerstone of psychiatric diagnosis began in the early 1970s with the publication of the Feighner (also called the St. Louis or Washington University) Criteria, which listed explicit rules for making psychiatric diagnoses based on signs and symptoms. The Research Diagnostic Criteria (or RDC), similar in approach and content to the Feighner Criteria, subsequently gained widespread acceptance in research settings. The RDC system had the added advantage of an accompanying structured interview that facilitated uniform data collection.

With the publication by the American Psychiatric Association in the early 1980s of the *Diagnostic and Statistical Manual of Mental Disorders,* Third Edition (DSM-III) and its more recent revision (DSM-III-R), the phenomenological approach to psychiatric disorders became widely accepted in clinical practice. In similar fashion to the RDC, a structured interview was recently developed for making DSM-III-R diagnoses. On the international scene, diagnostic criteria similar to those of DSM-III have been incorporated into the International Classification of Diseases (currently ICD-10). As the knowledge base expands, criteria for the DSM and ICD classifications are being updated, with DSM-IV to be issued shortly after publication of this text.

The current DSM-III-R criteria for major depression, the most common mood disorder, are summarized in Table 1. Two aspects of this classification deserve emphasis. First, a depressive episode represents a distinct, enduring decrement from normal mood and function; it is more than a transient dysphoric (unhappy) feeling, much as Freud pointed out almost a century ago. What is not effectively reflected in the phe-nomenological description of depression is the reality of the painful despair of a depressive episode. The gnawing emptiness experienced by depressed persons is made even more acute by the sense of pervasive hopelessness that makes the world seem bleak and their suffering interminable (see epigraph).

Second, while there is allowance for variability in the clinical picture of a depressive episode from person to person, multiple symptoms must be present. These symptoms and signs reflect changes in function on several fronts that may not at first glance seem related. Thus, depression may involve changes in mood, activity level, weight, and cognition, though the picture may be somewhat different for each person. One of the major contributions of psychopharmacological research in the 1960s was to provide convincing evidence that these functions were indeed linked in a common syndrome of depression, as these functions all improved with successful drug treatment of depression. The fascinating interplay of mood, cognition, and drive during depression has been the focus of substantial basic and clinical research by neurobiologists, psychiatrists, and psychologists.

TABLE 1. *Key features of major depressive episode*

Episode characteristics
  Must represent a distinct change from previous level of function and must be present for at least 2 weeks
  Not due to organic (physical) cause, normal grief reaction
  Not superimposed on certain psychotic disorders (e.g., schizophrenia)
Specific symptoms
  Must include either pervasive depressed mood or pervasive loss of ability to experience pleasure or interest in other things
  Must include at least five of the following:
    depressed mood
    loss of pleasure or interest
    weight change
    sleep disturbance
    fatigue or loss of energy
    psychomotor agitation or retardation
    feelings of worthlessness or guilt
    diminished concentration
    recurrent thoughts of death or suicide

Adapted from DSM-III-R.

In bipolar disorder, persons with depression also experience episodes of mania or hypomania. Some persons who experience a depressive episode also experience mania or its milder form, hypomania. These persons by definition have bipolar disorder, formerly known as manic-depressive disorder (Fig. 1). Classically, mania has been thought to be the opposite of depression in terms of mood: manics are often cheery, optimistic, self-confident, and energetic (see Table 2). However, recent research, which also has its roots in the original, careful observations of Kraepelin, indicates that manics may also be subjectively uncomfortable or irritable in mood. The core symptoms of mania, including increased speed of thoughts, increased drive to be active, increased energy, and decreased need for sleep, seem to have more to do with activity and energy than with mood.

Whether euphoric or dysphoric during a manic episode, such persons often get involved in dangerous or costly social situations. Irresponsible spending sprees, sexual encounters, and social commitments frequently lead to interpersonal and even legal difficulties. Substance abuse, and subsequently dependence, are frequent complications of all mood disorders, and bipolar disorder in particular. In its most florid form, mania can involve psychotic features (defined later in this section) and can be indistinguishable from a psychotic episode in schizophrenia. Hypomania is a milder form of mania, with fewer and less severe symptoms and without major social impairment. Nevertheless, the core symptoms of heightened activation and euphoric or irritable mood are similar. Judgment may still be impaired although to a lesser degree.

It has often been said that "a little bit of hypomania is good for you," since such persons can often be very self-confident, energetic, and productive. Some evidence does indicate that bipolar disorder occurs disproportionately in creative persons. There are accounts, supported by variable amounts of documentation, that a number of famous persons throughout history and on the contemporary political and cultural scene have had bipolar disorder. While there undoubtedly are valid aspects to this perspective, one must not lose sight of the fact that depressive and manic episodes are disruptive, debilitating, and often painful in both their experience and their consequences. To call bipolar disorder "the genius disease," as was recently done in a popular magazine, is to trivialize the very real suffering experienced by persons with the disorder, including the famous.

Dysthymia and cyclothymia are less severe forms of mood disorder. Some persons do not experience full-blown depressive or manic episodes, yet are impaired subjectively and often objectively by disordered mood. Dysthymic disorder is characterized by chronic, mild to moderate dysphoria. In a similar manner, persons with cyclothymia have a persistent pattern of mood instability, fluctuating from mild depressive symptoms to scattered manic symptoms or even hypomania over the course of several days.

Much less is known about these disorders, particularly cyclothymia, for at least two reasons. First, such persons come to caregivers (and researchers) less often than do persons with major mood disorders since they are usually less impaired by their symptoms. Second, the boundaries with normal mood variability are less distinct, so that it is more diffi-

TABLE 2. *Key features of mania*

Episode characteristics
  Must cause marked impairment in social role
  Not due to organic (physical) cause
  Not superimposed on certain psychotic disorders
    (e.g., schizophrenia)
Specific symptoms
  Must include abnormally elevated, expansive, or
    irritable mood
  Must include at least three (four if mood is irritable)
    of the following:
      inflated self-esteem
      decreased need for sleep
      increased rate and amount of speech
      racing thoughts
      distractibility
      increased goal-directed activity
      excessive involvement in pleasurable activities
        with high probability of painful consequences

Adapted from DSM-III-R.

cult to separate cyclothymics or dysthymics from normals. Nevertheless, family studies and studies of the natural history of the major mood disorders indicate that dysthymia and cyclothymia are closely related to the major mood disorders.

A variety of descriptors have been used to categorize mood disorders. While descriptive classification systems often appear etched in stone, they are in reality constantly evolving. The nosology, or categorization schemata, will continue to evolve until a series of unequivocal laboratory tests can identify separate or common pathophysiological mechanisms underlying the various mood disorders. This is what eventually happened in the study of syphilis, when the discovery of *Treponema pallidum* allowed codification of its diverse and confusing signs and symptoms into a single disease. Until such tests exist, we will be dependent on an imperfect nosological system.

Clear similarities exist between mood disorders and several other psychiatric illnesses. For instance, anxiety and panic symptoms can occur in depression as well as in the anxiety disorders. Persons can become psychotic, i.e., experience hallucinations or delusions, during many physical illnesses and during psychiatric illnesses such as schizophrenia. Similarly, depression can accompany various medical and psychiatric illnesses. Despite these complexities, however, accumulated evidence from the natural history of mood disorders, from their tendency to run in families, and from their specific treatment responses indicates that the mood disorders form a discrete group of syndromes.

Over the history of the study of mood disorders, various labels have been used to specify subtypes of depression. This is of more than historical interest, as many of these labels are used in different contexts today. Some labels describe areas of current research, while others are archaic holdovers best consigned to the scrapbook of psychiatric history. In the 1960s, several pairs of terms were used by various groups of researchers to dichotomize depression. These included *endogenous/reactive, endogenous/neurotic,* and *neurotic/psychotic.* The first pair was used to separate persons whose depressive episodes appeared to be stress-induced (reactive) from those for whom no stressor could be identified (and therefore presumably internally driven, or endogenous). The second pair was developed at about the same time to separate antidepressant-responsive (endogenous) from nonresponsive (neurotic) patients; the latter group appeared more frequently to have personality difficulties that were understood in terms of intrapsychic conflicts. The third pair, again contemporaneous in development, merely meant mild vs. severe.

Since that time, the terms *endogenous, melancholic,* and even *endogenomorphic* have evolved to denote those depressive episodes characterized by prominent "vegetative" symptoms and signs, including disruptions in appetite, sleep–wake cycle, and psychomotor activity, as well as a profound loss in reactivity of mood (in this context, reactivity refers to the ability of the depressed person to respond to pleasurable stimuli with a lightening of mood, as opposed to whether or not the episode itself is stress-induced). The term *neurosis* is still in use as an alternative to the term *dysthymia* (i.e., depressive neurosis), although it is unclear whether this terminology will be retained in further revisions of the DSM. Neurosis is still best understood when limited to its strict formulation as a descriptor of intrapsychic conflicts within the field of psychoanalysis.

Several distinctions are currently widely used, though not formally incorporated into DSM-III-R schemata. The *primary/secondary* distinction refers to whether an episode of depression occurs as a person's first psychiatric syndrome, or whether it is superimposed on another preexisting disorder, such as schizophrenia. A current area of active research focuses on whether *atypical* depression is separable as a distinct syndrome. Though without a really informative name, atypical depression, first described in the 1970s by the American psychiatrist Donald

Klein, is distinctive in its constellation of symptoms. Persons with atypical depressive episodes tend to sleep more, overeat, crave carbohydrates, and have a daily mood pattern that deteriorates in the evening. This is in contrast to persons afflicted with more *typical* depression, characterized by disrupted sleep, loss of appetite and weight, and heightened severity in the mornings with some mood lightening as the day goes on.

One often sees a distinction made between *bipolar* and *unipolar* depression. As outlined above, a person is considered to have bipolar disorder if he or she has an episode of mania or hypomania as well as depression; otherwise, the person is considered to have unipolar depression. However, it should be noted that the depressive episodes have a similar symptom profile in both unipolar and bipolar illness. Within bipolar disorder, an additional distinction is often made between *bipolar I* and *bipolar II*. This distinction is based on whether a person experiences full-blown mania (I) or the less severe syndrome of hypomania (II). While descriptively useful, it is not clear to what extent these two variants represent fundamentally different forms of bipolar disorder.

The terms *mixed* and *rapid cycling* are sometimes used as descriptors of episodes during bipolar disorder. Mixed episodes are characterized by the co-occurrence of prominent depressive symptoms during mania or hypomania. Rapid cycling refers to frequent, sometimes temporally linked, episodes of mania or hypomania and depression. Both mixed and rapid cycling patterns of bipolar disorder are receiving increasing attention, since they are often refractory to, and may in some cases even be caused by, standard therapies used to treat bipolar disorder.

Several modifiers have been incorporated into DSM-III-R for the description of mood disorders. These include *psychotic, melancholic,* and *seasonal* depression. Psychotic depression is defined by the presence of delusions or hallucinations during an episode of depression. Clearly, only the more severe episodes are characterized by psychosis. There is some evidence that psychotic depressions

will "breed true," that is, persons who have had an episode of psychotic depression will have psychotic symptoms in subsequent episodes. Psychotic symptoms can also occur in mania, as noted above, although the majority of persons with mania do not become psychotic. Melancholic depression refers to the endogenous subtype. Although various criteria based on symptom pattern have evolved from different research centers for the definition of melancholic/endogenous depressive episode, there is in general good agreement between schemata. Seasonal depression is a relatively recently described phenomenon, referring to depressive episodes that occur at the same time every year, usually in winter. This category is of increasing interest to researchers and clinicians alike, since recent studies have provided evidence that seasonal depression may respond to treatment with high-intensity light. However, it is not clear at present whether seasonal depression represents a distinct mood syndrome. For instance, it is not yet known whether such patients respond better to light therapy than to standard antidepressant treatment, or to what extent nonseasonal depression responds to light treatment. To complicate matters further, seasonality may also be a population trait, similar to height, weight, or eye color. There is evidence that prominent seasonal variations in energy, sleep, appetite, and mood may occur in a sizable percentage of persons, though without leading to clinical impairment.

NATURAL HISTORY

Mood disorders are common and tend to recur. Natural history refers to the evolution of a disease process over time. The patterns of age at onset of depression and bipolar disorder differ somewhat. While both can occur before puberty and have increased rates of onset around menarche or pubescence, the peak age of onset for unipolar depression is the mid to late 30s. In contrast, the peak age of onset for bipolar disorder is the early 20s, with a second, smaller peak for women in the 40s.

Approximately 10% to 30% of loss events (e.g., death of a loved one) are followed by a depressive episode. Conversely, many studies indicate that depressive episodes are stress-associated, and it has been hypothesized that such episodes may be stress-induced. However, methodological difficulties with these studies render much of the data inconclusive. What does seem clear, however, is that stress is associated with onset or worsening of many other psychiatric disorders (e.g., mania, schizophrenia) and medical illnesses (e.g., rheumatoid arthritis, hyperthyroidism). The relationship between stress and depression is therefore not specific. Further, it is important to note that, contrary to intuition, stress-associated depressive episodes respond to pharmacotherapy as well as do other episodes. It appears that the pathological process is the same, whether stress-induced or spontaneous.

What happens to persons who are depressed? Forty percent recover without further problems. An additional 30% recover but go on to experience at least one recurrence. Thirty-three percent of persons fully recovered from a depressive episode will relapse within a year; this figure doubles for persons whose major depressive episode is superimposed on dysthymia. Twenty percent of depressive episodes become chronic. Thus unipolar depression is cured without further problems in fewer than half the individuals initially diagnosed as having unipolar depression.

Bipolar disorder is by definition recurrent, with an average of seven to nine episodes over the course of a lifetime. In rapid cycling, which affects 15% to 20% of persons with bipolar disorder, more than four episodes per year and more than 50 episodes over the course of the illness are the rule.

EPIDEMIOLOGY

Mood disorders are common. Epidemiology is the study of patterns of disease occurrence in large populations. Its tools include survey techniques and sophisticated statisti-

cal analyses of complex datasets. While in-depth interviews by clinicians cannot be used in such large studies, well-validated structured interviews have been developed to ensure accurate diagnostic information. Because of their large-sample survey approach, epidemiological studies yield information not otherwise available about the pattern of occurrence of mood disorders. The most important information gained from epidemiological studies is that mood disorders are common throughout the world. In fact, symptoms of depression are remarkably consistent in transcultural studies of mood disorders across the continents of North America, Europe, Asia, and Africa. Particularly detailed information is available on the occurrence and clinical picture of mood disorders in the United States. Five to fourteen percent of American women will have an episode of major depression at some time in their lives, as will 2% to 4% of American males. Bipolar disorder affects 1% of the population. While major depressive episodes are twice as common in women as in men, bipolar disorder is evenly distributed across the sexes. There are no racial or social class differences in the occurrence of depression, and no racial differences in the distribution of bipolar disorder. Interestingly, bipolar disorder is more common in the upper socioeconomic classes, for reasons that are not yet clear. Several theories have been advanced to explain this "upward drift"; for example, certain aspects of bipolar disorder, such as the optimism, increased energy, and productivity seen in mild hypomania, may provide some competitive advantage in modern society. While there is some evidence for a tendency to underdiagnose bipolar disorder and to overdiagnose more severe disorders such as schizophrenia among the lower socioeconomic classes, this artifact alone cannot account for the upward drift of bipolar disorder.

Two recent sets of epidemiological observations have major public health implications. First, rates of depression have increased significantly over the course of the twentieth century, a trend that cannot be accounted for simply by increased awareness of the mood disorders. Second, as we study more carefully the deprived populations of the United States, such as inner-city youth, rates of depression as high as 15% are found —much higher than might be expected from the above figures. If indeed mood disorders are becoming more prevalent, we as a society will have to deal with tremendous costs due to increases in the attendant morbidity and mortality.

MORTALITY AND MORBIDITY

Mood disorders are serious illnesses. The risk of suicide in mood disorders is well recognized, and rightly so. Fifteen percent of persons with untreated depression die from suicide, and at least 50% of the 25,000 to 100,000 suicides per year in the United States occur during an episode of depression. Thus, well over 12,000 deaths per year can be attributed to depression. Many more suicides, reported as accidents, go unrecognized. No reliable figures are available for mortality associated with mania, although one would expect that suicide, accidents, and even death by homicide are common.

No age is exempt from the risk of suicide: 200 children *under 14 years of age* die by suicide each year in the United States. Suicide rates are highest in males in their early 20s, with a rate of 28 deaths by suicide per 100,000 persons in the population. There are some differences in suicide patterns across the sexes, with women three times as likely to attempt suicide, but males twice as likely to die from their attempts. Whether these disparities reflect differences in psychosocial factors (e.g., leading women to choose less lethal methods), differences in severity of depression, or differences in independent factors that augment the risk of each attempt (e.g., concurrent intoxication in men) is not clear. Nevertheless, mood disorders are clearly potentially fatal if not treated effectively.

Substantial, though underrecognized, morbidity is associated with mood disorders. A recent study by the Rand Corporation of over 11,000 persons attending general medical clinics showed that persons with major depression, and even persons with only scattered depressive symptoms, have significant decrements in their physical activities, functioning on their jobs, and social activities compared to nondepressed persons. Even though mood disorders are not usually considered physical illnesses, persons with major depression or depressive symptoms actually spend significantly more days in bed than controls. Equally impressive, persons with such mood pathology have levels of function on those indices mentioned above comparable to or worse than those of patients with several major medical disorders, including hypertension, diabetes, chronic lung disease, and arthritis. Only heart disease is equal to depression in terms of severity of decrements in work and social function, activity level, and days in bed. Clearly, mood disorders take their place beside these chronic medical conditions as major public health problems.

PSYCHOPHARMACOLOGICAL TREATMENT OF MOOD DISORDERS

New drug development is a time-consuming and highly regulated process. Before discussing specifically the drugs used to treat depression and mania, it would be useful to outline both the procedures involved in bringing any new drug to market and appropriate controlled conditions for conducting clinical studies of the effectiveness (or efficacy) of any drug.

Preclinical procedures or "screens" have been developed that detect the potential therapeutic efficacy of compounds, and newly developed compounds are evaluated initially in such tests. These screens may involve either behavioral testing in animals (e.g., "conflict tests" to detect anxiolytic activity) or tests conducted in vitro (i.e., in test tubes) using, for example, tissue samples obtained from an animal (e.g., radioligand binding tests to determine potency of compounds at receptors).

If a compound yields promising results in such "screens," its effects are then measured on all of the major organ systems of laboratory animals. Such studies are designed to detect any toxic effects of the compound. In addition, possible effects of the compound on the offspring of pregnant animals are studied to determine if the compound has teratogenic effects (i.e., causes fetal malformations).

If the compound passes such toxicity testing, it may then enter clinical evaluation. Clinical studies are carried out in sequential steps referred to as phase I, phase II, and phase III studies. Normal human volunteers are used in phase I studies in which factors such as the absorption and metabolism of the drug, dosage range, side effects, and toxicity are evaluated. If the drug is found to be safe in such studies, it then moves on to phase II trials. The purpose of phase II testing is to evaluate, in a limited number of patients, the efficacy of the drug in the condition for which it was developed under both noncontrolled and controlled conditions and an appropriate dosage range. If the compound continues to show promise during phase II trials, it then enters the final phase (III) where it is tested only under controlled conditions in a large number of patients; this enables both efficacy and safety to be evaluated in a large patient population.

If the safety and efficacy of the drug have been clearly established during phase III, the pharmaceutical company that developed the drug submits a report of all of its findings (both preclinical and clinical) to the Food and Drug Administration (FDA). The FDA has the responsibility to evaluate these data and to approve for clinical use only those drugs it considers both safe and effective. The FDA review is very thorough and, consequently, is usually very time consuming. Indeed, it is now estimated that it often takes 10 to 12 years from the time a compound is initially detected preclinically as having therapeutic potential until it is approved by the FDA as a marketable drug. Also, pharmaceutical companies estimate the cost of drug development as $200–250 million per new drug. This figure highlights an increasingly serious problem in drug development. Because costs are so high, the emphasis is on developing new drugs for common illnesses so that the volume of sales may be high. Drugs for serious but less common illnesses may become neglected in new drug development unless some mechanism is found to make it profitable for the pharmaceutical industry to develop such drugs, termed "orphan drugs."

As indicated above, there are several types of clinical studies. It is now a standard requirement for all such studies to obtain "informed consent" from all subjects prior to their inclusion in a study. This means that all aspects of the study are explained to the potential participant in lay language, including procedures to be done, drugs to be used, and, importantly, risks and side effects involved. In this process, no implicit or explicit pressure is to be placed on the subject to gain his or her consent. It is also now common practice to randomly distribute appropriate patients in the various treatment categories. Randomization is done to try to ensure that the characteristics of the patients (i.e., age, gender, severity of illness, etc.) are similar in all treatment groups.

To properly determine the efficacy of any drug, it is necessary to control the experimental conditions under which the study is carried out. Different types of standard "controlled" conditions are now in use. A study in which the patients do not know the identity of the drug they are receiving, but the physician does, is termed a *single-blind* study. There is less of a chance for bias if both patient and physician do not know the particular treatment being administered. In this type of study, termed *double-blind,* the different drugs (or placebo) being used are dispensed in a form that is identical in appearance for all drugs. The use of a placebo is a very important issue, particularly in psychopharmacology. A placebo is an inactive substance (e.g., a sugar tablet) or preparation given to satisfy the patient's symbolic need for drug therapy. If possible, it should be formulated to cause some of the side effects of the drug(s) being studied. The use of a placebo in controlled trials is necessary as it has been observed that some patients will respond to the administration of placebo as though given an active pharmacological agent. This may be due in part to the patient's having "expectations" about the drug he or she is to receive or the conditions under which the placebo is administered. A placebo can have marked effects in certain psychiatric illnesses, e.g., depression and anxiety, but usually has much less pronounced effects in other disorders, e.g., mania and obsessive-compulsive disorder. For those conditions in which placebo effects are prominent, it is especially important to compare the effects of the test drug(s) with those of a placebo in order to obtain a true estimate of the efficacy of the active medication(s).

Antidepressant Drugs

Three classes of antidepressant drugs are currently marketed. The most widely prescribed drugs are termed *tricyclic antidepressants (TCAs)* because of their chemical structure (Fig. 2). About the same time that TCAs

were developed, another class of drugs, referred to as *monoamine oxidase inhibitors (MAOIs),* was also found to have efficacy in the treatment of depression. These two classes of drugs have been referred to as "first-generation" or "typical" antidepressants. More recently, a third group of antidepressants has been developed that is heterogeneous with reference to the drugs' chemical structures and pharmacological effects; these drugs are called *"second-generation" or "atypical" antidepressants.*

Tricyclic Antidepressants

Chemistry

The structures of these compounds are shown in Fig. 2. They all have similar, but not identical, three-joined-ring structures—two benzene rings attached to a central seven-membered ring—which is why they are termed tricyclic antidepressants (TCAs). An amine-containing side chain is attached to the central ring. Those TCAs that contain non–hydrogen atom substituents on the nitrogen of the side chain are called tertiary amine tricyclics (amitriptyline, doxepin,

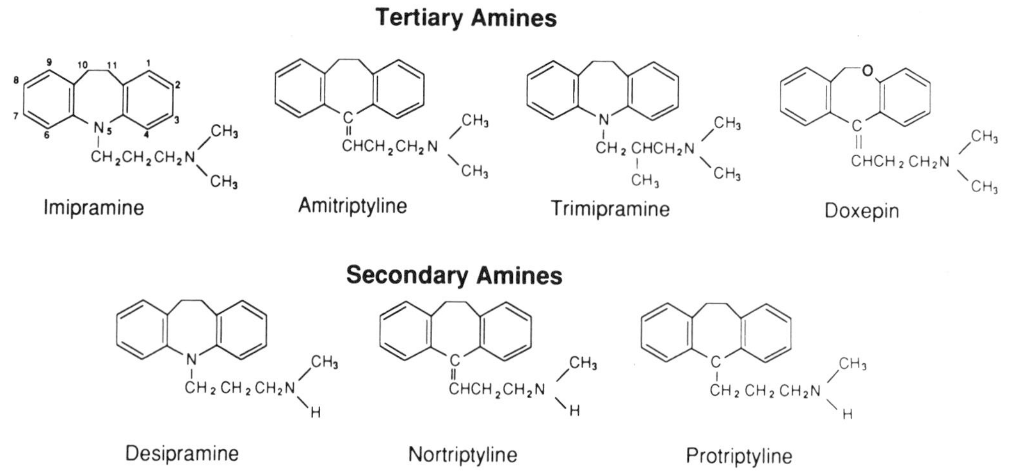

FIG. 2. Structures of various tricyclic antidepressants. Although these drugs have different ring structures, collectively they are termed tricyclic compounds because they all have three (tri) rings (cyclic).

imipramine, and trimipramine). Desipramine (also called desmethylimipramine), nortriptyline, and protriptyline have two non–hydrogen atom substituents attached to the side chain nitrogen and are referred to as secondary amine tricyclics. A major pathway for the metabolism of the tertiary amine tricyclics is their demethylation to the corresponding secondary amine. For example, imipramine is demethylated to desipramine and amitriptyline is metabolized to nortriptyline by liver enzymes. This means that patients treated with a tertiary tricyclic antidepressant will be exposed to a metabolite that itself may have antidepressant efficacy. Indeed, the extent of demethylation may be sufficiently great in some patients receiving a tertiary amine tricyclic that the predominant pharmacologically active compound in their body is the secondary amine metabolite.

History

In general, the development of psychotherapeutic drugs has been a serendipitous process. This is certainly true of the typical antidepressants. Imipramine, the prototypical TCA, was synthesized in 1948 as one of a number of structures (iminodibenzyl derivatives) to be tested as potential antihistamines, sedatives, or analgesics. The efficacy of chlorpromazine in the treatment of schizophrenia was evident by the mid-1950s, and imipramine is structurally similar to chlorpromazine (see Fig. 1 in Chapter 18). Consequently, the efficacy of imipramine in schizophrenia began to be evaluated. It was ineffective. However, an astute Swiss psychiatrist, Roland Kuhn, observed that in his schizophrenic patients with significant depressive symptomatology, the depressive symptoms improved upon treatment with imipramine even if the schizophrenic symptoms did not. Kuhn suggested that imipramine might be an antidepressant and performed the first clinical trial demonstrating this in the late 1950s. Kuhn's study not only showed that a chemi-

cal could have antidepressant efficacy but also, when taken together with its absence of utility in schizophrenia, demonstrated that drugs may have selective clinical effects.

Efficacy and Side Effects

Nondepressed individuals do not experience mood elevation with TCAs as they often do with stimulant drugs such as amphetamine or methylphenidate. Indeed, in normal subjects the TCAs often cause sedation and unpleasant effects such as dry mouth, blurred vision, and constipation. Probably because of this, the use or, more properly, abuse of TCAs as "street drugs" is very rare. By contrast, when given to depressed patients, even though unpleasant side effects may occur, over time the TCAs will produce a lightening of the entire depressive state. Recovery tends to be associated with improvement in all symptoms, even though their rates of improvement may not be identical, and certain symptoms may be more refractory to treatment than others in a particular patient. The therapeutic efficacy of all types of antidepressants, including the TCAs, usually takes about 2 to 3 weeks to become evident. This observation has given rise to the idea that there is a time delay in the onset of action of antidepressants. This may be so, but it is a very complex issue. What does seem clear is that maximal therapeutic benefit with all chemical classes of antidepressants usually takes 4 weeks or longer to occur. We still need to find a drug that produces maximal reduction of depressive symptomatology more rapidly.

The TCAs are efficacious. They were superior to placebo in 71% of studies comparing a TCA with placebo for the short-term treatment of nonpsychotic major depression. About 65% to 75% of depressives have a clinically significant response to TCAs but only about 20% to 40% show a comparable response to placebo. Not all depressives respond to TCAs equally well. As described originally by Kuhn, the best response is often seen in melancholic patients with symptoms such as early morning awakening, psychomotor retardation, loss of appetite, and weight loss, with the symptoms being worse in the morning and tending to improve during the day. Psychotic depressions (i.e., depressions accompanied by delusions or hallucinations) do not respond as well to TCAs. Finally, evidence is accumulating that the TCAs are effective in preventing or attenuating new episodes of depression, and they are being used increasingly as preventive treatments.

A basic tenet of pharmacology is that no drug has a single action. A consequence of this is that all drugs cause side effects and the TCAs are certainly no exception. Most commonly, they produce effects (e.g., dry mouth, blurred vision, constipation, urinary retention) due to their potency in blocking muscarinic cholinergic receptors of the parasympathetic nervous system (Table 3). Many of the TCAs are also sedative. They may have cardiovascular side effects; orthostatic hypotension (a fall of blood pressure upon standing) is the most clinically significant cardiovascular effect, but they can cause changes in cardiac conduction as well. This is particularly important because overdosage can cause fatal heart block and/or arrhythmias. As these drugs may be prescribed for some patients who are suicidal, the problem of overdosage is a serious one. Another side effect of the TCAs occurs in some depressives with bipolar disorder; in these depressives, treatment with TCAs can precipitate the transition from depression to mania or hypomania.

Monoamine Oxidase Inhibitors

Chemistry

Several monoamine oxidase inhibitors (MAOIs) are used clinically. The structures of three of them—isocarboxazid, phenelzine, and tranylcypromine—are shown in Fig. 3. Isocarboxazid and phenelzine are derivatives of hydrazine, but tranylcypromine is not. Tranylcypromine is related structurally to the stimulant amphetamine, so it is not surprising that tranylcypromine has some stimulant properties. The inhibition of MAO by

TABLE 3. *Side effect profiles of antidepressant drugs*

Generic name	Sedative or stimulant	Anticholinergic effect	Cardiovascular effects	
			Potential for orthostatic hypotension	Potential for conduction disturbance
Tricyclics				
Amitriptyline	Sedating	Marked	High	High
Desipramine	Stimulant	Moderate	High	High
Doxepin	Sedating	Marked	High	High
Imipramine	Sedating	Marked	High	High
Nortriptyline	Neither	Marked	Low	High
Protriptyline	Stimulant	Marked	High	High
Trimipramine	Sedating	Marked	High	High
MAOIs				
Isocarboxazid	Neither	None	High	None
Phenelzine	Neither	None	High	None
Tranylcypromine	Stimulant	None	High	None
Second-generation drugs				
Amoxapine	Sedating	Moderate	Moderate to high	Moderate to high
Bupropion	Stimulant	None	None	None
Fluoxetine	Stimulant	None	None	None
Maprotiline	Sedating	Moderate	Moderate to high	Moderate to high
Sertraline	Neither	None	None	None
Trazodone	Sedating	None	Moderate to high	None

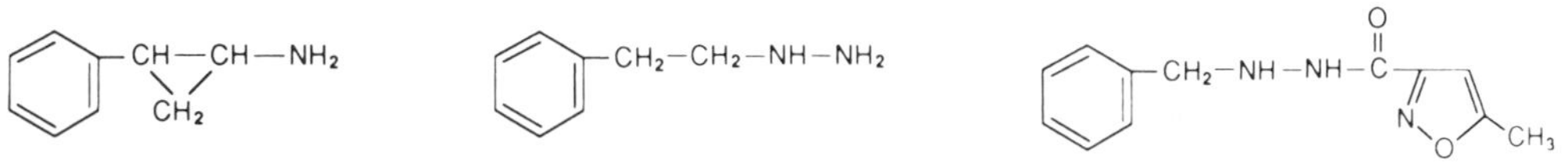

Tranylcypromine   Phenelzine   Isocarboxazid

FIG. 3. Structures of various monoamine oxidase inhibitors. Isocarboxazid and phenelzine are derivatives of hydrazine (NH_2NH_2). Tranylcypromine is a phenylalkylamine that is structurally similar to amphetamine.

these drugs is due to their forming covalent bonds at the active site of the enzyme. Phenelzine reacts with the flavin prosthetic group of MAO to inactivate the enzyme. Isocarboxazid acts similarly after its conversion to an active hydrazine intermediate. An activated intermediate of tranylcypromine seems to bind to the active site of MAO itself, resulting in inactivation of the enzyme. The binding of these drugs to MAO is essentially irreversible, so that inactivation of the enzyme exists even after the drugs themselves are metabolized and removed from the body. The recovery of MAO activity requires the synthesis of new MAO enzyme (i.e., protein synthesis), and it can take several weeks for MAO activity to return to normal after terminating the administration of an MAOI.

History

About the same time as the development of imipramine, two compounds, isoniazid and iproniazid, were developed for use in tuberculosis. It was noted that iproniazid caused euphoria and elation (essentially hypomanic-like behavior) in some of the tubercular patients but isoniazid did not. Further research revealed that iproniazid, but not isoniazid, inhibited the enzyme MAO. About this time, the drug reserpine was found to produce a state of psychomotor retardation (or lethargy or sedation) in laboratory rats that was considered by some to be an animal model of depression. It was found that administration of iproniazid prior to administration of reserpine prevented this behavioral state induced by reserpine; indeed,

the rats became hyperactive. This latter fact, coupled with the central stimulatory side effects observed in patients with tuberculosis, inspired the American psychiatrist Nathan Kline to suggest that iproniazid might have antidepressant or "psychic energizing" properties. This idea was further justified scientifically because iproniazid had been shown to inhibit MAO, which is involved in the catabolism of substances such as norepinephrine and 5-hydroxytryptamine (5-HT; serotonin) thought to be important in certain behavioral states. In 1957, Kline and his associates reported iproniazid to be efficacious in the treatment of depressives. Iproniazid has historical importance but is no longer used clinically because it produces hepatic toxicity.

Efficacy and Side Effects

In general, the efficacy of the MAOIs in depression is comparable to that of the TCAs and, therefore, superior to that of placebo. It has been widely believed that MAOIs work best in depressives with "atypical" features (see end of section "Diagnosis" above), such as increased eating and sleeping, sensitivity to rejection, reactivity of mood, and loss of energy. By contrast, depressives with more typical symptoms (e.g., weight loss, insomnia, feeling worse in the morning and better in the evening, agitation or retardation, guilt) were thought not to respond as well to MAOIs as they did to tricyclic antidepressants. However, studies conducted in the 1980s have found no difference in the response of either atypical or typical depressives to treatment with MAOIs.

Some side effects produced by MAOIs are similar to those caused by the tricyclic compounds although the mechanisms may be different. For example, orthostatic hypotension is caused by MAOIs as is the precipitation of hypomanic or manic symptoms in bipolar depressed patients. In contrast to the TCAs, the inhibitors of MAO do not seem to have important direct cardiac effects or to block muscarinic cholinergic receptors (Table 3).

The most publicized and perhaps alarming toxic effect of the MAOIs is hypertensive crisis. The high blood pressure may elicit a headache associated with sweating, pallor, nausea, and vomiting. Much more serious and even fatal syndromes can develop, such as intracranial hemorrhage due to the hypertensive crisis. Such a crisis, an acute and dramatic increase in blood pressure, is not a toxic effect of MAOIs alone but is more properly considered a drug (or foodstuff) interaction. The wife of a pharmacist, G. E. F. Rowe, was being treated with an MAOI, and he observed that she often had headaches after eating cheese. This phenomenon was then studied by Blackwell and his associates, who found that cheese could elicit a large increase in blood pressure in the presence of an MAOI, the so-called cheese reaction. In this case, the rise in blood pressure is caused by tyramine in cheese. Tyramine, an indirectly acting sympathomimetic amine, exerts its effect on blood pressure by releasing stored norepinephrine and epinephrine from sympathetic nerve terminals and the adrenal medulla. Normally, the tyramine in cheese is metabolized by MAO in the gastrointestinal tract and does not enter the circulation in appreciable amounts. If MAO is inhibited, tyramine can enter the circulation and release greater than normal amounts of the catecholamines, producing the hypertensive crisis. Foodstuffs containing indirectly acting sympathomimetic amines include certain aged and overripe cheese, chianti wine, chicken liver paté, sausages, pickled herring, broad bean pods, and certain yeast products. Consequently, patients being treated with MAOIs are restricted to diets that either eliminate completely or reduce substantially these foodstuffs. Equally important, many over-the-counter cold and sinus medications contain indirectly acting sympathomimetic amines, and their use must be avoided by patients being treated with MAOIs.

Since 1968, it has been known that there are at least two forms or isoenzymes of MAO, termed type A and type B monoamine oxidase. Studies of these isoenzymes revealed that they had selectivity for certain substrates. For example, tyramine is metabolized by the type A form much more avidly than by the type B form of the enzyme. Drugs have now been developed that inhibit each isoenzyme selectively; for example, clorgyline and maclobemide are selective inhibitors of type A, whereas deprenyl selectively inhibits type B. It has been demonstrated that administration of deprenyl is much less likely to precipitate a hypertensive crisis upon ingestion of tyramine than is administration of irreversible selective inhibitors of type A MAO. Unfortunately, type A MAOIs, such as clorgyline, more consistently have been found to have antidepressant efficacy than type B inhibitors, so that it might be difficult to separate the efficacy of irreversible MAOIs in depression from their ability to elicit a hypertensive episode.

Second-Generation Antidepressants

Chemistry

There are many second-generation antidepressants. Currently, six such compounds—amoxapine, bupropion, fluoxetine, maprotiline, sertraline, and trazodone—have been approved for use as antidepressants in the United States.[1] These drugs have diverse chemical structures (Fig. 4). Amoxapine is a dibenzoxapine derivative; it is the demethylated analog of loxapine, an antipsychotic drug. Maprotiline has a four-ring "bridged"

---

* Paroxetine was approved for use in early 1993. Its pharmacological profile is similar to that of fluoxetine and sertraline.

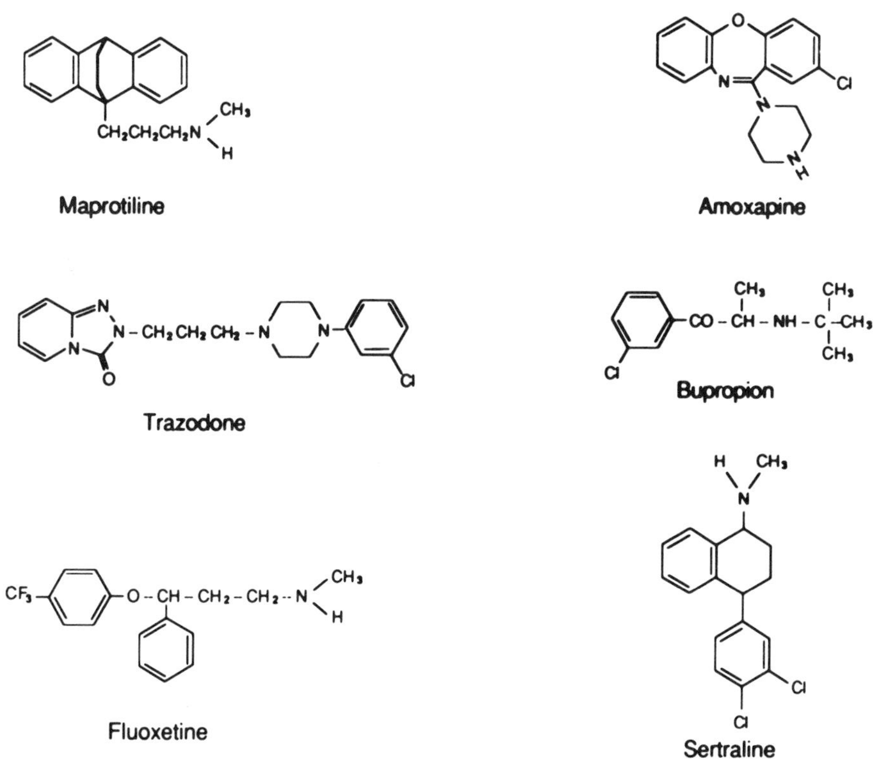

FIG. 4. Structures of various second-generation or atypical antidepressants.

structure rather than the three-ring structure of the TCAs; nevertheless, it is more closely related in structure to the TCAs than to any of the other second-generation compounds. Bupropion, fluoxetine, sertraline, and trazodone are clearly not related chemically to the other antidepressants.

Efficacy and Side Effects

The efficacy of these drugs in depression has been compared with that of the tricyclic compounds and placebo and found to be comparable to that of the TCAs, but no better. No consistent body of data has shown that these drugs produce improvement in a greater percentage of depressives than do TCAs or that patients respond more rapidly to the second-generation drugs.

What has made some of the second-generation drugs quite popular is that they elicit fewer side effects than do the first-

generation antidepressants. MAO is not inhibited by any of the second-generation antidepressants, so that there is little to no risk of patients treated with these drugs developing hypertensive crisis upon ingesting certain foodstuffs or over-the-counter medications. Also, bupropion, trazodone, sertraline, and fluoxetine are much weaker at blocking muscarinic cholinergic receptors than are TCAs, so that in general they produce no more anticholinergic side effects than placebo when administered to patients (Table 3). Amoxapine and maprotiline, however, do produce anticholinergic side effects when administered clinically. The cardiovascular side effect profile for amoxapine and maprotiline is, in general, similar to that of the TCAs, and they also produce sedation to a degree similar to that with amitriptyline or doxepin. By contrast, bupropion, fluoxetine, sertraline, and trazodone have little effect on the conduction system of the heart and the first three drugs produce little if any orthostatic hypotension (Table 3). Also in contrast to sedative TCAs, bupropion and fluoxetine may cause nervousness and insomnia and have more of a stimulant than a sedative profile. These drugs do, however, have some specific adverse effects that are either qualitatively or quantitatively unique. As many as 25% of patients taking fluoxetine or sertraline develop nausea and about 10% have diarrhea. Weight loss may occur with both fluoxetine and bupropion. Trazodone can cause priapism (protracted and painful penile erection), which may require corrective surgery or cause permanent loss of erectile function. Bupropion has a greater tendency to produce seizures than other marketed antidepressants.

Finally, among all the antidepressants, amoxapine is the only one that has neuroleptic activity in vivo, presumably due to its relatively high affinity for D_2 dopamine receptors. Consequently, treatment with amoxapine can cause many of the movement disorders (e.g., akathesia, akinesia, parkinsonism, and tardive dyskinesia) that are associated with antipsychotic treatments (see Chapter 18).

Mechanisms of Action

Antidepressants most probably act by affecting central noradrenergic and/or serotonergic neurotransmission. During the past 30 years, many pharmacological effects were found to be produced by antidepressants. The fact, though, is that we still do not understand how the neurochemical effects produced in brain by these drugs result in the beneficial behavioral effects they elicit. Indeed, if there is a particular area of brain most involved in their clinical effects, we still do not know what it is. Although this is clearly an unsatisfactory state, it must be viewed within the complexity of the human behavioral repertoire. We are just beginning to understand the anatomic and neurochemical bases of certain behaviors in simple organisms such as the snail *Aplysia* (see Chapter 13) and elementary behaviors in more com-

plex organisms such as the laboratory rat. Thus, there are as yet few concrete data regarding how a specific neurochemical effect of antidepressants can produce a behavioral change. However, improvements in both behavioral analysis and neuroanatomic localization of the effects of drugs in brain should make it possible to begin to study this type of association.

The first pharmacological effect ascribed to imipramine was reported in 1959 by Sigg, who found that it enhanced and prolonged certain peripheral effects produced by the catecholamine norepinephrine (NE). The ability to potentiate the effects of NE was subsequently shown to be a common feature of TCAs. This effect is a consequence of the ability of TCAs to block the neuronal reuptake of NE; the reuptake of NE into the presynaptic noradrenergic neuron from which it is released is the primary way in which the action of NE in the synapse is terminated (see Chapter 6). Inhibition of reuptake, then, raises and prolongs the concentration of NE in the synapse to allow greater than normal stimulation of postsynaptic noradrenergic receptors. The TCAs were shown not only to block the uptake of NE but also the uptake of the indolealkylamine serotonin (5-HT). Desipramine, protriptyline, and the second-generation drug maprotiline are relatively selective inhibitors of the uptake of NE in vivo. The other TCAs block the uptake of both NE and 5-HT at clinically relevant doses. Until recently, there were no drugs that selectively blocked the uptake of 5-HT in vivo. The second-generation antidepressants fluoxetine and sertraline do this (Table 4). Thus, these drugs have an initial pharmacological effect in the body different from that of the TCAs. If the monoamine uptake–inhibiting properties of these drugs are related to their clinical efficacy, then it seems that initial selective effects on either noradrenergic or serotonergic neurons can produce an antidepressant effect. Interestingly, another second-generation compound, trazodone, is not particularly potent at blocking the uptake of either NE or 5-HT, but rather is a potent antagonist of a

TABLE 4. *Potency of tricyclic antidepressants and second-generation antidepressants to block either monoamine uptake or receptors*

Generic name	IC_{50} values (nM)[a], monoamine uptake		K_i values (nM)[b], receptors		
	NE	5-HT	Histamine₁ histaminergic	Muscarinic cholinergic	α_1- adrenergic
Tricyclics					
Amitriptyline	50	150	1	20	25
Desipramine	2	800	100	200	130
Doxepin	400	1,500	0.25	80	25
Imipramine	30	150	10	90	90
Nortriptyline	10	600	10	150	60
Protriptyline	2	500	25	25	130
Trimipramine	5,000	10,000	0.25	60	25
Second-generation drugs					
Amoxapine	25	600	25	1,000	50
Bupropion	2,500	30,000	6,500	50,000	4,500
Fluoxetine	200	10	6,000	2,000	6,000
Maprotiline	50	30,000	2	600	90
Sertraline	200	1	10,000	20,000	4,000
Trazodone	20,000	750	350	300,000	40

[a] Values were taken from multiple sources in the literature. Values have been adjusted to reflect not only the absolute potency of the drug in blocking the uptake of NE or 5-HT but also their relative potencies in relationship to each other. Thus, for example, desipramine is 10–20 times more potent than imipramine in blocking the uptake of NE; similarly, desipramine is 200- to 500-fold more potent in blocking the uptake of NE than the uptake of 5-HT, i.e., the lower the IC_{50} value, the more potent the drug.

[b] Values from Richelson and Nelson (1984). The relationship between K_i values and IC_{50} values is given by the equation:

$$K_i = \frac{IC_{50}}{1 + L/K_D}$$

where L is the concentration of radioligand used in the experiment and K_D is the affinity of the radioligand for the receptor.

particular subtype of receptor for serotonin, termed the 5-HT₂ receptor (see Chapter 6). None of the first-generation or second-generation compounds is a potent inhibitor of the uptake of another catecholamine, dopamine (DA). The only antidepressant that is a reasonably potent inhibitor of the uptake of DA in vivo is bupropion.

As mentioned in more detail in Chapter 6, monoamine oxidase is responsible for the intraneuronal deamination of substances such as NE, DA, and 5-HT. Inhibition of this enzyme raises the content of these neurotransmitters in brain and this was speculated to enhance neurotransmission mediated by these substances.

When these pharmacological effects of the first-generation antidepressants became apparent, it was formally proposed by several groups of investigators in the mid-1960s that their clinical efficacy resulted from their enhancing noradrenergic transmission at key sites in brain. Several years later, the same concept was extended to serotonergic transmission. Indeed, it was speculated at the same time that depression itself was due to some type of deficiency of noradrenergic or serotonergic transmission. These latter ideas were called the monoamine (NE or 5-HT) hypotheses of depression. The possible clinical importance of these neurotransmitters stimulated much preclinical research on all aspects of their function in brain, for example, their neuroanatomic organization, physiological and pharmacological regulation, behavioral roles, and so on. Clinically, many creative strategies were employed to test the idea that depression was associated with a state of central monoamine deficiency: studies of the amines or their metabolites in body fluids;

postmortem studies of the amines themselves or of their uptake sites or receptors in the brains of depressives; sleep studies; psycho-pharmacological challenge studies in which a drug is used to elicit a response, usually a neu-roendocrine one, mediated by activation of either noradrenergic or serotonergic recep-tors. Also, it became apparent that if bi-ological alterations were to be found in depressives, it would only be evident if homo-geneous populations of patients were studied. Thus, these biological theories also stimu-lated research into improving the classifica-tion schemes for depression.

A detailed review of these clinical studies is beyond the scope of this chapter. No conclu-sive body of evidence has shown that depres-sion is related to a state of central mono-amine deficiency. In some subtypes of depression, for example, bipolar disorder, data have been obtained that are consistent with the noradrenergic hypothesis but similar data have not been found consistently for other types of depression. Part of the problem in attempting to test these ideas clinically is the limited access available to the brains of living patients. This problem may be over-come by the development of the newer imag-ing techniques (see Chapter 15). Neverthe-less, it is appropriate to point out that it may be fallacious to develop theories of the patho-genesis of an illness based on the pharmaco-logical effects of drugs useful in that illness, especially if there is no evidence that the drugs "cure" the disease.

Much research since the mid-1960s has continued to show a variety of potent and robust effects of antidepressants on central monoamine systems. Starting in the 1970s, attention focused on the longer term (usually 1 to 4 weeks) effects of antidepressants on nor-adrenergic or serotonergic function rather than on their acute effects. The rationale for such studies was that the drugs are given to patients chronically and there may be a time lag before their beneficial effects become evi-dent. Such research has shown that virtually all types of antidepressants produce numer-ous slowly developing effects on central nor-adrenergic or serotonergic neuronal systems. In general, these slowly developing effects may be viewed as an adaptational response of the neuronal system to the initial acute effect of the antidepressant (i.e., inhibition of up-take of NE or 5-HT or inhibition of MAO). For example, shortly after administration of uptake inhibitors, the soma in brain from which either noradrenergic or serotonergic neurons arise decrease their firing rates. This seems to be a consequence of the increased biogenic amine in the synapse, which occurs due to uptake inhibition, activating somato-dendritic "autoreceptors"; such stimulation leads to a decrease in the firing rate of the cell. MAOIs also produce this effect. Thus, very shortly after administration of antidepres-sants, there may be an exaggerated effect of either NE or 5-HT at postsynaptic receptors, but the neurons releasing these biogenic amines decrease their firing rate so as to cause less release of the transmitter into the synapse.

The acute inhibitory effect of antidepres-sants on the firing rate of noradrenergic or serotonergic soma does not persist after re-peated administration. Over time, the firing rate of these soma returns to normal. This appears to be a consequence of the autore-ceptors on these soma becoming subsensi-tive; that is, agonists such as NE or 5-HT are less potent and/or efficacious at lowering the firing rates of these soma in rats treated long term with antidepressants than they are in control rats. Thus, in animals treated for sev-eral weeks with antidepressants, the release of NE and 5-HT may be similar to that which occurs normally and this could cause greater than normal amounts of transmitter in the synapse due to the persistence of either inhibi-tion of uptake of NE or 5-HT or inhibition of MAO.

Compensatory effects caused by antide-pressants occur not only in noradrenergic or serotonergic neurons themselves but also in their postsynaptic neurons. For example, responses elicited by NE activating α_1-adrenoceptors are potentiated following re-peated administration of either TCAs or

MAOIs. By contrast, responses elicited by activation of β-adrenoceptors decrease after repeated administration of all types of antidepressants except, perhaps, those that are selective inhibitors of 5-HT uptake. Different types of responses elicited by activation of serotonin receptors can be either enhanced or inhibited after long-term administration of antidepressants. Using ligand-binding methodology, the antidepressant-induced decreases in β-adrenoceptor responsiveness have been shown to be a consequence of a decrease in the density or "down-regulation" of β-adrenoceptors. By contrast, no consistent picture has emerged to show that the changes in serotonergic responsiveness are accompanied by alterations in the density of serotonergic receptors.

It is thus apparent that the different types of antidepressants exert multiple effects over time on central noradrenergic and serotonergic neurons as well as on responses and receptors stimulated by either NE or 5-HT. Given this, it is difficult to make a general statement as to whether noradrenergic or serotonergic transmission is enhanced or diminished by the long-term administration of these drugs. Rather, effects may vary in different parts of the brain depending on, for example, the type of receptor present. Even if we do not know precisely how antidepressants modulate noradrenergic or serotonergic transmission in different parts of the brain, it is likely that some combination of the effects just enumerated is associated with their beneficial clinical effects. For example, in depressives treated successfully with a variety of antidepressants and maintained on these drugs, there is a rapid return of depressive symptomatology if procedures are carried out that deplete the brain of serotonin.

Drugs Used in the Treatment of Bipolar Disorder

As described above, persons who have bipolar disorder experience both episodes of depression and episodes of mania or hypo-mania. The acute depressive episodes are treated similarly to those that occur in major depressive disorder (i.e., with antidepressant drugs). However, several complications may occur with the use of such drugs, including abrupt switches to mania, the development of mixed manic and depressive states, or rapid cycling.

The mainstay of treatment for acute manic or hypomanic episodes is lithium. The therapeutic effects of lithium were first described by the Australian psychiatrist John Cade in 1949. Approximately 1,000 papers per year are published on this simple monovalent cation, yet its mechanism of action remains obscure. After administration, lithium is distributed widely throughout the brain and is handled similarly to the sodium ion in many cellular systems. Effects on norepinephrine-, serotonin-, and acetylcholine-containing neurons have been documented. Currently, one of the more attractive hypotheses is that lithium may exert its therapeutic effect via alterations of the phosphatidylinositol "second-messenger" system which, like the cyclic AMP system, is a key step in signal transduction in the postsynaptic cell (see Chapter 4).

Despite the lack of clarity in understanding the mechanism of action of lithium from a basic neurobiological perspective, clinical studies have shed light on three aspects of lithium's actions. First, the clinical effects of lithium are specific among monovalent cations, since others (e.g., rubidium) are not effective. Second, lithium is relatively specific for treatment of bipolar disorder, as other psychiatric syndromes such as schizophrenia do not respond as well. Lithium may also be an effective treatment for acute depressive episodes in bipolar illness, whereas it is less effective in unipolar depression. Third, lithium is an effective prophylactic, or preventive, treatment for bipolar disorder. Virtually all studies have shown lithium to be effective in decreasing the number of both manic and depressive episodes.

Substantial interest has arisen in the use of certain anticonvulsants in bipolar disorder. The anticonvulsant carbamazepine has been studied extensively. It is similar to lithium in that it is an effective antimanic agent and appears to have some prophylactic efficacy; however, its utility as an antidepressant has not yet been convincingly demonstrated. Also, as with lithium, its mechanism of action in bipolar disorder is unknown. Though also "tricyclic" in structure, carbamazepine has little effect on NE or 5-HT reuptake. Emerging evidence indicates that not all anticonvulsants share carbamazepine's effectiveness in the treatment of bipolar illness, though several other promising candidates, such as valproic acid, have been identified.

CONCEPTUAL ISSUES

Two sets of models have been used in the attempt to understand the mechanisms that underlie mood disorders. The two major approaches that have been taken in the effort to understand mood disorders are the following:

1. Mood disorders are a response to something that happens to an individual (*the psychological model*), and
2. Mood disorders are a manifestation of something wrong with the individual's brain (*the biomedical model*).

Of necessity this chapter, as part of a text on the biology of normal and abnormal brain function, has focused on the latter. However, the various psychological models are also of great importance.

Historically, the object loss theories of depression, theories of depression as misdirected aggression, and theories of depression as a sequela of loss of reinforcement have each focused on important clinical aspects of the syndrome and have developed schemata for their explanation. More recently, important controlled studies have shown that certain forms of structured psychotherapy (e.g., cognitive theory, interpersonal therapy) are equal in efficacy to antidepressants in the treatment of milder forms of major depressive disorder. Nevertheless, the evidence is incontrovertible that the major mood disorders have a biological component. Their syndromic nature and response to pharmacotherapy and the evidence for a genetic contribution to depression and bipolar disorder (see Chapter 16) strongly support this view.

How, then, is one to approach the study of mood disorders? While the complex intertwining of biological and psychosocial aspects humbles the student of mood disorders, one must be mindful that in both biomedical and social sciences the mysteries of many complex systems have yielded to the investigation of the individual components of those systems. The neural basis of mood disorders is clearly one such component. Neurobiological investigations have already contributed and will continue to contribute not only to the better understanding of major depression and bipolar disorder, but also to their more humane and effective treatment.

SUMMARY

Mood disorders are common and can often be quite severe. As indicated in the epigraph to this chapter, major depressive disorder is qualitatively distinct from "normal" sadness experienced as part of the vicissitudes of life. It can result in death—by suicide. The diagnoses of these disorders now occur through a phenomenological approach based on multiple signs and symptoms. There are different types of major depressive disorders and distinctions among them can have important therapeutic implications. Patients with bipolar depression have at some time experienced mania or hypomania in addition to depression. Unipolar depressives have recurrent depressive episodes without mania or hypomania. Other descriptors are currently in use and schemes for categorization are continuously evolving.

These disorders, even though severe in nature, can be treated successfully. A variety of pharmacological agents improve the signs and symptoms of depression. There are three major chemical classes of antidepressants: (1) tricyclic drugs, (2) monoamine oxidase inhibitors, and (3) second-generation or atypical antidepressants. The efficacy of these three classes of drugs in depression is comparable. About 65% to 75% of patients will have a substantial amelioration of depressive symptomatology; maximal therapeutic benefit often takes 6 to 8 weeks to occur. These drugs produce side effects that range in severity from being only mildly troublesome (e.g., dry mouth) to being clinically significant (e.g., orthostatic hypotension, development of seizures). The mainstay for the treatment of acute mania or hypomania is the lithium ion; more recently, evidence has been presented that anticonvulsants such as carbamazepine are effective also.

The mechanism of action of antidepressants is still not completely understood but most probably involves effects on central noradrenergic and/or serotonergic neurons. Initially, many antidepressants block the uptake of serotonin and/or norepinephrine or inhibit the catabolism of these biogenic amines by the enzyme monoamine oxidase. These initial pharmacological effects are followed by a variety of more slowly developing effects on noradrenergic or serotonergic neurons or on the nerves they innervate. It is likely that some combination of these effects is associated with their ability to ameliorate depressive symptomatology.

BIBLIOGRAPHY

Original Articles

Aghajanian GK, Foote WE, Sheard MH. Action of psychotogenic drugs on single midbrain raphe neurons. *J Pharmacol Exp Ther* 1970;171:178–187.

Delgado PL, Charney DS, Price LH, Aghajanian GK, Landis H, Heninger GR. Serotonin function and the mechanism of antidepressant action. *Arch Gen Psychiatry* 1990;47:411–418.

Frazer A, Pandey G, Mendels J, Neeley S, Kane M, Hess ME. The effect of tri-iodothyronine in combination with imipramine on [^{3}H]-cyclic AMP production in slices of rat cerebral cortex. *Neuropharmacology* 1974;13:1131–1140.

Klerman G, Lavori P, Rice J, Reich T, Endicott J, Andreasen N, et al. Birth-cohort trends in rates of major depressive disorder among relatives of patients with affective disorder. *Arch Gen Psychiatry* 1985;42:689–693.

Kline NS. Clinical experience with iproniazid (Marsilid). *J Clin Exp Neuropsychol* 1958;19(Suppl. 1):72–78.

Kuhn R. The treatment of depressive states with G

22355 (imipramine hydrochloride). *Am J Psychiatry* 1958;115:459–464.

Nybäck HV, Walters JR, Aghajanian GK, Roth RH. Tricyclic antidepressants: effects on the firing rate of brain noradrenergic neurons. *Eur J Pharmacol* 1975;32:302–312.

Richelson E, Nelson A. Antagonism by antidepressants of neurotransmitter receptors of normal human brain *in vitro*. *J Pharmacol Exp Therapeut* 1984;230:94–102.

Robins LN, Helzer JE, Weissman MM, Orvaschel H, Gruenberg E, Burke JD, et al. Lifetime prevalence of specific psychiatric disorders in three sites. *Arch Gen Psychiatry* 1984;41:949–958.

Sigg EB. Pharmacological studies with Tofranil. *Can J Psychiatry* 1959;4:S75–S85.

Wells KB, Stewart A, Hays R, Burnam A, Rogers W, Daniels M, et al. The functioning and well-being of depressed patients. Results from the Medical Outcomes Study. *JAMA* 1989;262:914–919.

Books and Reviews

American Psychiatric Association. *Diagnostic and statistical manual of mental disorders.* 3rd Ed., Rev. (DSM-III-R). Washington, DC: American Psychiatric Association Press; 1987.

Baldessarini RJ. Current status of antidepressants: clinical pharmacology and therapy. *J Clin Psychiatry* 1989;50:117–126.

Barchas JD. Biochemical hypotheses of affective disorders and anxiety. In: Siegel GJ, Agranoff BW, Albers RW, Molinoff PB, eds. *Basic neurochemistry,* 5th ed. New York: Raven Press; 1994 (in press).

Brotman AW, Falk WE, Gelenberg AJ. Pharmacologic treatment of acute depressive subtypes. In: Meltzer HY, ed. *Psychopharmacology: the third generation of progress.* New York: Raven Press; 1987:1031–1040.

Freud S. Mourning and melancholia. In: *Complete psychological works of Sigmund Freud.* Vol. 14. London: Hogarth Press; 1914, standard edition.

Goodwin FK, Jamison KR. *Manic-depressive illness.* New York: Oxford University Press; 1990.

Heninger GR, Charney DS. Mechanism of action of antidepressant treatments: implications for the etiology and treatment of depressive disorders. In: Meltzer HY, ed. *Psychopharmacology: the third generation of progress.* New York: Raven Press; 1987:535–544.

Hirschfeld R, Goodwin F. Mood disorders. In: Talbott J, Hales R, Yudofsky S, eds. *The American Psychiatric Association Press textbook of psychiatry.* Washington, DC: American Psychiatric Association Press; 1988:403–442.

Kraepelin E. *Manic-depressive insanity and paranoia.* Barclay R (Translator). Edinburgh: Livingston Press, 1919 (rereleased: Classics of psychiatry and behavioral sciences library, Carlson E [series ed.], Birmingham, AL: Gryphon Editions, 1989).

Prien RF. Long-term treatment of affective disorders. In: Meltzer HY, ed. *Psychopharmacology: the third generation of progress.* New York: Raven Press; 1987:309–314.

Schildkraut JJ. The catecholamine hypothesis of affective disorders: a review of supporting evidence. *Am J Psychiatry* 1965;122:509–522.

18

Schizophrenia

Raquel E. Gur

Strange! I seem to see two suns
and—two Thebes, yes,
two cities, two, each with seven gates. And you—
walking there before me—are you a bull?
I could wager that you are one,
with those horns
that have sprouted from your head!
Were you one before? An animal? I mean a bull,
decidedly a bull!

Euripedes,
The Bacchae, circa 405 B.C.
(passage spoken by Pentheus after being rendered mad under the spell of Dionysus)

- Schizophrenia is a major and severe psychotic disorder with significant impairment in mental functioning that interferes with an individual's ability to cope with the daily demands of life.

- There are five subtypes of schizophrenia: catatonic, disorganized, paranoid, undifferentiated, and residual.

- There is considerable variability in the course of the illness.

- Drugs are the cornerstone of treatment.

- Other factors besides medication can affect the treatment outcome.

- Many of the discrete clinical features of schizophrenia suggest a linkage to aberrant functioning in specific brain regions or networks.

- Schizophrenia is probably familial.

- Drugs that decrease dopamine neurotransmission decrease symptoms of schizophrenia.

- There is a growing literature linking certain neuroanatomic findings to schizophrenia.

- A range of physiological neuroimaging methods exists for assessing different parameters of brain function, and several of these methods have been applied to the study of schizophrenia.

This chapter first discusses the clinical manifestations of the disorder: clinical features, subtypes, prevalence, and course, as well as treatment and outcome. The chapter goes on to discuss the brain–behavior relationship and its pathophysiology. Finally, the pathophysiology of schizophrenia from neuroanatomic, neuropharmacological, and neurophysiological perspectives is reviewed.

Schizophrenia is a prevalent and severe psychotic disorder that affects about 1% of the population and has devastating consequences for individuals and their families. While aberrant behavior we see today as reflecting "mental illness" has been described for millennia, it was not until the late nineteenth century that delineation of symptoms was substituted by efforts to define syndromes that may constitute discrete disease entities. In Germany, Emil Kraepelin in 1896 coined the term *dementia praecox* to describe a disorder that begins in late adolescence or early adulthood and has a chronic deteriorating course. In 1911, the Swiss psychiatrist Eugen Bleuler introduced the term *schizophrenia* to denote the characteristic symptomatology of the disorder, emphasizing that it was not a true dementia but a "splitting" of mental capacities. He differentiated between primary symptoms (association, affect, ambivalence, and autism emphasizing loosening in thought processing, blunted affect, indecisiveness, and peculiar thinking) and accessory symptoms (delusions and hallucinations). Unlike Kraepelin's terminology, which emphasized a longitudinal perspective, Bleuler's focused on the cross-sectional, "here-and-now" presentation.

While concepts about the clinical features of schizophrenia have undergone refinement in the past 80 years, Kraepelin's and Bleuler's classic descriptions are still considered to convey the salient features of this challenging disease. Over the past 20 years, progress in clinical research methodology in psychiatry has led to a substantial emphasis on the use of clearly delineated, criterion-based diagnoses. This movement has stimulated the adaptation of standardized diagnostic procedures and the use of validated rating scales for evaluating patients suspected of having schizophrenia. Moreover, these developments have led to the formulation of more specifically defined criteria for making the diagnosis of schizophrenia, as described below.

CLINICAL MANIFESTATIONS

Clinical Features

Schizophrenia is a major and severe psychotic disorder with significant impairment in mental functioning that interferes with an individual's ability to cope with the daily demands of life. While heterogeneous in presentation, a number of common and essential features characterize schizophrenia. The presence, severity, and persistence of symptoms result in a general decline of functioning below premorbid levels. In particular, the individual's ability to care for himself or herself, perform effectively in school or at work, and maintain social and interpersonal relationships are all markedly impaired.

The *Diagnostic and Statistical Manual of Mental Disorders* of the American Psychiatric Association (DSM-III-R) lists the criteria necessary for making the diagnosis of schizo-

Biological Bases of Brain Function and Disease, edited by Alan Frazer, Perry B. Molinoff, and Andrew Winokur. Raven Press, Ltd., New York © 1994.

phrenia (see Table 1). One common presentation of the illness involves abnormalities in thought content with manifestations of delusional ideas. Delusions can be persecutory in nature, such as beliefs of being followed or beliefs of being the subject of elaborate plots. Other delusions may include thought broadcasting, the belief that others can pick up one's thoughts, or thought insertion, the belief that some thoughts do not originate from the self but are inserted without one's being able to control them. Patients may have *ideas of reference,* whereby commonplace events and situations are assigned particular significance and special meaning, as if taking place in relation to the individual. For example, a

---

TABLE 1. *DSM-III-R criteria for schizophrenia*

A. Presence of characteristic psychotic symptoms in the active phase: either (1), (2), or (3) for at least one week (unless the symptoms are successfully treated):
  (1) Two of the following:
    (a) delusions
    (b) prominent hallucinations (throughout the day for several days or several times a week for several weeks, each hallucinatory experience not being limited to a few brief moments)
    (c) incoherence or marked loosening of associations
    (d) catatonic behavior
    (e) flat or grossly inappropriate affect
  (2) Bizarre delusions (i.e., involving a phenomenon that the person's culture would regard as totally implausible, e.g., thought broadcasting, being controlled by a dead person)
  (3) Prominent hallucinations [as defined in (1b) above] of a voice with content having no apparent relation to depression or elation, or a voice keeping up a running commentary on the person's behavior or thoughts, or two or more voices conversing with each other
B. During the course of the disturbance, functioning in such areas as work, social relations, and self-care is markedly below the highest level achieved before onset of the disturbance (or, when the onset is in childhood or adolescence, failure to achieve expected level of social development).
C. Schizoaffective Disorder and Mood Disorder with Psychotic Features have been ruled out, i.e., if Major Depressive or Manic Syndrome has ever been present during an active phase of the disturbance, the total duration of all episodes of a mood syndrome has been brief relative to the total duration of the active and residual phases of the disturbance.
D. Continuous signs of the disturbance for at least six months. The six-month period must include an active phase (of at least one week, or less if symptoms have been successfully treated) during which there were psychotic symptoms characteristic of Schizophrenia (symptoms in A), with or without a prodromal or residual phase, as defined below.
  Prodromal phase: A clear deterioration in functioning before the active phase of the disturbance that is not due to a disturbance in mood or to a Psychoactive Substance Use Disorder and that involves at least two of the symptoms listed below.
  Residual phase: Following the active phase of the disturbance, persistence of at least two of the symptoms noted below, these not being due to a disturbance in mood or to a Psychoactive Substance Use Disorder.
  Prodromal or Residual Symptoms:
  (1) marked social isolation or withdrawal
  (2) marked impairment in role functioning as wage-earner, student, or homemaker
  (3) markedly peculiar behavior (e.g., collecting garbage, talking to self in public, hoarding food)
  (4) marked impairment in personal hygiene and grooming
  (5) blunted or inappropriate affect
  (6) digressive, vague, overelaborate, or circumstantial speech, or poverty of speech, or poverty of content of speech
  (7) odd beliefs or magical thinking, influencing behavior and inconsistent with cultural norms (e.g., superstitiousness, belief in clairvoyance, telepathy, "sixth sense," "others can feel my feelings," overvalued ideas, ideas of reference)
  (8) unusual perceptual experiences (e.g., recurrent illusions, sensing the presence of a force or person not actually present)
  (9) marked lack of initiative, interests, or energy
E. It cannot be established that an organic factor initiated and maintained the disturbance.
F. If there is a history of Autistic Disorder, the additional diagnosis of Schizophrenia is made only if prominent delusions or hallucinations are also present.

From American Psychiatric Association. *Diagnostic and statistical manual of mental disorders.* 3rd Ed., Rev. (DSM-III-R). Washington, DC: American Psychiatric Association Press, 1987.

patient may be traveling on a bus and believe that a passenger's leaving the bus at a particular stop has a special message for him. Thinking may be altered both in content and in form. During conversation, ideas are typically presented vaguely, with the person shifting from one thought to another without a logical connection. There is poverty in depth of information conveyed, and the listener often finds the conversation hard to follow.

Another characteristic feature of schizophrenia is the presence of *hallucinations,* reflecting disturbed perceptions such as hearing voices or seeing things. Auditory hallucinations are most commonly associated with schizophrenia, but other sensory modalities such as visual, tactile, and olfactory senses may also be implicated. Auditory hallucinations involve the perception of outside voices that comment on and discuss the behavior of the affected person, typically in a negative and derogatory manner.

In schizophrenia, *affect* (the outward expression of mood) can be altered in a number of ways. Affective expression can be minimal or absent in face, voice, or gestures, resulting in "flat" affect. A mismatch between affective expression and external circumstances, called *inappropriate affect,* often occurs. For example, a patient may talk about a painful event and smile or laugh while telling the story. Impairment of the capacity for social interactions is evident in a lack of interpersonal relatedness, social withdrawal, and detachment. Many other components of behavior are disturbed in schizophrenia. For example, disturbances in motor activity may be manifested by stereotypic repetitive movements or bizarre gesturing.

It thus seems that the very aspects of behavior that make us distinctly human are diminished in schizophrenia. Since the onset of this disorder typically occurs in adolescence or early adulthood, a period in life which is commonly associated with considerable academic, professional, and interpersonal challenges, individuals who develop schizophrenia are frequently placed at particular social and economic jeopardy.

Subtypes

There are five subtypes of schizophrenia. The disease as presented in DSM-III-R includes the *catatonic, disorganized, paranoid, undifferentiated, and residual subtypes.* The catatonic type, which is encountered infrequently, is characterized by severe psychomotor disturbance including stupor, rigidity, excitement, and posturing. The disorganized type is marked by incoherence, disorganized behavior, and flat or inappropriate affect. The paranoid type is noted for a preoccupation with systematized delusions or auditory hallucinations. The undifferentiated type includes pronounced psychotic symptoms that might not fit any other specific category or might fit more than one. In the residual type there has been at least one episode of schizophrenia with persistent signs of illness but without prominent psychotic features.

In the past decade there has been a revival of interest in categorizing symptoms in a manner that links them to brain function. This movement was stimulated by the classic studies of the British neurologist John Hughlings Jackson, who attempted to classify behavioral manifestations of brain damage into *negative* and *positive* categories. Negative symptoms are deficits in behavior manifested by a lack of a behavioral output, which are thought to reflect anatomic changes related to loss of brain tissue. Such behaviors include, for example, lack of initiation and lack of motivation. In contrast, positive or productive symptoms are manifested by increased behavioral output, suggesting physiological abnormalities. Since some symptoms of schizophrenia can be classified as negative (alogia, affective flattening, withdrawal, loss of motivation) and some as positive (delusions, hallucinations, thought disorder, and bizarre behavior), the existence of two types of schizophrenia has been postulated. Type I is speculated to have predominantly positive symptoms and no brain atrophy, whereas type II is characterized by negative symptoms and disturbed brain anatomy. However, most studies have reported that the majority of patients with schizophrenia have a mixture of negative and positive symptoms and cannot be categorized by this typology.

Prevalence and Course

Schizophrenia affects approximately 1% of the population, including approximately equal numbers of men and women, but with an earlier onset in men. It is more frequent in lower sociodemographic groups, suggesting a "downward drift" of affected individuals who cannot maintain their previous level of functioning.

There is considerable variability in the course of the illness. The active phase is usually marked by overt psychotic symptoms (as described above) that lead to the need for hospitalization and vigorous treatment. This active phase is often preceded by a period of gradual, insidious deterioration in functioning that affects all spheres of life: personal appearance, interests, and social relations. This prodromal phase is often hard to identify as a discrete psychiatric problem at the time and may only be appreciated in hindsight, following the development of the active phase. For example, a college freshman might have difficulties adjusting to the new environment, perform poorly in school, and have difficulty forming friendships. These behavioral patterns might simply reflect a problem in adjustment. Schizophrenia would be suspected if the student showed distinct signs of psychotic behavior in addition to the indications of gradual deterioration in function.

While recovery from the active phase of schizophrenia is variable, only about 10% of affected individuals return to the previous level of functioning. Patients with residual impairment typically suffer exacerbations (about 50%), and some go on to have a chronic course of illness, requiring long-term care and treatment (40%).

Treatment and Outcome

Drugs are the cornerstone of treatment. The introduction in the 1950s of anti-psychotic medication revolutionized the treatment of schizophrenia. The structure of the initial antipsychotic drug chlorpromazine is shown in Fig. 1. These agents are efficacious in reducing psychotic symptoms, and their use has resulted in shorter periods of hospitalization and better functioning of patients in the community. Treatment outcome is variable and can roughly be divided into three categories. About one third of patients respond well and recover fully from the first episode of illness with few recurrent episodes. Another third of patients continue to manifest exacerbations and remissions without significant decline between episodes. The final third never recover completely and progressive deterioration is evident.

Treatment with antipsychotic drugs is associated with a number of significant limitations. While their short-term effects on acute psychotic behavior such as agitation, thought disorder, or hallucination have been demonstrated, the time course of patients' responses to antipsychotic medication is not clear, nor is the drugs' role in the care of the chronically ill. Furthermore, antipsychotic drugs have early- and late-onset side effects, particularly of the extrapyramidal motor system (brain structures affecting body movements, excluding motor neurons, motor cortex, and the pyramidal tract). These abnormal movement disorders, including parkinsonism (rigidity of movement, mask-like faces), dystonia (abnormal tone), akathisia (inability to remain in a sitting posture, with motor restlessness), and dyskinesia (difficulty in performing voluntary movements), are thought to be related to the potency of the antipsychotic drugs in blocking dopamine receptors. Concurrent use of anticholinergic agents can

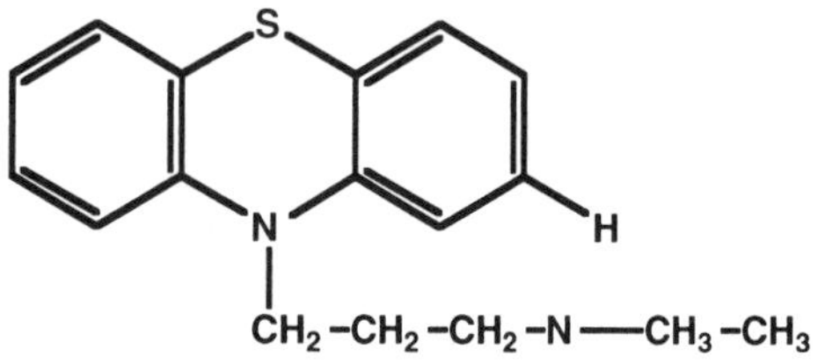

FIG. 1. Structure of the typical antipsychotic drug chlorpromazine.

ameliorate some of the extrapyramidal side effects. It is evident, however, that in most cases moderate doses of antipsychotic drugs are sufficient, and high doses are not more effective. Longitudinal studies suggest that about one third of patients relapse within a year while on medication, whereas two thirds of patients off medication relapse within that period.

Other factors besides medication can affect the treatment outcome. Outcome is affected not only by compliance with the medication regimen, but also by the aftercare program and support available to patients in the community. Also, patients who manifest less dysfunction and who have fewer negative symptoms during the active phase appear to have a better long-term prognosis.

The fact that some chronic schizophrenic patients do not respond to antipsychotic drugs and that these agents can produce neurotoxic effects has prompted a search for compounds with antipsychotic properties but without extrapyramidal side effects. Clozapine, which has serotonin receptor blockade effects and antinoradrenergic properties, was recently introduced in the United States for the treatment of patients with schizophrenia who do not respond adequately to treatment with typical antipsychotic drugs. The structure of clozapine is presented in Fig. 2. In a multicenter clinical trial it was found that 30% of patients who failed to respond to typical antipsychotic drugs showed improvement of both positive and negative symptoms after short-term treatment with clozapine. In Europe, where clozapine has had long-term use, studies indicate that about

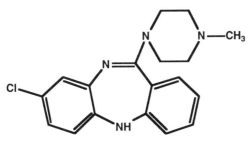

FIG. 2. Structure of the atypical antipsychotic drug clozapine.

two thirds of patients show moderate to substantial improvement after being on the drug for over 3 years. Patients treated with clozapine require close monitoring since a potential complication is agranulocytosis (suppression of the white blood cells, which can have fatal consequences). It is hoped that other novel agents will be developed that offer high benefits and lower risks.

BRAIN–BEHAVIOR RELATIONSHIPS

Many of the discrete clinical features of schizophrenia suggest a linkage to aberrant functioning in specific brain regions or networks. Brain regulation of behavior is examined in clinical populations by correlating behavioral deficits with clinical signs, postmortem findings, and, more recently, neuroimaging data (see Chapter 15). The surge of interest in examining the neurobiology of schizophrenia has resulted in increased application of neurobehavioral techniques in the search for brain networks and mechanisms that may be dysfunctional in schizophrenia. There is a large body of research on brain–behavior relations that can aid this endeavor.

Depending on location, brain lesions typically affect a functional system or network. Anterior lesions acting on the frontal brain system can disrupt most higher level cognitive operations by causing a disorganization of goal-directed behavior, particularly attentional processing and conceptual flexibility (see Chapter 15). Often identified as "executive" deficits, this impairment can affect multiple processes such as decision making and abstract thinking. In contrast, temporal lobe lesions, particularly of the medial temporal lobe region including the hippocampus and amygdala, are associated with deficits in memory and learning of new information. Subcortical systems, in particular the basal ganglia, have also been examined in imaging studies of schizophrenia. Perceptual-motor integration, fine motor skills, spatial ability, and procedural memory are putative neurobehavioral functions of the basal ganglia. Numerous dopamine pathways from the basal ganglia innervate regions of the two frontal lobes. Moreover, dopamine receptors in the basal ganglia are inhibited at the concentration of antipsychotic drugs used to treat schizophrenic patients. Such inhibition is responsible for the prominent neurological side effects (*extrapyramidal effects*) associated with antipsychotic drug therapy, as described previously.

Evidence supporting the link between aberrant brain functioning and abnormal behaviors seen in schizophrenia is based on similarities between behavioral consequences of brain lesions and abnormal behaviors seen in schizophrenia. For example, patients with frontal lobe lesions typically show impaired thought processes, lack of initiation of spontaneous behaviors, flat affect, and poor reality testing. Thus it seems reasonable to suggest that some schizophrenic patients with a pattern of such disorders also have frontal lobe dysfunction. Indeed, involvement of anterior brain systems, particularly the frontal lobes, has been suggested by studies demonstrating deficits in higher level abstraction and mental flexibility. Hallucinations, delusions, and positive thought disorder seem to be associated with temporolimbic structures. Poverty of speech and its content and form, as well as illogical thinking, are features suggestive of left hemisphere dysfunction (see Chapter 15). Involvement of the left hemisphere has also been implicated by deficits in verbal cognitive functions, for example, low verbal IQ relative to performance IQ and impairment on language tests. The positive symptoms (e.g., hallucinations and delusions) and pronounced decline in intellectual functioning (e.g., cognitive, perceptual, and attentional deficits) also suggest that subcortical-cortical modulation is impaired. Subcortical and cortical dysfunction have been implicated by studies of attention and information processing. The extensive interconnectivity between the frontal lobes and diencephalic limbic and reticular structures suggests that subcortical systems are potential sites for disruption of attentional processes via impaired selective gaiting of information. Mesulam has pro-

posed a neural network for attention that involves components of parietal, temporal, and frontal cortex as well as the cingulate gyrus and subcortical limbic regions. Some investigators have suggested that deficits in attention may provide a biological marker of schizophrenia. Interestingly, genetic studies of children of patients with schizophrenia have demonstrated attentional deficits that are similar in both the affected and unaffected children.

Application of a battery of tests that assess a range of behavioral functions and implicated brain regions permits evaluation of the relative involvement of frontal lobe and temporal lobe impairment by evaluating the performance of patients by means of testing procedures designed to measure functions associated with these brain regions. Specifically, the frontal lobe hypothesis predicts that patients are more impaired on abstraction relative to memory and learning tests, whereas the temporal lobe hypothesis predicts the reverse.

In a sample of schizophrenic patients and normal controls we found that patients were impaired on tests of both abstraction and memory. However, the impairment in memory and learning was significantly more pronounced than the impairment in abstraction. This effect, which supports a selective temporal lobe deficit in schizophrenia, existed for both men and women, across the age range (18 to 45), for all educational levels, and for both highly cooperative and less cooperative patients (Fig. 3).

While these findings implicate temporal lobe impairment in schizophrenia, they do not clarify the extent of involvement of the frontal lobe. Thus, it is important to determine how abstraction and memory compare with other functions. Conceivably, both could be superior or inferior to the general level of performance. We compared each to the other functions assessed by the neuropsychological battery and found that abstraction was significantly better in patients relative to their average neuropsychological performance, whereas memory and learning were

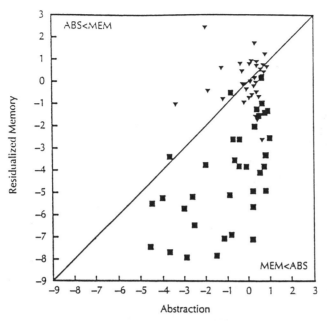

FIG. 3. Relationship of global memory and learning scores (MEM) to abstraction (ABS) for patients (squares) and controls (triangles). Memory data points are standardized residualized scores based on predicted scores given performance on abstraction. Scores below the diagonal identity line indicate worse performance for memory and learning than abstraction; points on the identity line, equal performance. From Saykin AJ, et al. Neuropsychological function in schizophrenia: selective impairment in memory and learning. *Arch Gen Psychiatry* 1991:48:618–624. Copyright 1991, AMA.

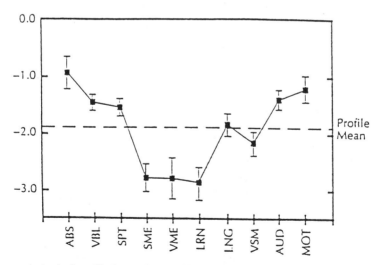

FIG. 4. Neuropsychological profile for patients with schizophrenia relative to controls whose performance is set to zero. Functions are abstraction (ABS), verbal-cognitive (VBL), spatial organization (SPT), semantic memory (SME), visual memory (VME), verbal learning (LRN), language (LNG), visual-motor processing and attention (VSM), auditory processing and attention (AUD), and motor speed and sequencing (MOT). From Saykin AJ, et al. Neuropsychological function in schizophrenia: selective impairment in memory and learning. *Arch Gen Psychiatry* 1991;48:618–624. Copyright 1991, AMA.

significantly worse than all other functions (Fig. 4).

But even this strong support for the temporal lobe hypothesis relative to the frontal lobe hypothesis does not settle the issue of identifying specific regional brain dysfunction. The memory deficit could be ubiquitous and robust and may indeed point to temporal lobe dysfunction, and yet a constellation of other deficits can suggest other brain regions that might be implicated as well. Thus, there is a need for systematic evaluation of a combined set of neuropsychological data in relation to current theories of brain-behavior regulation. This approach would permit the identification of impaired neural networks. The nature of the brain disease we expect to find in schizophrenia is not a focal lesion with circumscribed boundaries and effects but more likely a disorder involving neurotransmitter systems with distributed physiological effects. Given that, it would be a mistake to find an area of greatest abnormality and declare it the "site of schizophrenia." Rather, further studies are needed to explore systematically the functional state of central nervous system networks in schizophrenia. This objective requires the integration of neuropsychological testing with hypotheses linking them to the pathophysiology of the disorder.

PATHOPHYSIOLOGY

Schizophrenia is probably familial. The evidence is strong that schizophrenia is a familial disorder. Studies of relatives, twins, and adoptees suggest familial aggregation that is largely due to genetic factors (see Chapter 16). It is possible that genetic vulnerability interacts with other factors such as perinatal insult. Hypotheses regarding the pathophysiology of schizophrenia have been pursued vigorously as investigators in the field of biological psychiatry have developed a range of methodologies to investigate the neurobiology of the disorder. A complete account of these developments is beyond the scope of this chapter, but some salient progress that holds future promise is discussed below.

Neuropharmacology

Drugs that decrease DA neurotransmission decrease symptoms of schizophrenia. The involvement of dopamine (DA) in schizophrenia has received considerable attention. The DA hypothesis is based on evidence that pharmacological agents that increase synaptic levels of DA, such as amphetamine, exacerbate positive symptoms in schizophrenic patients and induce schizophrenic-type symptoms in some normal controls. Drugs that decrease synaptic levels of DA, such as reserpine, or that block DA receptors, such as the antipsychotic agents used in the treatment of schizophrenia, diminish these symptoms. Of note is that the positive symptoms respond to the antipsychotic drugs, and the clinical potency of these agents is related to their activity at the D_2 subtype of the DA receptor (see Chapter 4). Postmortem studies have shown increased D_2 receptor density (50% to 200%) in the striatum of patients with schizophrenia relative to controls. While treatment with antipsychotic drugs may account for some of these findings, it does not fully account for them since some of the patients in the studies were not treated with antipsychotic drugs. The role of the D_1 subtype of DA receptor, which is positively coupled to adenylyl cyclase, and the interactions between D_1 and D_2 receptors, are topics of current investigations. The interactions of DA with other neurotransmitters such as serotonin, norepinephrine, and γ-aminobutyric acid (GABA) are also being studied.

Neuroanatomy

There is a growing literature linking certain neuroanatomic findings to schizophrenia. Neuroimaging methods provide data on the neuroanatomic and neurophysiological substrates of behavior. Regarding anatomy, there is a large body of literature on the application of computed tomography (CT) to the study of brain structure in schizophrenia. Several reports suggest that some patients with schizophrenia have more cerebrospinal fluid (CSF) in the brain ventricles than normal controls. Most studies have examined the lateral ventricles since they contain the largest body of CSF that can be identified accurately and reliably. The technique of magnetic resonance imaging (MRI) is a recent addition to schizophrenia research, offering better resolution and the capacity to examine brain volume and CSF volume in ventricles and sulci of the brain. Sample MRIs from a normal control (Fig. 5A) and from two patients with schizophrenia of the same age (Fig. 5B and C) are illustrative.

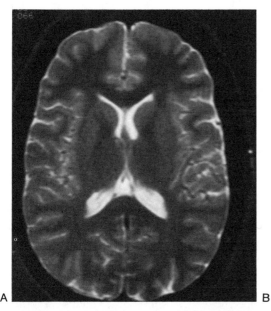

A

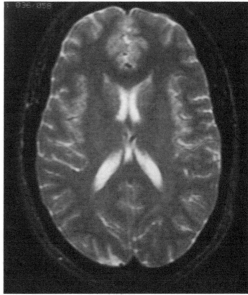

B

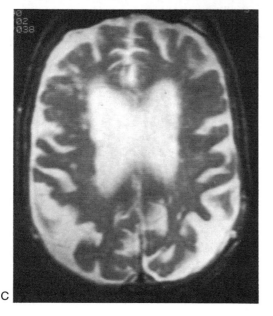

C

FIG. 5. (A) MRI of a normal control. Note the CSF in ventricles and sulci (white) where it is barely visible. **(B, C)** MRI of two patients with schizophrenia. Note greater prominence of CSF in **(B)** and marked prominence in **(C)**.

The literature on brain structure in schizophrenia is growing rapidly. In addition to separation of brain tissue from CSF (see Chapter 15), CSF can be examined in ventricles and in sulci (Fig. 5C). Examination of volumes of specific structures is feasible, and reduced volume of the left temporal lobe has been reported in schizophrenic patients. This ties in with the findings of impaired memory described above. Thus, the ability to measure the volume of specific brain structures permits examination of hypotheses on the relationship between abnormalities in these regions and the aberrant behavior manifested in schizophrenia. Moreover, changes in brain volume can also be related to neuropathological investigations of brain abnormalities in postmortem tissue. Indeed, a number of recent studies have found abnormalities in the hippocampus and related limbic structures in brains of patients with schizophrenia.

Associations between structural abnormalities and clinical variables such as premorbid level of functioning, symptoms, response to treatment, and course of illness have received attention. While no firm conclusions can yet be drawn, it appears that the abnormalities observed are not a result of treatment since they are evident in newly diagnosed patients with schizophrenia who have not received treatment. Furthermore, there is no evidence that these abnormalities are progressive. The changes observed are more likely to be static lesions that relate in part to pregnancy and birth complications.

Neurophysiology

A range of physiological neuroimaging methods exists for assessing different parameters of brain function, and several of these methods have been applied to the study of schizophrenia. Neuroimaging methods applied to schizophrenia include electroencephalography (EEG) and evoked potentials, for measuring the electrical activity of the brain; regional cerebral blood flow (rCBF) determination with xenon-133; single-photon emission computed tomography (SPECT), for measuring rCBF as well as the density of neuroreceptors; and positron emission tomography (PET) for measuring glucose metabolism, rCBF, and density of neuroreceptors. Except for EEG, these methods rely on the administration of a radioactive ligand whose brain activity can be measured via a scanner with special detectors that count radioactivity in the brain.

To illustrate the application of these methods in advancing the understanding of brain function in schizophrenia, a few avenues of research can be summarized. Physiological studies examining regional brain abnormalities in schizophrenia have usually been conducted under resting conditions. Initial reports suggested diffusely reduced cerebral blood flow (CBF) and metabolism and evidence for *hypofrontality,* a relatively decreased activity in the frontal lobes. In studies with the xenon-133 method for measuring rCBF (see Chapter 15) that tested young patients who were never medicated or who were treated for a relatively short period, resting rCBF was normal or even higher than normal. This underscores the importance of considering such factors as age and medication in studies attempting to evaluate disease-specific effects on measurements of brain activity.

The application of physiological neuroimaging techniques to psychiatric populations may be enhanced when combined with activation procedures or neurobehavioral probes (see Chapter 15). Since the behavioral abnormalities of schizophrenia may occur in response to environmental triggers, regional abnormalities in brain activity may be undetected at rest but may become apparent in the pattern of changes in activity produced by task activation. Few studies have examined both resting and activated conditions in schizophrenia. We have initially concentrated on examining the laterality hypothesis (suggesting an abnormal pattern of hemispheric activity) by using verbal and spatial tasks that normally activate the left and right hemispheres, respectively. We found pronounced abnormalities in the asymmetry of activation for the tasks. Schizophrenics failed to show the normal left hemispheric activation for a defined verbal task and showed a "paradoxical" left hemispheric activation for a spatial task. This supports the hypothesis, based on previous behavioral studies, that schizophrenia is associated with left hemispheric dysfunction and overactivation of the left dysfunctional hemisphere. In addition, greater activity of the left hemisphere was associated with increased severity of symptoms. At the National Institute of Mental Health, Weinberger and colleagues, also using the xenon-133 inhalation technique for measuring rCBF, examined the hypothesis of disturbed frontal lobe function in schizophrenia. They reported that schizophrenics failed to show the normal increase in dorsolateral frontal activity during the performance of an abstraction task. Performance on this test is affected by frontal lobe damage.

Most PET studies in schizophrenia have used the ligands [^{18}F]fluorodeoxyglucose (FDG) for measuring cerebral glucose metabolism and ^{15}O-labeled water for measuring CBF (see Chapter 15). More recently, several ligands have been used to examine the density of DA receptors in the brain. Studies conducted to date have included somewhat varied patient samples as well as different conditions of uptake and image and data analysis. In addition, most reports have been based on relatively small samples. Different studies have reported abnormalities in three major brain dimensions: anterior-posterior (lower frontal activity ratios), lateral (higher left activity associated with severity of disease), and cortical-subcortical (lower ratios). Most of these studies were performed during a resting state.

Although the majority of PET studies in schizophrenia have used FDG, as pointed out, no consistent body of data has emerged to date. This circumstance is explained by several factors including the heterogeneity of the disorder, small sample size, variable medications, cross-sectional designs, and limited resolution of the PET scanners. Few PET FDG studies have attempted to address the relationship between pharmacological intervention and cerebral metabolism. Figure 6 presents an example of glucose metabolism in a single patient and in a single normal control.

The ability to study receptor density with PET provides the opportunity to test the dopamine hypothesis and find out, as new ligands are developed, whether other receptor systems are implicated. Two research groups have reported findings using D$_2$ receptor ligands. Investigators at Johns Hopkins University found an increase in the density of D$_2$ receptors in antipsychotic drug-naive patients, whereas in Sweden investigators at the Karolinska Institute, using a different D$_2$ ligand, did not find differences between drug-

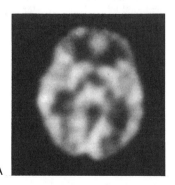 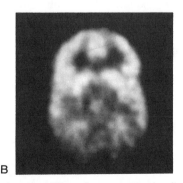

A   B

FIG. 6. PET glucose metabolism of a young normal control (**A**) and an untreated patient with schizophrenia (**B**) who is presenting for the first time. The basal ganglia appear more prominent in the patient.

naive patients and controls. The studies differed in many other ways including patient characteristics and analysis methods. The methodological differences among studies limit comparisons.

Thus, while progress has been made in the study of schizophrenia using neuroimaging methods, such studies should become more productive as the techniques undergo further development and their application broadens.

SUMMARY

Schizophrenia is a prevalent and devastating psychiatric disorder that afflicts the young and has lifelong consequences. Developments in the neurosciences have made it possible to identify brain abnormalities in what was previously considered a functional disorder. We are not yet at the state of knowledge where firm conclusions can be drawn regarding the specific brain structures or systems that are dysfunctional. Work to date has consistently suggested that schizophrenia is associated with diffuse brain abnormalities, with greater involvement of left hemisphere and frontotemporal regions. However, this is only the beginning of what is likely to be a far-reaching effort in upcoming decades. Most likely, given the complexity and heterogeneity of schizophrenia, an integration will be needed of genetic, neuroanatomic, neurochemical, neuropharmacological, and neurophysiological data, from a developmental perspective, to explain the behavioral manifestations.

BIBLIOGRAPHY

Original Articles

Baldessarini RJ, Cohen BM, Teicher MH. Significance of neuroleptic dose and plasma level in the pharmacological treatment of psychosis. *Arch Gen Psychiatry* 1988;45:79–91.

Gur RE, Mozley PD, Resnick SM, Levick S, Erwin R, Saykin AJ, et al. Relations among clinical scales in schizophrenia: overlap and subtypes. *Am J Psychiatry* 1991;148:472–478.

Kane J, Honigfeld G, Singer J, Meltzer H. Clozapine for the treatment-resistant schizophrenic. *Arch Gen Psychiatry* 1988;45:789–796.

Saykin AJ, Gur RC, Gur RE, Mozley D, Mozley LH, Resnick SM, et al. Neuropsychological function in schizophrenia: selective impairment in memory and learning. *Arch Gen Psychiatry* 1991;48:618–624.

Weinberger DR. Implications of normal brain development for the pathogenesis of schizophrenia. *Arch Gen Psychiatry* 1987;44:660–669.

Books and Reviews

American Psychiatric Association. *Diagnostic and statistical manual of mental disorders.* 3rd Ed., Rev. (DSM-III-R). Washington, D.C.: American Psychiatric Association Press; 1987.

Andreasen NC. The diagnosis of schizophrenia. *Schizophr Bull* 1987;13:9–22.

Barchas JD. Biochemical aspects of the psychotic disorders. In: Siegel GJ, Agranoff BW, Albers RW, Molinoff PB, eds. *Basic neurochemistry,* 5th ed. New York: Raven Press; 1994 (in press).

Carpenter WT. Approaches to knowledge and understanding of schizophrenia. *Schizophr Bull* 1987;13:1–8.

Crow TJ. Molecular pathology of schizophrenia: more than one disease process? *Br Med J* 1980;280:66–68.

Gur RE, Gur RC, Saykin AJ. Neurobehavioral studies in schizophrenia: implications for regional brain dysfunction. *Schizophr Bull* 1990;16:445–451.

Meltzer HY. Biological studies in schizophrenia. *Schizophr Bull* 1987;13:77–111.

Schizophrenia Bulletin. Frontal lobes, basal ganglia, temporal lobes. Three sites for schizophrenia? (issue theme: neuroimaging) 1990;16(3).

19

Anxiety Disorders

Andrew Winokur

It was an unhappy life that I lived, and its one dominant anxiety, towering over all its other anxieties like a high mountain above a range of mountains, never disappeared from my view. Still, no new cause for fear arose. Let me start from my bed as I would, with the terror fresh upon me that he was discovered; let me sit listening as I would with dread, for Herbert's returning step at night, lest it should be fleeter than ordinary, and winged with evil new; for all that, and much more to like purpose, the round of things went on. Condemned to inaction and a state of constant restlessness and suspense, I rowed about in my boat, and waited, waited, waited, as I best could.

Charles Dickens,
Great Expectations, 1861

- Clinically significant anxiety typically produces pronounced effects on emotional state, behavior, cognitive function, and a variety of physiological parameters.

- There are several rating scales for the assessment of anxiety.

- Currently there are five recognized subgroups of anxiety disorder: panic, generalized, obsessive-compulsive, phobias, and post-traumatic stress disorders.

- Panic disorder is characterized by the abrupt onset of intense symptoms of anxiety.

- Generalized anxiety disorder is characterized by gradually developing, persistent patterns of anxiety.

- Obsessive-compulsive disorder is characterized by recurrent obsessions and/or compulsions that cause significant distress and interfere with the individual's functioning.

- A phobia is characterized by strong fear of a specific situation.

- Post-traumatic stress disorder involves the development of characteristic symptoms of anxiety, fears, or terror in the aftermath of exposure to an intense, psychologically stressful event.

- The delineation of discrete subgroups of anxiety disorders has made specific therapeutic recommendations possible.

- The benzodiazepines were the first class of drugs to show widespread applicability in the treatment of anxiety.

- The abrupt discontinuation of a benzodiazepine can bring on severe withdrawal.

- Buspirone has an efficacy similar to that of the benzodiazepines, but has a different structure, different speed of onset, and fewer side effects.

- The discovery of the presence of benzodiazepine receptors in the brain was important in defining the mechanism of action of these compounds.

- Benzodiazepines act on receptors located on a macromolecular complex in conjunction with GABA receptors and chloride ion channels.

- Techniques of molecular biology are now being applied to investigation of drug-receptor interactions.

- Animal fight-or-flight experiments suggested a causal link between secretion of adrenalin (epinephrine) and anxiety.

- Serotonin has been implicated as a factor in obsessive-compulsive disorder.

This chapter begins with a discussion of the manifestations and clinical assessment of anxiety. There follows a review of the current definitions of anxiety disorders and a discussion of the pharmacological therapies available to treat these disorders. Finally, the biological theories proposed to explain the origins of the anxiety disorders are discussed.

This chapter deals with a heterogeneous group of psychiatric illnesses referred to as the anxiety disorders. While the term *anxiety* is widely used by both physicians and the lay public, this expression may be employed in a number of different ways. Thus, anxiety may be used to describe (1) a normal and expectable human emotion (e.g., a student who feels tense and apprehensive prior to an important examination), (2) a symptom commonly observed in conjunction with other psychiatric or medical illnesses, or (3) a set of specific psychiatric illnesses. The fact that the term anxiety has several different connotations potentially creates considerable confusion around this topic.

Because anxiety is such a universal human experience, most people have at least an intuitive sense of what is meant by this term. Nevertheless, developing a consistent, clear definition of anxiety and distinguishing this entity from closely related concepts such as fear represents a more challenging task. Prototypically, fear pertains to a state of physiological arousal and heightened behavioral responsivity in the context of environmental conditions that are threatening to the organism's survival. In contrast, the term anxiety is generally used to describe a state of mental distress and physiological arousal in the absence of threatening environmental circumstances.

It is of interest that human anxiety represents an outgrowth of basic instinctual behaviors in very primitive species. The expression *fight-or-flight response* was used by the American physiologist Walter Cannon to describe the complex array of physiological responses that animals across the phylogenetic spectra demonstrate as a means of surviving threatening situations. These physiological arousal mechanisms maximize the organism's chances to survive threatening situations, either by fleeing and escaping or by mounting an aggressive response. In humans, numerous symptoms reflecting arousal of the sympathetic component of the autonomic nervous system are observed at times of stress, threat, or anxiety. Such symptoms as rapid pulse, palpitations, sweating palms, tremulousness, and butterflies in the stomach that are of little or no survival value for man represent evolutionary vestiges of the fight-or-flight response. Yet these and other related symptoms are often experienced as being extremely unpleasant and intrusive. In some individuals, these symptoms may become chronic and enduring, they may interfere significantly with the subject's functioning, and in some cases they may be associated with the development of significant psychological impairment, medical dysfunction, or even suicide.

MANIFESTATIONS OF CLINICAL ANXIETY

Clinically significant anxiety typically produces pronounced effects on emotional state, behavior, cognitive function, and a variety of physiological parameters. Since anxiety is a ubiquitous human emotion, a physician faces the challenge of determining when its manifestations represent a clinically signifi-

Biological Bases of Brain Function and Disease, edited by Alan Frazer, Perry B. Molinoff, and Andrew Winokur. Raven Press, Ltd., New York © 1994.

cant problem. There is no single symptom or laboratory finding that makes it possible to establish the diagnosis of an anxiety disorder. Rather, identification of a complex array of symptoms existing over a period of time provides the basis for arriving at a discrete diagnosis.

ASSESSMENT OF ANXIETY

There are several rating scales for the assessment of anxiety. Anxiety is a symptom that is present in many patients seen by clinicians in various medical and psychiatric settings, and it can represent a considerable diagnostic challenge. In some situations, the presence of clinically significant anxiety is not recognized, as the patient is preoccupied with specific physiological symptoms such as cardiac palpitations or gastrointestinal discomfort, which appear to indicate a purely medical problem. Such a patient may undergo many complicated medical diagnostic tests but never receive appropriate treatment for the anxiety. In other instances, symptoms of anxiety represent the primary focus of the patient's concern, yet these symptoms may represent only a part of a broader psychiatric syndrome, such as depression.

In recent years, several rating scales have been developed to facilitate the assessment of anxiety. Using one such scale, the Self-Rating Anxiety Scale, Zung and coworkers found that clinically significant levels of anxiety were observed in 9% of a normal adult population, 32% of patients seen in a medical general practice setting, 52% of patients with diagnosed heart disease, and 71% of a heterogeneous group of psychiatric patients. The results of this study provide an indication of the variation in the frequency of symptom levels of anxiety across different populations.

In another study, Mallinger and coworkers employed a symptom checklist self-rating scale to obtain information on symptoms of *psychic distress* in a group of 2,552 subjects selected from diverse communities across the United States. In this survey of randomly selected American adults, 27% indicated that they had experienced significant levels of psychiatric distress during the year prior to the interview, with the incidence of significant emotional symptomatology being almost twice as high in women as in men. These findings emphatically underscore that symptoms of emotional distress (frequently involving manifestations of anxiety) occur in a significant proportion of adults. Rating scale scores, however, do not provide a reliable basis for establishing discrete diagnoses. Thus, while the symptoms of anxiety are frequently encountered, considerable care is needed to establish specific diagnoses of anxiety disorders.

DIAGNOSIS

Currently there are five recognized subgroups of anxiety disorder: panic, generalized, obsessive-compulsive, phobias, and post-traumatic stress disorders. Descriptions of individuals apparently suffering with anxiety disorders have appeared in the literature for many centuries, dating back at least to the writings of the ancient Greeks. The term *neurasthenia* was employed by Beard in 1869 to describe the illness of a group of patients that would correspond reasonably closely to current concepts of anxiety disorders. In the latter part of the nineteenth century, Freud provided detailed descriptions of clinical anxiety disorders. An important component of Freud's theory involved distinguishing between anxiety deriving from external sources and anxiety emanating internally as a consequence of intrapsychic conflicts. He used the expression *anxiety neurosis* to describe the latter condition, and this term became the most commonly applied diagnosis of anxiety disorders for the next 80 years.

A limitation to the diagnostic expression anxiety neurosis was the fact that it was applied to a heterogeneous cross section of patients who had in common certain clinical features of anxiety. However, employing a very broad diagnostic approach can potentially obscure the existence of significant subsets of patients within that category. In recent years, a major development in the diagnosis and treatment of anxiety disorders has been the pronounced increase in attention to the process of arriving at careful, systematic diagnoses. In 1980, the *Diagnostic and Statistical Manual,* Third Edition (DSM-III) was published. This text is the officially recognized reference for psychiatric diagnoses in the United States. DSM-III reflected advances in the process of making reliable and meaningful diagnoses based on clearly delineated criteria. This refined approach to the process of making psychiatric diagnoses had a major impact on concepts about the anxiety disorders. In particular, it provided a basis for identifying distinct subgroups of anxiety disorder patients who may differ in a number of important ways, including clinical symptoms, family history, recommended forms of treatment, and biochemical and neurobiological characteristics.

The DSM-III-R (revised edition), published in 1987, describes the overarching clinical features of these disorders as symptoms of anxiety and/or avoidance behavior. Five general categories of anxiety disorders are included: panic disorder, generalized anxiety disorder, obsessive-compulsive disorder, phobic disorders, and post-traumatic stress syndrome. A brief review of each of these disorders follows.

Panic Disorder

Panic disorder is characterized by the abrupt onset of intense symptoms of anxiety. In addition to the central symptom of fast-onset anxiety, panic disorder may include feelings of fear, terror, or dread; a sense of losing control or impending death; shortness of breath; dizziness; a choking sensation; palpitations; sweating; flushing; trembling; numbness; nausea; and a sense of unreality. Typically, a panic attack will last for minutes to hours and then gradually subside. Some panic attacks occur within the context of a situation that is stressful for the individual

(e.g., being stuck in traffic or caught in a crowd), but it is also common for a panic attack to occur without any known trigger. Many individuals are able to recall vividly the first panic attack they ever experienced. Following the initial attack, the subject may not experience any subsequent problems for weeks or months. Eventually, however, a second panic attack is likely to occur, often followed more quickly by a third. The panic attacks may occur with greater frequency over time. DSM-III-R criteria require a frequency of three panic attacks in a 3-week period, but the rate may be much higher than that. In addition, the subject may become preoccupied with concerns about subsequent attacks and thus develop anticipatory anxiety. Some individuals manifest an associated condition referred to as *agoraphobia,* which literally means "fear of the marketplace." They become extremely apprehensive about being in public places in which they feel they are not in control or from which they may not readily be able to escape. Such individuals may have great difficulty in going out of the house and may do so only when accompanied by someone they trust. In extreme cases, an individual may become completely housebound.

Panic disorder is typically a disease affecting young people (i.e., persons in their mid-20s), and it occurs approximately twice as often in women as in men. Family studies and twin studies have suggested that panic disorder represents a separate or distinct entity from other forms of anxiety disorder, such as generalized anxiety disorder. For example, in a study by Crowe and coworkers, first-degree relatives of patients with panic disorder had a much higher incidence of panic disorder (25%) than did relatives of normal controls (2%). In contrast, relatives of patients with generalized anxiety disorder did not show a significant increase in panic disorder.

Generalized Anxiety Disorder

Generalized anxiety disorder is characterized by gradually developing, persistent pat-

terns of anxiety. Generalized anxiety disorder is defined in DSM-III-R on the basis of unrealistic or excessive anxiety about two or more life circumstances for 6 months or longer. Thus, in order to qualify for this diagnosis, an individual must have significant concerns about more than a single situation, and the symptoms must persist for a considerable period of time. In addition, the subject must demonstrate signs of motor tension (trembling, shaking, restlessness), autonomic hyperactivity (shortness of breath, palpitations, rapid heart rate), and vigilance and scanning (feeling keyed up, exaggerated startle response, trouble concentrating, insomnia, irritability).

It is apparent that many of the symptoms of generalized anxiety disorder overlap with those seen in panic disorder. However, a key point of distinction between panic disorder and generalized anxiety disorder involves the intense periods of anxiety that characterize panic disorder, whereas generalized anxiety disorder is manifested by slower onset, persistent patterns of anxiety. Patients with generalized anxiety disorder may demonstrate intermittent or chronic, continuous periods of anxiety. As noted above, family studies have also suggested that panic disorder and generalized anxiety disorder represent distinct illnesses in terms of genetic predisposition.

Obsessive-Compulsive Disorder

Obsessive-compulsive disorder is characterized by recurrent obsessions and/or compulsions that cause significant distress and interfere with the individual's functioning. The term *obsession* refers to a persistent idea or impulse. It is important to note that these ideas or impulses are experienced by the subject as being foreign, intrusive, and senseless. Examples of obsessions include thoughts of violence or concerns about contamination by germs or dirt. The term *compulsion* refers to an intentional, repetitive behavior that is performed in an effort to deal with an obsession and reduce the anxiety it causes. Examples of

compulsive behaviors include handwashing, counting, and repeated checking of prior actions (e.g., locking the door, turning off the stove).

Obsessive-compulsive disorder (OCD) is frequently associated with manifestations of depression and/or anxiety. Family studies have provided data suggesting a genetic aspect to this disorder. For example, monozygotic twins have been reported to show a higher concordance rate for OCD than dizygotic twins. Additionally, first-degree family members of patients with OCD show an increased incidence of obsessionality and of depression.

Phobias

A phobia is characterized by strong fear of a specific situation. Phobias may involve fear of one or more situations, typically leading to avoidance behavior. Social phobia is characterized by concerns about being under the scrutiny of others. Common examples of this condition include fears of public speaking or eating in public. Simple phobias are defined as fears of specific stimuli or situations, such as animals, heights, or enclosed spaces. Typically, a phobic individual in the feared situation experiences a rapid onset of intense symptoms of anxiety.

Post-traumatic Stress Disorder

Post-traumatic stress disorder involves the development of characteristic symptoms of anxiety, fears, or terror in the aftermath of exposure to an intense, psychologically stressful event. Particularly characteristic stressful events that may precipitate post-traumatic stress disorder (PTSD) include threat to the individual's life or observing severe injury or death of others. This disorder was particularly noted and attracted attention among veterans returning from the Vietnam War. For the individual suffering from PTSD, the traumatic event is reexperienced, often in vivid detail, through intrusive thoughts while awake and, frequently, through intense, distressing dreams (see Chapter 10).

TREATMENT

The delineation of discrete subgroups of anxiety disorders has made specific therapeutic recommendations possible. Indeed, the recognition of distinct disorders has led to the demonstration of treatments that offer selective efficacy in specific populations. Thus, the ability to match the most effective treatment to a defined subgroup has markedly enhanced the clinical management of this heterogeneous group of patients.

For one of the anxiety disorders, phobic anxiety, medication approaches are rarely recommended. This is especially true for simple phobias (monophobias). The best established treatment for this condition is a form of behavior therapy referred to as systematic desensitization. The patient is initially given instructions about a deep-muscle relaxation technique. Then a hierarchy is constructed of progressively more anxiety-provoking scenes related to the individual's feared situation. Thus, a subject who has a phobia related to flying might rank speaking to an airline agent to make reservations as relatively mildly anxiety provoking, getting into a cab to go to the airport as being considerably more stressful, and sitting on the plane fastening the seatbelt as being intensely uncomfortable. In the systematic desensitization approach, the subject is first instructed to assume a thoroughly relaxed state using the deep-muscle relaxation technique. The therapist then instructs the patient to imagine as vividly as possible the scene from the hierarchy that is least stressful. This process is repeated until the subject is able to maintain a sense of true physical relaxation while imaging the evocative scene. Over a series of sessions, the patient will be encouraged to work up the hierarchy of threatening scenes while simultaneously maintaining a relaxed state. This office technique is often coupled with gradually encouraging the patient to encounter feared situations in real life. Interestingly, there appears to be a strong relationship between learning to associate a sense of relaxation with imaging a feared situation and actually being able to tolerate that situation in reality. It is important to reemphasize that medication is rarely recommended for the treatment of this form of anxiety disorder.

PTSD can be intensely discomforting to the individual and highly disabling. Unfortunately, efforts to provide relief for this condition have generally been only minimally to moderately effective. As was described for phobic disorders, psychotherapeutic interventions often represent the most effective form of treatment. Some improvement with antidepressant drugs, both tricylic antidepressants and monoamine oxidase inhibitors (MOAIs), has been reported in patients with PTSD, but the results have generally been modest at best, and far from satisfactory.

In contrast to the aforementioned anxiety disorders, the other three major categories of anxiety disorders have been shown to be responsive to treatment with medication. Interestingly, each of these three disorders has been shown to respond preferentially to different pharmacological therapies. Thus, in the treatment of generalized anxiety disorder, a class of drugs referred to as the benzodiazepines (referring to the basic chemical structure, as shown in Fig. 1) has been shown to be quite efficacious in alleviating the symptoms of anxiety.

In contrast, panic disorder is generally not thought to respond well to most benzodiaze-

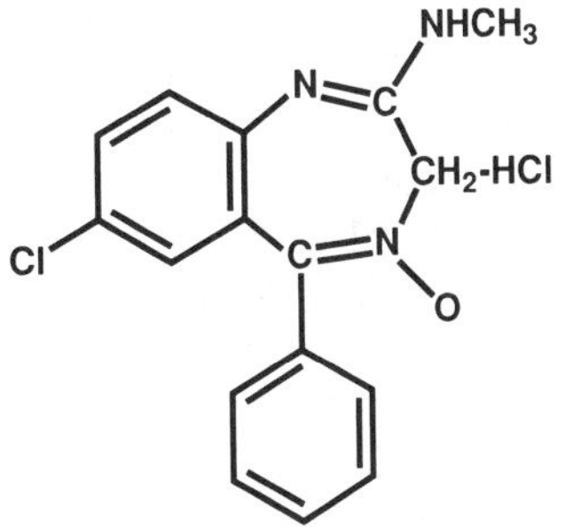

FIG. 1. Structure of a typical benzodiazepine antianxiety compound.

pines. Rather, antidepressant drugs, including both the tricyclic antidepressants and the MAOIs (see Chapter 17), have been reported to produce significant amelioration of panic attacks. Recently, a benzodiazepine derivative, alprazolam, was also approved for use in the treatment of panic disorder.

Finally, OCD appears to be reasonably selectively responsive to a specific tricyclic antidepressant compound, chlorimipramine. Chlorimipramine has a distinctive pharmacological profile among the tricylic antidepressant compounds. It is a highly potent inhibitor of the presynaptic uptake of serotonin, although it also has prominent norepinephrine uptake inhibitor effects as well (see Chapter 17 for a discussion of the mechanism of action of the antidepressant compounds). The fact that chlorimipramine seems to be more effective than other tricyclic antidepressants in treating OCD has prompted suggestions that effects on serotonin release or uptake may represent an essential component of its mechanism of action. Recent studies with the new antidepressant drug fluoxetine, a serotonin-selective uptake inhibitor, have also indicated efficacy in the treatment of OCD. Additionally, the observation that drugs such as chlorimipramine and fluoxetine ameliorate obsessive compulsive symptoms has contributed to the formation of a hypothesis about the role of serotonin in the pathophysiology of OCD (see below).

To reiterate, the delineation of discrete categories of anxiety disorders, as outlined in DSM-III-R, has provided a basis for establishing specific treatment recommendations. Two of the classes of anxiety disorders (i.e., phobias and PTSD) are generally treated with some form of psychotherapy, while the efficacy of pharmacotherapy is less well established. For several of the anxiety disorders (generalized anxiety disorder, panic disorder, and PTSD), medication has been shown to provide considerable benefit. It should also be emphasized that optimal treatment approaches for these conditions frequently involve a combination of pharmacotherapy and psychotherapy. The fact that different psychotropic drugs or drug classes appear to be preferentially effective for these conditions raises the possibility that they may be associated with different underlying neurobiological etiologies, though such speculation requires considerable further investigation.

CLINICAL PHARMACOLOGY

Clinical Profile of Drugs

The benzodiazepines were the first class of drugs to show widespread applicability in the treatment of anxiety. The first of the benzodiazepines, chlordiazepoxide, was synthesized in 1957. Studies with chlordiazepoxide in monkeys demonstrated a "taming" effect, and this observation led to the suggestion that it might exert calming effects in human subjects. Indeed, in literally hundreds of clinical trials, the benzodiazepines have been demonstrated to produce a reduction in symptoms of anxiety in patients suffering from anxiety disorders. Many of these studies were conducted under double-blind, placebo-controlled conditions (see Chapter 17). Patients tend to respond rapidly to benzodiazepine administration with reduction in symptoms. After 6 weeks of therapy, typically 65% to 70% of patients demonstrate significant clinical improvement, and this improvement is generally maintained with continued treatment for several months. Another important and consistently observed finding is that a number of patients with significant clinical anxiety (typically ranging from 25% to 40%) demonstrate improvement in association with the administration of placebo. This finding underscores the point that improvement from anxiety disorders often represents a complex interaction of physiological and psychological factors. Moreover, the observation that some patients suffering from a significant clinical disorder may improve following administration of a pharmacologically inactive pill underscores the importance of conducting rigorously controlled clinical trials to evaluate the true efficacy of a new therapeutic agent.

Benzodiazepines are now well established as effective drugs for the treatment of anxiety, and these agents have become widely used for this purpose. Among the DSM-III-R anxiety disorder, generalized anxiety disorder appears to represent the major indication for benzodiazepine use. In patients with panic disorders, benzodiazepines may not be effective in alleviating the acute pain attacks, but may be of help in diminishing anticipatory anxiety that can occur between acute panic attacks. Additionally, the benzodiazepines can be used to relieve anxiety associated with other states such as medical disorders, other psychiatric conditions such as depression or schizophrenia, or situational stress. It should also be noted that the benzodiazepines have a number of clinical uses in addition to the treatment of anxiety. Thus, these compounds are frequently employed as anticonvulsant agents and as sedative-hypnotic drugs (i.e., "sleeping pills"). In addition, the benzodiazepines are often used as preoperative medications prior to anesthesia and to provide relief of muscle spasms. This diverse range of clinical uses reflects the broad spectrum of actions of the benzodiazepines on the central nervous system.

The benzodiazepines have been in common clinical use for over 30 years. In light of this considerable history, they have a generally very positive safety record. Thus, there is little evidence of organ toxicity (e.g., liver, kidney, or cardiovascular problems) with benzodiazepine administration, even when the drugs are taken for considerable periods of time. Another significant advantage of the benzodiazepines is the fact that they are rarely fatal when taken in overdose. However, as is the case with all medications, some problems can be encountered with benzodiazepine administration. The most common side effects produced by the benzodiazepines are sedation and dizziness. Some impairment in memory, in particular the consolidation of new information, can be observed in association with benzodiazepine use. Loss of coordination and reflex response time may compromise driving ability or safety in operating

heavy equipment. A significant warning must be given to patients with regard to the combined use of benzodiazepines and alcohol. Accidental or intentional fatalities can occur as the result of combined administration of large amounts of alcohol and benzodiazepines, primarily as a consequence of suppression of the brain stem respiratory drive center.

The abrupt discontinuation of a benzodiazepine can bring on severe withdrawal. One other important problem associated with benzodiazepine use has been recognized within the past decade. Carefully controlled clinical studies have clearly demonstrated that patients who take a benzodiazepine compound daily for a considerable period of time (e.g., more than 6 months) and then abruptly discontinue therapy may experience prominent withdrawal reactions.

Figure 2 presents data from a patient who had been taking modest doses of diazepam (15 mg/day) for approximately 4 years. This patient was studied in a protocol in which, on a double-blind basis, he received diazepam or placebo in an alternating pattern for 4-day periods. As illustrated in Fig. 2, during the periods in which the diazepam capsules were replaced with placebo, the patient exhibited

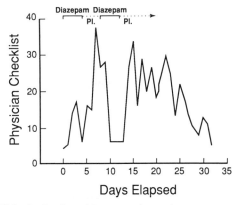

FIG. 2. Profound increase in anxiety symptoms associated with withdrawal symptoms when diazepam therapy was replaced by placebo pills. The patient had been receiving diazepam (15 mg/day) for 4 years. From Winokur A, Rickels K, Greenblatt DJ, Snyder PJ, Schatz NJ. *Arch Gen Psychiatry* 1980;37:101–105.

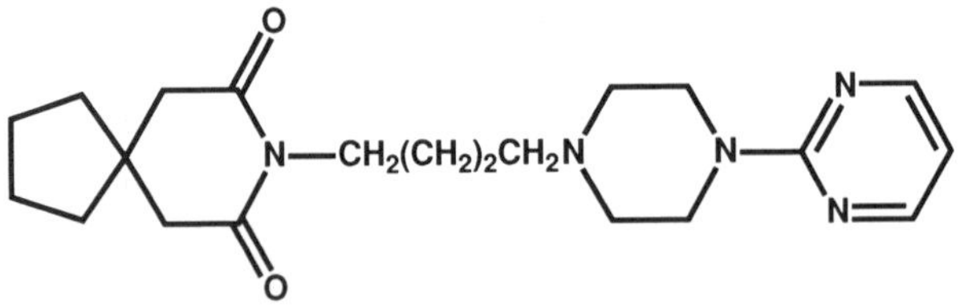

FIG. 3. Structure of buspirone.

rapid and pronounced increases in symptoms, and these symptoms promptly remitted following reinstitution of diazepam. Through such studies, the characteristic symptoms of benzodiazepine withdrawal reactions have been well described. Such symptoms include a rapid and pronounced increase in anxiety, tremulousness, and agitation; a "flu-like" syndrome including gastrointestinal symptoms and muscular aches and pains; hyperactivity of sensory perceptions, such as increased sensitivity to sounds, light, odors, or touch; feelings of unreality; and perceptual distortions. In light of the recent recognition that long-term benzodiazepine therapy can lead to problems with dependence and withdrawal, it is now generally recommended that most patients be kept on these agents for limited periods of time (e.g., less than 6 months) and that treatment be terminated through gradual reduction of dose.

Buspirone has an efficacy similar to that of the benzodiazepines, but has a different structure, different speed of onset, and fewer side effects. Buspirone is a recent addition to the pharmacological armamentarium for anxiety with a chemical structure very different from that of the benzodiazepine compounds (Fig. 3). As is the case with the benzodiazepines, buspirone appears to work most effectively in patients with generalized anxiety disorder. Figure 4 illustrates two observations from clinical research studies regarding the characteristics of buspirone in the treatment of anxiety.

Buspirone tends to have a much slower onset of action than is seen with the benzodiazepines, such as clorazepate, the comparative drug included in the study illustrated in Fig. 4. Indeed, the time course for buspirone to demonstrate clinical efficacy is much more comparable to that normally seen with the antidepressant drugs. Understandably, this relatively slow onset of action may be a highly undesirable feature for some patients with generalized anxiety disorder, particularly those who have previously experienced prompt relief with benzodiazepine therapy. In general, it does appear that buspirone has an efficacy approximately equivalent to that of the benzodiazepines in the treatment of generalized anxiety disorder. Moreover, buspirone exhibits two features that may be highly advantageous for some patients. First, it appears that interactions between alcohol and buspirone occur infrequently, in contrast to the situation previously described for interactions between alcohol and benzodiaze-

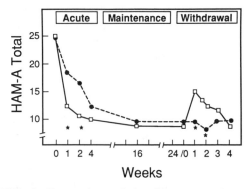

FIG. 4. Comparison of the time course to response, efficacy with maintenance therapy, and withdrawal reactions in anxious patients treated with the benzodiazepine compound clorazepate (solid line) or buspirone (dotted line). HAM-A Total refers to the rating of severity of symptoms of anxiety on the Hamilton Anxiety Rating Scale. From Rickels K, Schweizer E, Csanalosi I, Case WG, Chung H. *Arch Gen Psychiatry* 1988;45: 444–450.

pines. Additionally, as illustrated in Fig. 4, long-term administration of buspirone does not seem to lead to withdrawal reactions following termination of treatment. Thus, buspirone may be particularly well suited for patients with longstanding generalized anxiety disorder who would require extensive periods of continuous treatment with medication.

MECHANISMS OF ACTION

The discovery of the presence of benzodiazepine receptors in the brain was important in defining the mechanism of action of these compounds. In recent years, substantial advances have been made in delineating the mechanism of action of the antianxiety drugs. The most significant finding has been the demonstration of the presence of benzodiazepine receptors in brain tissue. Regions of particularly high receptor localization include limbing structures (e.g., amygdala and hippocampus), periaqueductal gray region, brain stem, and some areas of cerebral cortex. Benzodiazepine receptors have been characterized as demonstrating stereoselectivity and saturability, properties consistent with physiologically relevant binding sites (see Chapter 4). The demonstration of receptors for benzodiazepines in the central nervous system has prompted some investigators to speculate that the brain may contain natural substances (also called *endogenous compounds*) that act as agonists on these receptors. Intense efforts are under way to isolate such endogenous benzodiazepine receptor agonists. The identification of such hypothesized compounds might provide important insights about the neurochemical mechanisms underlying anxiety states.

Benzodiazepines act on receptors located on a macromolecular complex in conjunction with GABA receptors and chloride ion channels. Considerable information has been obtained in recent years about the manner in which benzodiazepine compounds act on these receptors. As shown in Fig. 5, benzodiazepine receptors are located on a large structure, referred to as a macromolecular complex. Also located on this complex are receptors for GABA (see Chapter 7), the important inhibitory neurotransmitter agent, and for other drugs, in particular barbiturates. The benzodiazepine and GABA receptors are located in close proximity to chloride ion channels. The actions of a benzodiazepine agonist on a benzodiazepine receptor

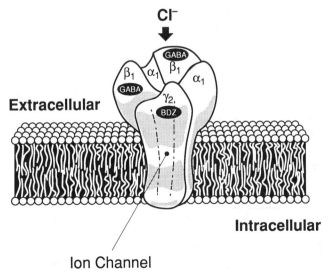

FIG. 5. Schematic depiction of the benzodiazepine-GABA macromolecular complex. From Zorumski CF, Isenberg KE. *Am J Psychiatry* 1991;148:162–173.

potentiate the effects of GABA on the GABA receptor. This potentiated effect leads to an enhanced hyperpolarization of the postsynaptic neuron. Thus, the clinical properties of the benzodiazepines in alleviating anxiety, producing sedation, and exerting anticonvulsant protection would also seem to be directly attributable to enhancement of the actions of GABA on chloride ion influx.

Recently, a potent benzodiazepine receptor antagonist, flumazenil, has been developed. Animals treated continuously with a benzodiazepine compound for several weeks and then given flumazenil demonstrate pronounced withdrawal symptoms. Flumazenil is now available for clinical use, and it may be of value in reversing the effects of excessive central nervous system depression associated with benzodiazepine overdosage. Additionally, some investigators have speculated that the availability of a benzodiazepine receptor antagonist may be of value in the treatment of dependence on benzodiazepine compounds.

Another class of compounds was recently discovered that exerts interesting effects on the benzodiazepine macromolecular complex. The compound β-carboline-3-carboxylate ethyl ester (BCCE) has been demonstrated to have very high affinity for the benzodiazepine binding site on the benzodiazepine/GABA macromolecular complex. Initially, BCCE was shown to antagonize the effects of benzodiazepines. Subsequently, it was recognized that BCCE not only functioned as an antagonist at the benzodiazepine receptor, but it also exerted pharmacological actions at this site that were opposite to those produced by the benzodiazepines. Thus, BCCE is described as an *inverse agonist* at the benzodiazepine receptor. When administered to primates, BCCE has been noted to produce effects of behavioral agitation and autonomic hyperactivity (such as increased heart rate and blood pressure). Thus, the effects produced by BCCE appear to resemble an anxiety response in humans. A compound closely related to BCCE has been administered to a limited number of human subjects. Interest-

ingly, in humans, as in the primate studies, symptoms of behavioral agitation and autonomic hyperactivity were observed. Additionally, these subjects reported feelings of pronounced apprehension and fear. These findings raise the possibility that naturally occurring compounds in brain with BCCE-like properties could play a role in the generation of anxiety. Currently, research is under way to demonstrate the presence of such compounds in brain tissue. One candidate for such a role is a peptide called diazepam-binding inhibitor, a compound that has been shown to inhibit the effects of GABA. Whether such compounds play an important role in mediating anxiety responses is a subject awaiting further investigation.

Techniques of molecular biology are now being applied to investigation of drug–receptor interactions. Work in the field of molecular biology (see Chapter 5) is progressing rapidly, as illustrated by the following observations. The existence of two distinct benzodiazepine receptor subtypes had been hypothesized for several years. The type I benzodiazepine receptor was characterized to be a high-affinity binding site for a subset of benzodiazepine-related compounds, while the type II benzodiazepine receptor was characterized as a low-affinity site for these compounds.

Application of molecular cloning technology has led to the identification of a much larger number of benzodiazepine/GABA receptors. Several subunits of the GABA$_A$ receptor (the form of GABA receptor associated with benzodiazepine binding sites) have been described, including α, β, γ, δ, and ϵ subunits. In addition, several forms of a particular subunit have been described. For example, using cloning techniques, at least six different forms of the α subunit have been shown to exist. Benzodiazepine/GABA receptor subtypes are composed of different combinations of the various subunits. These receptor subtypes have been shown to be differentially concentrated in different brain regions, to demonstrate differential responsiveness to GABA in terms of electrophysiological activity, and to demonstrate discrete pharmacological profiles to benzodiazepine compounds. Progress in this field raises the possibility of developing new, therapeutically relevant compounds with even more specific effects on GABA inhibitory systems in the central nervous system.

In the discussion of clinical features of the antianxiety agents, some prominent differences were pointed out between the benzodiazepine anti-anxiety drugs and buspirone. In light of these pronounced clinical differences, it has also been of interest to learn that the two classes of antianxiety compounds work through distinctly different neurochemical mechanisms. Thus, buspirone does not exert effects on the benzodiazepine receptor. Rather, the major neurochemical actions of buspirone appear to be exerted on the serotonin system, where it functions as an agonist on the 5-HT_{1A} receptor subtype (see Chapter 6).

BIOLOGICAL THEORIES OF ANXIETY DISORDERS

Animal fight-or-flight experiments suggested a causal link between secretion of adrenalin (epinephrine) and anxiety. Many investigators have speculated about biological mechanisms underlying the anxiety disorders. Both animal behavioral studies and clinical investigations have provided data implicating discrete brain regions and specific neurochemical systems in their pathophysiology. A few specific examples will be reviewed to illustrate the types of studies that are being pursued in this field.

As noted earlier, Cannon drew attention to the fight-or-flight response that was consistently associated with situations of extreme threat to the animal's survival. He emphasized that the secretion of adrenalin (also known as epinephrine) was a key hormonal component of this fight-or-flight response. Shortly thereafter, Karplus and Kreidel conducted studies in which they implanted electrodes into the hypothalamus of laboratory animals. Electrical stimulation of this region

produced physiological and behavioral effects of arousal that strongly resembled the fight-or-flight response described by Cannon. This finding provided the first indication that the central nervous system played a role in mediating the fight-or-flight response.

Over the years, considerable evidence has implicated an important role for brain norepinephrine systems in the mediation of anxiety. As reviewed in Chapter 6, the site of origin of the majority of norepinephrine-containing neurons is the locus coeruleus. From this site, some norepinephrine fibers descend into the spinal cord, while others ascend into higher brain regions, where they innervate structures such as the hypothalamus, amygdala, hippocampus, and many cortical regions. These neuroanatomic areas are widely believed to be involved in the regulation of emotional state and cognitive activity.

Redmond and his colleagues at Yale conducted a series of studies utilizing a primate model to examine the role of the locus coeruleus–norepinephine system in anxiety. When monkeys studied under experimental conditions were exposed to threatening stimuli, they demonstrated signs of physiological arousal (e.g., increased heart rate, blood pressure, and respiration) and behavioral distress (e.g., struggling, startling, hand wringing) that seemed to indicate a fear response. While it is not possible to prove that these types of behavioral responses represent a fully valid analog of human anxiety, the similarities in presentation are striking.

When lesions were introduced into the locus coeruleus of an experimental animal, presentation of threatening stimuli no longer elicited fear-like responses. In contrast, monkeys that were electrically stimulated through electrodes implanted in the locus coeruleus demonstrated a markedly increased fear response to the same threatening stimuli. These findings suggest that the locus coeruleus represents a critical anatomic component of the fear–response mechanism. Since the locus coeruleus contains a large proportion of the norepinephrine cell bodies, these findings are compatible with the suggestion that norepinephrine systems are involved in the fear response (and perhaps in human anxiety as well). However, these findings provide no direct evidence for the involvement of norepinephrine in the fear response. To examine this hypothesis more directly, these investigators employed neuropharmacological research techniques using drugs known to stimulate or inhibit norepinephrine neurons in the locus coeruleus. In particular, drugs that act on the α_2-adrenergic receptor were used. As described in Chapter 6, activation of this autoreceptor produces a slowing of firing rate of locus coeruleus neurons and a reduction of norepinephrine activity. In contrast, inhibition of the α_2-adrenergic receptor increases locus coeruleus neuronal firing rate and norepinephrine activity. Administration of clonidine, an α_2-receptor agonist, to monkeys studied in this paradigm resulted in a pronounced reduction in the response to a threatening stimulus. On the other hand, when the α_2-receptor antagonist yohimbine was administered, fear responses were markedly accentuated. Thus, utilization of pharmacological strategies that specifically alter norepinephrine activity allowed the investigators to obtain information implicating norepinephrine systems in the fear response. While this association seems compelling, it should be emphasized that much additional information is needed to confirm that the norepinephrine system plays a central role in human anxiety states.

Another approach to investigating neurobiological aspects of anxiety disorders has involved administration of treatments intended to provoke panic attacks in susceptible individuals. Conditions that have been reported to precipitate panic attacks or intense anxiety reactions include administration of sodium lactate (lactic acid is a metabolic breakdown product of glucose in the process of glycolysis), inhalation of carbon dioxide, and administration of the α_2-receptor antagonist yohimbine. This type of study is designed to identify procedures that are effective in producing panic reactions in a large percentage of patients with a prior history of panic attacks, but that rarely produce panic attacks in normal subjects (i.e., individuals with no prior history of panic attacks). All three treatments mentioned above have been reported to provoke panic attacks in at least some at-risk individuals. It thus becomes a challenge to explain the neural mechanisms involved in the precipitation of these panic attacks. While more work is needed to clarify the underlying mechanisms, Gorman, an investigator at Columbia University, has proposed a theory that lactate infusion, carbon dioxide inhalation, and yohimbine administration all stimulate panic reactions through actions exerted at brain stem sites. As illustrated in Fig. 6, activation of sensitive brain stem regions is thought to result in heightened autonomic function (e.g., increased pulse rate, rapid respirations) and stimulation of neurotransmitter systems arising in brain stem regions (e.g., locus coeruleus–norepinephrine pathways, raphe nucleus–serotonin pathways).

Activation of aminergic pathways would be expected to have significant functional effects in limbic and cortical regions. Thus, while this theory postulates an important role for brain stem sites in the generation of panic attacks, it is important to recognize that several brain regions are likely to be involved, in an integrated manner, in the mediation of anxiety reactions.

Brain-imaging techniques, as described in Chapter 15, have been employed by some investigators to explore the neurobiological substrates of anxiety in human subjects. For example, Reisman and coworkers from Washington University utilized positron emission tomography (PET) to study regional cerebral blood flow in patients with panic disorder and in normal control subjects. Cerebral blood flow is thought to provide an indication of neuronal activity in discrete brain regions. Panic patients studied during neutral (i.e., nonpanic) conditions demonstrated some significant alterations in cerebral blood flow when compared with appropriately matched control subjects. Pa-

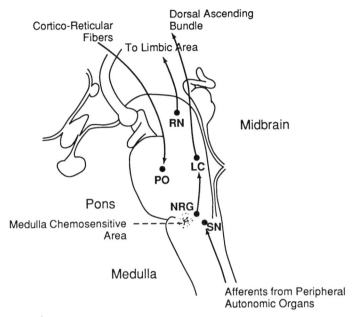

Cortico-Reticular Fibers

Dorsal Ascending Bundle

To Limbic Area

RN

Midbrain

LC

PO

Pons

NRG

Medulla Chemosensitive Area

SN

Medulla

Afferents from Peripheral Autonomic Organs

FIG. 6. Schematic diagram illustrating the origin of panic attacks in the brain stem, with transmission to higher limbic and cortical sites. RN, raphe nucleus; PO, pontis oralis; LC, locus coeruleus; NRG, nucleus reticularis giganotocellularis; SN, solitary nucleus. From Gorman JM, Liebowitz MR, Fyer AJ, Stein J. *Am J Psychiatry* 1989;146:148–161.

tients with a history of panic attacks demonstrated an unusual asymmetry of blood flow, blood volume, and metabolic rate for oxygen in the parahippocampal gyrus, a cortical region bordering on the hippocampus. Compared to control subjects, the panic patients had less blood flow in the parahippocampal gyrus of the left hemisphere than of the right.

The investigators then employed the lactate infusion technique to identify subjects susceptible to the provocation of panic attacks. In this study, a number of patients with a history of panic attacks but none of the normal controls developed an anxiety attack during the lactate infusion. In conjunction with the episode of induced anxiety, the subjects demonstrated a significant increase in blood flow bilaterally in a region of the temporal cortex referred to as the temporal pole. Interestingly, a similar increase in blood flow in the temporal pole was observed in normal subjects studied in a behavioral paradigm designed to induce high levels of anticipatory anxiety. These findings suggest that a common neuroanatomic site (the temporal poles)

is activated in anxiety attacks experienced by patients with panic disorder and in normal subjects who are induced to experience substantial anticipatory anxiety. In addition, the panic disorder patients were noted to manifest unusual features of cerebral blood flow in the temporal lobes while at rest in a nonpanic state. Additional research is needed to clarify whether such alterations in brain function may explain why these individuals are susceptible to developing panic attacks.

Serotonin has been implicated as a factor in obsessive-compulsive disorder (OCD). In recent years, biological theories of obsessive-compulsive disorder have focused on the role of serotonergic mechanisms. This interest has been stimulated to a large extent by advances in the field of clinical psychopharmacology. In particular, the tricyclic antidepressant clomipramine has been demonstrated to have considerable efficacy in the treatment of OCD. As noted above, among the tricyclic antidepressant compounds, clomipramine is characterized by its highly potent effects in blocking the presynaptic uptake of serotonin.

Evidence suggesting that the serotonergic effects of clomipramine are implicated in its mechanism of action in OCD is provided by the observation that other tricyclic antidepressant compounds that have less potency in blocking presynaptic uptake of serotonin are less effective in relieving symptoms of OCD. On the other hand, preliminary studies suggest that the potent and selective serotonin uptake inhibitor fluoxetine does have significant efficacy in the treatment of OCD.

Another pharmacological strategy has been used to link serotonergic systems with OCD. The compound *meta*-chlorophenylpiperazine (m-CPP), a metabolite of the antidepressant drug trazodone, has direct agonist effects on postsynaptic serotonergic receptors. When m-CPP was administered to remitted OCD patients in one study, a pronounced exacerbation of OCD symptoms was observed.

SUMMARY

Anxiety is a commonly observed symptom in our society. Since the term is subject to a number of interpretations, it has proven to be essential to develop well-defined, standardized diagnostic criteria to identify discrete patient groups. The development of DSM-III-R provided valuable guidelines for classifying the anxiety disorders, with five specific disorders being defined: panic disorder, generalized anxiety disorder, OCD, phobias, and PTSD. An important aspect of accurate diagnostic classification is the ability to identify more specific, effective treatment modalities. As described above, several of the anxiety disorders are associated with specific treatment recommendations, which further underscores the value of this classification system.

Medication plays a prominent role in the treatment of some of the anxiety disorders, in particular panic disorder, generalized anxiety disorder, and OCD. For panic disorder, tricyclic antidepressants and MAOIs are frequently effective. Patients with generalized anxiety disorder are often treated successfully with benzodiazepine compounds and, more

recently, with buspirone. For OCD, the tricyclic antidepressant chlorimipramine has been reported to demonstrate considerable efficacy. Each of these classes of drugs can produce some side effects, and physicians must weigh the benefits against these potential liabilities in deciding how to treat a patient. The use of psychotherapy, either in combination with or as an alternative to pharmacotherapy, is often of value in the treatment of anxiety disorders.

Considerable progress has been made in clarifying the mechanism of action of the antianxiety drugs. Of particular importance has been the demonstration of receptors for benzodiazepine compounds in the central nervous system and clarification of the mechanisms by which this class of drugs produces suppression of neuronal activity. Experimental evidence suggests that several neurotransmitter systems and neuroanatomic regions are involved in the pathophysiology of anxiety disorders. The results of continued research efforts should provide us with a more comprehensive understanding of the relevant neurochemical alterations associated with the various important anxiety disorders. Furthermore, such insights may provide opportunities for developing more effective, specific pharmacological agents to treat these prevalent and often highly disabling conditions.

BIBLIOGRAPHY

Original Articles

Mellinger GD, Balter MB, Uhlenhuth EH. Prevalence and correlates of the long-term regular use of anxiolytics. *JAMA* 1984;251:375–379.

Ninan PT, Insel TM, Cohen RM, Cook JM, Skolnick P, Paul SM. Benzodiazepine receptor-mediated experimental "anxiety" in primates. *Science* 1982;218: 1332–1334.

Pritchett DB, Lüddens H, Seeburg PH. Type I and type II GABA$_A$-benzodiazepine receptors produced in transfected cells. *Science* 1989;245:1389–1392.

Reiman EM, Fusselman MJ, Fox PT, Raichle ME. Neuroanatomical correlates of anticipatory anxiety. *Science* 1989;243:1071–1074.

Rickels K, Case WG, Downing RW, Winokur A. Long-term diazepam therapy and clinical outcome. *JAMA* 1983;250:767–771.

Rickels K, Schweizer E, Csanalosi I, Case WG, Chung H. Long-term treatment of anxiety and risk of withdrawal: prospective comparison of clorazepate and buspirone. *Arch Gen Psychiatry* 1988;45:444–450.

Books and Reviews

Barchas JD. Biochemical hypotheses of affective disorders and anxiety. In: Siegel GJ, Agranoff BW, Albers RW, Molinoff PB, eds. *Basic neurochemistry*, 5th ed. New York: Raven Press; 1994 (in press).

Gorman JM, Liebowitz MR, Fyer AJ, Stein J. A neuroanatomical hypothesis for panic disorder. *Am J Psychiatry* 1989;146:148–161.

Paul SM, Marangos PJ, Skolnick P. The benzodiazepine-GABA-chloride ionophore receptor complex: common site of minor tranquilizer action. *Biol Psychiatry* 1981;16:213–229.

Redmond DE Jr. Studies of the nucleus locus coeruleus in monkeys and hypotheses for neuropsychopharmacology. In: Meltzer HY, ed. *Psychopharmacology: the third generation of progress.* New York: Raven Press; 1987:967–975.

Sheehan DV. Panic attacks and phobias. *N Engl J Med* 1982;307:156–158.

Vicini S. Pharmacological significance of the structural heterogeneity of the GABA receptor–chloride ion channel complex. *Neuropsychopharmacology* 1991;4:9–15.

Zohar J, Insel TR. Obsessive-compulsive disorder: psychobiological approaches to diagnosis, treatment and pathophysiology. *Biol Psychiatry* 1987;22:667–687.

Zorumski CF, Isenberg KE. Insights into the structure and function of GABA-benzodiazepine receptors: ion channels and psychiatry. *Am J Psychiatry* 1991;148:162–173.

20

Substance Abuse

Karen M. Kumor and Charles P. O'Brien

Sherlock Holmes took his bottle from the corner of the mantelpiece and his hypodermic syringe from its neat morocco case. . . . "Which is it to-day?" I asked. "Morphine or cocaine?" He raised his eyes languidly from the old black-letter volume which he had opened. "It is cocaine," he said; "a seven per cent solution. Would you care to try it?" "No, indeed," I answered brusquely. . . . He smiled at my vehemence. "Perhaps you are right, Watson," he said. "I suppose that its influence is physically a bad one. I find it, however, so transcendently stimulating and clarifying to the mind that its secondary action is a matter of small moment."

"But consider!" I said earnestly. "Count the cost! Your brain may, as you say, be roused and excited, but it is a pathological and morbid process, which involves increased tissue-change, and may at least leave a permanent weakness. You know, too, what a black reaction comes upon you. Surely the game is hardly worth the candle. Why should you, for a mere passing pleasure, risk the loss of those great powers with which you have been endowed?"

". . . .But I abhor the dull routine of existence. I crave for mental exaltation. . . ."

A. Conan Doyle,
The Sign of Four

- Drug variables include rewarding properties, pattern of tolerance, cost and availability, pattern of withdrawal, mode of administration, and speed of onset.

- User variables include metabolism and sensitivity to drugs, overall mental and emotional well-being, and response to stress.

- Environmental variables include peer influence and conditioned environmental response.

- Animal self-administration experiments have been an important source of information on drug abuse potential.

- The modes of treatment for addiction are common for all drugs of abuse.

- Drug dependence must be considered a chronic disease.

- Cocaine—especially crack—has the highest addiction potential of any drug in the United States.

- The opiate drugs are potent analgesics.

- It has been demonstrated that the active substance after heroin injection is not heroin itself but its metabolite, morphine.

- In early work it was noted that all opiate/opioid receptors were antagonized by the unique opioid drug naloxone.

- Subsequent discoveries revealed the presence of three families of natural opioid peptides—enkephalins, dynorphins, and endorphins.

- Treatment with methadone, a long-acting opiate drug, suppresses opiate withdrawal symptoms.

- Of all the many sedatives, alcohol is the most commonly used.

- The benzodiazepines are the most commonly prescribed drugs in the world.

- The cannabinoids are associated with a feeling of mild euphoria, decreased cognitive abilities, and a relatively mild withdrawal.

- The psychoactive constituents of the cannabinoids found in the cannabis plant are the tetrahydrocannabinols.

- Tetrahydrocannabinols suppress nausea and vomiting and are useful in the treatment of vomiting induced by cancer chemotherapy.

- Nicotine has all of the features of an addictive drug.

- Nicotine is a cholinergic drug that stimulates ganglionic neurons.

This chapter begins by discussing some common properties of drugs of abuse as well as ways of predicting the abuse potential of new compounds. General principles of treatment of drug addiction are covered, followed by systematic discussions of specific drugs of abuse. The chapter emphasizes the biological and pharmacological aspects of the problem, but a comprehensive discussion of substance abuse requires sociological, political, psychological, and economic considerations as well.

Substance abuse is a complicated biological, psychological, and social problem that has at times been epidemic in the United States in the last century, waxing and waning in response to poorly understood forces. It is arguably the most important psychiatric/social ill of the nation by virtue of the number of addicts, the serious impact on families, the economic burden to industry reflected in the loss of workers and efficiency, the growth of crime, and the detrimental effects on the mental and physical health and safety of addicts.

The definition of drug dependence or addiction agreed on by the American Psychiatric Association in collaboration with the World Health Organization and listed in the DSM-III-R is given in Table 1. It emphasizes that addiction is a problem in which involvement with a drug becomes a large or even central focus of an individual's existence. The first six of the nine criteria note *lack of control* of drug use or drug use that is the *first priority among activities.* Only the last three criteria focus on pharmacological tolerance and withdrawal. Thus, overall, the emphasis in the diagnosis is on behavior. The presence of withdrawal symptomatology or tolerance (see below) is neither sufficient nor necessary for the diagnosis.

The diagnosis of drug abuse is made when a maladaptive pattern of psychoactive substance use exists. The necessary criterion for drug abuse is either use of a psychoactive substance in situations in which it is physically hazardous or its use despite persistent or recurrent social, occupational, psychological, or physical problems caused or exacerbated by the psychoactive substance. It contrasts with *drug dependence* in that the driven, compulsive drug-taking quality is absent. The drug-abusing individual retains substantial control over the use of the drug. Clearly, the drug abuser is at risk for the development of dependence. At times, the line between drug abuse and dependence is unclear. Both problems warrant treatment.

COMMON PROPERTIES OF DRUGS OF ABUSE

Any substance can be abused if taken to excess. An extreme example is compulsive water drinking, a behavioral disorder that can produce intoxication even to the point of death. Of course, people normally don't use water excessively, but substances such as drugs that produce immediate pleasurable effects may result in excessive use in anyone. A large number of variables influence the taking of drugs to excess. These variables can be classified under three categories: the drug, the user, and the environment.

Drug Variables

Drug variables include rewarding properties, pattern of tolerance, cost and availability, pattern of withdrawal, mode of adminis-

Biological Bases of Brain Function and Disease, edited by Alan Frazer, Perry B. Molinoff, and Andrew Winokur. Raven Press, Ltd., New York © 1994.

TABLE 1. *Criteria for diagnosis of drug or alcohol dependence*[a]

Any three of the following are sufficient for the diagnosis.
1. The substance is often taken in larger amounts or over a longer period than the person intended.
2. Persistent desire or one or more unsuccessful efforts to cut down or control substance use.
3. A great deal of time spent in activities necessary to get the substance, taking the substance, or recovering from its effects.
4. Frequent intoxication or withdrawal symptoms when expected to fulfill major role obligations at work, school, or home, or when substance use is physically hazardous.
5. Important social, occupational, or recreational activities given up or reduced because of substance use.
6. Continued substance use despite knowledge of having a persistent or recurrent social, psychological, or physical problem that is caused or exacerbated by the use of the substance.
7. Marked tolerance, i.e., the need for markedly increased amounts of the substance to achieve intoxication or a desired effect, or markedly diminished effect with continued use of the same amount of substance.
8. Characteristic withdrawal symptoms, depending on the individual drug, upon stopping its use.
9. Substance often taken to relieve or avoid withdrawal symptoms.

[a] As listed in the DSM-III-R.

tration, and speed of onset. All drugs of abuse have in common the ability to elevate mood state. Drugs vary in their rewarding properties. Cocaine produces an immediate, intense euphoria, sometimes termed a "rush." Thus, a person who tries cocaine is likely to repeat the experience. A less rewarding drug such as diazepam (Valium) carries a lower risk of abuse. A drug that produces disagreeable effects would tend not to be taken again even if needed for long-term benefits.

Most drugs of abuse demonstrate the property of *tolerance,* that is, a pattern of declining response to repeated administration of drug. Tolerance is one of the criteria for drug dependence and an important determinant of the dose of drug taken. Abusers increase the dose of drug taken over time in an effort to regain the effect obtained when the drug was taken in a naive or less tolerant state. Thus, tolerance may offer the user some physiological protection from toxic doses; however, the development of tolerance may also cause individuals to take higher doses of drug, leading to problems associated with drug overdose.

When a rewarding drug is readily available and cheap, the risk of abuse increases significantly. Cocaine, for example, was expensive until the 1980s and was thought by many to be a relatively harmless drug. Then cocaine became cheap and, therefore, was used more regularly and in higher doses. Subsequently, the dangers of cocaine became obvious.

When some drugs, both drugs of abuse and others, are taken chronically, there is a withdrawal syndrome associated with the abrupt interruption of drug administration as the result of a temporary loss of homeostasis. The pattern of physiological and psychological changes and the time course for reestablishment of homeostasis in the drug-free state are characteristic of each class of drug. The physiological changes found are generally opposite in direction to the pharmacological actions of the drug. For example, when administration of some medicines used in the treatment of high blood pressure is stopped suddenly, an elevation of blood pressure higher than the patient's baseline status is observed temporarily. In the case of drugs of abuse associated with a withdrawal syndrome, physiological changes may be seen (e.g., in heart rate, blood pressure, bowel function, and skin temperature). Withdrawal syndromes associated with drugs of abuse are always accompanied by unpleasant mood states and distress, which are thought to be part of the withdrawal itself. The distress of withdrawal is one factor that makes breaking the cycle of drug use so difficult and sometimes even dangerous.

The mode of administration is another important drug variable affecting the potential for abuse. Drugs can be taken by mouth and absorbed via the gastrointestinal tract; they can be chewed and absorbed through the lining of the mouth (oral mucous membranes); they can be injected into a vein, under the skin, or into a muscle. They may be taken by rectum, by skin patch, or smoked and absorbed through the lungs into the pulmonary circulation. The mode of administration influences the time it takes for a drug to reach the target organ, which, for drugs of abuse, is the brain. The speed of onset of effect is one factor that influences a drug's potential to be abused. Generally, the more rapidly the drug reaches the brain and produces the desired effect, the more likely the substance is to be abused.

User Variables

User variables include metabolism and sensitivity to drugs, overall mental and emotional well-being, and response to stress. Another set of variables pertains to differences among individual users. The metabolism of a drug depends on enzymes whose activity is controlled by genes. Thus, heredity may influence the absorption, disposition, and elimination of prescribed and illegal drugs and alcohol. For example, some individuals have inherited insensitivity to alcohol that is evident at the time of first use. Others are very sensitive to alcohol. Some, particularly people of Asian descent, may routinely develop an immediate adverse effect from alcohol called a "flushing reaction."

Generally, people with mental disorders have a higher rate of addiction than those not afflicted. Mental disorders known to increase the risk of drug addiction include depression, schizophrenia, post-traumatic stress disorder, anxiety disorders, and personality disorders. Many investigators believe that drug-taking behavior may start as a result of an effort by the person to self-medicate to feel better.

Persons who experience stress may have an increased vulnerability to addiction. One type of stress is poverty. Poverty depletes personal, economic, and emotional resources and support, causing anxiety and despondency. Drug administration temporarily relieves the distress associated with poverty. Of course, drug addiction worsens poverty, but the initial motivation is to experience a pleasant mood state when good mood states are difficult to achieve naturally. Another example is the severe stress experienced by soldiers at war; during the Vietnam War, many soldiers without previous drug-taking experience became drug-dependent, probably as a result of the intense stress of waiting for combat and the easy availability of drugs.

Environmental Variables

Environmental variables include peer influence and conditioned environmental response. Because social acceptability of drug use is very important, drug use is influenced by factors such as peers who may be using drugs or may be opposed to their use. Drug use may be established as normal behavior in some populations and, therefore, drug use becomes almost universal. One example is the use of drugs by jazz musicians in the 1950s and 1960s. Here the example of older musicians admired by younger performers may have had a particularly strong influence on drug use in the younger set. Conversely, drug use may be seen as an antagonistic political statement (e.g., the use of coffee was at one time considered rebellious behavior). In the 1960s, the use of marijuana became identified with antiestablishment causes.

An important environmental feature influencing drug abuse is conditioned environmental response. Seeing people with whom one had used drugs or experiencing sights, sounds, and smells that are linked or associated with drug use induces an increase in desire and the probability of using drugs. Sometimes this is expressed as an increase in drug "craving." Laboratory studies have shown that patients can experience these conditioned drug responses and even conditioned drug withdrawal symptoms if the setting is arranged suitably. Studies in animals have indicated that dopamine, a neurotransmitter in the brain (see Chapter 4), may be involved in conditioned environmental responses. For example, dopamine is released in the brains of animals just *upon their exposure to drug-associated environments* in animals self-administering drugs. These findings support the importance of drug-associated environments in relapse and aid our understanding of the processes involved.

PREDICTING THE ABUSE POTENTIAL OF NEW DRUGS

Animal self-administration experiments have been an important source of information on drug abuse potential. Four classes of data give us information on which to base a prediction of the likelihood that a drug will be abused. First are reports from people who have tried it. Did they like it? Would they like to take it again? Clinical reports could have predicted the cocaine epidemic during the 1980s because patient surveys consistently reported that cocaine was highly desired by drug abusers but that they could not obtain sufficient quantities. A second type of information comes from law enforcement agencies. Which drugs are being stolen from pharmacies or smuggled into the country? A third method of predicting the abuse potential includes the interpretation of double-blind studies of the drug's subjective effects in human volunteers. A new drug of unknown abuse potential can be compared with a standard drug of abuse and with a placebo using rating scales to quantify the subjective effects of the drugs. Volunteers with a history of drug abuse often place a different value on a drug's effect than do normal volunteers who have never abused drugs. Therefore, the participation of drug users is important and necessary for such studies to be valid. Finally, a fourth type of data comes from studies of the self-administration of drugs by animals.

The development of animal self-administration studies rests on two sets of observations. In the 1950s, James Olds, an American psychologist, determined that animals implanted with brain electrodes would repeatedly press levers to obtain electrical stimulation when the electrodes were placed in certain areas of the brain. These regions of the brain included the hypothalamus, tegmentum, and limbic system (see Chapter 1), areas known to be involved in appetitive behaviors such as eating, drinking, and sexual activity. In other experiments it was found that epileptic patients receiving focal electrical brain stimulation in an effort to identify the sites of origin and control their seizures reported pleasurable experiences upon stimulation of certain areas of the brain including the hypothalamus, tegmentum, and amygdala. Subsequently, it was found that animals would press levers in their cages to receive drug injections into the brain in much the same way as they would to obtain electrical stimulation. These findings were important to the development of animal models of drug dependence (see Chapter 14). It has been found that animals will also press levers for rewards of stimulants or opiates delivered orally, intravenously, or by air (absorbed by the lungs). The intensity of behavioral motivation produced by the drug is quantified by the rate and amount of lever pressing the animal will perform to obtain the drug. These results are a quantification of the desirability of the drug, termed *reinforcement.*

MODES OF TREATMENT

The modes of treatment for addiction are common for all drugs of abuse. Drug addiction is best treated in facilities specializing in chemical dependency, for three reasons. First, it has been found that addicts respond positively in a therapeutic milieu in which others who are recovering from addiction support each other. Second, these patients tend to be drug-seeking, demanding, and manipulative, especially during the early stages of recovery; thus, having a facility with specialized staff skilled in setting limits while maintaining a genuine concern for these patients works best. Lastly, drug-related conditioned environmental responses (mentioned above) influence relapse profoundly, and specialized counseling and support for avoiding cues to use drugs are useful in recovery. These findings support the importance of drug-associated environments in drug-seeking behavior.

The general form of treatment entails detoxification followed by rehabilitation. Detoxification is a period of treatment in either an in-patient or out-patient setting during which the focus is to promote recovery from pharmacological drug withdrawal and develop an initial period of abstinence. Once this is established, it is necessary for all addicts to participate in some form of rehabilitation which is a long-term period of treatment following detoxification that focuses on supporting abstinence and permanently changing behavior. It is almost universal for patients to do poorly and relapse after a 30-day in-patient detoxification period that is not followed by rehabilitation. Drug dependence is a chronic disorder and requires a long-term commitment to treatment for success in altering behavior.

Several forms of rehabilitation treatment are used commonly: drug counseling, group therapy, and individual therapy. The most important variable is the duration of rehabilitation. In general, a period of about two years of involvement in rehabilitation is recommended. The type of therapy should be tailored to the individual patient's needs because there are many different types of patients with different patterns of problems complicating the drug-taking. An example of this is a heroin-dependent individual who also suffers from schizophrenia and is unable to grasp social structure and convention. Such a patient would do better with a combination of methadone and one-on-one therapy than with methadone and group therapy. Group therapy would be inappropriate as such patients are rejected by the others in the group because they are so different. Patients with depression or an anxiety disorder may need specific behavioral or pharmacological treatment in addition to treatment for alcoholism or cocaine dependence. For some pa-

tients, family therapy is essential because family difficulties may be a source of enormous distress and thus a contributing factor to the patient's lack of control.

Drug dependence must be considered a chronic disease. As is the case with arthritis, heart disease, and diabetes, there are very few cures for drug dependence. Unfortunately, the general tendency is to think of addiction as a time-limited, curable illness analogous to pneumonia or a broken leg. When these latter disorders are successfully treated, the patient is considered cured. With chronic disorders, the patient needs continued medical contact and often continuing medication such as insulin for diabetes. Periodically, there may be a return of symptoms, but these usually respond to another course of more intensive treatment. In the sense of a chronic disorder, addiction responds very well to treatment. The vast majority of patients improve as a result of treatment, at least to the level of their functioning before they became involved with drugs. Of course, a drug addict with a poor education, long criminal history, and chaotic family background has a poor prognosis even if she or he becomes drug-free. On the other hand, patients who have achieved some success prior to becoming involved with drugs are likely to return to a much higher level of functioning in response to treatment of their addiction. For example, more than 80% of physicians treated for drug or alcohol dependence are able to return to medical practice. Patients with a high-school education who come to the Philadelphia Veterans Affairs Medical Center for treatment of cocaine dependence have a 60% chance of remaining free of cocaine 4 months after beginning treatment. Both of these examples include all patients who begin treatment, not simply those who complete the program successfully. Also, none of these people are considered "cured" because all continue to have various types of psychological problems and are likely to have to struggle against returning to drug abuse for months or years to come. If they do relapse, however, it is likely that they will respond better to treatment the next time as a result of the insights and experience gained from the prior treatment and the therapeutic analysis of the causes of the relapse.

SPECIFIC DRUGS OF ABUSE

While drugs of abuse have in common the ability to produce euphoria or a "high," each causes a distinct type of euphoria and has a characteristic time course of action, pattern of use, withdrawal syndrome, toxicity, and neuropharmacological effect. To illustrate this, one important drug from each of six classes of drugs of abuse is discussed below. Represented are the stimulants, opiates/ opioids, alcohol, benzodiazepines, cannabinoids, and nicotine. Not included are miscellaneous sedatives, barbiturates, hallucinogens, and inhalants, which are currently less important drugs of abuse.

Psychostimulant Drugs: Cocaine

Cocaine—especially crack—has the highest addiction potential of any drug in the United States. Cocaine is ecgonine methylester benzoate (Fig. 1). It is obtained from the leaves of *Erythroxylon coca,* the coca plant.

History

For centuries, coca leaves were chewed by Indians living in the Andes mountains of South America. The effects were enhanced by combining the leaves with lye (sodium hydroxide) to increase the pH and improve absorption. Because only modest blood levels of cocaine can be achieved by absorption through the lining of the mouth, the stimulation produced was mild. There is no evidence that significant abuse occurred; rather, this society used cocaine to enhance work performance at high altitudes.

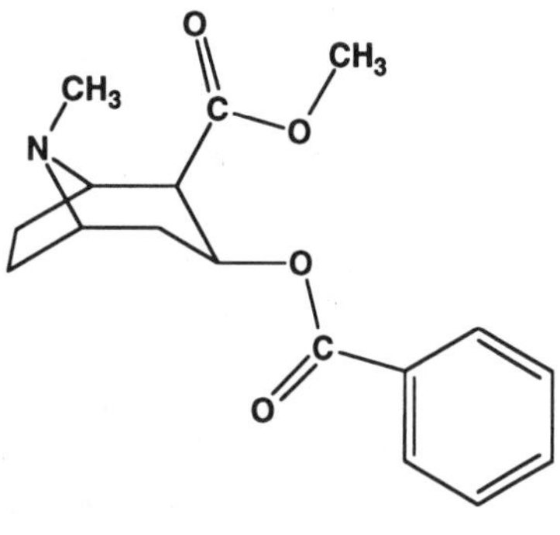

In the nineteenth century, the active ingredient in coca leaves, cocaine hydrochloride, was extracted and purified. This form of cocaine was subsequently used as a medication and as an additive in alcoholic drinks. Cocaine in powder form was also used in the manner of snuff and placed on the nasal membranes. The absorption was more rapid than by mouth, and higher blood levels were obtained. Thus, the stimulation produced by intranasal cocaine hydrochloride was much more intense than that produced by chewing coca leaves. While nineteenth century physicians initially thought that the stimulant properties of cocaine had medical value, it soon became obvious that its use via the nasal route was accompanied by serious problems of abuse and addiction.

The opportunity to inject drugs occurred when fine-bore hypodermic needles came into general medical practice in the latter half of the nineteenth century. Injecting drugs directly into a vein produces a more rapid onset of euphoria than does placing them on a mucous membrane such as the inside of the nose. It is not surprising, then, that intravenous cocaine induces a more rapid onset of abuse and addiction. In the early twentieth century, the risks of cocaine dependence became known in the United States, and laws were passed to limit supplies of the drug. Cocaine became scarce and expensive on the black market. Few people could afford to take it regularly; thus, physicians saw few patients with problems of cocaine abuse or dependence.

In the 1980s, large supplies of cheap cocaine became widely available; this was a new, smokable preparation of cocaine, the al-

FIG. 1. Structure of cocaine.

kaloid or "free base" form. Cocaine hydrochloride cannot be smoked because its vapor point is very high, and it is inactivated and carbonized before it reaches a volatile state. Alkaloidal cocaine, on the other hand, vaporizes at a lower temperature and remains pharmacologically active when heated and inhaled. This form produces a crackling sound during heating, thus the street name *crack.* Crack combines all of the most dangerous features of a drug of abuse because, when it is inhaled, high blood concentrations, comparable to those after intravenous use, are achieved rapidly. The rapid absorption causes an intense pleasure, or rush, that is not present when coca leaves are chewed or the drug is snorted. It is not surprising, therefore, to find that even in South America, the descendants of the same Indians who used cocaine without problems for centuries are now plagued with serious abuse problems caused by cocaine in this new form.

Medical Use

Cocaine is a local anesthetic as well as a drug of abuse. Like other local anesthetics, cocaine blocks nerve conduction. For most of this century, cocaine was used as a topical (surface) anesthetic for surgical procedures of the eye and nasal passages. It is still used for anesthesia of the nose by some practitioners, but its use is limited by its abuse potential and its toxicity.

Addiction

The addiction potential of crack is not only a property of its pharmacology but also of environment and conditioning. In the United States, populations at risk for cocaine addiction often have some experience with smoking marijuana prior to exposure to cocaine. This experience may give a false sense of safety in smoking other drugs since marijuana is a drug associated with a low rate of addiction. Further, injecting a drug is associated with being a "junky," and self-injection is repugnant to many people. The necessity of injecting a drug into a vein is a barrier to use and tends to lower the addiction potential. Thus, the ability to smoke cocaine enhances its abuse potential.

Cocaine probably has the highest addiction potential of any drug. Laboratory studies involving drug self-administration in animal models often use cocaine initially to train the animal in the study procedures and then switch to the drug of interest. This is an indication of the ease with which cocaine self-administration develops and is a measure of its addicting potential. Other drugs, even heroin, require drug "priming" or involuntary administrations before the animal will self-administer the drug. Cocaine usually does not require priming.

Patterns of Use

The pattern of drug administration for cocaine is distinctive. The most common pattern for both intravenous injection and smoking crack via a pipe apparatus is repeated administrations as injections or inhalations at intervals of 5 to 30 min. The user administers drug repeatedly for hours to a few days. The amount of drug taken and the length of time of the binge are usually determined by the amount of drug or money to buy drug that is available. Some cocaine addicts report stopping sessions after feeling ill or paranoid or being frightened by chest pains or palpitations (disturbingly forceful heart beats). However, there are also cocaine users who use small amounts of the drug daily. These individuals probably represent abusers who are not addicted or individuals with poor control of their addiction who cannot save enough money at a time to finance a binge.

Pharmacokinetics and Metabolism

The pharmacokinetics of cocaine provide a clue to its toxicity. In studies of cocaine undertaken in human volunteers, nonlinear kinetics have been observed, i.e., the rate of metabolism expressed as a percentage of total drug present is not constant (similar to alcohol). With most drugs, a constant percentage of the total drug present is eliminated per unit of time; this demonstrates first-order kinetics. For example, approximately 23% of morphine in the blood is metabolized hourly. This rate is independent of the concentration of morphine in blood: the rate is 23% of 1 μg/ml or 23% of 1000 μg/ml (Fig. 2). By contrast, cocaine does not have a constant half-life. The rate of metabolism as a percentage of total amount of drug in the body decreases as more cocaine is accumulated because there is a limit to the absolute rate of cocaine metabolism (Fig. 2). Thus, it is easy to accumulate cocaine, and once a high concentration accumulates in the body, its concentration may stay elevated for a long period before returning to baseline. This is an important consideration in the cocaine-intoxicated or poisoned individual and can explain why drug effects can last for many hours.

Behavioral Effects

The pleasurable mood induced by intravenous or smoked cocaine generally lasts from 1 to 2 hr. However, the initial period of euphoria (i.e., the rush) lasts about 10 min. Rush is described as having a speeding or explosive quality. It can be experienced simultaneously with unpleasant sensations induced by cocaine such as palpitations and paranoia. Cocaine users report that rush is the motivating factor for using intravenous and smoke delivery routes of cocaine administration. Intranasal use of cocaine powder does not induce rush and has a lower addiction potential. The pleasurable sensation following rush, lasting as long as 2 hr after dosing, has no unique name other than "high," a term that is used to describe any pleasurable change from a baseline mood state. In human laboratory experiments, rush and the less intense high can be blocked independently, indicating that the two effects may be independent responses to cocaine.

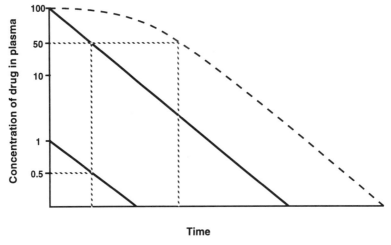

Time

FIG. 2. Linear and nonlinear pharmacokinetics. In first-order or linear kinetics, a constant fraction of drug is removed from plasma per unit of time regardless of the plasma concentration (solid lines). Thus, the time for drug to be reduced from 100 to 50 units is the same as the time to reduce the drug from 1 to 0.5 unit. For nonlinear kinetics, the rate of removal from plasma is concentration-dependent (dashed line). Thus, it takes longer to reduce the concentration in plasma from 100 to 50 units than it does to reduce concentration from 1 to 0.5 unit.

Toxicity

Overdoses of cocaine have caused death, generally as the result of cocaine's effects on the heart, blood vessels, and brain. Cocaine has caused myocardial infarctions resulting in death in young persons who did not have abnormalities of the coronary arteries. Coronary spasm has been observed in patients overdosing with cocaine; it can also cause dangerous arrhythmias. Cocaine-induced arrhythmias and infarction are not necessarily linked to one another and may occur independently. Cocaine causes increases in heart rate and blood pressure. In patients overdosed with cocaine, it can cause hypertensive crises. It is not surprising, therefore, that cocaine has been associated with stroke and ruptured aneurisms.

Neuropharmacology

Brain areas important in the self-administration of stimulants are the ventral tegmental area, nucleus accumbens, lateral hypothalamus, and, perhaps, the prefrontal cortex (see Chapter 1). These brain areas contain the neurotransmitter dopamine (see Chapter 6). Numerous experiments interrupting dopamine pathways or blocking dopaminergic activity in these regions have demonstrated an important role for dopamine in the self-administration of stimulant drugs, i.e., dopamine must be present for cocaine to elicit self-administration. In particular, the nucleus accumbens has been considered a vital part of the brain's "reward" system, that part of the brain involved in reinforcement of activity. Just how this system participates in supporting and maintaining chronic drug use is unknown, but is an active focus of research.

The role of dopamine in the self-administration of other classes of abused drugs is not known, in part because self-administration of drugs in animals is not a perfect pharmacological model for human use. Animals generally do not self-administer cannabinoids, hallucinogens, or nicotine, and alcohol self-administration requires special conditions. Thus, where the animal model is less applicable, the mechanism linking complex behaviors to neurochemistry and neuroanatomy is less well understood.

Both cocaine and another psychostimulant, amphetamine, act to increase the amount of dopamine in synapses including synapses involving brain reward pathways. Amphetamine causes release of dopamine from dopaminergic neurons and inhibits the reuptake of dopamine by the presynaptic dopamine transporter back to the nerve terminal. Cocaine binds with high affinity to the dopamine transporter, inhibiting the uptake of dopamine, but does not cause the release of dopamine. As a consequence of these actions, cocaine and amphetamine increase the effect of dopamine at postsynaptic dopaminergic receptors. Although animals will self-administer drugs that act as dopamine agonists by direct action on postsynaptic dopamine receptors (e.g., apomorphine, bromocriptine), these drugs are not potent in animal self-administration assays nor are they abused by humans. Drugs that bind to the presynaptic dopamine transporter molecule are self-administered in direct proportion to their affinity for the transporter (Fig. 3). Taken together, these findings indicate that dopamine is very important in stimulant-taking behavior and that specifically the presynaptic dopamine transporter molecule plays a major role.

The addiction potentials of cocaine and amphetamine are probably comparable. Both amphetamine and cocaine can be injected, smoked, and taken orally. Currently, in the United States, addiction to amphetamine (or "speed") is at a low ebb, while cocaine addiction is relatively high. However, in Japan, amphetamine addiction problems have been very severe since the 1960s and continue to be a big problem. These observations suggest that cultural factors may play a role in the observed difference in addiction

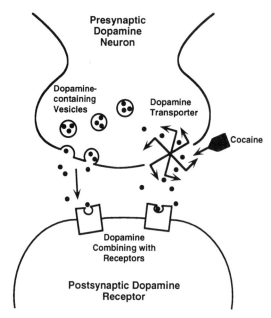

Presynaptic
Dopamine
Neuron

Dopamine-
containing
Vesicles

Dopamine
Transporter

Cocaine

Dopamine
Combining with
Receptors

Postsynaptic Dopamine
Receptor

FIG. 3. Schematic of dopaminergic neuron with dopamine release, postsynaptic coupling with receptor and dopamine transporter, showing blockade of the dopamine transporter by cocaine.

rates between the two drugs. It is possible that there will be future U.S. epidemics of amphetamine addiction as fashion and supply change.

Withdrawal and Treatment

Although cocaine is clearly addicting and in the behavioral sense has dependence liability, the existence of a cocaine withdrawal syndrome is unclear. One study reported clinical observations of a *crash,* which is a period of sleep, a period of low craving and anhedonia (inability to experience pleasure), and a period of intense craving for drug following abstinence. Another study failed to confirm this in a double-blind, controlled, inpatient study of cocaine abstinence.

In recent years, in addition to psychotherapy and counseling (see Modes of Treatment), a number of drugs have been suggested for the treatment of cocaine addiction.

Some were proposed as candidates to block the effects of cocaine, others to provide a cocaine-like effect combined with blockade of cocaine's intense mood state effects, and still others as having effects on drug craving. Among these drugs are bromocriptine, haloperidol, amantadine, desipramine, carbamazepine, calcium-channel blockers, and bupropion. At this writing, bromocriptine and haloperidol have been discarded. Carbamazepine was reported to reduce craving for cocaine in an uncontrolled trial but was ineffective in a placebo-controlled study. The remaining drugs continue to be investigated. Thus far, there are no effective pharmacological treatments for cocaine dependence, but research is continuing on effective aids to treatment.

Opiates and Opioids: Heroin

The opiate drugs are potent analgesics. Opiate dependence has been a problem in the United States for over 100 years. During that time it has involved different opiates and different classes of users. Currently, heroin is the most important abused drug in this class, although almost all drugs in this class are abused. Heroin (Fig. 4A) is diacetylmorphine hydrochloride and is derived from morphine (Fig. 4B), a drug obtained from the juice of the Oriental poppy *Papaver somnifera.* Opium is the air-dried milky exudate from incised, unripe seed capsules of certain species of poppy. It contains over 20 opiate drugs including morphine, codeine, papaverine, noscapine, and thebaine. Opium and other drugs that are derivatives of naturally occurring plant substances are termed *opiates,* whereas drugs having similar properties of analgesia and addiction liability that are synthesized and have different basic chemical structures are termed *opioids.*

History

Opiate drugs have been known since at least the third century B.C. Theophrastas, Ar-

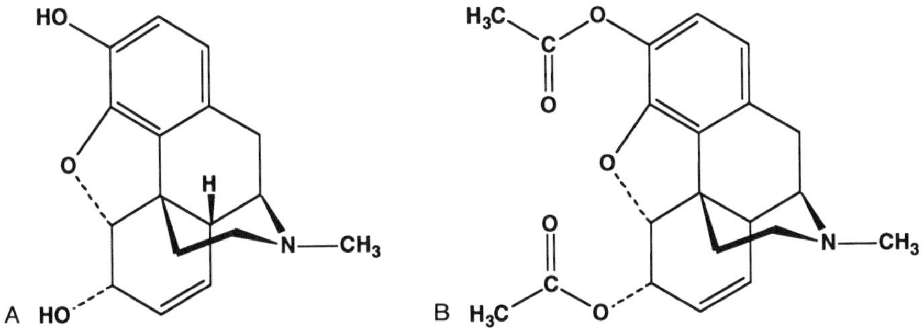

FIG. 4. Structure of **(A)** heroin and **(B)** morphine.

istotle's successor at the Lyceum, wrote a history of plants in which he mentions poppy juice. Arab physicians used opium in medicine for analgesia, and Arab traders introduced it to the East. Early practitioners knew about the problems of toxicity caused by opium, and throughout history the use of opiates has risen and fallen in response to the appreciation of its benefits and risks. In the nineteenth century, European traders profited from the opium trade and defeated an attempt by the Chinese to stop marketing of the drug. Subsequently, addiction became a severe problem in China. Addiction to opiates occurred in Europe and America as well, though to a lesser degree than in Asia. The invention of the hypodermic needle and the use of purified opiate compounds such as morphine and codeine increased the abuse of opiates in a way that is analogous to the recent history of cocaine.

Medical Use

Because the opiate drugs are potent analgesics, their use in a medical setting for relief from pain is certainly one of the most important advances in pharmacology. Morphine, a natural plant alkaloid, remains the most important analgesic for serious pain but all opiate drugs including heroin relieve pain. Heroin is still prescribed for pain relief in the United Kingdom but in the United States there is no legal supply of heroin except for research purposes.

Methadone is a synthetic opioid (Fig. 5)

that is used principally for the treatment of opiate addiction. Patients are given a daily dose of this long-acting opioid to maintain a high level of drug tolerance that prevents the patient from experiencing euphoria from heroin use.

Patterns of Use

Heroin is by far the most abused opiate drug despite the fact that in a study of heroin-using research subjects, the subjects could not detect a difference between injected heroin and other potent opiates such as hydromorphone. Heroin is generally injected intravenously, although it is possible to snort it or inject it under the skin (i.e., "skinpopping"). Heroin's effect lasts for 3 to 12 hr after injection. The usual pattern of use is to inject the drug one to three times daily. Such injection results in physical dependence. Some people "chip" heroin; that is, they attempt to use it only once a week or only every second or

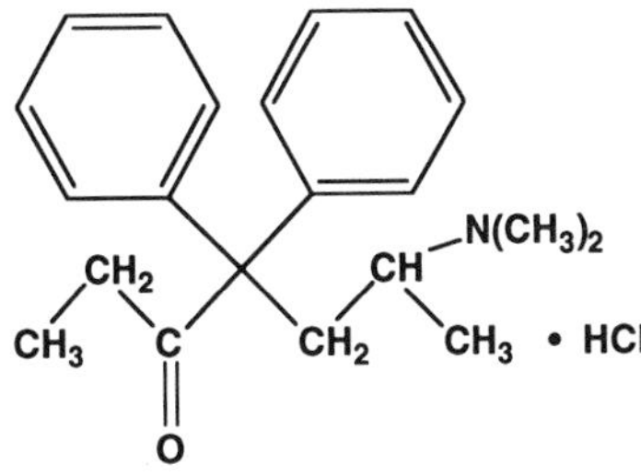

FIG. 5. Structure of methadone, a synthetic opioid.

third day to avoid strong physical dependence. Based on patient reports, many, if not most, of these "chippers" graduate to daily use.

Pharmacokinetics and Metabolism

Heroin is a highly lipid-soluble opiate. *It has been demonstrated that the active substance after heroin injection is not heroin itself but its metabolite, morphine.* Heroin is hydrolyzed rapidly in the brain to morphine. Shortly after injection of heroin, the concentration of opiate in the brain is higher than its concentration in the blood. Thereafter, the drug is redistributed, and the brain concentration falls as the drug concentration rises in other tissues. The initial high brain concentration attained after drug administration may be the mechanism of the heroin rush, the intense sensation felt soon after drug injection and differing in quality from later sensations.

Drug Effects

A heroin rush is short-lived, as with cocaine, in the range of 15 to 20 min, and is followed by a milder pleasurable sensation lasting 5 to 8 hr. However, the quality of the heroin rush differs from that of cocaine. Addicts describe a peaceful, warm sensation of rush. Many heroin addicts become sleepy and nod for a while after injecting heroin, but lower doses of heroin and/or use of heroin in subjects with high levels of heroin tolerance may not interfere with the ability to perform work in an efficient and orderly fashion.

The common physiological changes that occur after heroin injection are miosis (pupil constriction), small changes in blood pressure and heart rate, and decreases in respiratory rate and temperature. Since there is little tolerance to miosis, it is a particularly useful and reliable clinical sign of drug activity. There is also little tolerance to the respiratory depression caused by opiates, so that respiratory depression becomes a serious problem with overdoses.

Toxicity

Overdoses with opiates can cause serious toxicity and death. The mode of death is usually respiratory depression progressing to coma, hypotension (abnormally low blood pressure), and cessation of breathing. In acute overdoses from injection, there is often pulmonary edema, a condition in which the air spaces of the lung fill with fluid.

Neuropharmacology

In 1943, Klaus Unna, director of the U.S. Addiction Research Center in Lexington, Kentucky, observed that some opiate drugs demonstrated the interesting property of antagonizing opiate poisoning. This work repeated and expanded the observation by the German physician J. Pohl in 1915 that *nor-allylcodeine could reverse opiate poisoning.* Later, these drugs were shown to precipitate withdrawal symptoms in morphine-dependent addicts. In 1964, the clinical pharmacologist, William Martin, and his colleagues reported that three drugs from the opiate/opioid class had distinctly differing properties and each of the drugs failed to cross-suppress opiate withdrawal in animals dependent on one of the other two drugs. These scientists concluded that more than one receptor must exist to account for these results. Subsequently, three groups of scientists, working independently, determined that these postulated receptors did exist. Today it is generally agreed that there are at least three classes of opiate receptors: μ, κ, and δ. *In early work it was noted that all opiate/opioid receptors were antagonized by the unique opioid drug naloxone.* By convention, it has been decided that antagonism by naloxone is a defining characteristic of opiate receptors, i.e., receptor actions not antagonized by naloxone are not opiate-mediated.

It is now clear that in humans μ receptors are associated with analgesia and euphoria. Activation of κ receptors also causes analgesia, though of a different type from that associated with μ analgesia. In addition, κ-receptor activation elicits dysphoria, giddiness, and hallucinations. The effects of drugs activating κ receptors in humans differ distinctly from those in animals, which has caused some confusion in the interpretation of experiments. For example, activation of κ receptors causes sedation in dogs, whereas in humans κ activation is stimulatory. In mice morphine is a stimulant but in humans it has sedative properties. Thus, although the classes of opiate receptors are the same in humans and animals, they are associated with different actions.

The development of agonist-antagonist drugs at μ or κ receptors was intended to provide drugs that offered analgesic properties without the potential for abuse. Many drugs such as pentazocine, nalbuphine, butorphenol, and buprenorphine act as antagonists or partial agonists (see Chapter 4) at μ or κ receptors, sometimes interacting with both types of receptors. Because the intrinsic activities of these drugs at μ receptors are weak relative to those of full agonists, they have the property of acting as antagonists in the presence of full agonists. Fatal overdoses with these drugs are rare because their maximum pharmacological effects, particularly on respiratory depression, are less than those caused by full agonists such as heroin. However, the maximum analgesia attained is also less than that with full agonists.

The anatomic sites associated with opiate self-administration in animals overlap with those for cocaine. Damage to the nucleus accumbens in rats causes impairment of heroin or cocaine self-administration in the animals without impairing movement or appetite. However, after some time, lesioned animals will resume self-administration of heroin but not cocaine. It has also been shown that drugs that block opiate receptors block self-administration of opiates but not of cocaine.

It would appear that the nucleus accumbens is important for both opiate and cocaine reward but that it may be activated through different pathways by cocaine and by exogenous opiates.

In 1975, the German-born physiologist Hans Walter Kosterlitz and his colleagues working in Scotland isolated peptides from pig brain that bound to opiate receptors. These were the first endogenous opioid peptides discovered. *Subsequent discoveries revealed the presence of three families of natural opiate peptides—enkephalins, dynorphins, and endorphins.* These peptides are derived from the peptide precursors proopiomelanocortin, proenkephalin, and prodynorphin (see Chapter 8). Release of endogenous opioids has been observed in response to physical stress in both animals and humans. In humans, increases in the release of opioid peptides that have preferential μ-agonist properties are thought to cause a sense of well-being and euphoria. The release of endogenous opioids has also been reported to increase during acupuncture analgesia.

Withdrawal and Treatment

Withdrawal from opiate drugs induces a very distinctive syndrome. The length of time of the withdrawal syndrome depends on the half-life of the opiate drug. The active metabolite of heroin, morphine, has a half-life of about 3 hr, and withdrawal from heroin peaks at 24 to 60 hr after the last dose of the drug. In contrast, methadone, the drug used for maintenance treatment of opiate-dependent patients, has a half-life of 36 hr and a withdrawal syndrome that peaks at 7 to 10 days after stopping the drug and lasts about 30 days. The patient experiencing methadone withdrawal after a period of methadone treatment and stabilization feels weak and will complain of a flu-like syndrome. The peak of distress for methadone withdrawal is less than that for heroin withdrawal. However, patients find the comparatively long duration of withdrawal from methadone difficult to endure.

The symptoms of opiate withdrawal include mild elevations in blood pressure, temperature, and pulse; sweating; mydriasis (pupil dilation); nasal congestion; runny nose; "goose flesh"; shivering; and diarrhea. A prominent sign is the bent, drawn-up position of the patient in bed or while walking. Associated with this sign is the symptom of severe cramping pains most prominent in the lower back, joints, and back of the legs. Opiate withdrawal is treated with tapering doses of other opiate/opioid drugs such as methadone and propoxyphene. Clonidine, an α_2-adrenergic agonist, relieves many symptoms of withdrawal. Severe, untreated opiate withdrawal has resulted in death that may have been due to inanition because of sickness.

Most heroin addicts opt for a period of methadone maintenance instead of drug-free treatment. *Treatment with methadone, a long-acting opiate drug, suppresses opiate withdrawal symptoms* (Fig. 5). Thus, although the patient is still physically dependent on opiates, he or she is no longer required to seek opiate supplies to suppress sickness. Methadone treatment also causes substantial tolerance to the effects of opiates including heroin: the patient may inject heroin but feel little of the opiate effect. Methadone is given as a single, oral, individually adjusted, daily dose to satisfy the patient's physical need for opiates. In order to receive this treatment, patients must come to a special clinic daily and must receive counseling and other health services.

Some people object to the use of methadone on philosophical grounds because patients transfer their dependence from an illegal opiate, heroin, to a legally prescribed opioid, methadone. However, the difference can be life saving. Patients on methadone usually diminish and then cease illegal opiate use with all of the attendant risks of criminality and infections. On an appropriate dose of methadone, patients can function normally, including attending school, operating a business, or practicing law or medicine. There is no sedation or impairment. Patients may be treated for a period of years and then be gradually tapered off the drug to become drug-free. Results of one long-term study are given in Fig. 6. Some patients opt to remain on methadone indefinitely, and many physicians feel that methadone can be considered a kind of hormone replacement therapy similar to lifelong treatment with thyroxin, insulin, or cortisone.

Sedatives: Alcohol

Of all the many sedatives, alcohol is the most commonly used. Sedatives are generally defined by their ability to produce central nervous system depression manifested by decreased alertness and, with higher doses, sleep, coma, and death. The sedatives comprise several different pharmacological categories and consequently produce their effect by various mechanisms of action. The most commonly used and abused sedative is alcohol. The fluid commonly termed *alcohol* is ethyl alcohol or ethanol (Fig. 7), a product of the fermentation of sugars, starches, or other carbohydrates.

History

Alcohol imbibed in the form of wine or beer has been documented in the earliest human written histories, myths, and art. Wine and beer are produced by the fermentation of grapes, grain, or honey during which yeast enzymes convert sugar to ethyl alcohol. Wine, the fermented product of grapes or other fruits, was made in Egypt by the year 3000 B.C. Homer, living in the ninth century B.C., used the words "wine-dark sea" to describe the Mediterranean Sea. Beer, the fermented product of grain or honey, originated in places where grapes do not grow. Its use is more ancient than that of wine and has been documented in Babylon in 4000 B.C. Both wine and beer technology passed sequentially from the Near East (Mesopotamia) to the empires of Egypt, North Africa, Greece, and

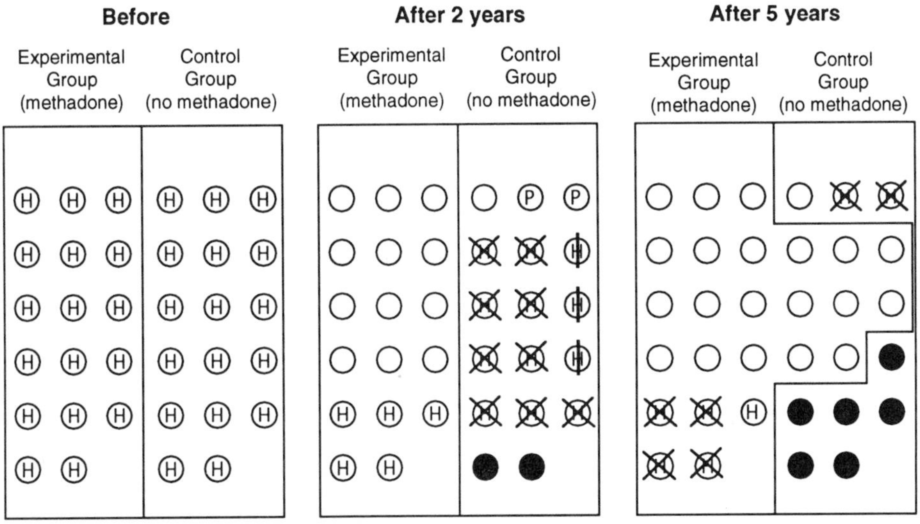

FIG. 6. Methadone treatment and relapse rate. Clinical trial of methadone maintenance vs. outpatient nonmethadone treatment for heroin addiction conducted through the Swedish Methadone Maintenance Program. The left half of each box represents the group assigned to methadone maintenance; the right half represents the control group. Before admission (**left box**): each circle represents an individual 20 to 24 years old. H indicates regular intravenous heroin abuse. Two years after admission (**middle box**): O, no drug abuse; H, abuse of heroin; P, subject in prison; ●, subject deceased; X, subject expelled from program; |, subject hospitalized for drug abuse–related condition. Five years after admission (**right box**): 10 persons who had been expelled from the original control group were accepted into methadone maintenance. Modified from Grönbladh L, Gunne L. Methadone-assisted rehabilitation of Swedish heroin addicts. *Drug Alcohol Depend* 1989; 24:31–37.

Rome, to Western Europe, and to China and Japan.

Liquors are fermentation products of grapes, grains, molasses, or other starches and sugars in which the fermentation process is followed by distillation, which concentrates the alcohol. Distillation of alcoholic beverages was known by the Romans and was practiced in China by 800 B.C.

Patterns of Use

There are many misconceptions about alcoholism, the most dangerous being that it always involves heavy, daily use of alcohol.

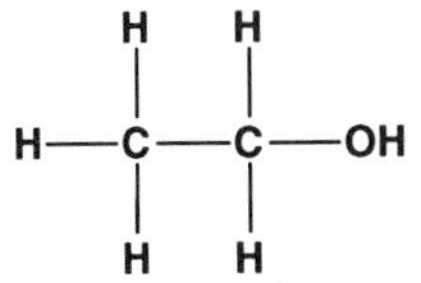

FIG. 7. Structure of ethyl alcohol.

This leads to a delay in diagnosis until the condition is very severe and most difficult to treat. Alcoholism is diagnosed using the same criteria as for other types of drug dependencies. The essential characteristic of the disorder is loss of control. Increased tolerance to the effects of alcohol may be present and withdrawal symptoms when alcohol is stopped may be part of the clinical picture, but the diagnosis of alcohol dependence can be made without these elements. An episodic user who cannot control quantity and whose use of alcohol interferes with work or family responsibilities would qualify as being alcoholic.

Pharmacokinetics and Metabolism

Alcohol is metabolized by alcohol dehydrogenase, catalase, and microsomal oxidizing enzymes to acetaldehyde and then to acetate. Alcohol dehydrogenase is the most important enzyme, accounting for a large portion of the conversion. Alcohol taken chronically induces enzymes in the liver, thereby increasing its rate of metabolism; this may account for the increased tolerance to alcohol observed in heavy drinkers. As with the disposition of cocaine, alcohol metabolism is nonlinear, that is, the rate of metabolism expressed as a percentage of total drug present is not constant (Fig. 2). As alcohol is accumulated, the rate of its metabolism slows down. This predisposes people to alcohol accumulation and toxicity when multiple drinks are taken in one session. It also substantially prolongs the duration of the effects of the drug.

Drug Effects

The initial effects of low doses of alcohol appear to involve depression of neuronal pathways that are inhibitory to behavior. Thus, the effects observed typically include relaxation of inhibitions, increased talking, and increased probability of engaging in certain behaviors deemed unacceptable to the drinker in a completely sober state.

As with all drugs, the effects of alcohol vary across individuals. Some people lose inhibitions and become extremely excited by even a low dose of alcohol, and some become aggressive. This is known as pathological intoxication. Others show very little of the excitation phase and move directly into a sedated phase. Still others, most often people of Asian ancestry, show a vasodilation or flushing reaction that can be quite unpleasant; it is the result of the accumulation of the alcohol metabolite acetaldehyde.

Toxicity

Since the effects of alcohol show such individual variation, it may seem surprising that the legal definitions of intoxication are so precise. In most states of the United States, a person is considered to be "legally drunk" at a blood alcohol level of 0.1 g/100 ml. In fact, most people show significant impairment on tests of vigilance and reaction time at levels half as great. Others are naturally tolerant to higher plasma levels, and some acquire tolerance by repeated heavy use of alcohol. While a single episode of alcohol consumption can produce intoxication to the point of overdose and death, chronic alcohol use even in moderate doses can produce toxic effects on many organs and behavioral toxicity known as alcohol abuse or alcohol dependence (alcoholism).

In the United States, alcoholism is the most common cause of thiamine (vitamin B_1) deficiency. Symptoms of thiamine deficiency are polyneuritis, an inflammation of nerves with motor and sensory deficits, or Wernicke–Korsakoff syndrome, brain lesions characterized clinically by ophthalmoplegia (paralysis of eye movements), nystagmus (repeated horizontal eye movement), and ataxia (unsteady gait, loss of coordination), along with confusion, memory loss, and confabulation (fabrication of details).

Neuropharmacology

Alcohol (ethyl alcohol) is a small molecule with a molecular weight of 46 (Fig. 7). It is water-soluble and enters all tissues of the body. The effect of alcohol on membranes is similar to that of anesthetics—it increases membrane fluidity and causes membrane expansion. Among the consequences of this action are effects on membrane proteins and ion channels. *Alcohol potentiates the effects of GABA (γ-aminobutyric acid), a neurotransmitter, at the GABA/receptor complex, and increases the influx of chloride ions into the neurons* (see Chapter 19). *This raises the threshold for excitation of the membrane.* Interestingly, benzodiazepine receptor inverse agonists block this action and also reverse some of the pharmacological effects of alcohol, directly linking the effects of alcohol with actions at the benzodiazepine receptor complex site. Inverse agonists are drugs that interact with a receptor, not only blocking agonist-like effects but causing actions opposite in kind to those of agonists.

Withdrawal and Treatment

Alcohol withdrawal is a dangerous syndrome with the potential to cause death. Withdrawal symptoms generally begin to appear from 8 to 12 hr after the patient's last drink. Reliable signs of withdrawal are increases in blood pressure, temperature, and pulse. Sweating also occurs. A body tremor is present that is sometimes so severe that patients are unable to walk or feed themselves. Patients complain of sensations of tension and anxiety that may be very severe. They may develop alcohol withdrawal psychosis with hallucinations. The most serious consequences of alcohol withdrawal are seizures or cardiac arrhythmias with death.

Treatment of alcohol withdrawal always includes thiamine, either injected or given orally. Many alcoholic patients can be safely and economically detoxified as outpatients with daily visits, daily doses of benzodiazepines, and daily breathalyzer testing to ensure that the patient is not continuing to use alcohol. However, severely dependent or sickly patients need to be detoxified in the hospital using benzodiazepine treatment.

Disulfiram (Antabuse; Fig. 8) is a useful medication for the maintenance of abstinence among alcoholics provided it is taken daily and is prescribed as part of an overall rehabilitation program. It inactivates aldehyde dehydrogenase, the enzyme that metabolizes acetaldehyde formed from alcohol, allowing acetaldehyde to accumulate in the body (Fig. 9). Thus, if the patient drinks alcohol while taking disulfiram, he or she will suffer symptoms such as vasodilation, hypotension, headache, vomiting, sweating, weakness, vertigo, and confusion. Severe drinking while using disulfiram can be dangerous, and its use is recommended only for healthy, motivated patients who are able to understand the consequences of drinking alcohol while taking this medication. It can be very useful for patients trying hard to abstain but with a history of impulsive drinking leading to relapse in prior drug-free treatments.

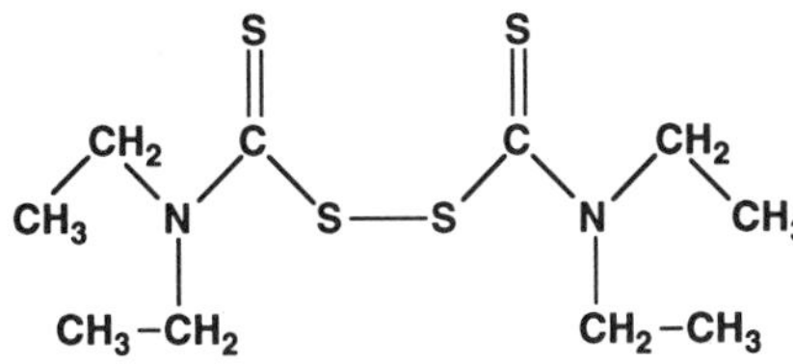

Recently, there has been active inquiry into the use of the opiate receptor antagonist naltrexone to aid alcoholic patients. This work is based on the observation that rats who learn to drink alcohol under certain conditions will reduce consumption or stop drinking alcohol if they are treated with naltrexone. This may be related to the observation that alcohol produces an increase in the release of endorphins in the brain. It appears that in the presence of naltrexone a portion of the reward induced by alcohol is blocked. Two double-blind treatment trials have shown that outpatient alcoholics receiving naltrexone relapse less often than those receiving placebo.

Inherited and Environmental Influences

A variety of genetic studies implicate heredity in up to 50% of cases of alcoholism. Some of the strongest data come from follow-up studies of people who were adopted at birth and raised apart from their biological parents. In these studies, the risk of alcoholism developing in men by age 35 was related to the presence of alcoholism in the biological but not the adoptive father. The risk was several times higher than that of adoptees whose biological fathers were not alcoholic, whether or not the adoptive household contained an alcoholic. Studies comparing monozygotic twins with dizygotic twins (see Chapter 16) have also reported a genetic component in early, severe alcoholism. However, there is still some controversy about these studies since not all researchers have found the same results using similar methodology. It is also true that genetic influence typically accounts for only 10% to 20% of the variability in the

FIG. 8. Structure of disulfiram.

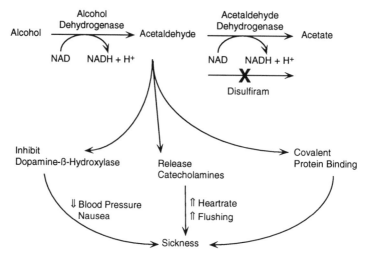

FIG. 9. Alcohol metabolism and the biochemical action of disulfiram. Alcohol is converted to acetate via the action of two enzymes, alcohol dehydrogenese and acetaldehyde dehydrogenase. Disulfiram inhibits the action of acetaldehyde dehydrogenase, resulting in an accumulation of acetaldehyde that results in manifestations of toxicity.

expression of alcoholic outcome. Therefore, patients should not be given deterministic ideas about the inevitability of developing alcoholism.

Despite the focus on genetics, it is clear that a large portion of the variability in the potential for developing alcoholism and recovery from alcoholism is related to environment and treatment or the interaction between the two. The influence of these variables should not be underestimated. Improvement of high-risk environments and early intervention and treatment have the potential to realize enormous gains in the prevention and treatment of alcoholism.

Benzodiazepines: Diazepam

The benzodiazepines are the most commonly prescribed drugs in the world. Benzodiazepines are widely used to treat the symptoms of anxiety. Of this class, diazepam is the most commonly used (Fig. 10). Abuse of these drugs is infrequent in relation to the large number of prescriptions written.

History

The first benzodiazepine, chlordiazepoxide, was synthesized in 1955 by the working group of Leo Sternbach, a chemist working at the pharmaceutical company Hoffmann–La Roche Inc. Two years later, the capacity of drugs in this class to reduce anxiety, cause sedation, and act as a muscle relaxant became evident in animal models. Chlordiazepoxide (Librium) was marketed in early 1960. By 1972, its cousin, diazepam (Val-

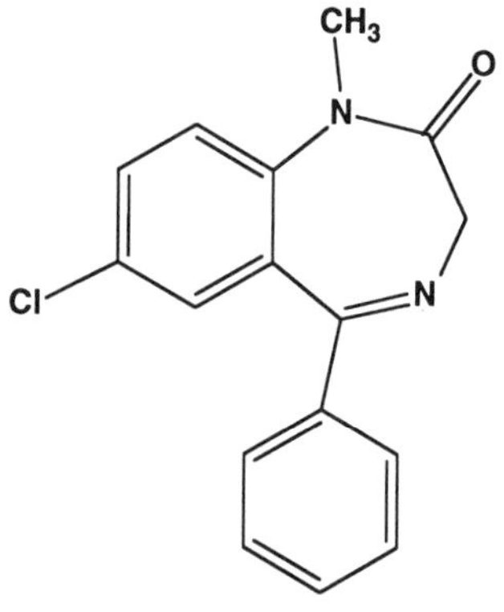

FIG. 10. Structure of diazepam.

ium) was the number one selling drug in the United States.

Clinical Use

The main use of benzodiazepines is in the treatment of anxiety disorders, although they have sedative effects as well (see Chapter 19). There is a very high demand for these drugs by patients, who often want to use them to blunt the problems of everyday life, to escape discomfort. Escaping from normal anxiety is not an appropriate use of this medication, and may lead to excessive use of this class of drugs.

The sedative and anxiolytic properties of benzodiazepines make them useful preanesthesia medications. They reduce the patient's anxieties and impair remembrance of the events just prior to surgery.

Diazepam and several other benzodiazepines can suppress epileptic seizures (see Chapter 22). It is used to treat alcohol withdrawal seizures and to stop serious, unrelenting seizures called status epilepticus. However, upon repeated use, the ability of diazepam to suppress seizures declines, i.e., tolerance to the antiseizure activity develops, and thus it is not useful in the long-term treatment of epilepsy. Other benzodiazepines are useful in the treatment of specific types of seizures.

Diazepam and other benzodiazepines are also important muscle relaxants. They can be used in muscle disease to relieve debilitating, painful muscle spasms and after routine muscle trauma.

Abuse and Dependence

Benzodiazepines including diazepam are commonly used by substance abusers to self-treat anxiety occurring after cocaine use, promote sleep, substitute for opiates when they are scarce, or treat withdrawal from other drugs. Some substance abusers take benzodiazepines such as diazepam or triazolam in high doses to experience a kind of high, but this euphoria is not as intense as that produced by cocaine or opiates.

It is rare for patients to intentionally abuse benzodiazepines. However, it is common for physical dependence to develop when these drugs are taken regularly for greater than 6 to 8 months even in moderate or low doses for appropriate medical reasons such as a chronic anxiety disorder. Long-term users of benzodiazepines develop tolerance to the sedating effects typically produced by this class of drugs.

Pharmacokinetics and Metabolism

Diazepam is very well absorbed into the body from the gastrointestinal tract; peak blood concentrations occur about 1 hr after ingestion. It is a long-acting drug, with a half-life of approximately 30 hr. It has an unusual metabolic profile (Fig. 11). Diazepam is metabolized to *N*-desmethyldiazepam (a methyl group is removed from the parent compound). This metabolite is also an active benzodiazepine with a half-life of 51 hr, even longer than that of diazepam. Both diazepam and *N*-desmethyldiazepam are further metabolized to another active metabolite, oxazepam, which has a half-life of 5 to 15 hr.

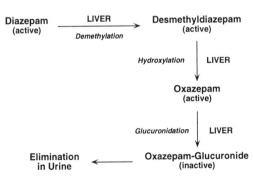

FIG. 11. Schematic diagram of the metabolism of diazepam. Metabolism of diazepam occurs in the liver, where it is both demethylated and oxidized to metabolites that have pharmacological activity. Oxazepam is not only a metabolite but is also prescribed as an antianxiety medication.

Toxicity

Diazepam and all benzodiazepines have very little acute toxicity. An overdose may cause sleep for long periods of time and discoordination. Little depression of respiratory or cardiovascular function is seen even at high doses. However, elderly people are often quite sensitive to the effects of diazepam and may become confused. Benzodiazepines do potentiate the effects of alcohol, and the use of benzodiazepines and alcohol together may result in serious unexpected overdoses because of the tendency of alcohol and benzodiazepines to potentiate each others' effects.

Withdrawal and Treatment

If benzodiazepine treatment or abuse is stopped suddenly, the appearance of withdrawal symptoms is likely. These symptoms are the opposite of the effects of benzodiazepines: irritability, exaggerated reflexes, insomnia, and, in some cases, seizures. This withdrawal syndrome resembles that seen after alcohol withdrawal, but with the addition of hyperacusis (excessive acuteness of the sense of hearing), paresthesias (pins and needles, abnormal prickling or itching), and other unusual sensory phenomena. It is important to taper benzodiazepine doses over time to avoid withdrawal symptoms. During detoxification treatment, most withdrawal symptoms occur when the dose has been tapered to less than 25% of the original dose.

For the patient who has been abusing large doses of benzodiazepines, treatment consists of gradually reducing the drug of abuse or transferring the patient to the long-acting barbiturate phenobarbital. There is cross-tolerance between barbiturates and benzodiazepines. Large initial doses of phenobarbital are given and tapered while the patient abstains from benzodiazepine use. This permits immediate abstinence from the rewarding effect of the benzodiazepines, breaking the cycle of addiction and preventing serious withdrawal symptoms.

Persons who have been dependent on benzodiazepines should have a careful psychiatric evaluation once they are detoxified as they sometimes have an underlying anxiety disorder that requires further treatment. These patients, like other drug-dependent patients, should enter a rehabilitation program after detoxification.

Cannabinoids

The cannabinoids are associated with a feeling of mild euphoria, decreased cognitive abilities, and a relatively mild withdrawal. Cannabinoids is the class name given multi–ring aromatic compounds that are derived from the hemp plant *Cannabis sativa. The psychoactive constituents of the cannabinoids found in the cannabis plant are the tetrahydrocannabinols* (Fig. 12). These psychoactive materials are present in all parts of the plant although concentrations differ. The flowering tops (female plant) have the highest concentration of tetrahydrocannabinols whereas the stems and leaves have less.

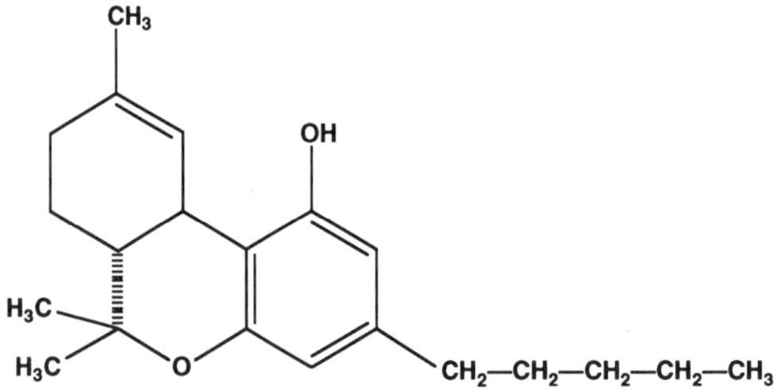

FIG. 12. Structure of Δ-9-tetrahydrocannabinol.

The drug products that are concentrated in the resinous secretions coating the plant are called *hashish, cannabis, charas,* or *kif.* The dried leaves and stems are termed *bhang, ganja,* or *marijuana.*

History

The first recorded reference to the use of the cannabis plant is in a Chinese book of pharmacy written in 2737 B.C. by Emperor Shen Nung, who called it the "liberator of sin" and also recommended it for its medicinal value. Later references to cannabis plant use appear in China, India, and the Middle East. Western Europeans attributed its discovery to the Arabic world, possibly because it was introduced in Europe via contact with Moslems during the Crusades. In the twelfth century its use was considered epidemic among Moslems. Marco Polo related accounts of the Hashishiyya Cult who murdered for political reasons and used hashish. The word *assassin* is derived from the name of the cult.

Napoleon prohibited the use of cannabis by his soldiers during the Egyptian campaign. The French writers Dumas, Gautier, and Baudelaire experimented with the use of hashish as an aid to creativity. Some of the most vivid and accurate descriptions of the effects of cannabis were recorded by Baudelaire in his book *Artificial Paradise.*

Clinical Use

Tetrahydrocannabinols suppress nausea and vomiting and are useful in the treatment of vomiting induced by cancer chemotherapy. Related synthetic pharmaceuticals are now licensed for this purpose. Tetrahydrocannabinols also decrease intraocular pressure and therefore have therapeutic potential in the treatment of glaucoma.

Drug Abuse and Dependence

The abuse potential of the tetrahydrocannabinols is substantially less than that of co-caine, opiates, or alcohol. However, they are so-called gateway drugs. Although surveys show that most marijuana users never go on to use cocaine or heroin, those who do use hard drugs almost always begin with tobacco, alcohol, or marijuana.

Patterns of Use

The drug can be ingested or smoked, with the latter the most common route of administration, often via a water pipe. The pattern of use is to smoke an amount that gives the desired effect; in heavy users this may be repeated hourly or more to maintain a high throughout the day.

Pharmacokinetics and Metabolism

Among the 60 cannabinoids found in the plant, the major compounds responsible for the psychoactive effect are Δ-9-tetrahydrocannabinol (THC; Fig. 12) and Δ-8-tetrahydrocannabinol. THC is metabolized quickly to an active metabolite, 11-hydroxytetrahydrocannabinol. The half-lives of the active cannabinols are long, on the order of 1 to $2\frac{1}{2}$ days, because these drugs dissolve in body fats, slowly leach out, and are eliminated over a long period. There is documentation that these substances can accumulate in the lipid reservoirs of heavy chronic users. Complete elimination from the body can take as long as 45 days. This means that a urine test for marijuana metabolites may be positive 4 to 6 weeks after the last use of marijuana in a heavy user, but this does not imply that the metabolites are pharmacologically active.

The onset of drug effect is within 10 min of smoking tetrahydrocannabinols or within an hour of their ingestion. The psychoactive effects peak 20 to 30 min after smoking and 2 to 3 hr after ingestion, and last 3 to 5 hr. There are reports of some impairment of coordination and eye movements lasting up to 11 hr.

Drug Effects

The tetrahydrocannabinols cause mild euphoria, relaxation, and slowed and distorted perception, thinking, and judgment. Emotions may be intensified, and a sensation that the changes in perception are significant and meaningful develops. The sense of time passing is slowed; sensory awareness is heightened and distorted, and depersonalization occurs. With large doses, dysphoria, paranoia, and temporary psychosis may appear. Tolerance does develop to the sedative effects of the tetrahydrocannabinols. In contrast, a kind of reverse tolerance has been reported for some of the subjective effects of marijuana. Some experienced users are able to accurately detect doses below those detectable by naive users. Some people appear to be more vulnerable to the adverse effects of the tetrahydrocannabinols and report paranoia at low doses. Physiologically, tetrahydrocannabinols increase heart rate, sometimes markedly, and cause vasodilation of the blood vessels of the eye membranes, which is commonly seen as bloodshot eyes.

Toxicity

Tetrahydrocannabinol intoxication impairs performance. Laboratory tests of motor and cognitive function as well as field tests of driving and piloting performance have established impairment. Some studies have reported that tetrahydrocannabinols impair eye tracking and performance on flight simulators for up to 24 hr after a single dose, although not all investigators have been able to detect effects for such a long duration.

Neuropharmacology

For a long time the mechanism of action of tetrahydrocannabinols was believed to be a nonspecific membrane interaction with the active drugs. The drugs are highly lipid-soluble and cell membranes are lipid-rich structures. Since the tetrahydrocannabinols and alcohol demonstrate some cross-tolerance and there is substantial evidence that alcohol changes the physical properties of membranes, it was reasoned that tetrahydrocannabinols must function through membrane interactions. More recently, evidence has been found of a specific G protein–linked receptor (see Chapter 4) that binds cannabinoid compounds. This receptor has been synthesized from rat DNA maps of G-protein peptides. The tetrahydrocannabinols bind to the synthesized receptor with affinities that have the same rank order as the potencies of naturally occurring psychoactive tetrahydrocannabinols found in the cannabis plant. The properties of the binding conform to the criteria for a drug/receptor interaction. Furthermore, in vivo the distribution of tetrahydrocannabinol binding is similar to the distribution of the receptor. The existence of these highly specific receptors raises questions as to their normal function and the possibility of the existence of endogenous cannabinoid-like substances. After the discovery of the opiate receptor, this line of reasoning led to the successful search for endogenous opioids (endorphins).

Withdrawal and Treatment

Cessation of chronically administered large doses of tetrahydrocannabinols results in withdrawal symptoms similar to those of sedative withdrawal: irritability and nervousness with tremor, chills, and insomnia. This syndrome lasts for 4 to 5 days and is mild.

Tetrahydrocannabinol withdrawal does not require medical treatment. Compulsive users meet criteria for dependence and this is treated by rehabilitation in a drug treatment program. No unique treatment is necessary.

Nicotine

Nicotine has all of the features of an addictive drug. Nicotine is a plant alkaloid that occurs in the tobacco plants *Nicotiniana tabacum* and *Nicotiniana rustica* (Fig. 13).

History

Tobacco is a New World plant unknown to the Old World until the end of the sixteenth century. It was introduced into Europe by either John Hawkins or Sir Francis Drake, English sea captains. Sir Walter Raleigh introduced the practice of smoking to the English.

The use of tobacco is ancient. A Mayan stone sculpture shows a god smoking a cigar. The Amerindians used tobacco medicinally by smoking it, chewing the leaves, drinking tea, or applying ointments or hot leaves to the skin to heal many ailments. Amerindian priests used tobacco smoke as a hallucinogen in religious rituals to obtain sacred visions. North American Indians developed many important rituals around smoking tobacco, which was considered a gift from the gods.

Although nicotine has always been a legal drug in the United States, it has not always been legal in other countries. In the seventeenth century, the Russian, Turkish, Chinese, and Japanese empires outlawed the use of tobacco and levied severe penalties including torture and death (Russia and Turkey) and heavy fines and loss of lands (China and Japan) on those found using it. Despite this, tobacco use spread, finally becoming accepted and legal in the second half of the seventeenth century as new leaders and their royal courts became users of tobacco themselves. The kings of England, France, and Prussia and Pope Urban VIII opposed the use of tobacco and taxed its use heavily rather than banning it. All of these countries, including the United States, eventually found that taxation of tobacco was a lucrative source of government funds. Eventually each of these nations actively sought control of supplies and developed protectionist policies.

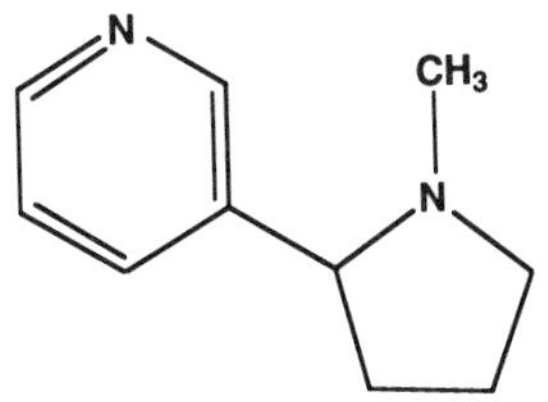

Drug Abuse and Dependence

Nicotine possesses all the features of a drug of addiction including the ability to cause euphoria, physical dependence and withdrawal, use despite knowledge of physical damage and even death, difficulty in stopping, and using more than intended (Table 1). In 1942, the American physician Lennox Johnston found that intravenous injections of nicotine were pleasurable to smokers but not to nonsmokers. Experimenting on himself, he reported that injections gave more pleasure than smoking itself. Studies of human smokers have demonstrated evidence of physical dependence on nicotine because a characteristic withdrawal syndrome ensues upon cessation of nicotine administration. Since most nicotine users are physically dependent, some have argued that nicotine, not cocaine, is the most addictive drug.

Patterns of Use

The interval of smoking nicotine is characteristic of an individual and may vary from one cigarette every 10 min to one every 6 to 8 hr. Even the interval between cigarette puffs is a stable characteristic of the user. The user, by varying the puff frequency and depth, maintains stable blood concentrations of nicotine. This is done unconsciously as smokers make adjustments without knowledge of the nicotine content of the cigarette.

Pharmacokinetics and Metabolism

Nicotine is metabolized to cotinine and nicotine-1'-*N*-oxide in liver, kidney, and lung. The half-life of nicotine is about 2 hr. How-

FIG. 13. Structure of nicotine.

ever, nicotine has a short duration of action because it undergoes rapid body redistribution after absorption from the lung. Thus, the nicotine in the smoke is absorbed into the blood and rapidly transported into lipid-rich body tissues including the brain. The drug continues to be distributed to other body tissues from the blood and the lipid-rich tissues at a rate only a little slower than the initial transportation to the lipid-rich tissues. This redistribution results in rapidly decreasing brain concentrations, consequently ending the effect of the drug.

Drug Effects

The effect of nicotine smoking is a mild stimulation. Nicotine administered intravenously in research studies has been likened to low doses of cocaine by drug-experienced research subjects. It is calming, relaxes muscles, and has subjective effects interpreted as desirable and pleasant (mild euphoria). Nicotine use does not impair performance. In some instances it may enhance performance by decreasing irritability and aggression although tremors and difficulty with sleep may evolve. The drug has both stimulant and depressant phases of action.

Toxicity

Nicotine is a plant poison. The alkaloid protects the plant from ingestion by animals and insects. Some pesticides contain nicotine. Smoking too much (more rapidly, deeply, or longer than usual) can cause severe nausea, vomiting, headache, and tremor. Ingestion of nicotine-containing insecticides (usually by accident) or ingestion of tobacco products by mouth can cause high drug concentrations in body tissues and can result in hallucinations, respiratory stimulation followed by respiratory arrest, convulsions, severe slowing of the heart, and death.

Contrary to popular belief, nicotine does not cause cancer or emphysema. These diseases are caused by exposure of the respira-

tory tract to complex cancer-causing chemicals produced by the burning of tobacco. Smoking is also related to an increased risk of heart attack and stroke. The mechanism by which smoking increases these risks is uncertain but nicotine itself may play a role by causing constriction of blood vessels.

Neuropharmacology

Nicotine is a cholinergic drug that stimulates ganglionic neurons. The likelihood of abuse of nicotine may be related to its causing cholinergic ganglionic stimulation since mecamylamine, a ganglionic blocking drug, interferes with nicotine-induced subjective effects. In addition to ganglionic nicotine receptors, there are nicotine receptors in the central nervous system, and some of nicotine's effects are mediated there, including nausea and tremor. Cholinergic activity is probably essential for the addicting properties of nicotine since taking another naturally occurring cholinergic alkaloid, arecoline, found in betel nuts, is pleasurable; betel nuts are used by millions of people in Africa, Asia, and the Pacific.

Withdrawal and Treatment

Interruption of nicotine dosing causes a withdrawal syndrome that may include decreases in blood pressure and pulse, decrements in psychomotor performance and vigilance, weight gain, diarrhea, headache, and nausea. People withdrawing from nicotine may become hostile, aggressive, and anxious. Sleep is impaired. EEG changes have been found that can be reversed with administration of nicotine. Withdrawal symptoms may ensue within 4 to 6 hr of cessation of smoking. The worst symptoms occur within a week, but some symptoms may last for months. The dysphoria experienced during withdrawal enhances the probability of relapse.

Cessation of tobacco use is difficult to achieve and even more difficult to maintain, especially for individuals who began smoking under the age of 20. Nicotine's legality and ease of access and the relative social acceptability of its use make permanent abstinence difficult. Persons addicted to other drugs often seek and maintain abstinence motivated by the huge personal losses sustained by their addictive behavior. Nicotine generally does not cause such losses immediately, and abstinence is more difficult to achieve.

Nicotine addiction can be treated with a tapered schedule of nicotine administered as a gum preparation or as a skin patch. The patient is stabilized on nicotine treatment for 1 to 2 months. During this time, smoking abstinence should be accomplished. It is common for patients to continue their nicotine dependency with nicotine gum (the patch studies are still pending). Such use should be discouraged, even though chronic use of nicotine gum is less a health problem than smoking since cancer and emphysema are related to chemicals from burned tobacco and not nicotine. However, the risk of heart attack and stroke rapidly diminishes upon cessation of smoking. These health problems may be caused by the nicotine itself though this has not been proven.

Rehabilitation treatment is useful for nicotine addiction as it is for other addictions. Rehabilitation usually consists of group therapy involving only nicotine-dependent subjects and excluding patients with other chemical dependencies.

SUMMARY

Drug abuse is a complex biosocial problem that comprises sociology, pharmacology, psychiatry, medicine, public health, economics, and political and forensic science and must be addressed using multidisciplinary approaches. The diagnosis of drug dependence advanced by the World Health Organization depends heavily on a pattern of loss of control over drug use and evidence that drug use has become the first priority in the life of the person. Tolerance and withdrawal may also be features of drug dependence but are not necessary nor sufficient to make the diagnosis.

A large number of variables influence drug use. All drugs of abuse induce a state of euphoria. The abuse potential of a drug is proportional to its ability to induce euphoria. In general, drugs providing more intensely pleasurable states cause both a higher frequency of addiction and a more intense addiction than those resulting in milder changes. Methods of taking the drug into the body that enhance the intensity of the euphoria also increase abuse potential. Easy availability and low cost increase drug usage; this is true for legalized drugs as well as illegal drugs. The social acceptability of drug use is an extremely important but often underrated variable that plays a key role in the experimentation and establishment of drug use by individuals. Nearly all addicts are introduced to drug use by friends or family.

Some groups of people are more vulnerable to drug addiction than others. There is a mounting body of evidence that some people have a genetic vulnerability for addiction problems. People with mental illnesses, including depression, bipolar disease, schizophrenia, post-traumatic stress disorder, and some personality disorders, are at a higher risk for chemical dependency than people without such problems. In general, people who are subjected to severe increases in stress or have inadequate means of escaping stress have an increased risk for addiction. Thus, poverty without opportunity, poor family situations, and war coupled with drug availability can be expected to result in increased substance abuse and addiction.

There are 10 broad classes of drugs of abuse, each with unique pharmacology, all sharing the property of being pleasurable to at least some people but not necessarily all or even most people. Despite differences among drug mechanisms, effects, and withdrawal, treatment is similar for all drug addictions. Treatment includes a period of detoxification during which the patient may experience drug withdrawal signs and symptoms which, if severe or serious, can be treated with medication. After drug detoxification, the patient enters rehabilitation that may take any of several forms, including drug counseling, group therapy, and individual psychiatric therapy. Various treatment modes benefit some patients more than others and therefore patients are assigned to treatments maximizing the potential for the individual's recovery. The evidence available suggests that the longer the treatment period the better the outcome. Treatment of addiction is best understood as a lifelong condition requiring behavioral change that induces a remission and periodic treatment after relapse once remission is obtained. Despite the enormous difficulties in treating addiction disorders, there is abundant evidence that treatment does have a profound positive influence on patients' lives.

BIBLIOGRAPHY

Original Articles

Devane WA, Dysarz FA III, Johnson MR, Melvin LS, Howlett AC. Determination and characterization of a cannabinoid receptor in rat brain. *Mol Pharmacol* 1988;34:605–613.

Dole VP, Joseph H. Long-term outcome of patients treated with methadone maintenance. *Ann NY Acad Sci* 1978;311:181–196.

Moskowitz H, Burns MM, Williams AF. Skills perfor-
mance at low blood alcohol levels. *J Studies Alcohol* 1985;46:482–485.

Sheren MA, Kumor KM, Jaffe JH. *Psychiatry Research* 1989;27:117–125.

Weddington WW, Brown BS, Haertzen CA, Cone EJ, Dax EM, Herning RI, et al. Changes in mood, craving, and sleep during short-term abstinence reported by male cocaine addicts: a controlled, residential study. *Arch Gen Psychiatry* 1990;47:861–868.

Woody GE, Luborsky L, McLellan AT, O'Brien CP, Beck AT, Blaine J, et al. Psychotherapy for opiate addicts. *Arch Gen Psychiatry* 1983;40:639–645.

Books and Reviews

Brownstein MJ, Usdin TB. Molecular targets of abused drugs. In: Siegel GJ, Agranoff BW, Albers RW, Molinoff PB, eds. *Basic neurochemistry,* 5th ed. New York: Raven Press; 1994 (in press).

Collins RL, Leonard KE, Searles JS, eds. *Alcohol and the family: research and clinical perspectives.* New York: Guilford Press; 1990.

Jaffe JH. Drug addiction and drug abuse. In: Gilman AG, Rall TW, Nies AS, Taylor P, eds. *The pharmacological basis of therapeutics.* 8th Ed. New York: Pergamon Press; 1990:522–573.

Jasinski DR. Assessment of the abuse potentiality of morphine-like drugs (methods used in man). In: Martin WR, ed. *Drug addiction.* Vol. I. New York: Springer-Verlag; 1977:197–258.

Pomerleau OF, Pomerleau CS, eds. *Nicotine replacement: a critical evaluation.* New York: Alan R Liss; 1988.

Roy-Byrne PR, Cowley DS, eds. *Benzodiazepines in clinical practice: risks and benefits.* Washington, DC: American Psychiatric Press; 1991.

Vaillant GE. The natural history of narcotic drug addiction. *Semin Psychiatry* 1970;2:486–498.

21

Obesity

Daryth D. Stallone and Albert J. Stunkard

*Leave gourmandizing; know that the grave doth
for thee gape thrice wider than for other man.*

William Shakespeare,
Henry IV, Part II (Henry IV to Falstaff)

- Obesity is almost certainly a heterogeneous disorder with multiple causes.

- The ability to store fat has been important in human evolution.

- Obesity is a condition characterized by an excess of body fat.

- In general, obesity is on the rise in the developed world.

- The distribution and quantity of body fat are disease risk factors.

- Despite controversy, overeating and psychopathology appear to be more common among obese than nonobese persons.

- Psychopathology among the obese appears to be secondary to their obesity.

- The hypothalamus is an integration center for the regulation of feeding behavior.

- Gastrointestinal peptides, especially cholecystokinin, are involved in the regulation of feeding behavior.

- Peptidergic and nonpeptidergic neurotransmitters act in specific brain areas to influence feeding behavior.

- Genetic factors are important determinants of body size.

- Clues to the causes of obesity lie in adipose tissue.

- Obesity may result from regulation of body weight at an elevated level.

- Lifestyle, not diets, is the key to treatment of mild and moderate obesity.

- Although it afflicts only 0.5% of obese persons, severe obesity (>100% overweight) is very often associated with major medical problems.

- Most drugs that decrease appetite act centrally through dopaminergic, noradrenergic, or serotonergic mechanisms.

This chapter presents an overview of the clinical aspects of obesity. Starting with the evolutionary hypothesis of fat storage, the chapter proceeds to discussions of the definition, assessment, epidemiology, health consequences, and etiology of obesity. Human biological and genetic mechanisms are explored, as is the set point theory of body weight. Finally, the chapter explores the current status of treatment.

─────────────────────────────────────

Obesity is one of the most prevalent but least understood health problems in Western society. In one sense, the cause of obesity is known (i.e., an energy intake that exceeds energy expenditure for a significant period of time), but very little is known about why this imbalance occurs. One thing that has become clear is that most cases of obesity are not, as was long believed, the manifestation of an eating disorder. When obese persons eat in a disordered manner, it is more often a result of their efforts to control their obesity. *Obesity is almost certainly a heterogeneous disorder with multiple causes.*

FAT STORAGE AND HUMAN HISTORY

The ability to store fat has been important in human evolution. In recent years the evolutionary significance of the human capacity for fat storage has become clearer, as has the nature of the medical complications of obesity. The mammalian capacity for fat storage varies widely from the limited stores of hunters, such as wolves, to the massive capacity of whales. The position of any mammal within this wide range of fat storage appears to be determined by the relative needs for mobility and energy reserves. The hunter-gatherer backgrounds of recent hominids places humans closer to the limited capacity of hunters, whose need for mobility takes precedence over the need for energy storage.

Gender dimorphism provides a useful perspective on the balance between mobility and energy storage. From the point of view of the individual, the benefits of increased energy storage are readily outweighed by the limitation on mobility. From the point of view of the species, however, the need for mobility shifts in favor of storage, particularly in women. Fat stores enable a woman (and a man) to survive a period of food scarcity and in addition favors survival of her fetus. Accordingly, nature should favor increased storage for women and, in fact, that is what is found. A "normal weight" man has 18% body fat while a "normal weight" woman has 28% body fat, and pregnancy brings with it an increased capacity for fat storage.

This evolutionary hypothesis is supported by the existence of a highly developed hormone-enzyme system that regulates fat storage during pregnancy. The overall result of this system is an efficient mechanism for storing fat during pregnancy and then transferring this fat to the breasts for lactation. If this complex fat storage mechanism were developed in the interests of survival of the species, it should not present health hazards and, in fact, it does not. Lower body fat, which is characteristic of women, confers little health risk. Societal concern with fat hips and thighs is based solely on issues of style and fashion, and not at all on medical concerns. In striking contrast, the typical pattern of obesity in men, upper body abdominal obesity, which confers no evident evolutionary benefit, car-

Biological Bases of Brain Function and Disease, edited by Alan Frazer, Perry B. Molinoff, and Andrew Winokur. Raven Press, Ltd., New York © 1994.

ries very significant health risks as discussed below.

Before the industrial revolution the lot of most of humanity was little better than that of our prehistoric ancestors. Only in recent years have entire populations had more than enough to eat for any prolonged period of time. For this reason, throughout history, as in many developing areas today, obesity existed only among the wealthy, and it became a well-established symbol of status.

Art has shown that body fat was considered a virtue as long ago as neolithic times. The Venus of Willendorf, a fertility symbol over 20,000 years old (Fig. 1), is the earliest known representation of the human form. This ideal-

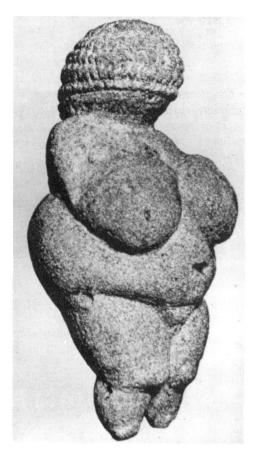

FIG. 1. The Venus of Willendorf, a fertility symbol over 20,000 years old, is the oldest known representation of the human body.

ization of obesity continued in the ancient world, in Shakespearean England, and as recently as the turn of the twentieth century when the buxom Gibson Girl was the feminine ideal on both sides of the Atlantic.

In the United States and Europe moderate obesity was considered a sign of sustained youth and good health until the early 1900s. As food became more plentiful and palatable, and as machines such as automobiles and television reduced our need and desire to move, obesity became more prevalent. As a result, the health risks of obesity became more obvious. It was probably status rather than health, however, that formed modern society's attitudes toward body weight. As the American sociologist Thorstein Veblen postulated in 1899, status symbols must be restricted to the "leisure class." Obesity had once been a prerogative of the wealthy, but when it became accessible to entire populations, it lost its appeal. Instead, thinness among women became the fashion, and this trend has continued for nearly two generations. As discussed below, adiposity among American and European women is inversely related to socioeconomic status.

CLINICAL PERSPECTIVE

Definition and Assessment of Obesity

Obesity is a condition characterized by an excess of body fat. Since fatness is a continuum, any cutoff point that separates obese from nonobese individuals must be arbitrary and related to some standard of what is normal.

The standards of normality used until recently were the so-called tables of desirable weight, derived from data collected by life insurance companies from insured populations. Although easy to understand, the periodic changes in "desirable" or "ideal" weight have discouraged their use, and they are being displaced by the *body mass index* (BMI), which is weight in kilograms divided by the square of height in meters (kg/m^2). The upper range of normality is considered to be a BMI of 26.4 for men and 25.8 for women.

Although measures of weight adjusted for height are strongly correlated with adiposity, they cannot account for differences in body composition. For example, a body builder with large amounts of muscle tissue and very little adipose tissue will have a high BMI and be classified as overweight. Thus, a high BMI really reflects overweight, not necessarily overfat.

The actual quantity of fat in the body can be estimated by several methods. Two commonly used methods are the determinations of body density (densitometry) and total body water. Both techniques require special equipment and expertise, and their use is primarily restricted to research.

Densitometry is considered the "gold standard" in the determination of body composition. Body density is determined according to Archimedes's principle, by weighing the subject while he or she is completely submerged in water. The percentage of body weight that is fat is calculated from body density based on the difference between the density of adipose tissue (0.90 g/ml) and fat-free mass (1.10 g/ml).

The principle underlying the measurement of total body water to obtain fat mass is that stored fat is anhydrous in nature, and approximately 73% of lean tissue, or fat-free mass, is water. Thus, knowledge of total body water content allows calculation of fat mass. Total body water is determined by measuring the dilution in the body of a traceable water-soluble substance, such as deuterium (^2H_2O) or tritium (^3H_2O).

Epidemiology

In general, obesity is on the rise in the developed world. Over the last century the populations of most industrialized countries have become fatter. In the United States an estimated 34 million adults between 20 and 74 years of age are obese. The National Health and Nutrition Examination Survey (NHANES II) of 1976–1980 found that 26% of adult Americans were overweight, with almost 1 in 10 (9.3%) weighing more than 95% above "accepted" weight norms. More women of all races (27%) were overweight than men (24%). The difference in prevalence rates between men and women became especially pronounced after age 50 because of the higher mortality rate among obese men after that age.

Age is strongly correlated with adiposity. There is a monotonic increase in the prevalence of obesity between preadolescence and age 50 in men and age 60 in women, after which prevalence declines.

As discussed above, the prevalence of obesity is strongly influenced by social factors. Over 32 studies in the United States and Europe have shown that the prevalence of obesity among women is inversely related to socioeconomic status: prevalence rates for obesity are higher among women of low socioeconomic status than among women of high socioeconomic status. The relationship of socioeconomic status to obesity in men in the United States and Europe is less clear. In some populations it is inverse; in others it is direct. Parents' socioeconomic status is almost as strong a predictor of adiposity as is current socioeconomic status.

The relationship between socioeconomic status and body weight for both men and women in developing countries is as strong as it is for women in developed countries, but in the opposite direction; men and women of high socioeconomic status are more overweight than those of lower socioeconomic status. In developing countries adiposity is an outward sign of wealth, since only the wealthy are able to buy enough food to become obese.

Ethnic factors and immigration to other countries also influence adiposity. NHANES II found the percentage of overweight blacks to be greater than that of overweight whites, particularly for black women, 45% of whom were overweight—almost twice the figure for white women (25%). Even when corrected for differences in socioeconomic status and education, black women were at a considerably higher risk of obesity than other members of the U.S. population. Interestingly, rates for black and white men were about equal (26% vs. 24%). In the first generation of seven European ethnic groups that settled in the United States, there was a marked increase in the prevalence of obesity over that found in their native land. The prevalence of obesity then decreased with succeeding generations, from 24% to 5% between the first and fourth generations in the United States. Similarly, the body weight of Japanese rose substantially among immigrants to Hawaii, and further still in the move from Hawaii to the U.S. mainland.

Health Consequences

The distribution and quantity of body fat are disease risk factors. Increasing body weight and duration of obesity are directly related to both mortality and morbidity. As shown in Fig. 2, the mortality ratio, the number of deaths among people of a certain weight class expressed as a percentage of expected deaths for the total population (i.e., 100 for people of normal or somewhat less

than normal weight), increases from 110 among people 5–15% overweight to 227 among people 40–45% overweight.

Obesity increases the risk of several serious diseases, such as hypertension, diabetes, and cardiovascular disease. Other serious conditions associated with obesity include dyspnea upon mild exertion, sleep apnea, gallstones, and a variety of orthopedic problems including aggravation of osteoarthritis and low back pain. Weight loss reverses or ameliorates most of these conditions.

Cardiovascular disease and diabetes are much more common among obese men than among obese women. Obese men are at a greater health risk than obese women because of the difference between the sexes in the distribution of body fat. As discussed earlier, the obesity of most men is characterized by fat in the upper part of the body, particularly abdominal fat (i.e., beer belly), a fat distribution referred to as *android* obesity. The obesity of most women, by contrast, is of the *gynoid* type in which fat is primarily located in the hips and thighs. Android obesity poses a far higher risk of cardiovascular disease and diabetes than does gynoid obesity. The ratio of waist circumference to hip circumference (W/H) gives a good estimate of upper vs.

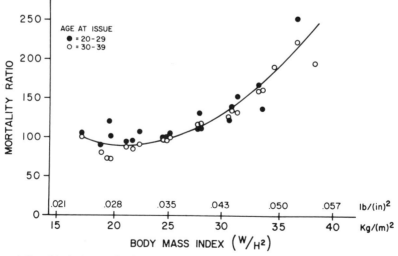

FIG. 2. The relationship between body mass index and excess mortality. Note that the upper range of normality is considered to be a BMI of 26.4 for men and 25.8 for women. Reprinted with permission from Bray GA. *The obese patient.* Philadelphia: WB Saunders; 1976:219.

lower body obesity and is therefore a predictor of risk that can be easily assessed in a clinical setting.

Very recently, modern imaging techniques, such as computed tomography (CT), have greatly advanced our understanding of the deleterious effects of upper body obesity. They have revealed that fat distribution *within* the abdomen is critical in disease risk. Abdominal fat is stored in two distinct depots: the visceral depot, located beneath the abdominal muscles within the abdominal cavity, and the subcutaneous depot, between the skin and the abdominal muscles. Figure 3 shows CT scans of the abdomen of two obese patients: the abdominal fat deposition of the patient on the left is primarily of the visceral type whereas that of the patient on the right is largely subcutaneous. We now know that it is largely visceral fat that confers the increased risk of disease. Subcutaneous abdominal fat does not appear to confer significant health risk.

ETIOLOGY

On the simplest level, obesity is a consequence of a sustained energy imbalance, i.e., obesity results when more calories are taken in than are expended. The underlying causes of this imbalance, however, are not completely understood. Several factors probably contribute to obesity and to body weight in general: (1) overeating and psychopathology, (2) brain neuropeptides and neurotransmitters, (3) heredity, (4) body weight set point, and (5) adipose tissue metabolism. No one of these factors is capable of explaining all obesity and several may interact to determine an individual's body weight.

Overeating and Psychopathology

Despite controversy, overeating and psychopathology appear to be more common among obese than nonobese persons. For years obesity was viewed solely as the consequence of overeating. Although overeating relative to energy expenditure is, in a simplified sense, the cause of obesity, it is not known whether obese persons consume more calories than do persons of normal weight.

Laboratory studies of food intake generally support the findings that obese people eat no more than people of normal weight. However, observations of eating behavior in restaurants and other natural environments give mixed results; some studies indicate that obese people *do* eat more than normal weight people, whereas others report no differences.

Studies of self-reported food intake have consistently indicated that obese people eat no more, and perhaps even less, than nonobese people. For example, the reported calo-

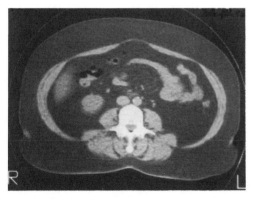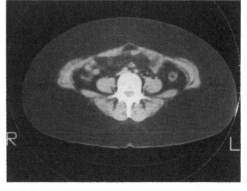

FIG. 3. CT scans of the abdomens of two obese women at the level of the umbilicus. Note the difference in the distribution of abdominal fat. Fat in the woman on the left is primarily visceral in nature; that of the woman on the right is primarily subcutaneous.

ric intakes of over 6,200 men and women interviewed in NHANES I did not correlate with degree of obesity. However, recent studies that compared self-reported caloric intake with actual food intake and/or energy expenditure have shown that overweight individuals consistently underreport their food intake by as much as 40%, suggesting that overeating may contribute to the development of obesity.

Psychopathology among the obese appears to be secondary to their obesity. The belief that obesity results from overeating secondary to psychopathology was a predominant thesis for many years. One characteristic article by Becker declared: "We must consider obesity as the presenting symptom of a basic personality problem or disorder. It is a particular way of handling one's difficulties in human relationships, and even more one's poor relationship to one's self."

Since the time of this pejorative statement it has been established that obese people suffer no more general psychopathology than do people of normal weight. They do, however, present psychopathology specific to their obese state. One such problem is disparagement of the body image: some obese persons see their bodies as grotesque and believe that others despise them because of their appearance. Persons who hold these beliefs are preoccupied with their body weight and feelings of self-loathing. When one considers the overt prejudice and discrimination suffered by obese people in our society, it is not surprising that disparagement of body image exists among some obese individuals. In fact, one might expect that all obese people would loathe their physical appearance, but this is not the case. Emotionally healthy obese persons suffer no disturbance of body image. Those afflicted are generally young women of middle or upper-middle socioeconomic status, groups in which obesity is less prevalent and social pressures to be thin are strong. Psychopathology does not appear to be a significant cause of obesity. Rather, psychopathology among the obese appears to be a consequence of their obesity and of the preju-

dice and discrimination to which they are subjected.

Another form of psychopathology prevalent among obese individuals is the newly defined *binge eating disorder* (BED). This disorder, which is characterized by recurrent episodes of binge eating (at least twice per week) without subsequent vomiting or laxative use, afflicts approximately 30% of all obese individuals enrolled in weight control programs. BED is more common in women than in men and is associated with the degree of adiposity and with a history of weight fluctuations.

Role of the Brain

The hypothalamus is an integration center for the regulation of feeding behavior. In the 1940s it was discovered that the brain plays a key role in feeding behavior, and hence indirectly in the etiology of obesity. The *hypothalamus* (see Chapter 1), a brain organ of the limbic system that controls basic functions such as temperature regulation and endocrine function, was found to be an important area for control of ingestive behavior. Destruction or stimulation of neurons in two areas of the hypothalamus, the *ventromedial hypothalamus* (VMH) and the *lateral hypothalamus,* has profound effects on food intake. Electrolytic or chemical lesions of the VMH produce hyperphagia and obesity whereas similar lesions in the lateral hypothalamus result in aphagia and weight loss. Stimulation of the VMH inhibits feeding; stimulation of the lateral hypothalamus promotes feeding. These types of results led to the designation of the VMH as the "satiety center" and the lateral hypothalamus as the "feeding center" in a dual-center hypothesis of feeding behavior. According to this theory, the lateral hypothalamus initiates eating when signals it receives indicate a state of energy depletion within the body. As feeding progresses, the VMH, detecting rising nutrient levels, inhibits the feeding signals. This dual-center hypothesis proved to be too simple to explain the complexities of the neuroregulation of feeding, and it has been expanded into more complex models of feeding behavior.

The hypothalamus remains the focus for the study of feeding behavior, although interest has shifted from the lateral hypothalamus and the VMH to the *perifornical region* of the lateral hypothalamus (PFH) and the *paraventricular nucleus* of the medial hypothalamus (PVN). These regions are viewed as integrating centers for a complex system of excitatory and inhibitory influences that come into and leave the brain and that drive hunger and feeding and invoke satiety. Evidence suggests that PFH integrates signals that initiate feeding while the PVN integrates signals that mediate satiety. Information is relayed to and from these integration centers and other brain areas by a wide variety of neurotransmitters and neuropeptides. The identification of these neurotransmitters and neuropeptides, their sites of action, and their interactions are now a central focus of research (see Chapters 6 and 8).

One model of the neuroregulation of feeding views feeding behavior as the result of the coordinated efforts of two separate systems: a peripheral satiety system and a central feeding system. Within the peripheral system, peptide hormones released from the gastrointestinal tract in response to ingested food initiate neural satiety signals that result in termination of the meal. The central feeding system serves as a central integrator of signals involved in feeding behavior and ultimately controls feeding (Fig. 4).

Most conclusions about the role of specific neurotransmitters involved in the neuroregulation of feeding derive from observations of eating behavior in laboratory animals following administration of neurochemical substances in the periphery or in specific brain areas. Although these studies have been valuable in identifying systems involved in feeding behavior, the doses of the agents used are often very high, at pharmacological levels, making extrapolation to physiological doses crude at best. Recently developed microdialysis techniques, which allow measurement in vivo of neurotransmitters in specific brain regions in free-living animals, are providing clearer data regarding specific changes in central neurotransmitters involved in feeding behavior.

THE PERIPHERAL SATIETY SYSTEM

Gastrointestinal peptides, especially CCK, are involved in the regulation of feeding behavior. A host of gut peptides have been shown to inhibit feeding when administered exogenously: cholecystokinin (CCK), glucagon, somatostatin, and bombesin (see Chapter 8). CCK, long known for its action in stimulating contraction of the gallbladder, is the most thoroughly studied of these gut peptides. Exogenous CCK administered at the time of a meal decreases meal size and, in laboratory animals, produces a set of behaviors associated with natural satiety. Growing evidence suggests that endogenously released CCK is involved in satiety. CCK inhibits food intake at physiological doses, and antibodies to CCK and CCK antagonists increase food intake. The neural pathway for CCK-induced satiety is fairly well established. CCK transmits satiety signals to the hypothalamus via the afferent fibers of the vagus and *nucleus of the tractus solitarius* (NTS). Abdominal or selective gastric vagotomy or selective lesions of the afferent vagal roots at the point where they enter the medulla attenuate inhibition of feeding by CCK. Gastric fibers of the vagus terminate within the medial and caudal NTS, which relays information from the vagus to the PVN of the hypothalamus. Lesions of the NTS, PVN, or fibers of the ventrolateral and dorsal tegmental areas, which link the NTS and the PVN, block the satiety effect of CCK, indicating that this is indeed the neuronal circuit involved in CCK-induced satiety. The PVN appears to be the central site that ultimately receives CCK's satiety signals. Injection of minute quantities of CCK into the PVN inhibits feeding, suggesting that CCK may itself transmit the satiety message. Other data suggest that the ultimate effector of

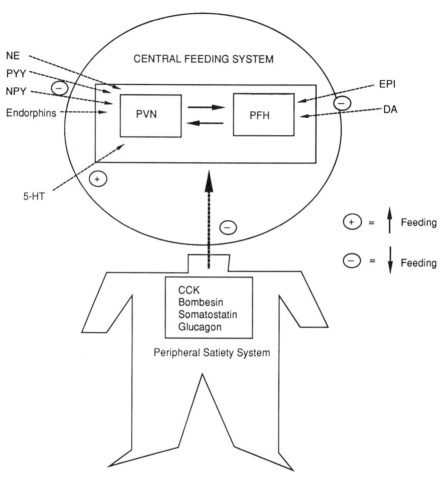

FIG. 4. Simplified overview of the peripheral and central neurotransmitter/peptide systems involved in the modulation of feeding behavior. PVN, paraventricular nucleus of the medial hypothalamus; PFH, perifornical region of the lateral hypothalamus; NE, norepinephrine; PYY, peptide YY; NPY, neuropeptide Y; EPI, epinephrine; DA, dopamine; 5-HT, serotonin; CCK, cholecystokinin.

CCK-induced satiety in the PVN may be norepinephrine (NE) or serotonin (5-HT).

In humans, as in rats, CCK and CCK analogs administered intravenously or subcutaneously decrease food intake in a single meal. For this reason, CCK has been touted as a potential treatment for obesity. However, CCK is not active in oral form and thus must be administered intravenously, making it unsuitable for long-term treatment of obesity. Further, chronic infusion of CCK to rats does not lead to weight loss. CCK has a short duration of action. When administered at each meal it decreases meal size, but there is a compensatory increase in the number of meals

eaten. Thus, CCK may be effective as a treatment for obesity only when a long-acting orally active analog is developed.

CENTRAL FEEDING SYSTEM

Peptidergic and nonpeptidergic neurotransmitters act in specific brain areas to influence feeding behavior. Peptides modulating food intake include the opioids, neuropeptide Y (NPY), peptide YY (PYY), and galanin. The major nonpeptidergic neurotransmitters that affect food intake are NE, dopamine (DA), and 5-HT (see Chapters 6 and 8).

A role for opioids in the stimulation of feeding was first suggested by studies showing that the opioid antagonist naloxone decreases food intake in rats. Further studies showed that opioid antagonists decrease meal size in a number of animal species. The opioid receptors most involved in modulating feeding behavior are the κ receptors, although μ and δ receptors have also been implicated. Dynorphin and α-neo-endorphin, which are endogenous κ ligands, stimulate feeding when administered centrally, whereas antibodies to neo-endorphin have been shown to attenuate feeding. Evidence points to the PVN as a site of opioid-mediated modulation of feeding behavior, as physiological doses of endogenous opioids administered there stimulate feeding. Other brain areas implicated in opioid-induced feeding are the amygdala, nucleus accumbens, and ventral tegmental areas.

In humans, the opioid agonist butorphanol tartrate stimulates hunger while several studies have shown that naloxone decreases meal size in both lean and obese humans. Prolonged administration of opioid antagonists, however, has been ineffective in producing weight loss in obese subjects.

The pancreatic polypeptides NPY and PYY, named for the tyrosine residue at both ends of the molecules (tyrosine = Y), are the most potent of the endogenously occurring peptides that stimulate feeding. Doses of NPY as low as 78 pmol (i.e., 78×10^{-12} mol) injected into the PVN of rats produce dramatic increases in water and in food intake—specifically intake of carbohydrates. Chronic administration of NPY into the PVN produces sustained increases in food intake, body weight, and body fat in rats. PYY is an even more potent stimulator of feeding than NPY.

NE was the first amine found to affect food intake. Central administration of NE, particularly into the PVN, increases food intake. NE-induced feeding is characterized by an increase in meal size, not meal frequency, and a preference for carbohydrate over fat or protein. Physiological doses of NE injected into the PVN elicit feeding in satiated rats, an effect mediated through stimulation of α_2-adrenergic receptors. Daily injection into the PVN of NE or α_2 agonists, such as clonidine, enhance daily food intake and weight gain in rats. Since the PVN is involved in the inhibition of food intake and its destruction increases food intake and body weight, the effect of α_2-adrenergic stimulation in the PVN appears to involve a release of the inhibition to feed.

A physiological role for brain monoamines in the control of satiety was hypothesized from the observation that drugs such as amphetamine and fenfluramine, which act through catecholaminergic and serotonergic systems, respectively, inhibit food intake. DA appears to be the most important catecholamine involved in the inhibition of feeding, although in one extrahypothalamic area, the neostriatum, DA increases motivated behavior, including feeding. Microinjections of DA into the hypothalamus decrease feeding whereas DA antagonists injected into the hypothalamus increase feeding.

The perifornical region of the lateral hypothalamus (PFH) is the site most responsive to the inhibitory effects of the catecholamine. When administered acutely into the PFH of hungry animals, DA significantly suppresses food intake. Chronic infusion of DA into the PFH decreases food intake and body weight, similar to the effect of electrolytic lesions of the PFH. Other catecholamines, epinephrine, and to a lesser extent NE also decrease feeding when injected into the PFH. The inhibition of food intake produced by peripheral administration of amphetamine or administration of amphetamine or catecholamine into the PFH is characterized by a delay in meal onset and a preferential decrease in protein intake. The effect of catecholamine in the PFH is mediated through stimulation of β-adrenergic receptors.

The observation from recent microdialysis studies that levels of DA increase in the nucleus accumbens and prefrontal cortex suggests that DA in other brain regions may be involved in the regulation of feeding.

The earliest notions about the control of feeding implicated NE and DA as the principal mediators. Over the last 10 years, however, the role of 5-HT has received considerable attention. Changes in 5-HT metabolism have clear effects on food intake and body weight. Centrally administered 5-HT and peripherally administered drugs that enhance serotonergic activity, such as fenfluramine and fluoxetine, inhibit feeding. The medial hypothalamus appears to be especially sensitive to 5-HT. Injection of 5-HT into the PVN decreases food consumption in food-deprived rats offered a meal and antagonizes the stimulatory effects of NE on food intake. Lesions of the PVN attenuate 5-HT-induced anorexia. Recent microdialysis studies showing that feeding induces a rise in extracellular 5-HT in the medial hypothalamus strengthen the hypothesis that hypothalamic 5-HT plays a physiological role in the control of food intake.

The anorexia induced by 5-HT is characterized by decreased meal size and duration and decreased rate of eating. In contrast to the effects of DA within the PFH, 5-HT does not affect the latency to meal onset; the inhibition of food intake is secondary to the induction of satiety. In addition, whereas DA induces a preferential decrease in protein consumption, 5-HT spares protein by causing a preferential decrease in carbohydrate consumption.

The serotonergic and catecholaminergic systems within two closely associated sites in the hypothalamus, the PFH and PVN, seem to work antagonistically to control food intake and selection of protein, carbohydrate, and fat. The catecholamines appear to exert control over hunger, whereas the serotonergic system is involved in satiety. The interplay between the two systems may regulate the ratio of carbohydrate to protein in the diet.

Do any of the centrally or peripherally active neurotransmitters discussed above have a role in the etiology of obesity? This question is not easy to address, especially in humans, due to the difficulty in measuring levels of these substances within the brain. In experimental animal models of obesity, brain levels of some neurotransmitters appear to be abnormal. Elevated levels of β-endorphin have been found in the pituitary of obese rodents. The concentrations of NE and 5-HT, but not DA, have been reported to be increased in the brains of genetically obese mice and rats. However, since nutrient intake may itself alter the synthesis of neurotransmitters, whether such alterations are a cause or effect of the obesity is not clear.

Data on the role of neurotransmitters in obesity in humans are just beginning to appear. For example, one study reported elevated levels of β-endorphin in obese preadolescents, adolescents, and adults. Whether abnormal levels of neurotransmitters play a role in the etiology of human obesity is at present largely speculative. However, the knowledge gained through the study of these neurotransmitters has been applied to the development of treatments for obesity.

HEREDITY

Genetic factors are important determinants of body size. Millennia of experience with farm animals had pointed to a genetic basis for obesity, but systematic evaluation of genetic factors in obesity began relatively recently with studies of obese rodents such as the yellow obese mouse (1927) and the ob/ob mouse (1950). The first suggestion that human obesity may be inherited came from studies of similarities in body weight within families. These studies showed that obesity runs in families and that children of obese parents have a greater chance of becoming obese than children of lean parents. Figure 5 shows that most offspring of two obese parents are obese as adults and most offspring of two lean parents are lean as adults. Although family studies support the idea of a parental influence on body weight, they can not differentiate the effects of environmental factors from heredity. Until recently, much of the evidence suggested that a person's environ-

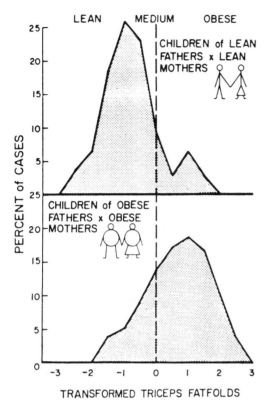

FIG. 5. Relationship between parental obesity and the distribution of the fatfold thickness (a clinical measure of adiposity) of their adult offspring. On the horizontal axis the extent of leanness or adiposity is shown by the normalized *z* scores of the fatfold thickness (−3 lean, 3 most fat). Most of the offspring of thin parents were thin; most of the offspring of fat parents were fat. Reprinted with permission from Garn SM, Clark, DC. *Pediatrics* 1976;57:443–456.

ment, particularly socioeconomic status, was the more important of these two factors.

In the last few years we have learned that genetics play an important part in human obesity, as in other diseases (see Chapter 16). This information has been derived from the study of two special types of populations—twins and adoptees. The rationale of twin studies is simple: identical, or monozygotic (MZ), twins share both a common environment and common genes. Fraternal, or dizygotic (DZ), twins share a common environment but, on average, only half of their genes. Since the environments of twins of either

type are presumably similar, any difference between the intrapair correlations of the two types of twins should be due to genetic influences.

Traditional twin studies indicate that about 80% of the variation in body mass index can be explained by genetic factors. Traditional twin studies, however, may overestimate the influence of genetic factors since the two types of twins may not, in fact, share completely similar environments: the environment in which MZ twins are raised may make them more alike than DZ twins. Any such environmentally induced similarity would be attributed to genetic factors and thus exaggerate the importance of heredity.

This problem can be obviated by the study of an unusual population—identical twins reared apart. Such a population has been identified by the Swedish Adoption/Twin Study of Aging. Since they have not shared any environmental influences, heritability can be estimated for this population by the intrapair correlation. Estimated in this manner, heritability of the body mass index is about 70%, suggesting that traditional twin studies overestimated heritability only slightly.

Studies of adopted individuals and their biological and adoptive parents have confirmed and extended the findings of twin studies. In adoption studies of heredity, adoptees are compared with both their biological and their adoptive parents for the trait under consideration. A significant relationship between the biological parents and the adoptees indicates a genetic influence whereas a relationship between the adoptive parents and the adoptees indicates an environmental influence.

One such adoption study compared the BMI of 540 adult Danish adoptees with the BMI of their biological and adoptive parents. The results, illustrated in Fig. 6, show that the BMI of the adoptees corresponded to that of their biological parents but bore no relation to that of their adoptive parents. The BMI of the adoptees was more strongly related to the BMI of their biological mothers than to that

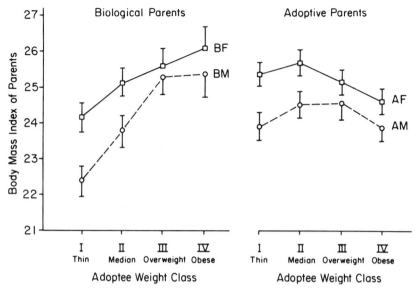

FIG. 6. Relationship between the weight class of adoptees and the body mass index of their biological and adoptive parents. The weight class of the adoptees was strongly related to the body mass index of their biological parents, and it bore no relation to the body mass index of their adoptive parents. BF and BM indicate females and males, respectively, in comparison to biological parents. AF and AM indicate females and males, respectively, in comparison to adoptive parents.

of their biological fathers. Similar findings have since been made in a study of adoptees in Iowa. Thus, studies of adoptees have confirmed the findings of twin studies that genetic factors are important in determining adiposity.

What exactly is the role of genetics in human obesity? Are people born to be fat just as they are born with blue eyes or brown hair? The answer is no! Fatness is not determined at conception. What is inherited is a vulnerability to obesity that requires a suitable environment in order to permit its expression. Genetic makeup may predispose one to become obese, but the obesity may not manifest itself except under certain conditions. The conditions that cause a predisposition to obesity to be expressed are now under investigation; a sedentary lifestyle and an abundance of high-fat food are two prime candidates. The current American diet contains sufficient fat to produce obesity in thin rats, and our labor-saving devices are so efficient that we now become fat on a diet that contains 1,000

fewer calories than at the turn of the century. The issue in human obesity is not one of heredity or environment, or heredity vs. environment, but of heredity and environment or genetic vulnerability and environmental challenge.

ADIPOSE TISSUE

Clues to the causes of obesity lie in adipose tissue. Excess adipose tissue relative to lean body mass is the *sine qua non* of obesity. Not surprisingly, then, the growth, development, and metabolism of adipose tissue constitute a major area of interest. Morphologically, obesity can be characterized by adipocyte (fat cell) hypertrophy (*hypertrophic obesity*), adipocyte hyperplasia (*hyperplastic obesity*), or both (*hypertrophic-hyperplastic obesity*). Fat cell number is largely established early in life and appears to be genetically determined. Increases in adipocyte number occur most rapidly in the last trimester before birth and in preadolescence. In most individuals, fat cell number remains fairly stable from adolescence through adulthood. In very overweight individuals, however, fat cell number can increase when the lipid storage capacity of the existing fat cells is surpassed. Although fat cells may be added, they can never be lost. A person of average weight has about 30 billion fat cells; in hyperplastic obesity, this number may rise as high as 180 billion.

Following puberty, changes in body fat content take place primarily through increases or decreases in the triglyceride volume of adipocytes. Thus, most people who become obese as adults suffer hypertrophic obesity, whereas those whose obesity began in childhood most often suffer hyperplastic or hyperplastic-hypertrophic obesity. It was once believed that the increased number of fat cells found in people with childhood onset obesity was caused by overfeeding during infancy or childhood. However, recent research has shown that overfeeding early in life does not predict later obesity, nor does underfeeding in early life protect against increased adipocyte cellularity or obesity. Furthermore, neonatal adiposity is not a good predictor of later adiposity.

The possibility that obesity may result from an error in metabolism that results in abnormally high rates of lipid storage has stimulated a great deal of research on factors that affect adipose tissue metabolism. Lipoprotein lipase (LPL), an enzyme found in adipose tissue that plays a critical role in lipid storage, has become a focus of such research. LPL directs the uptake of triglycerides from the blood into adipocytes for storage. High levels of adipose tissue LPL have been implicated in the propensity of genetically obese animals, such as the Zucker fatty rat, to accumulate large fat stores, even when faced with caloric restriction. At high levels of LPL so much triglyceride is diverted into fat cells that other tissues, such as muscle, are deprived of energy. This energy deficit is believed to trigger hunger and compensatory increases in food intake. Human obesity has been attributed to abnormally high rates of LPL production, but data are sparse and inconsistent. Some researchers have reported an elevation of LPL in the adipose tissue of obese persons who are losing weight and have suggested that the high levels of LPL are responsible for the difficulty obese people have in maintaining weight loss. Others, however, have seen no change in LPL level in obese persons during weight loss. Resolution of this issue is currently the topic of vigorous research which should clarify whether LPL has a role in the etiology of human obesity.

A SET POINT THEORY OF BODY WEIGHT

Obesity may result from regulation of body weight at an elevated level. The theory that body weight or body fat is regulated about a particular level, or *set point,* arose from the study of weight changes in normal and overweight humans and experimental animals. Three major types of observations have provided evidence for this theory: (1) the weight of humans and animals from other species remains relatively stable throughout adulthood despite large fluctuations in food intake; (2) following periods of food restriction or overeating, the body weight of both humans and experimental animals returns to this level; and (3) following surgical removal of adipose tissue (lipectomy) from laboratory animals, the size of the remaining fat depots increases until total body fat returns to its presurgery level.

Two studies have become classics of research on the regulation of body weight in humans. One examined the effects of prolonged caloric restriction, the other the effect of sustained overeating. The first was conducted during the Second World War, when the pioneering American nutritionist Ancel Keys subjected a group of young male conscientious objectors to prolonged semistarvation. These men lost one third of their body weight, but as soon as they were allowed to eat freely they became hyperphagic and their body weight returned to its prediet level. The second study examined a group of lean male prison inmates who voluntarily agreed to overeat until they had gained 20 pounds. The men consumed two to three times their normal caloric intake but did not easily get fat. Not all of the men were able to gain the desired 20 pounds, and those who did required an average of 5,000 kilocalories a day just to maintain their new body weight. When these men were allowed to eat freely, their body weight fell without difficulty to its initial level.

Such observations in humans and animals suggested that the body has a mechanism for detecting its level of either body weight or body fat. When body weight/fat climbs above or drops below the regulated level, or set point, the detection system sends out physiological signals that direct changes in metabolic rate and/or hunger that act to return body weight to its regulated level. Insulin is hypothesized to be one signal that relays information to the brain, via the cerebrospinal fluid, about the quantity of body fat.

Many studies examining the effects of caloric restriction or caloric excess on the metabolic rate and body weight of normal-weight subjects are consistent with the set point theory of weight regulation. During periods of overeating, metabolic rate increases, slowing weight gain. Conversely, during periods of food deprivation, metabolic rate decreases, limiting weight loss. Following food deprivation, hunger remains high (and indirect evidence suggests that metabolic rate stays low), until weight is regained to the set point level.

This evidence for regulation gave rise to a set point theory of obesity. According to this theory, obesity is the result of a body weight set point that is higher than normal. Obesity is viewed not as a dysfunction in regulation but rather as the result of regulation of body weight around an elevated set point. According to this view, the difficulty obese people have in reducing their weight and maintaining weight loss is the consequence of the same regulatory mechanisms that operate to keep the weight of normal weight people at a "desirable level." The metabolic response of many obese persons during weight loss, and the rapid regain of weight following dieting, have been cited as evidence for an elevated set point in obesity. The metabolic rate of obese women can drop by as much as 20% within the first 2 weeks of a low-calorie diet. Although metabolic rate rises after food intake increases, there are reports that the metabolic rate of formerly obese persons who maintain their weight loss is significantly lower than that of never-obese persons of the same height and weight. According to other reports, however, the metabolic rate of previously obese persons is normal for their new body size. Resolution of this empirical question will go a long way toward establishing, or refuting, the set point theory of obesity. Although considerable data support the existence of a body weight set point, the theory is too loosely formulated to be readily testable in humans, and it has been vigorously contested. Opponents of the set point theory argue that body weight is not regulated, and one theory is that the degree of adiposity one attains is simply the net result of efforts to maintain a socially acceptable body weight.

TREATMENT

Lifestyle, not diets, is the key to treatment of mild and moderate obesity. The basis of weight reduction is utterly simple—establish a caloric deficit by reducing intake below output. All of the treatment regimes have as their goal this simple task. How they achieve this goal, however, varies greatly. The chief approaches to the treatment of obesity involve behavior change related to diet and physical activity, surgical or mechanical methods designed to reduce food intake or absorption, and pharmacological methods to reduce hunger or increase satiety.

In theory, weight loss should be accomplished easily by dieting, but in practice, traditional diet therapy has had only limited success. People who lose weight tend to gain it back.

The most important recent development in the treatment of obesity has been the change in who delivers it. The traditional role of the physician has been largely supplanted by commercial organizations. Today most treatment of obesity in America, and a growing proportion in the developed countries, occurs under commercial auspices. There are advantages to this development. Behavior therapy for obesity and nutritional science have both advanced to a point where they can be standardized for administration to large numbers of persons. Industry is better equipped than individual physicians to manage the logistics of programs that today enroll 2 million persons and to incorporate new research findings into these programs. One problem faced by patients is how to choose a program. A classification based on the severity of obesity helps in making this choice.

Three levels of severity of obesity have been defined: mild, moderate, and severe. They are characterized by body weights that are 20% to 40% overweight, 41% to 100% overweight, and more than 100% overweight, respectively. The percentage of obese persons falling into these three categories is 90.5%, 9%, and 0.5%, respectively.

Treatment of Mild Obesity

Mild obesity, which afflicts 90% of the obese population, is best treated by moderate changes in lifestyle and personal habits. The basis of these changes is an extensive program of behavior modification designed to improve eating behavior and increase physical activity. The goal is to create a small negative caloric balance until weight loss is achieved and then to maintain this loss. The idea of a formal diet is currently in disfavor. "Going on" a diet implies "going off" it and the resumption of old eating habits. Instead of a diet, many programs favor a gradual change in eating habits and a shift to foods that the patient can continue to eat indefinitely—fruits, vegetables, and cereals—and

few fats. Such a change gives the best chance of maintaining a healthy weight level, and it is safe. A diet based primarily on sensible eating habits does not require medical supervision and is particularly well suited to use by the lay-led commercial organizations that treat mild obesity.

Some of these organizations have excellent treatment plans, and they are generally safe. However, a large number are poorly administered, have very high drop-out rates, and consequently are ineffective. Under these circumstances, those who care for obese patients can render them a major service by selecting the most effective weight-loss programs in their area and by encouraging their patients to remain in them.

Treatment of Moderate Obesity

Moderate obesity (40% to 100% overweight) is far less prevalent than mild obesity, affecting only 9% of the obese population. Nonetheless, this means that several million persons in the United States are moderately obese, and the medical indications for treatment are more urgent. The rationale of treatment is the same as that for mild obesity. The greater severity of the disorder, however, has led to the use of very-low-calorie diets, which provide from 400 to 700 calories a day, in order to achieve more rapid weight loss. Weight losses may reach 3 to 5 pounds a week, great enough to require medical monitoring with frequent electrocardiograms and measurement of electrolytes. Under such medical supervision these diets are safe for moderately obese persons for periods as long as four months; they should not be used by mildly obese persons.

Programs for the treatment of moderate obesity are better managed than those for mild obesity, but they are also more expensive, costing between $2,000 and $3,000 for a 6-month treatment program. Their major problem is maintenance of patients' weight losses beyond a period of 1 year.

Treatment of Severe Obesity

Although it afflicts only 0.5% of obese persons, severe obesity (>100% overweight) is very often associated with major medical problems. Surgery to restrict the size of the stomach can control most such problems, as it produces weight losses of from 30% to 70% of excess weight—as much as 150 pounds. Given the high surgical risk of these patients, surgery is surprisingly safe, with an operative and perioperative mortality rate of less than 1%.

The psychosocial benefits of the surgical treatment of obesity are as impressive as are its physical benefits. Many incapacitated patients return to work or resume domestic responsibilities. Whereas weight losses achieved by dieting are often associated with anxiety and depression, those achieved by surgical treatment are associated with improved mood and feelings of well-being. Body image disparagement is greatly reduced, and food preferences shift from fatty foods to foods of low caloric density.

Pharmacological Treatments of Obesity

The goal of pharmacological treatment of obesity is to decrease feelings of hunger or invoke early satiety in order to make adherence to diet therapy easier for the obese patient. *Most drugs that decrease appetite act centrally through dopaminergic, noradrenergic, or serotonergic mechanisms.* The anorectic effect of the two prototypic agents amphetamine and fenfluramine, discussed earlier, is a result of their ability to potentiate the catecholaminergic and serotonergic systems, respectively. Both drugs increase weight loss by about half a pound per week compared to diet therapy alone.

Because of the potential for addiction with certain of these drugs and because of the development of tolerance to their anorectic effects, pharmacotherapy for obesity has traditionally been used for only short periods.

However, once the drug is withdrawn, patients regain almost all of the weight they lost through pharmacotherapy. Since weight loss can be considered a successful outcome of treatment only if it is maintained, short-term drug therapy is useless in the treatment of obesity. Recent studies indicate that although the anorectic effect of these drugs is short-lived, they have a suppressive effect on body weight that is long-lasting, and thus their chronic use may be warranted. Patients treated with fenfluramine and diet for periods of up to a year are better able to maintain their weight loss than those who lost weight through diet alone. The chronic use of certain of these drugs is, however, limited by side effects.

The development of new pharmacological treatments for obesity that lack the side effects and addiction potential of conventional agents is being vigorously pursued by many pharmaceutical companies. Several compounds not yet available to physicians have given encouraging results in clinical trials. However, the long-term safety and efficacy of such treatments will not be known for some time to come.

SUMMARY

Obesity is a condition of excess body fat that increases the risk of premature mortality and morbidity. The distribution of the excess fat is a good predictor of risk; excess intra-abdominal fat conveys a considerable risk of cardiovascular disease and diabetes. Weight loss improves or reverses most of the adverse health effects of obesity.

Although the causes of obesity have not been clearly ascertained, current research is coming closer to identifying factors important in its etiology. The parts played by genetics, adipose tissue metabolism, mechanisms of body weight regulation, and the neurobiology of eating behavior have become clearer in recent years.

Treatment of obesity is a challenge for the obese patient and the physician alike. The goal of treatment is to induce a sustained negative energy balance. Diet therapy, behavior modification, exercise, surgery, and pharmacotherapy are the tools used to achieve this negative balance. The choice of treatment is based on the severity of the obesity. The development of safe, effective pharmacological agents holds special promise in the long-term treatment of obesity.

BIBLIOGRAPHY

Original Articles

Becker BJ. The obese patient in group psychoanalysis. *Am J Psychother* 1960;14:322–337.

Cohn C, Joseph D. Influence of body weight and body fat on appetite of "normal" lean and obese rats. *Yale J Biol Med* 1962;34:598–607.

Sims EAH, Goldman RF, Gluck CM, Horton ES, Kelleher PC, Rowe DW. Experimental obesity in man. *Trans Assoc Am Physicians* 1968;81:153–170.

Stunkard AJ, Foch TT, Hrubec Z. A twin study of human obesity. *JAMA* 1986;256:51–54.

Stunkard AJ, Sørensen TI, Hanis C, Teasdale TW, Chakraborty R, Schull WJ, et al. An adoption study of human obesity. *N Engl J Med* 1986;314:193–198.

Books and Reviews

Bray GA. Definitions, measurements and classification of the syndromes of obesity. *Int J Obes* 1978;2:99–112.

Greenwood MRC, Savard R, West DB, Kava R. Energy metabolism and nutrient 'gating' in pregnancy and lactation. In: Berry E, Blondheim SH, Eliahou HE, Shafrir E, eds. *Recent advances in obesity research.* Vol. 5. London: John Libbey, 1987;258–263.

Keesey RE. A set-point theory of obesity. In: Brownell KD, Foreyt JP, eds. *Handbook of eating disorders,* New York: Basic Books, 1986;63–87.

Keys A, Brozek J, Henschel A, Mickelsen O, Taylor HL. *The biology of human starvation.* Minneapolis, MN: University of Minnesota Press, 1950.

Leibowitz SF. Brain monoamines and peptides: role in the control of eating behavior. *Fed Proc* 1986;45: 1396–1403.

Morley JE, Blundell JE. The neurobiological basis of eating disorders: some formulations. *Biol Psychiatry* 1988;23:53–78.

Poissonnet CM, LaVelle M, Burdi AR. Growth and development of adipose tissue. *J Pediatrics* 1988; 113:1–9.

Sobal J, Stunkard AJ. Socioeconomic status and obesity: a review of the literature. *Psychol Bull* 1989;105: 260–275.

Stallone D, Stunkard AJ. The regulation of body weight: evidence and clinical implications. *Ann Behav Med* 1991;13:220–230.

Van Itallie TB. Health implications of overweight and obesity in the United States. *Ann Intern Med* 1985;103:983–988.

22

Epilepsy

Marc A. Dichter

He was thinking, incidentally, that there was a moment or two in his epileptic condition almost before the fit itself, when suddenly amid the sadness, spiritual darkness and depression, his brain seemed to catch fire . . . his sensation of being alive and his awareness increased tenfold . . . his mind and heart were flooded by a dazzling light . . . culminating in a great calm, full of serene and harmonious joy and hope, full of understanding and the knowledge of the final cause. The "fit" (which followed) was, of course, unendurable. . . .

Fyodor Dostoyevsky,
The Idiot, 1868
Trans. by David Magarshack (New York: Penguin Classics, 1955)

- Epilepsy is a symptom of neurological dysfunction characterized by seizures.

- Seizures occur in many different forms.

- Classification of seizure types is based on the EEG patterns and on the behavioral phenomena that occur during the seizure.

- The electroencephalogram (EEG) allows us to record the electrical activity generated by the underlying cortex.

- The normal EEG is characterized by several different patterns, depending on the physiological state of the individual.

- Different seizure types have different natural histories.

- Brain regions can be hyperexcitable even when seizures are not occurring.

- Seizures develop in an area of hyperexcitability and then spread throughout the brain.

- Hyperexcitability of the cortex can develop in several ways.

- Epilepsy must be treated.

- Most seizures are treated with medication.

- Some forms of seizures can be effectively treated by brain surgery.

- Behavioral disturbances that are independent of seizures may occur in individuals with epilepsy.

- Unusual personality characteristics may occur in individuals with complex partial seizures.

- Some individuals with epilepsy develop affective disorders.

- Very few persons with epilepsy are psychotic.

- Some individuals with epilepsy experience endocrine dysfunction or disorders of sexuality.

- Antiepileptic drugs can produce behavioral changes.

This chapter discusses seizures: their etiology, classification, and natural history. Starting with a discussion of the electroencephalogram, the chapter details the nature of different seizure disorders along with their diagnosis and treatment regimens. Also covered are cellular mechanisms and psychological syndromes associated with epilepsy.

Epilepsy is a condition in which individuals experience sudden and unprovoked (paroxysmal) changes in behavior caused by abnormalities in the electrical activity of the brain. Each specific behavioral/electrophysiological event is referred to as a *seizure,* and these seizures can take many forms. They may consist of a sudden loss of consciousness and repetitive movements of all four limbs, a brief lapse in attention, or a change in an individual's interaction with his or her environment.

Epilepsy is a common neurological problem affecting between 0.5% and 2% of the population. It has been present in the medical "literature" from almost the beginning of written descriptions of human behavior; seizures were described in ancient Egyptian and Mesopotamian writings and were the subject of whole treatises in the Greek literature. Some of history's most famous figures were known to have epilepsy, including Alexander the Great, Julius Caesar, Napoleon, Beethoven, and Dostoyevsky, among many others. Indeed, three of Shakespeare's four great tragic figures—King Lear, Macbeth, and Othello—were said to have epileptic seizures. Epilepsy thus is neither rare nor confined to individuals of limited accomplishments.

ETIOLOGY OF SEIZURES

Epilepsy is a symptom of neurological dysfunction characterized by seizures. The circuitry to sustain an epileptic seizure appears

Biological Bases of Brain Function and Disease, edited by Alan Frazer, Perry B. Molinoff, and Andrew Winokur. Raven Press, Ltd., New York © 1994.

to be part of the normal structure of the brain; normal individuals, and essentially all vertebrate animals, can be induced to have seizures with relatively small perturbations of normal brain function. Similarly, the mechanisms by which seizures are generated and spread throughout the brain appear to depend on normal synaptic physiology, as discussed below.

In some individuals, seizures occur with no apparent cause; these are called *idiopathic.* Many idiopathic seizures in childhood appear to have a genetic origin. Thus, such individuals will often have close relatives with epilepsy, or, if electroencephalograms (EEGs) are performed on parents and siblings, abnormal excitability will be seen, even in people who have never had a seizure! The degree of genetic influence on the development of epilepsy can be quite variable among different epilepsy syndromes. Some forms of genetically determined epilepsy appear to have a very direct inheritance pattern, whereas others seem to have a more variable penetrance (i.e., not everyone who carries the gene demonstrates the phenotypic trait) or may be inherited based on more than one gene. In three forms of epilepsy specific chromosomal localization of an abnormal gene has been accomplished. The gene for juvenile myoclonic epilepsy is located on chromosome 6, for benign neonatal convulsions on chromosome 20, and for progressive myoclonic epilepsy of the Unverricht–Lundborg type, on chromosome 21. How abnormalities at each of these genes can produce epilepsy is still not known.

In other individuals, seizures are directly attributable to an underlying structural or biochemical lesion in the brain. For example, brain tumors, pressing on normal brain and distorting normal architecture, can cause seizures. Areas of brain damaged by trauma or a stroke can become hyperexcitable and give rise to seizures (e.g., become *epileptogenic*). Abnormalities in cell migration (cortical *dysplasias*), differentiation during embryonic development, or other brain malformations that occur during development can also be epileptogenic. In addition, brain infection, chemical imbalance in the body, drug intoxication, and low blood sugar can all cause seizures. Thus, both the normal brain and brain made abnormal by a variety of disturbances appear to have the capacity to develop seizures.

CLASSIFICATION OF SEIZURES

Seizures occur in many different forms. Epilepsy is a family of disorders that have distinct behavioral and EEG manifestations, different life histories, different underlying provocations, and different cellular mechanisms. Moreover, different forms of epilepsy require different medications or treatment strategies. Thus, to better understand this group of disorders, a classification scheme is needed. This could be based on a description of the seizures themselves or on whole syndromes (e.g., a combination of the age of the individual, kind of seizures that are occurring, EEG findings, family history, cause of the epilepsy, etc.) Classification of either seizures or syndromes, however, is sometimes easier said than done, as epilepsy in any given individual can be a complicated combination of seizure types. In this chapter we will classify only seizure types, not syndromes.

Classification of seizure types is based on the EEG patterns and on the behavioral phenomena that occur during the seizure. The seizure discharge can begin in an isolated region of the brain (*partial* or *focal* seizures) or may appear to begin diffusely throughout both hemispheres (*primary generalized seizures*) (Table 1).

Partial or Focal Seizures

Partial or focal seizures originate in specific parts of the cortex and either remain confined to those areas or spread to other parts of the brain. These seizures most often

---

TABLE 1. *Classification of seizure types (simplified)*

1. Partial or focal seizures—Seizures originating from a localized area of brain
   a. Simple partial seizures—A partial seizure with no alteration in consciousness
   b. Complex partial seizures—A partial seizure with alteration in consciousness
   c. Partial seizure with secondary generalization—Spread of seizure activity from one focal area to multiple brain regions resulting in loss of consciousness and possibly a tonic-clonic seizure
2. Primary generalized seizures
   a. Tonic-clonic seizures (Grand Mal)—Abrupt loss of consciousness without warning, followed by tonic contraction of all muscle groups (leading to an arched back and extensor posturing), followed by rhythmic jerks of arms and legs (clonic contractions)
   b. Absence seizures (Petit Mal)—Brief lapses of attention without loss of consciousness or loss of body tone, associated with a 3-Hz spike-and-wave pattern in the EEG
   c. Myoclonic seizures—Brief contractions of muscle groups, involving a limb, the face, an entire side of the body, or the entire body, unassociated with a loss of consciousness
   d. Other (akinetic, tonic, clonic)—Seizures that consist of falling to the floor due to abrupt loss of body tone, without loss of consciousness (akinetic) or of fragments of the tonic-clonic seizure pattern (tonic or clonic seizures)
3. Status epilepticus
   a. Tonic-clonic status—Continuous tonic-clonic seizure activity or recurrent tonic-clonic seizures without the individual's regaining consciousness between seizures
   b. Absence status—Prolonged or continuous lapses of consciousness associated with continuous generalized spike-and-wave activity in the EEG
   c. Epilepsia partialis continua
   d. Complex partial status

originate in limbic cortical structures (e.g., hippocampus, orbital frontal cortex, amygdala) and are often associated with an identifiable structural lesion at the site of origin. The behavioral aspects of these seizures are related to the area of the cortex in which the seizures start, how widely they are propagated, and how long they last. Consciousness may or may not be altered; however, changes of consciousness provide the basis for a classification into simple and complex partial seizures.

Simple Partial Seizures (SPSs)

Simple partial seizures are seizures that do not alter the individual's conscious interaction with the environment. They may consist of motor, sensory, visceral, or psychic phenomena and are usually brief (seconds to 1–2 min) but may be prolonged. They are caused by synchronous electrical discharges of neurons confined to one area of the cortex. If the discharges occur in the motor cortex, the seizures consist of repetitive contractions of muscle groups in the appropriate contralateral body area. If the discharges occur in the sensory cortex, the seizures may consist of abnormal sensory phenomena, such as auditory hallucinations or unformed or formed visual hallucinations. If the seizures occur in the limbic cortex, they may consist of abnormal emotional reactions, such as sensations of fear, or disturbances in autonomic function, such as nausea or a rising feeling in the abdomen.

Individuals with partial seizures often have spike discharges in their EEGs, signifying an area of the brain with abnormal electrical excitability. If the spikes are consistently well localized to one area, it is likely that the brain underlying that area is abnormal and is responsible for the epileptic activity. In other individuals, spikes will not be seen, despite multiple recordings, and in these individuals the diagnosis of epilepsy may be difficult to confirm.

During a seizure, large repetitive spikes and spike–wave complexes will be seen to originate in a cortical area that corresponds to the area involved in the clinical seizure. Thus, focal motor seizures will show repetitive discharges in the contralateral motor cortex whereas sensory seizures will show repetitive discharges in the sensory cortex.

Complex Partial Seizures (CPSs)

Complex partial seizures are partial seizures in which consciousness is impaired. They often originate in the limbic cortex but can also begin in neocortical areas. Consciousness is not necessarily lost. Rather, the individual may remain conscious and even appear relatively normal to an inexperienced observer. However, the individual may not be able to answer questions coherently or carry on an intelligible conversation. These seizures are usually associated with amnesia for events occurring during the seizure. The electrical discharges underlying these seizures usually spread beyond a local area of origin into other limbic structures that are involved in an individual's conscious interaction with the environment. However, the exact structures involved in conversion of an SPS to a CPS are not known.

The behavioral repertoire that can be activated during a CPS is extensive. Some individuals engage in complicated, skilled tasks, such as playing musical instruments or driving a car, and have no awareness of the events afterward. Other individuals carry out slightly bizarre behaviors, such as disrobing in a public place, venturing into traffic, or walking aimlessly around a room picking up and putting down objects. Occasionally, individuals may even develop different "personalities" during a CPS while appearing otherwise relatively normal, except for a postictal amnesia. Thus, some of these behavioral changes could be mistaken for a psychiatric disorder rather than a manifestation of an abnormal electrical discharge in the brain. CPSs are often distinguishable from pure psychiatric disorders by the paroxysmal nature of the symptomatology and the abnormal EEG that accompanies the events.

Secondary Generalization of Partial Seizures

When a seizure involves diffuse and bilateral brain areas it is considered generalized. Our classification scheme assumes that some seizures are generalized at onset (see below) but that others start in a local area of brain and spread to many other parts of the brain, or "secondarily generalize." Both SPSs and CPSs can spread from local areas of the cortex to involve the entire cortex and subcortical structures. This often occurs over a period of seconds or even minutes, but can also occur more rapidly. The individual then loses consciousness and experiences a tonic-clonic seizure (see below). This kind of secondary generalization occurs by the spread of the seizure discharge over normal synaptic pathways, the exact direction and speed of spread depending on the site of origin of the seizure discharge and connections to other brain regions.

Primary Generalized Seizures

Primary generalized seizures cannot be localized to one area of the brain but appear to start simultaneously in multiple regions on both sides. The pathophysiology of generalized seizures is less well understood than that of focal seizures; generally, these seizures are not associated with single focal lesions in one or another brain region but may occur in an individual with no detectable pathology or an individual with multifocal brain abnormalities. Whether primary generalized seizures actually commence simultaneously in many parts of the brain or are generated from deeper, more localized structures that have widespread bilateral connections remains to be determined.

Tonic-Clonic Seizures (Grand Mal)

Tonic-clonic seizures begin with a sudden and abrupt loss of consciousness. All muscle groups appear to contract simultaneously (*tonic* contraction) and since extensors tend to be more powerful than flexors, the individual arches his or her back, with arms and legs extended, and falls to the floor. Sudden contraction of expiratory muscles often leads to a "cry" as air is expelled through the vocal cords. After several seconds, the motor activity becomes more rhythmic and the limbs flex and extend, the *clonic* part of the tonic-clonic seizure. The seizure may continue for seconds to a minute or two but then usually subsides. The individual slowly regains consciousness, most often with a period of confusion and disorientation, as well as amnesia for the seizure and often for a short period of time preceding the seizure. When these seizures occur without any warning and in the absence of any focal brain lesions or focal seizures, they are called primary generalized tonic-clonic seizures.

The EEG during primary generalized tonic-clonic seizures can show various features. Often the EEG is obscured by muscle artifact generated by the motor component of the seizure. When recordings are done in specialized ways to avoid such artifacts, the EEG may show low-voltage, fast activity or high-voltage, synchronized activity. The surface EEG reflects the activity of neurons in the immediate underlying cortex, and its pattern is determined by where the seizures are originating and how they are being propagated to the surface.

Primary Generalized Absence Seizures (Petit Mal)

Absence seizures are different from seizures that have major motor manifestations. These seizures consist of a lapse of attention, accompanied by a brief staring spell and, occasionally, by a fluttering of the lips or a slight movement of the hands. These seizures are usually brief, lasting less than 1 min, sometimes for only several seconds. Occasionally, absence seizures are prolonged and convert to either generalized tonic-clonic seizures or even a "complex absence" resembling a CPS. Absence seizures are accompanied by characteristic 3-Hz spike-and-wave discharges. Often individuals with absence seizures have multiple episodes of brief 3-Hz spike-and-wave discharges in the EEG that do not have any behavioral consequences (e.g., do not interfere with consciousness.) Interestingly, relatives of individuals with primary absence epilepsy may also demonstrate brief episodes of spike-and-wave discharges in their EEGs without any manifestations of epilepsy. Absence seizures almost always begin in childhood, between the ages of 5 and 10 years. Some children will also have tonic-clonic seizures. At puberty, approximately one third of individuals with absence seizures will stop having them, one third will continue to have absences, and one third will continue to have tonic-clonic seizures.

Primary Generalized Myoclonic Seizures

Myoclonic seizures consist of brief jerks of a limb, facial muscles, or the entire body, without alteration in consciousness. They may occur singly or in groups. If prolonged, they may progress to loss of consciousness and tonic-clonic seizure activity. The movements are accompanied by spike-and-wave discharges in the EEG.

Other Forms of Primary Generalized Seizures

Seizures may consist of sudden loss of body tone without loss of consciousness (akinetic or atonic seizures), or isolated tonic or clonic activity. Some individuals, especially children with preexisting brain damage or injury, may have multiple forms of seizures.

Status Epilepticus

When seizures are continuous or when they occur repetitively at short intervals such that an individual does not regain consciousness between seizures, the condition is called *status epilepticus.* As there are different kinds of seizures, there can be different kinds of status epilepticus. Tonic-clonic status epilepticus can be a life-threatening condition, absence status epilepticus may consist of a continuous trance-like state, and epilepsia partialis continua may be manifest as a continuous twitching of a finger or hand without any alteration in consciousness.

THE ELECTROENCEPHALOGRAM

The electroencephalogram allows us to record the electrical activity generated by the underlying cortex. Seizures are described on the basis of their behavioral phenomenology, but they are understood in relation to their electrophysiological manifestations at the level of the whole brain, the neuronal network, and the single neuron. The cellular mechanisms underlying seizure activity are discussed later in this chapter, but at this point it is appropriate to describe one of the more important clinical tools for investigating epilepsy, the *electroencephalogram.*

The EEG is generated by the currents that flow in the extracellular spaces of the cortex. These currents are generated by synaptic potentials of neurons in the underlying cortex. The predominant neuron in the cortex is the pyramidal cell. Pyramidal cells occur in several cortical layers, they are large- or medium-sized neurons, and they are aligned in columns, perpendicular to the surface of the cortex. The extracellular current flow around these neurons occurs mostly in a direction perpendicular to the surface so that the surface of the cortex will be positive when the depth of the cortex is negative, and vice versa. If the current generated is to be detected at the scalp, neurons must be synaptically activated in groups with some degree of synchrony. During restful wakefulness and during various stages of sleep, normal EEG activity reflects some degree of rhythmic synchronous activation. During more active thought or cerebral activity, EEG rhythms are desynchronized, and the EEG demonstrates lower voltage, faster activity.

The normal EEG is characterized by several different patterns, depending on the physiological state of the individual. When awake but in a relaxed state, the EEG consists of relatively rhythmic, 8- to 12-Hz activity, with a posterior predominance, called α waves (Fig. 1). When the individual is alerted, the EEG consists of lower voltage, faster activity, β waves. As the relaxed individual begins to enter sleep, the EEG expresses intermittent, slower (4–7 Hz), higher amplitude activity, called θ waves. As sleep deepens, θ waves become more prominent and then even larger amplitude, slower (less than 4 Hz) activity is seen, called δ waves. During normal sleep, at fairly regular intervals, δ activity is interrupted by low-voltage fast activity resembling β waves but accompanied by several other physiological phenomena, including rapid eye movements (REM), loss of body muscle tone, and autonomic discharges, the so-called REM stage of sleep (see Chapter 10).

Epileptic seizures are caused by abnormal hypersynchronous activation of neurons in the brain. The EEG can reflect this abnormal activity in two ways: it can reflect the *propensity* to develop hypersynchronous activation of neurons or it can reflect the *event* itself (the seizure or *ictus*) when it occurs. Thus, during the *interictal* period between seizures, the EEG may show some manifestation of hyperexcitability; during the seizure, the EEG will show the abnormal electrical activity that underlies the altered behavior.

The hallmark of hypersynchronous activation of a population of neurons is a sharp wave in the EEG (Fig. 1). The more neurons involved, the closer they are to the surface electrode, and the more synchronous their activation, the larger and sharper the po-

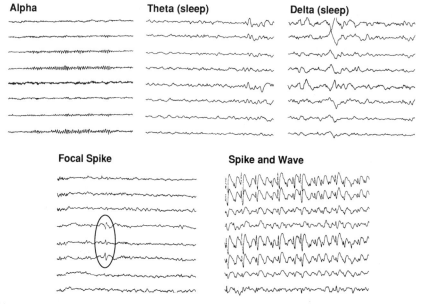

FIG. 1. Normal EEG patterns and epileptic EEG patterns. The top three traces represent normal α (**left**), θ (**middle,** during drowsiness), and δ (**right,** during deep sleep) activity recorded in the EEG. The bottom two traces illustrate a focal "spike discharge" (circled) and a sudden burst of spike-and-wave activity seen simultaneously in all the leads.

tential. Events with a duration of approximately 70 to 80 msec on the EEG appear very sharp and are called spikes. Somewhat slower events are called sharp waves. When these occur in one or only a few EEG locations, they are called focal. Sharp waves that occur in many EEG locations simultaneously, on both sides of the brain, are called generalized.

Spikes or sharp waves are often followed by slow waves, signifying a different kind of synchronous activity of neurons in the underlying cortex. Such complexes are called spike/wave complexes and they can occur locally or diffusely (Fig. 1). Spike and wave activity may also occur repetitively.

Electroencephalographic manifestations of a seizure can vary widely. The different types of seizure activity seen in the EEG and the significance of these patterns are discussed elsewhere in relation to the type of seizure.

NATURAL HISTORY OF SEIZURES

Different seizure types have different natural histories. The occurrence of a single seizure does not mean that an individual has epilepsy. Epilepsy only exists when seizures are repetitive and unprovoked. Isolated tonic-clonic seizures can occur after a minor head injury, after an episode of hypoglycemia, during a fainting attack (e.g., "at the sight of blood"), or even after one or two nights of sleep deprivation. These seizures are not likely to recur if the provoking cause is eliminated, and individuals who experience these kinds of seizures do not have epilepsy.

Some kinds of seizures occur repetitively, but still represent a relatively mild problem. For example, many young children between 6 months and 5 years of age have tonic-clonic seizures with high fevers (*febrile convulsions*). If there is no other complication, these children will outgrow this tendency and not develop epilepsy later in life. Similarly, children have some specific seizure syndromes that are known to be associated with a very good outcome in that the children outgrow these seizures. Unfortunately, many seizure types are associated with serious problems; seizures will continue to occur throughout life and may even become more frequent and more severe, or more difficult to control with medication, as children grow into adulthood. These seizures need to be treated more aggressively.

A difficult problem arises when an individual has a single, unprovoked seizure. Studies show that approximately 50% to 60% of such individuals will not have additional seizures; it is not always easy to predict which individuals will go on to have seizures and which will not. When the situation is in doubt, some physicians will not start treatment after only one seizure whereas others will.

CELLULAR MECHANISMS OF EPILEPSY

As noted above, almost any insult or damage to cerebral grey matter, especially the cortex, can produce a hyperexcitable state that manifests itself as a seizure or recurrent seizures. In addition, the normal anatomy and physiology of mammalian brain appear to contain the necessary ingredients for a seizure to occur with only a very slight provocation. Thus, the "mechanisms of epilepsy" in many cases are exaggerations of the normal physiological mechanisms by which the brain functions.

Brain regions can be hyperexcitable even when seizures are not occurring. EEG interictal spike discharges are manifestations of hypersynchronous activation of a group of pyramidal neurons underlying the area in which the discharge is observed. The underlying cellular event that generates the EEG spike is a large depolarizing potential that occurs synchronously in many pyramidal neurons within the epileptic focus (Fig. 2). This has been called the *depolarizing shift* (DS). It is usually followed by a large, prolonged hyperpolarization (post-DS HP). Neurons are alternately excited during the DS and inhibited during the post-DS HP. The DS represents a combination of synaptic currents

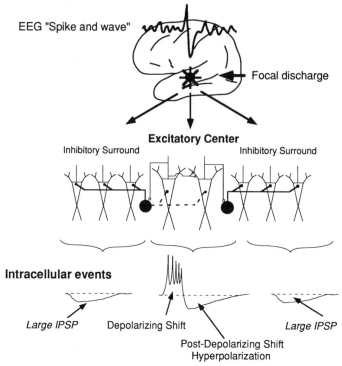

EEG "Spike and wave"

Focal discharge

Excitatory Center

Inhibitory Surround   Inhibitory Surround

Intracellular events

Large IPSP   Depolarizing Shift   *Large IPSP*

Post-Depolarizing Shift
Hyperpolarization

FIG. 2. Diagrammatic representation of the interictal discharge. The EEG records a spike-and-wave from a focal area of temporal lobe. This is produced by an area of hyperexcitability within that temporal lobe, where neurons in the center (excitatory center) are undergoing a large depolarizating shift (DS) followed by a hyperpolarization (the post-DS hyperpolarization). These neurons activate, via their axon collaterals, inhibitory interneurons (black) which send axons to local neurons surrounding the excitatory focus. These interneurons produce inhibitory postsynaptic potentials (IPSPs) in the neurons onto which they synapse. Thus, in the "inhibitory surround" regions, the pyramidal neurons are inhibited while the neurons in the center of the focus are excited.

(presumably mediated by the excitatory neurotransmitters glutamate and aspartate) flowing through neuronal dendrites arranged perpendicular to the cortical surface and voltage-dependent depolarizing currents (Fig. 3). [Voltage-dependent currents are currents due to opening of membrane channels when cells depolarize. The best understood of these is the sodium current that is responsible for the action potential in nerve and muscle, but voltage-dependent calcium currents are also plentiful in both the cell bodies and dendrites of brain neurons (see Chapter 2).]

Neurons become synchronized by several mechanisms. Local recurrent excitatory circuits are enhanced, either chronically because of reorganization of synaptic circuits after a lesion or acutely because of increases in the strength of excitatory synapses produced by high-frequency activation of neurons. The increase in synaptic strength may involve the recruitment of N-methyl-D-aspartate (NMDA) receptors (see Chapter 7). These glutamate- or aspartate-activated receptor/channel complexes are relatively quiescent during normal synaptic transmission, as they are blocked at normal neuronal resting potentials by ambient concentrations of magnesium. However, as neurons depolarize, the block by magnesium becomes less effective, and more depolarizing channels can be activated by a given amount of excitatory neurotransmitter. Thus, a positive feedback

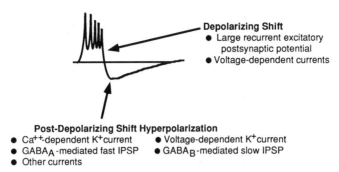

FIG. 3. Cellular mechanisms underlying the depolarizing shift and postdepolarizing shift hyperpolarization. The depolarizing shift seen in pyramidal neurons in the center of an epileptic focus is generated by both excitatory postsynaptic potentials, probably mediated by recurrent axon collaterals, and voltage-dependent depolarizing currents. The following hyperpolarizing potential is also generated by a variety of both synaptic currents and intrinsic membrane currents.

system is established by both the circuitry and the nature of excitatory synaptic actions. In addition, as neurons depolarize, one or more classes of voltage-dependent calcium channels are activated. The depolarization produced by current flow through these channels can also contribute to the DS. All of these mechanisms are present in normal neurons within the cortex. They presumably are activated at relatively low levels during normal activity of brain, and excessive activation is kept in check by powerful inhibitory mechanisms. When, for whatever reason, such inhibition is reduced, these positive feedback events in the excitatory pathways are brought into play, and a focal epileptic discharge develops. If inhibitory control mechanisms break down further, or excitatory buildup continues, a full seizure can develop.

The hyperpolarization that follows the DS (and which contributes to the wave of the spike–wave complex in the EEG) is thought to be produced by a variety of mechanisms (Fig. 3). Synaptic inhibition, especially that mediated by γ-aminobutyric acid (GABA), is very powerful and ubiquitous in the cortex, producing both feedforward and feedback inhibition. As pyramidal cells discharge, they activate inhibitory interneurons that relay inhibition back to the originating neurons and to surrounding areas. Thus, synaptic inhibition can shut off the discharge and limit its spread within the cortex. In addition,

voltage-dependent hyperpolarizing currents (mostly potassium currents), which also limit the duration of the discharge, are activated during the DS. Finally, the large influx of calcium that occurs during the DS can activate calcium-dependent currents generated by ion channels (potassium and possibly chloride) that are turned on when intracellular calcium rises to specific levels (see Chapter 2) that further limit the duration of excitatory events.

Neurons can also be synchronized by large currents that flow extracellularly around their dendrites, by the changes in their external environment during excessive activity (increases in extracellular potassium and decreases in extracellular calcium), and by electrical coupling, which may be present within some areas of cortex.

Thus, the DS occurs when a group of neurons in the cortex is excessively excited, leading to a synchronous depolarization mediated by both recurrent synaptic and voltage-dependent inward currents. The depolarization itself and subsequent calcium influx produce activation of outward currents that contribute to the cessation of the activity. Simultaneously, activation of recurrent inhibitory connections also limits the duration of the depolarizing shift and its spread to nearby and distant areas of the cortex.

Seizures develop in an area of hyperexcitability and then spread throughout the brain. When inhibitory mechanisms break down or when excitatory mechanisms become enhanced, a relatively limited interictal discharge can be converted to a full seizure. This transition involves an "escape" of the local discharge and the spread of the discharge to nearby and distant areas of brain. The development of seizure activity and the spread of seizure activity to normal areas of the brain appear to involve normal synaptic pathways and physiological mechanisms. Discharges travel down axons and invade projection areas and are fed back to the actively discharging areas by recurrent excitatory connections. High-frequency discharges produce potentiation of excitatory synapses. In addition, as the postsynaptic neuron depolarizes, more NMDA receptors become active, more depolarization occurs, and more calcium enters the cell.

At the same time that excitation is being potentiated, inhibitory circuits diminish their function. GABA is the main inhibitory neurotransmitter in mammalian forebrain (see Chapter 7). It acts via GABA$_A$ and GABA$_B$ receptors to hyperpolarize neurons and decrease excitability. GABA also acts presynaptically to reduce neurotransmitter release. Although the action of GABA can be very powerful, the strength of synaptic inhibition appears to be sensitive to high-frequency activation. Therefore, activation patterns that enhance excitation will also decrease inhibition and lead to the development and spread of epileptic activity (Fig. 4).

As excitation is enhanced and inhibition diminished, more and more areas will be incorporated into the seizure. In addition to "downstream" spread, axon terminals in a primary area of discharge can become activated, presumably because of neurotransmitters being released and the accumulation of extracellular potassium. These axons will fire antidromically (backward, toward the cell bodies from the terminals), activating areas of brain "upstream" from the focus and, via recurrent collaterals, multiple additional areas. Thus, seizure activity can spread rapidly from a focal area of abnormality to many other areas that are not part of the epileptic focus. The speed and extent of spread will depend on connections from a primary area of abnormality, the intensity of the primary discharge, and the "receptive" state of other regions of brain.

The last factor may conceptually explain how certain systemic events can cause indi-

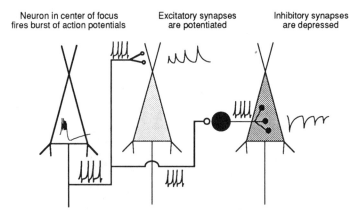

FIG. 4. Spread of seizure activity. The neuron on the left represents a group of neurons in the center of an epileptic focus undergoing a depolarization and burst of action potentials. The high-frequency burst of action potentials produces an enhancement of the strength of excitatory synapses onto neurons connected to the bursting neurons (**middle**), while at the same time, inhibitory connections are becoming depressed (**right**). Although the exact mechanisms for these two opposite effects are not completely understood, it is apparent that such changes in strength of excitatory and inhibitory connections can lead to increased excitability in the neuronal network.

viduals with a seizure propensity to develop a seizure at a given point in time. For example, some women will have seizures only at specific times in their menstrual cycles. This could be due to the actions of estrogen on the epileptic focus itself or its actions on the excitability of normal areas of brain into which the primary epileptic focus is projecting. Similarly, stress, illness, or other factors could "facilitate" seizures via a variety of physiological changes related to secretion of stress hormones and cytokines (agents originally described as operating on white blood cells but now known to affect brain excitability as well). None of these factors will produce epilepsy by itself, but each may facilitate the de-velopment of seizures in someone with an underlying excitable lesion or predisposition.

Hyperexcitability of the cortex can develop in several ways. Areas of hyperexcitability can develop acutely (e.g., if drugs are administered that block inhibition or enhance excitation). Alternatively, epileptogenic areas of brain may develop over time after some form of brain injury. Under these circumstances, it appears that injury evokes a reaction in surviving neurons such that their axons sprout collaterals that "fill in" for missing synapses (Fig. 5). These new synapses tend to be excitatory and increase the local recurrent excitatory connections in an area. In addition, there may be an alteration in NMDA recep-

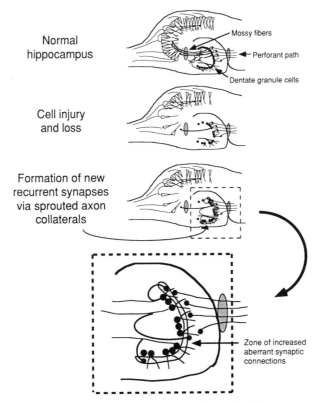

FIG. 5. Development of new recurrent excitatory connections after hippocampal injury. **Top:** Schematic diagram of some of the normal connections of the mammalian hippocampus; **Middle:** When injury and cell loss occur throughout the hippocampus, many connections are disrupted; **Bottom:** Axons deprived of their normal targets may regenerate and grow toward areas of dendrites that are denuded of their normal inputs, thereby forming aberrant connections. The insert in the box illustrates aberrant recurrent connections between dentate granule cell axons and dendrites of nearby granule cells. It is hypothesized that these new recurrent excitatory connections may be responsible for the hyperexcitability of damaged hippocampus.

tors in such regions to make them more likely to be activated by synaptic activity. Thus, the stage is set for the development of hyperexcitability. Under certain circumstances, inhibitory interneurons may be particularly susceptible to hypoxia or injury and this may lead to a selective loss of inhibitory elements after some forms of brain injury—again leading to a hyperexcitable area of cortex. The mammalian hippocampus appears to be especially vulnerable to hypoxia and injury and is strongly epileptogenic (perhaps because of the close packing of neurons in this structure.) It is not surprising, therefore, that many individuals with acquired focal epilepsy have abnormalities in their hippocampi. In fact, this is the most common cause of complex partial seizures.

Some individuals with epilepsy have no detectable lesion, even at postmortem examination. As mentioned above, many of these individuals have a genetic predisposition to develop epilepsy. As yet, no known specific lesion in humans or in animals has been established as the cause of epilepsy. However, in several animal models of epilepsy abnormalities have been reported, although how specific genetic defects cause epilepsy remains to be worked out. As almost any disturbance in brain function can produce epilepsy, the possibilities are almost limitless. Epilepsy could be produced by small alterations in the function of one or another voltage-dependent current, a synaptic recep-

tor, a metabolic pump, the concentration of any of a large number of neurotransmitters, or even a change in vascular or glial function. As syndromes with specific genetic components are characterized and the genes isolated, it may be possible to work backward to find a physiological lesion that produces the hyperexcitability.

TREATMENT

Epilepsy must be treated. Almost all forms of seizures produce significant disruptions of normal brain function and need to be treated. If a specific cause is found, such as a tumor, treatment may consist of removing the cause. In many circumstances, however, this is not possible and the seizures need to be suppressed with medication. It is important that the seizure type be identified correctly so that the appropriate medication can be chosen. In general, about 50% of individuals have their seizures well controlled with medication, 25% to 30% have occasional seizures, and 20% to 25% of individuals with epilepsy have continuous major problems despite attempts at treatment.

Most seizures are treated with medication. Three medications are commonly utilized for focal or partial seizures: carbamazepine, phenytoin, and phenobarbital (or its related barbiturate, primidone) (Fig. 6). Either carbamazepine or phenytoin is usually

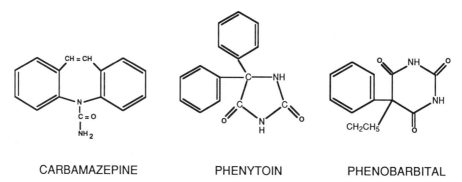

CARBAMAZEPINE   PHENYTOIN   PHENOBARBITAL

FIG. 6. Chemical formulas for carbamazepine, phenytoin, and phenobarbital. These agents are widely used for partial seizures and generalized tonic-clonic seizures.

tried first, as neither produces significant sedation. They both appear to produce antiepileptic effects by blocking voltage-dependent sodium channels in a use-dependent manner, i.e., the more the channels open, the more effective are these drugs at blocking the channel. This may account for these drugs' abilities to suppress epileptic activity while having very little effect on normal brain activity. The exact mechanism(s) of action may be more complicated, however, as phenytoin has also been shown to have effects on calcium currents and metabolic pumps.

Phenobarbital and other barbiturate medications also suppress sodium currents, but they have another important mechanism of action. These agents can potentiate brain inhibition mediated by GABA and at high concentrations may even mimic GABA. The latter effects may be related to the barbiturates' sedating side effects.

Primary generalized tonic-clonic seizures are also treated with carbamazepine, phenytoin, and phenobarbital, and in addition can be very effectively treated with sodium valproate. The mechanism by which this drug works is not known, although it can also block sodium currents in a use-dependent manner.

Primary generalized absence epilepsy is very effectively treated by sodium valproate and ethosuximide. Ethosuximide appears to have a unique mechanism of action by blocking one class of voltage-dependent calcium currents. These currents (T currents) are very large in neurons in deep diencephalic structures and may be partially responsible for the 3-Hz spike-and-wave activity seen in the EEG during absence seizures. Other forms of primary generalized seizures, including myoclonic seizures and complex absence seizures, are best treated by sodium valproate, although phenytoin may also be effective.

Another class of medications that is very effective for stopping seizures while they are occurring is the benzodiazepines. These agents are commonly employed as antianxiety medications or as sleep-promoting agents (see Chapter 19). They work by enhancing GABA-mediated inhibition, but they utilize a different mechanism than do the barbiturates. The benzodiazepines increase the amplitude of inhibitory potentials by increasing the frequency of opening of GABA-activated chloride channels. The barbiturates, on the other hand, increase the duration of inhibitory potentials by keeping chloride channels open longer.

Some of the medications used to treat epilepsy may cause behavioral disturbances in a minority of individuals. As mentioned, barbiturates may cause sedation or intellectual dulling and may cause depression. Carbamazepine and phenytoin do not usually cause cognitive or memory problems, unless they are given in very high doses. Ethosuximide, commonly used in children with absence seizures, can cause changes in behavior and in sleep patterns. Valproic acid (VPA) usually does not produce overt behavioral changes, but a minority of patients on VPA develop significant weight gain, most likely because of increased appetite (Fig. 7).

Some forms of seizures can be effectively treated by brain surgery. If seizures are intractable to medication and appear to emanate from a localized area of brain that can be safely removed, surgery can "cure" or render almost seizure-free between 70% and 90% of appropriate candidates. The most common form of surgery for focal epilepsy is temporal lobectomy. In many individuals with CPSs, the seizures emanate from one temporal lobe, usually the hippocampus or amygdala. The seizures may be caused by hippocampal sclerosis or a temporal lobe tumor, or they may originate from the site of a previous injury. If the contralateral temporal lobe is functioning well and seizures do not appear to originate bilaterally, the diseased temporal lobe can be removed with good success, i.e., an elimination or dramatic reduction in the seizures and improvement in a variety of neurological/cognitive functions. The latter result may be from the ensuing reduction in antiepileptic medication or from the removal of a diseased and chronically discharging area

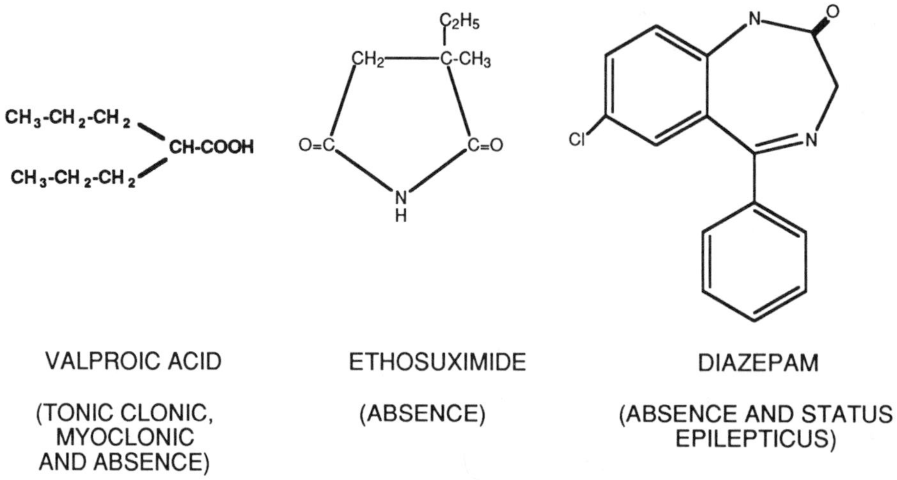

VALPROIC ACID

(TONIC CLONIC,
MYOCLONIC
AND ABSENCE)

ETHOSUXIMIDE

(ABSENCE)

DIAZEPAM

(ABSENCE AND STATUS
EPILEPTICUS)

FIG. 7. Chemical formulas for valproic acid, ethosuximide, and diazepam. Note the difference between the simple structure of valproic acid and the complex ring structures of the other antiepileptic drugs illustrated in this figure and in Fig. 6.

of brain that was interfering with the function of normal brain tissue. Interestingly, however, even when seizures are completely eliminated, underlying personality difficulties tend to persist.

Another form of brain surgery used to control very difficult seizures is corpus callosum section. In this procedure the large bundle of axons that connects the two cerebral hemispheres is cut. Surprisingly, this produces relatively little detectable change in personality or neurological or intellectual functioning. Occasionally, a "disconnection" syndrome can be seen, usually only for a short time during which the two hands (each controlled by only one half of the brain) may want to do different things. One individual tried to smoke with her left hand while her right hand tried to put out the cigarette! This kind of surgery can be used to reduce the severity of seizures by stopping the spread of the abnormal electrical activity from one side of the brain to the other.

DISORDERS THAT MAY ACCOMPANY EPILEPSY

Behavioral disturbances that are independent of seizures may occur in individuals with epilepsy. Many individuals with epilepsy are of normal intelligence and do not suffer from any specific psychological disorder. However, since various forms of brain dysfunction, both genetic and acquired, can produce epilepsy, these conditions may also produce other problems with brain function, notably mental retardation, a loss of intellectual ability, a decrease in memory, and changes in personality. Thus, problems that develop as a consequence of the brain damage that produced the epilepsy need to be distinguished from those that may be due more specifically to the seizures or the epileptogenic lesion itself. This is most difficult when attempting to deal with personality disturbances in an individual who has normal intelligence and intellectual function. If, for example, such an individual develops a psychosis, it may be difficult to determine whether the psychosis is due to an underlying neurological lesion, the seizures, the secondary consequences of the seizures, the medication the individual is taking, or the psychosocial consequences of epilepsy. In this section, some of the behavioral syndromes that have been associated with epilepsy are described, and pathophysiological mechanisms that may explain these conditions are identified.

Unusual personality characteristics may

occur in individuals with complex partial seizures. Some individuals with CPSs of presumed temporal lobe origin develop a series of personality traits that occur commonly enough to appear to constitute a syndrome. These include a peculiar interpersonal "stickiness" and overintellectuality, which may be associated with hyperreligiosity or strong concern with "cosmic" issues. These individuals may also develop *hypergraphia* (a tendency to write a lot), keeping excessively detailed journals, writing long and sometimes incoherent letters, and occasionally writing large amounts of fiction or poetry. In addition, many individuals with CPSs appear to be relatively hyposexual, having little interest in normal heterosexual activity. The latter symptom may be part of a general social withdrawal or may be the only behavioral change in an otherwise normally functioning individual.

It is not known why these characteristics develop in some individuals and not in others with similar seizure disorders. The neuroanatomic basis for these characteristics is also not known. The hyposexuality may be related to subtle endocrine disturbances known to exist in many individuals with CPSs (see below), but the exact mechanisms remain to be determined.

Some individuals with epilepsy develop affective disorders. Individuals with epilepsy tend to become depressed. This may be a natural consequence of the limitations that epilepsy imposes; alternatively, it could be related to the underlying cause of the seizures or a consequence of the seizure activity on the brain. No specific affective syndrome, such as a bipolar affective illness, has been identified in these individuals. However, individuals may develop a borderline personality disorder that mimics some features of a primary affective disorder and is commonly misdiagnosed. In addition, some antiepileptic medications, especially barbiturates, can induce depression.

Unfortunately, individuals with CPSs have a relatively higher rate of suicide than an age-matched control group. Why this occurs is not clear, but it has been documented in several studies. The suicide rate seems to be independent of the severity of the seizure disorder itself and in fact the likelihood of suicide does not seem to change even for individuals whose seizures are eliminated by temporal lobe surgery.

The relation between serious depression and epilepsy is not fully understood. The induction of generalized seizures is actually an accepted treatment for severe depression (electroconvulsive shock treatment), although the mechanism by which this treatment helps the depression is unknown.

Very few persons with epilepsy are psychotic. A long, old, and rather nonilluminating literature exists about the relationship between psychosis and epilepsy. Although few individuals with epilepsy are also psychotic, some components of CPSs are similar to psychotic symptoms (e.g., hallucinations), and it is clearly possible to confuse the two diagnoses in some individuals. It has been suggested that the two conditions are actually "antagonistic" and that individuals with both epilepsy and schizophrenia will go through periods where the schizophrenia gets better as the seizures get worse, and vice versa. However, the evidence for this is very poor. Since both epilepsy and schizophrenia are relatively common disorders, especially in the late teenage and young adult age group, they may coexist simply because of statistical probability. Good epidemiological studies have not demonstrated either a specific link or exclusion between these conditions.

Some individuals with epilepsy experience endocrine dysfunction or disorders of sexuality. A variety of difficulties with endocrine and sexual function have been reported in individuals with specific forms of epilepsy. Some women have difficulties with menstruation or conception. Other individuals with CPSs, both men and women, appear to develop a hyposexuality or lack of interest in sexual activities, as mentioned earlier. Others with no known endocrine dysfunction may demonstrate abnormal endocrine regulation when examined with provocative tests. How widespread these changes are has never been determined in a prospective study. However, it is not difficult to relate some behavioral changes commonly seen in individuals with chronic epilepsy to the kinds of endocrinological dysfunctions that have been documented. Many of the areas of the cortex that are most susceptible to chronic focal seizures are also involved in regulation of the hypothalamus and the peripheral endocrine system. The amygdala in particular has connections to the hypothalamus and is frequently involved early in complex partial seizures. The hippocampus and orbital frontal cortex also have connections to the hypothalamus. Both interictal and ictal discharges in these structures could produce disturbances in the control of delicate cyclic functions, such as the menstrual cycle. In addition, chronic recurrent disturbances in hormone secretion could lead to disturbances in sexual or reproductive function.

Antiepileptic drugs can produce behavioral changes. Individuals with epilepsy generally require medication to control their seizures. In general, it is believed that these medications are safe, but several have been shown to have effects on behavior or on brain development. Phenobarbital and related barbiturates are brain depressants; they produce sedation and drowsiness at high doses. Interestingly, in young children, barbiturates can produce paradoxical hyperactivity. In adults, barbiturates can also produce depression and since some epilepsy patients are prone to depression even in the absence of barbiturates, the medication can worsen the depression. In young animals, administration of high doses of barbiturates can produce delayed and retarded brain development. This has not been clearly demonstrated at clinical dosages in humans, but some studies suggest that children maintained on chronic barbiturate medication may have lower IQs than age-matched controls.

Most other antiepileptic drugs do not cause this kind of sedation, except when administered at toxic levels. However, it is common for individuals on any chronic medication to feel "spacey" or "washed out" or to complain of problems with concentration or memory. It is often difficult to determine if these feelings are true side effects of the drugs, are effects of the underlying epilepsy, or are part of a psychological reaction to the chronic illness.

SUMMARY

Epilepsy is a manifestation of a hypersynchronous and repetitive discharge of neurons in the brain, either starting focally and spreading to other areas, or starting in a more diffuse, bilateral pattern. The anatomic location of the activated neurons and the duration of their synchronized activity determine the behavioral nature of the seizure. Epilepsy can have a variety of manifestations, depending on what part and how much of the brain is involved. In all cases, normal brain function is disrupted by the abnormal activity. The cellular phenomena that occur during epileptic events appear to be driven by perturbations in normal cellular mechanisms of neuronal excitability and synaptic function. Many of these mechanisms are now being identified, and strategies are being developed to counteract some of the manifestations of hyperexcitability. As neuroscientists learn more about normal brain mechanisms, these new mechanisms are likely to be as important for epileptic events as they are for normal brain functioning. Thus, the study of epilepsy and the study of normal brain function at both the cellular/molecular and the behavioral levels are intimately entwined. The more we learn about how the brain works, the more likely we are to understand epilepsy, and the more we learn about epilepsy, the more likely we are to understand how the brain works.

BIBLIOGRAPHY

Original Articles

Dichter MA, Ayala GF. Cellular mechanisms of epilepsy: a status report. *Science* 1987;237:157–164.

Macdonald RL. Antiepileptic drug action. *Epilepsia* 1989;30(Suppl 1):S19–S28.

Malenka RC, Kauer JA, Perkel DJ, Nicoll RA. The impact of postsynaptic calcium on synaptic transmission—its role in long-term potentiation. *Trends Neurosci* 1989;12:444–450.

Mattson RH, Cramer JA. Epilepsy, sex hormones, and antiepileptic drugs. *Epilepsia* 1985;26(Suppl. 1): S40–S51.

Books and Reviews

Daly D, Pedley T, eds. *Current practice in clinical electroencephalography.* 2nd Ed. New York: Raven Press; 1990.

Delgado-Escueta AV, Ward AA Jr, Woodbury DM, Porter RJ, eds. *Basic mechanisms of the epilepsies: molecular and cellular approaches.* Advances in Neurology, Vol. 44; 1986.

Dichter MA. Cellular mechanisms of epilepsy and potential new treatment strategies. *Epilepsia* 1989; 30(Suppl 1):S3–S12.

Dichter MA. The epilepsies and convulsive disorders. In: Wilson JD, Braunwald E, Isselbacher KJ, Petersdorf RG, Martin JB, Fauci AS, Root RK, eds. *Harrison's principles of internal medicine.* 12th Ed. New York: McGraw-Hill; 1991:1968–1977.

Dichter MA. Modulation of inhibition and the transition to seizures. In: Dichter MA, ed. *Mechanisms of epileptogenesis: the transition to seizure.* New York: Plenum Press; 1988.

Engel J Jr. *Seizures and epilepsy,* Philadelphia: FA Davis; 1989.

Meldrum B. Epileptic seizures. In: Siegel GJ, Agranoff BW, Albers RW, Molinoff PB, eds. *Basic neurochemistry,* 5th ed. New York: Raven Press; 1994 (in press).

Zucker RS. Short-term synaptic plasticity. *Annu Rev Neurosci* 1989;12:13–31.

23

Neurodegenerative Disorders

Jeffrey N. Joyce and Howard I. Hurtig

Before concluding these pages, it may be proper to observe once more, that an important object proposed to be obtained by them is, the leading of the attention of those who humanely employ anatomical examination in detecting the causes and nature of diseases, particularly to this malady [Parkinson's disease]. By their benevolent labours its real nature may be ascertained, and appropriate modes of relief, or even of cure, pointed out.

C. Gardner-Thorpe,
James Parkinson 1755–1824: An Essay on the Shaking Palsy (printed by Whittingham and Rowland, London (Goswell Street), for Sherwood, Neely, and Johnes, Paternoster Row, 1817)

- Premature death of selected neurons in the human central nervous system (CNS) is a common theme of several chronic neurological diseases, all of which are characterized by progressive clinical disability.

- Parkinson's disease (PD) is clinically distinguished by slowed voluntary movement and tremor at rest.

- PD exists everywhere in the world, and the pathology is now known to be due to a selective loss of dopamine-containing neurons.

- An understanding of the neurochemical deficiency associated with the pathology of PD led directly to an effective pharmacotherapy for PD.

- Animal models of PD have helped scientists to develop new treatments for PD and have provided evidence of an environmental cause.

- The promise of a revolutionary treatment of PD, the transplantation of dopamine-expressing cells into the brains of PD patients, has not yet been fulfilled.

- Alzheimer's disease (AD) is defined on the basis of severe memory loss and the presence of plaques and tangles on microscopic examination of the brain.

- There is a direct correlation between the extent of impairment and the number of neurofibrillary tangles in the brain.

- Genetic studies of AD have established a link to chromosome 21 and Down's syndrome.

- The molecular neuropathology of AD is being clarified and is focused on the structure of plaques and tangles.

- Neurochemical deficiencies in the brains of AD patients are providing clues about the pathology of the disease.

- The clinical signs of Huntington's disease (HD) are diverse, but the most common are choreiform involuntary movements and dementia.

- Pathogenesis of HD involves the loss of neurons in the corpus striatum, a region involved in the control of movement.

- The molecular pathology of HD is being clarified by focusing on the selective vulnerability of neurons of the corpus striatum.

- Genetic studies have established the specific location of the gene responsible for this disease on chromosome 4.

This chapter highlights the current knowledge of three chronic neurological diseases: Parkinson's, Alzheimer's, and Huntington's. Each major section begins with a discussion of the clinical features of the disease and its pathogenesis. Sections conclude with coverage of biochemistry and molecular pharmacology.

Premature death of selected neurons in the human central nervous system (CNS) is a common theme of several chronic neurological diseases, all of which are characterized by progressive clinical disability. The three disorders chosen for examination in this chapter—Parkinson's disease (PD), Alzheimer's disease (AD), and Huntington's disease (HD)—have been investigated extensively during the last two decades. Parkinson, Alzheimer, and Huntington were great physicians of the nineteenth and early twentieth centuries whose names were immortalized by others in tribute to their seminal early descriptions of the important clinical and pathological features of these disorders. Recent scientific advances have not diluted the impact of their landmark studies that originally defined the distinctive parameters of each disease as we know it today. In each disease a particular subset of neurons is the target of selective cell death leading to readily recognizable clinical disorders. Although the cause of each has remained elusive, the pathological anatomy and physiology have become well known. In the case of PD, effective if not curative treatment has evolved rationally from an understanding of the effects of neuronal death on the biochemistry of synaptic transmission. Treatments for AD and HD have been largely disappointing despite application of promising biochemical discoveries to experimental therapeutics (Table 1).

Biological Bases of Brain Function and Disease, edited by Alan Frazer, Perry B. Molinoff, and Andrew Winokur. Raven Press, Ltd., New York © 1994.

PARKINSON'S DISEASE

James Parkinson, an English physician, described the clinical characteristics of this common disorder in his classic *Essay on the Shaking Palsy* in 1817 (see epigraph). If not the first to write about it (Leonardo DaVinci described the tremor at rest of parkinsonism in the fifteenth century), Parkinson gave the disorder its first comprehensive analysis. Few modern chroniclers of this disease have surpassed the lucid clinical description of the six patients he portrayed in his monograph. It was another 75 years before Jean Martin Charcot, the distinguished French neurologist and mentor of Sigmund Freud, attached Parkinson's name to the disease. By the end of the nineteenth century, physicians around the world recognized PD as a common neurological disorder of mid- to late life.

Clinical Features

Parkinson's disease (PD) is clinically distinguished by slowed voluntary movement and tremor at rest. The most visible evidence of Parkinson's disease is the *tremor,* a rhythmic (5- to 8-Hz) oscillation of opposing muscle groups of various parts of the body, present at rest and dampened or abolished by postural manipulation. Approximately 70% of patients will notice tremor as the earliest prominent sign of the disease, usually in the hands and fingers, but arms, legs, lips, tongue, and chin can become involved. The tremor often starts on one side of the body and can either remain confined to that side or progresses to

TABLE 1. *Hallmark features of Parkinson's, Alzheimer's, and Huntington's disease*

Clinical disorder	Clinical symptoms	Neuropathological hallmarks	Treatment
Parkinson's disease	Bradykinesia Rigidity Tremor Age of onset after 50 Subset will develop dementia	Lewy bodies in neurons of substantia nigra Cell loss in substantia nigra Loss of dopamine in striatum	L-Dopa/carbidopa to increase levels of dopamine in brain
Alzheimer's disease	Dementia Personality disorder Age of onset after 60 Subset will develop parkinsonism	Plaques, tangles, and amyloid deposits in association cortex and temporal cortex Loss of cholinergic input to the cortex and hippocampus	None are effective for dementia
Huntington's disease	Choreiform movements Dementia Age of onset after 20	Substantial loss of neurons in the striatum Some loss of neurons in cortex	Initially responds to drugs that block dopamine receptors

the other side. Since purposeful action tends to reduce the tremor, most patients find early on that the tremor by itself does not interfere with the functional motor activities of daily living. However, it is the other symptoms of PD—rigidity and akinesia (absence or poverty of movements)—that eventually develop to compromise function. Tremor and mild rigidity may be the only clinical signs early in the course of the disease, but as the disease unfolds, generalized slowing of all voluntary movements occurs, as does stooping of the shoulders, forward flexion of the neck, involuntary flexion of the knees in the standing position, and shuffling, bloc-like walking. In the later stages of the disease, most but not all patients with PD will notice that their feet freeze when they take the first step, approach a doorway, or turn.

The most striking characteristic of disturbed motor function in PD is *bradykinesia* (slowed movement), which all PD patients experience as the disease advances. Infrequent eyeblinking, slowed swallowing, softly articulated speech (hypophonia), sluggish bowels, slow initiation of any purposeful movement, even slowed thinking (bradyphrenia) are classic examples of bradykinesia. Loss of postural stability in standing and walking is the single most burdensome and functionally restricting problem in PD. In late stages of the disease the majority of patients will easily lose their balance and fall if unaided.

The signs, symptoms, and disability of PD tend to increase with time, but the rate of progression is highly variable. A number of factors may influence the natural history of the disease for a given individual, including age of onset (progression tends to be slower in young people), early clinical pattern (some will have tremor-dominant disease without the other, more disabling aspects), and response to pharmacotherapy, but for the majority the course of PD is unpredictable. Many patients will respond dramatically to treatment with the drug levodopa; others will not. A minority—perhaps 20%—will develop progressive loss of cognitive function and become clearly demented, especially after 20 or more years of illness and as the patient moves into the eighth and ninth decades of life.

Pathogenesis

PD exists everywhere in the world, and the pathology is now known to be due to a selective loss of dopamine-containing neurons. Although PD is prevalent worldwide, it is more common in developed countries with older populations. Since prevalence increases with age, especially after 60, age-related neuronal senescence could have a pivotal role in the pathogenesis of the disease. Parkinson's disease is common; approximately 1% of people over 60 are affected. An environmental cause of PD related to chemical pollution is favored by recent epidemiological data, but data on mortality and prevalence of PD dating back to the mid-nineteenth century (early in the industrial revolution) show little change in the occurrence of PD in England and the United States. PD is not a genetically transmitted disease by usual standards (e.g., low concordance in identical twins), although an active debate surrounds this issue. Some experts believe that genetic predisposition is important, perhaps through a polygenetic influence, since familial aggregation of PD may approach 25%.

Pathologists actively searched for the exact location of the pathology of PD until the early 1950s, when most accepted the substantia nigra in the mesencephalon (see Chapter 1) as the principal site of neuronal death. In 1912 Frederick Lewy, a German neuropathologist, discovered the eosinophilic inclusion body that bears his name within the cytoplasm of neurons near the substantia nigra, but he was not impressed by the relationship of the loss of nigral neurons to the profound akinesia that is the hallmark of PD. The dopaminergic pathway that projects to the corpus striatum (caudate and putamen) from the substantia nigra (Fig. 1) degenerates as a result of the progressive death of nigral neurons and their projecting axons (Fig. 2); the end result is a severe loss of dopamine input to the striatum. Neurons in the pontine raphe and locus coeruleus and their neurotransmitters (serotonin and norepinephrine) are moderately depleted, but their clinical importance is minor compared with the severe loss of dopamine. The substantia nigra is one of the few regions of the brain where melanin can be found in the cytoplasm of neurons that synthesize dopamine. The reason why

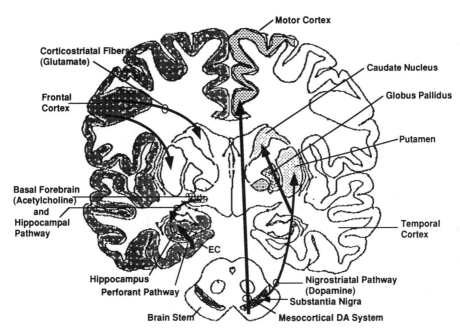

FIG. 1. Diagrammatic representation of neurotransmitter pathways in human brain. Several important transmitter systems are depicted: the nigrostriatal and mesocortical dopamine pathways that utilize dopamine and are affected in Parkinson's disease; the corticostriatal fibers that utilize glutamate and may be involved in Huntington's disease; the pathway from the basal forebrain to the hippocampus that utilizes acetylcholine and is affected in Alzheimer's disease. The perforant pathway that arises from the entorhinal cortex, innervates the hippocampus, and utilizes glutamate may also be involved in Alzheimer's disease.

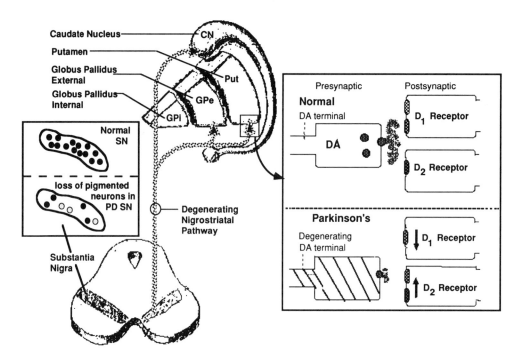

FIG. 2. Diagrammatic representation of the nigrostriatal dopamine system and the dopamine synapse in Parkinson's disease. Degeneration of the nigrostriatal dopamine system following loss of neurons in the substantia nigra (left side box, SN) results in the loss of dopamine in the synapse (see box on right of figure) and compensatory changes in the density of dopamine receptors in the striatum (caudate nucleus and putamen). The ability of levodopa (converted to dopamine) to reverse parkinsonian symptoms in this disease may depend in part on the compensatory changes in dopamine receptor densities.

these neurons are singled out for destruction in PD is unknown. Although neuronal loss is confined to a few distinctive sites, the clinical effect of the pathology is widespread and global because of the important role of dopamine in the execution of normal movement.

The cause of dementia in PD is unknown; there may even be many causes. A significant number of demented parkinsonians will have pathological evidence of coexisting AD, suggesting that PD and AD share a common etiology. Alzheimer's disease and PD are both common disorders of late life and may coexist in the same person as a result of chance alone. Conventional staining procedures can be used to visualize eosinophilic Lewy inclusion bodies in the cytoplasm of neurons in the substantia nigra of parkinsonian brains.

Lewy bodies appear to be abnormally expressed aggregates of cytoskeletal neurofilaments in the soma. New staining techniques have revealed an accumulation of Lewy bodies in neurons of the cerebral cortex of demented PD patients that cannot be seen on routine histopathological analysis. In AD, abnormal neurofilaments are expressed in the form of "neurofibrillary tangles" inside the cytoplasm of degenerating neurons of the hippocampus. Age-related attrition of neurons creates an important background on which either AD or PD pathology may be superimposed. Some investigators, however, have deduced from postmortem studies of the pathology of PD that a unique, non-Alzheimer's dementia exists and is associated with a combination of neuronal loss, Lewy bodies, and related biochemical deficiencies of dopamine, acetylcholine, and other neurotransmitters.

Biochemistry and Molecular Pharmacology

An understanding of the neurochemical deficiency associated with the pathology of PD led directly to an effective pharmacotherapy for PD. In the late 1950s, Arvid Carlsson and his colleagues in Sweden reported that administration of reserpine to animals produced a Parkinson-like syndrome of akinesia (catatonia) by depleting the brain of various neurotransmitters, including serotonin and dopamine. Carlsson and his coworkers also showed that treatment with levodopa, the precursor in the catecholamine synthesis pathway that is decarboxylated by dopa decarboxylase in the brain and converted to dopamine (Fig. 2) (see Chapter 6), could reverse the behavioral and neurochemical defects induced by reserpine. While it would appear to make more sense to replace dopamine directly by giving dopamine, levodopa was used because dopamine does not cross the blood–brain barrier. It was proposed that the loss of dopamine might be the underlying chemical deficiency in PD. In 1960 Ehringer and Hornykiewicz obtained conclusive evidence that this was the case by showing a remarkable loss of dopamine in the striatum of parkinsonian brains when compared with age- and sex-matched controls. It is worth noting that these investigators hypothesized the existence of a dopamine pathway connecting the substantia nigra with the striatum prior to the development of techniques that could visualize the dopamine-containing nigrostriatal fibers. In recent years another important dopamine pathway from the ventral tegmental area to the motor cortex has been described (Fig. 1). Moreover, Gaspar and associates at INSERM in Paris determined that degeneration to this cortical dopamine system also contributes to the motor symptoms of Parkinson's disease. Clinical trials with dopamine replacement therapy were initiated and by 1967 the results of treatment were consistent and dramatic.

Replacement pharmacotherapy, utilizing exogenous levodopa as a dopamine precursor, relieved the symptoms and signs of PD and represented a revolutionary concept in the treatment of degenerative diseases of the central nervous system. Although beneficial to most patients, levodopa has not altered the progressive natural history of PD and also has been associated with numerous undesirable side effects (e.g., nausea, confusion, involuntary movements). These problems have been ameliorated to some extent (Fig. 3) by the development of newer drugs that (1) improve the efficiency of the delivery of levodopa to the brain by inhibiting dopa decarboxylase (with carbidopa) in peripheral tissues outside the brain; (2) supplement levodopa's action by directly activating the dopamine receptor (dopamine agonists) without first requiring decarboxylation; (3) block reuptake of dopamine into the terminal and thereby prolong its pharmacological effect at the synapse; and (4) block the enzyme-driven oxidative metabolism of dopamine (monoamine oxidase inhibitors) at the nerve terminal and thereby enhance its pharmacological effect at the synapse.

Animal models of PD have helped scientists to develop new treatments for PD and have provided evidence of an environmental cause. Reliable animal models of human disease are rare, but when they are available, either in nature or by human creative ingenuity, major advances in understanding human disease usually follow. One of the earliest models for PD was produced by the intra-cerebral injection of the neurotoxin 6-hydroxydopamine (6-OHDA), which destroys the dopamine-rich nigrostriatal pathway. When administered intracerebrally, 6-OHDA is taken up into terminals of dopamine and norepinephrine neurons and causes an oxidative reaction that leads to degeneration of the neurons. Appropriate pretreatment of the animals with inhibitors of norepinephrine uptake allows selective up-

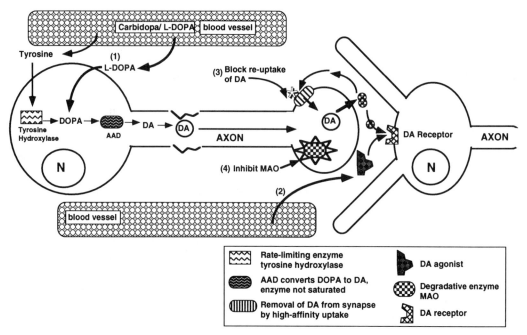

FIG. 3. Diagrammatic representation of the nigrostriatal dopamine (DA) system and the dopamine synapse in Parkinson's disease. Therapeutic intervention to increase dopamine release in the remaining neurons and reverse parkinsonian symptoms in this disease occurs at four sites. (1) Normally, tyrosine is converted to dopa by the rate-limiting enzyme tyrosine hydroxylase. The enzyme amino acid decarboxylase (AAD) converts dopa to dopamine and is not saturated. Consequently, the treatment with carbidopa plus levodopa (L-dopa) allows direct conversion of L-dopa to dopamine. (2) Treatment with dopamine agonists that directly stimulates dopamine receptors (DA receptors). (3) Blockade of reuptake of DA into terminals allows for higher concentration in the synapse. (4) Inhibition of the degradative enzyme monoamine oxidase (MAO) will also allow for increased levels of dopamine.

take of 6-OHDA into dopamine terminals and subsequent dopamine cell loss. Animals, usually rodents, lesioned by this technique develop severe loss of spontaneous movement, the equivalent of bradykinesia in PD. Investigators using the 6-OHDA model have been able to show that (1) severe depletion (>90%) of nigrostriatal dopamine is necessary for the appearance of clinical signs of disordered movement; (2) nigral neurons that survive treatment with 6-OHDA increase dopamine synthesis as one compensatory mechanism; and (3) a second compensatory mechanism, postsynaptic "denervation hypersensitivity," also follows degeneration of the nigrostriatal pathway. After 6-OHDA-induced lesioning of the nigrostriatal dopamine pathway on one side of the brain, animals show an exaggerated pharmacological (increased firing of postsynaptic neurons in the basal ganglia) and behavioral (contraversive circling) response to the administration of dopamine or dopamine agonists. The enhanced behavioral and pharmacological response to dopamine is correlated with an increase in the number of dopamine receptors (primarily the D_2 subtype) in the striatum of the lesioned (denervated) side. This increase in the number of dopamine D_2 receptors following degeneration of dopamine terminals is also observed in PD (Fig. 2), and it may explain the dramatic response to stimulation by dopamine that many patients with PD experience when they take levodopa for the first time, compared with normal volunteers who never experience such effects.

Dopamine receptors classically have been divided into two subtypes, D_1 and D_2, based on pharmacological and biochemical data (see Chapter 6). All current antiparkinsonian agents that are direct dopamine receptor agonists (e.g., bromocriptine and pergolide) are active at the D_2 but not the D_1 receptor. The contribution of the D_1 receptor to the reversal of parkinsonian symptoms with dopamimetic drugs remains unclear, but recent evidence suggests an important contributory role. Stimulation of the D_1 receptor by endogenous dopamine (e.g., levodopa) may permit or facilitate expression of D_2 receptor–mediated behavioral responses. Thus, even in advanced stages of PD, where levodopa treatment is ineffective without the use of direct D_2 agonists, levodopa appears necessary for the full benefit of D_2 agonists to be apparent. Recent molecular studies have discovered genes that code for many more receptors that respond to dopamine than the two classically defined subtypes (see Chapter 6). The contribution of these other purported dopamine receptor subtypes to the pathophysiology of PD is not yet known.

By the 1970s it had become clear that not all dopamine-containing neurons in the mesencephalon were affected in PD. Neurons containing melanin were known to be most susceptible to pathological change, whereas nonpigmented neurons in regions near the substantia nigra were relatively unaffected. The importance of the susceptibility of melaninized neurons was sharply focused in the early to mid-1980s as a result of an extraordinary misfortune that befell a group of young drug addicts, and subsequent experimental work that led to the creation of a better animal model of PD. The misfortune occurred in 1982 in northern California, where a small group of young intravenous drug abusers suddenly and coincidentally developed signs and symptoms of severe PD. Dr. William Langston, the neurologist who first observed these patients, showed that most of the patients responded dramatically to levodopa. He and his team of investigators discovered that all patients had used a synthetic heroin-like compound (made illegally) that was contaminated with the meperidine congener 1-methyl-4-phenyl-1,2,3,6-tetrahydropyridine (MPTP). Within a year, several researchers had reported that MPTP could produce parkinsonism in monkeys and mice, that the pathology in these animals was confined to the pigmented neurons of the substantia nigra, and that the toxicity of exposure to MPTP was not caused by MPTP itself but by the enzymatic conversion of MPTP to the neurotoxic compound 1-methyl-4-phenylpyridinium (MPP^+) in astrocytes (Fig. 4). Further investigation demonstrated that MPTP toxicity to nigral neurons could be completely blocked in experimental animals by pretreatment with drugs that inhibit monoamine oxidase, the enzyme that converts MPTP to MPP^+. It is now believed that MPP^+ is taken up into the dopamine-containing neurons through the high-affinity dopamine uptake system where it acts on the mitochondria that provide the "energy factory" for the neuron. MPP^+ poisons the respiratory chain, eventually leading to cell death. A single autopsied human case of MPTP parkinsonism in a young drug addict showing loss of nigral neurons had been reported in 1979 but had gone unnoticed. The importance of this case was not appreciated until after the California accident and subsequent experimental developments showing that MPTP could produce a "pure" model of PD.

The sequence of discoveries brought about by the fortuitous synthesis of MPTP has had a great impact on current thinking about the cause of PD. If a highly specific neurotoxin can cause parkinsonism in humans and experimental animals by destroying the very same neurons that degenerate in PD, a related but as yet unidentified environmental toxin might contribute to the causation of PD itself. Parallel research had focused on the likelihood that normal aging produces a

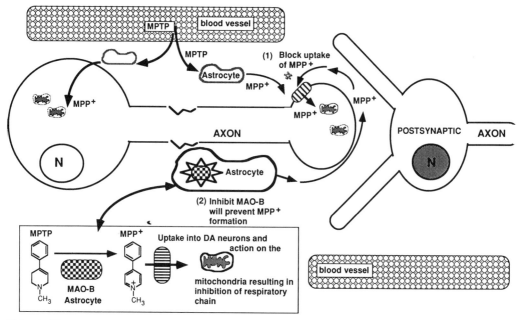

FIG. 4. Diagrammatic representation of the nigrostriatal dopamine (DA) system and the sites of action of the neurotoxin 1-methyl-4-phenyl-1,2,3,6-tetrahydropyridine (MPTP). MPTP is converted by the enzyme MAO-B to 1-methyl-4-phenylpiridinium (MPP$^+$), predominantly in astrocytes (see inset). MPP$^+$ is taken up into DA neurons through the dopamine uptake site and poisons the mitochondria (inhibition of the respiratory chain). This in turn blocks the ability to provide the appropriate energy sources for the neuron, which leads to cell death. Drugs that block uptake of MPP$^+$ into neurons effectively reduce the neurotoxicity of MPTP (1) and those that inhibit MAO-B reduce conversion of MPTP to MPP$^+$ (2). N = nucleus.

steady, "natural" attrition of cells in the brain and that certain brain regions are more vulnerable than others to accelerated aging or to unknown environmental or endogenous neurotoxins in genetically predisposed people. Normal oxidative metabolism is known to generate oxygen-free radicals that peroxidize and damage the lipid bilayer of cell membranes. Stimulation of free radical formation by external or intrinsic mechanisms could destabilize the normal homeostatic system for disposing of harmful oxidation products. Evidence to support this complex hypothetical construct is still incomplete, but the age-related prevalence of PD and the higher-than-chance aggregation of PD in some families are two lines of evidence to support a theory of aging linked to genetic predisposition. Furthermore, if an MPTP-like substance is present in the environment to trigger a chain reaction that ultimately results in

selective neuronal death in a genetically susceptible, aging host, such a multifactorial pathogenesis of PD, if validated, would become a model for research into the causes of other neurodegenerative diseases. The recent discovery that the drug deprenyl (phenylisopropylmethyl-propynylamine), a type B monoamine oxidase inhibitor and potent antioxidant, may slow the pace of clinical deterioration among patients treated early in the course of PD, possibly by blocking the toxic effect of an unknown substance on nigral neurons, lends additional strength to the logic of the three-pronged etiological hypothesis.

The promise of a revolutionary treatment of PD, the transplantation of dopamine-expressing cells into the brains of PD patients, has not yet been fulfilled. The notion that recovery from brain damage might be effected by transplantation of neuronal tissue into the brain was first suggested in the 1890s in a report by W. Gilman Thompson describing the effects of removing a piece of a cat's brain and implanting it into the brain of a dog. The grafted tissue did not survive, but interest in transplantation resurfaced in the 1970s. Workers from several universities, but most notably from the University of Lund in Sweden, showed that adrenal medulla chromaffin cells, transplanted into a central nervous system environment (e.g., the iris of the eye), could be transformed into neuronal-like cells that secreted dopamine. Furthermore, it was shown that embryonic neuronal tissue transplanted into a similar environment produced massive outgrowth of axons from the transplant into the host nervous tissue. This set the stage for experiments in animals for testing the ability of transplantation technology to produce behavioral recovery in animals with brain damage. Animals treated to make them parkinsonian were given transplants of either dopamine-rich embryonic mesencephalic tissue containing the substantia nigra or catecholamine-producing adrenal medulla cells.

The goal of transplantation therapy in the latter case was to transfer healthy catecholamine-producing cells from the adrenal medulla to the dopamine-depleted striatum, where the fresh cells would sprout, grow, and differentiate into a functionally effective and regenerative new source of dopamine. Because there was some suggestion of benefit in these animals, Backlund and his colleagues in Sweden in the early 1980s carried out surgical autografts of adrenal medullary chromaffin cells into the right striatum of four patients with advanced PD. Cell suspensions of adrenal medulla were grafted into the body of the caudate nucleus in two patients and into the putamen in two others. All operations were technically successful, but the patients showed only slight, transitory improvement.

Although the results of these early human experiments were disappointing, research on rodents and nonhuman primates has continued. Results in parkinsonian animals suggested that neurological improvement occur-

ring after transplantation might happen because of a stimulating or trophic effect of the surgical procedure on surviving dopamine terminals in the surrounding striatum, i.e., since the transplanted adrenal tissue usually did not survive but dopamine levels were raised in the striatum, surviving fibers might be sprouting in response to trophic substances.

The spotlight returned dramatically to the human stage in 1987 with the publication of a report from Mexico by Madrazo and colleagues of two severely parkinsonian patients whose disability was almost completely abolished within weeks after adrenal medullary autografting. The response of these two patients to transplantation was so startling that investigators in medical centers around the world immediately launched independent programs to duplicate the results. Within a year of Madrazo's report, over 200 patients with PD had received adrenal autografts but with comparatively unfavorable outcomes. A few had significant but temporary improvement, but most were not better, and an important minority experienced serious postoperative morbidity; some died as a direct result of the transplantation procedure.

In 1989 a number of reports of cases with adrenal autograft fatalities with histopathology of the graft sites accumulated in the neurological literature. Most of the patients showed no evidence of a postoperative clinical benefit. In all cases, the grafted tissue was completely necrotic (nonviable) and the host striatum exhibited no ingrowth of dopamine fibers, with three exceptions: two cases showed a few viable chromaffin cells surrounded by macrophages and inflammatory cells; a third showed a necrotic graft surrounded by a network of neural fibers that stained positive with monoclonal antibodies to tyrosine hydroxylase. None of the patients improved after grafting. By the beginning of 1990, adrenal medullary autografting had all but stopped because of the demonstrated lack of efficacy in the face of a significant risk of serious perioperative complications.

Grafting of human fetal dopamine-rich

mesencephalic neuronal tissue into the striatum of patients with PD began in 1988: the 50 patients treated by implantation in both the United States and Europe have shown encouraging, but modest, clinical improvements. However, fetal dopamine neurons (in contrast to adrenal chromaffin cells) implanted into the striatum of experimental MPTP-treated parkinsonian animals survive and induce abundant sprouting of dopamine fibers into the denervated striatum surrounding the graft. Moreover, neurological improvement is more pronounced and lasting in the fetally transplanted animals. These more dramatic effects have been confirmed with 200 patients having MPTP-induced Parkinsonism. The consistently positive results of the fetal experiments provide a strong foundation for cautious optimism that human trials of fetal implantation of mesencephalic grafts will eventually be successful.

ALZHEIMER'S DISEASE

Dementia in late life has become a major public health problem in developed nations as people live longer. The pathology of the disorder that is commonly known as Alzheimer's disease (AD) was first described by the German pathologist Alois Alzheimer in 1907. He examined the brain of a middle-aged woman who died after a 4-year history of progressive loss of memory and other cognitive abilities. The brain was small (atrophic) with severe cell loss, and the cerebral cortex contained the distinctive microscopic abnormalities—neurofibrillary tangles (NFTs) and smudge-like senile plaques (SPs; also known as neuritic plaques)—that have become the official pathological signature of the disease that bears Alzheimer's name. Neurofibrillary tangles are abnormal neuronal soma in which the cytoplasm is filled with microscopic filamentous structures wound around each other (paired helical filament). Senile plaque consists of clusters of degenerating nerve endings with a central core that usually contains amyloid protein. Successive generations of neuro-

pathologists have found little that alters Alzheimer's original description of the typical pathological anatomy. Most of the scientific advances in research on AD have occurred in the areas of molecular pathophysiology and clinical nosology.

Clinical Features

Alzheimer's disease is defined on the basis of severe memory loss and the presence of plaques and tangles on microscopic examination of the brain. Dementia is an abnormal mental state characterized by disturbances of memory, language, judgment, and abstract thinking, sufficient to interfere significantly with social and occupational functioning. The first symptom of dementia is usually forgetfulness, which tends to have a benign onset (absentmindedness) before taking on more ominous qualities such as environmental dislocation and compulsive questioning. The acuity of memory deteriorates with normal aging in most people, so that many who reach the eighth and ninth decades experience "age-associated memory loss," a relatively mild, circumscribed deficiency that may or may not evolve into the more global cognitive impairment typical of fully expressed dementia. The most devastating features of dementia occur later in its progressive course, when personality changes occur and abstract reasoning and judgment are disrupted. Patients with AD often lose the ability to identify members of their nuclear family and usually suffer significant loss of expressive and comprehensive language function.

As with PD, the clinical expression of AD is highly variable. The average duration of the disease is 8 to 10 years from onset to death. Death usually results from complications of the immobilized and vegetative condition that evolves in the final stage of the disease. The spectrum of cognitive and behavioral problems in AD ranges from mild to severe, depending on several factors. The rate of progression depends on the age of onset; unlike PD, AD tends to follow a more accelerated course in young-onset AD (like HD; see below) than later onset disease. The presence of other complicating medical problems and the social skills of the patient before onset of AD (people with antisocial tendencies have more serious behavioral problems than those whose premorbid social skills are highly developed) add to the complex spectra of altered behavior that can be expressed in AD patients. However, these factors do not completely explain why some patients are confused and placid, while others are psychotic and violent. In addition, dementia resulting from multiple ischemic infarctions (strokes) of the brain can mimic all the signs of AD; postmortem examination of the brain may be the only way to differentiate the two disorders.

Pathogenesis

There is a direct correlation between the extent of impairment and the number of neurofibrillary tangles in the brain. Until the 1970s there was disagreement as to whether AD was a neuropathological disorder separable from dementia associated with increasing age. The seminal work of Tomlinson, Blessed, and Roth in 1970 inaugurated a new era of thinking on the subject of late-life dementia. It was they who found a linear correlation between the severity of the dementia and the number of NFTs in the brain. These investigators also showed that the pathology in the majority of cases with dementia was compatible with AD and that ischemia from occlusive vascular disease of cerebral arteries was responsible for dementia in only 10% of cases. Moreover, previously established age distinctions in nomenclature (e.g., senile vs. presenile) were held to be completely artificial, since the configuration or abundance of the classic plaques and tangles did not differ with respect to the age of the demented patient at the time of death. Because aging itself can produce plaques and tangles in small quantities without the occurrence of dementia, the pathological diagnosis of AD depends on the delineation of a quantitative threshold

above which the correlation between clinically documented dementia and the number of plaques and tangles is strong. However, the quantitative threshold for diagnosis does need to be age-corrected, since the number of plaques and tangles in the brains of normal old people, mostly confined to the hippocampus, increases linearly with age. It is likely, however, that "age-associated memory loss" is related to this subthreshold accumulation of plaques and tangles in the entorhinal cortex and hippocampus (Fig. 5).

Biochemistry and Molecular Pharmacology

Genetic studies of AD have established a link to chromosome 21 and Down's syndrome. Estimates of incidence and prevalence of AD vary around the world, but there is general agreement that AD is primarily a disease of aging with an important but as yet ill-defined genetic basis. According to recent surveys, the risk of becoming demented increases from 5% at 65 to 45% at 85. Since the diagnosis is currently confirmed only by postmortem analysis of brain tissue, clinical diagnosis is imprecise despite the impressive efforts to codify and standardize clinical diagnostic criteria. Recent clinicopathological investigations indicate that approximately 80% of patients bearing a diagnosis of AD during life will have it confirmed pathologically after death. Cerebrovascular disease (multi-infarct dementia), Creutzfeldt–Jakob disease, alcoholism, PD, and other less common degenerative diseases account for the remainder of the cases.

AD has a more strongly expressed genetic basis than PD but is less clearly a single-gene defect than HD (see below), which follows a strict pattern of autosomal dominant inheritance. Recent data suggest that 20% to 40% of AD is transmitted as autosomal dominant, the rest occurring as sporadic cases. In one study of AD in identical twins, 40% were concordant, but with variable modes and times of disease expression. Ascertainment of diagnosis is especially difficult in a disease like AD, which characteristically does not appear

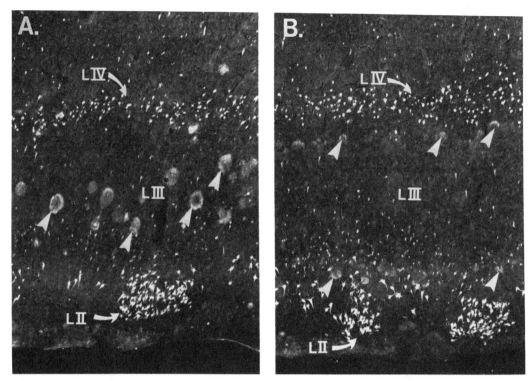

FIG. 5. Photomicrographs of a section through the entorhinal cortex of an Alzheimer's case. The section has been stained with thioflavin S to reveal the presence of neurofibrillary tangles in the islands of neurons in layer II (LII→) and layer IV (LIV→). These neurons would not be visible with conventional histochemical stains as the cells have died but are filled with the neurofibrillary tangles. The large arrows point to neuritic plaques that can be located in layer III (LIII) as shown in **A** or in deeper layers as shown in **B**. Figure published with the permission of Van Hoesen GW, Hyman BT, Damasio AR. Entorhinal cortex pathology in Alzheimer's disease. *Hippocampus* 1991;1:1–8.

until late in life. In many instances of potential familial expression of the disease, those at risk may die of other causes before the symptoms of AD can become apparent. However, the aggregation of affected members in those families with an autosomal dominant phenotype has been sufficient to permit genetic linkage studies (see Chapter 16). Work on the localization of the gene for AD is incomplete, but preliminary data have identified chromosome 21 as a strong suspect. Plaques and NFTs accumulate prematurely in the brains of people with Down's syndrome (trisomy 21), so that by age 35 most will have abundant Alzheimer pathology. Moreover, high abundance of the amyloid precursor protein is evident in the brain of younger Down's pa-

tients. The gene encoding the precursor protein for the amyloid found in neuritic plaques (see below) has also been located on chromosome 21; production of β-amyloid protein in Down's is increased by virtue of an extra copy of the gene on the trisomy. Chromosome 21 has been further implicated in the pathogenesis of AD by the finding in some studies that Down's syndrome is more common in families of patients with AD. On the other hand, several studies have failed to show that the β-amyloid protein gene is overexpressed in familial or sporadic AD. Therefore, if the gene for familial AD is definitively localized to chromosome 21, it occupies the same address as the precursor protein by coincidence and not by linkage. Work on the genetic basis of AD is just beginning, but early results are important and tantalizing.

The molecular neuropathology of AD is being clarified and is focused on the structure of plaques and tangles. The molecular pathophysiology of AD has been partly clarified in the last decade, although much work remains to be done. Abnormalities of cytoskeletal proteins have been identified and catalogued. The structural integrity of cells in the body is maintained by the presence and healthy function of cytoskeletal proteins, which maintain the cell's shape and are responsible for moving molecules around the inside of the cell. The three principal cytoskeletal proteins—microtubules, microfilaments, and intermediate neurofilaments—and their subunits have been well characterized with the use of monoclonal antibodies and other immunocytochemical techniques. The classic intraneuronal NFT of AD is composed of paired helical filaments (PHFs). PHFs are visible only with electron microscopy and accumulate in the soma of the cells. The PHFs are abnormally configured proteins unique to NFTs but also found in other diseases in which NFTs are pathological markers, such as particular variants of parkinsonism (postencephalitic parkinsonism, Parkinson–dementia complex of Guam, progressive supranuclear palsy), "dementia pugilistica" of boxers, and Down's syndrome. The senile (SP) or neuritic plaque, the other microscopic hallmark of AD, appears as a spherical cluster of dystrophic neurites (axons and dendrites) surrounding a central core that contains amyloid. Unlike NFTs, SPs are found only in AD and normal aging, and they correlate in number with severity of dementia. SPs and, to a lesser extent, NFTs accumulate mainly in the limbic (hippocampal), temporal, and association cortices (parietal) of the cerebral hemispheres, sparing the primary sensory and motor regions (Fig. 5). Within the affected region, populations of neurons are differentially affected, with the large pyramidal neurons most affected. Positron emission tomography (PET), a computerized technique that uses radioisotopes to create images of brain function (see Chapter 15), has consistently demonstrated in vivo hypometabolism (decreased utilization) of glucose in parietal association cortex in patients with mild to moderate clinical AD.

Sophisticated studies of the behavior and distribution of amyloid in normal and Alzheimer brain have illuminated certain aspects of the pathogenesis of AD. Amyloid is an abnormal proteinaceous extracellular material that has been known to pathologists for decades by its histochemical response to staining with Congo red and thioflavin S (Fig. 5). In AD, amyloid staining is found in the core of the plaque, in the NFT, and in the walls of cerebral arterioles and capillaries. Recent studies using monoclonal antibodies have demonstrated that amyloid has a much wider distribution throughout the brain in AD than was previously suspected from traditional microscopic analysis with Congo red, thioflavin S, or silver stains. These results suggest that amyloid or its precursor protein may accumulate inside neurons and blood vessels as the brain ages. In normal old people the effect is modest and neuronal function is minimally disrupted. For unknown, perhaps genetically determined, reasons, accumulation of amyloid is more rapid and widespread in vulnerable regions of the brain in AD, and the associated disruption of neuronal function is the source of clinical dementia. The latest research on the cause of the accumulation of amyloid suggests that the major component of amyloid and NFT is the protein A68. Virginia Lee and John Trojanowski at the University of Pennsylvania determined that A68 appears to accumulate in exaggerated amounts through the increased phosphorylation of a normal constituent of the microtubule assembly, tau (Fig. 6). Determining how this enhanced phosphorylation occurs may provide an important clue to the pathogenesis of the disease.

Neurochemical deficiencies in the brains of AD patients are providing clues about the pathology of the disease. Degeneration of specific neurons in brain may occur in AD, and

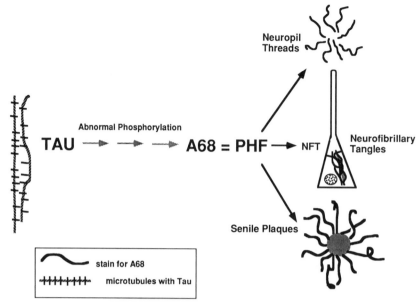

FIG. 6. Diagrammatic representation of the possible mechanism leading to the generation of the protein A68 and paired helical filaments (PHFs). The presence of the protein A68 in PHFs of neuropil threads, neurofibrillary tangles of pyramidal neurons, and the corona of senile plaques (which contain amyloid) is shown. Tau, which is a normal constituent of axonal microtubules and provides stability to their structure, may be abnormally phosphorylated into A68. Modified from Lee VM-Y. Unraveling the paired helical filaments of Alzheimer's disease. *J NIH Res* 1991;3:52–54.

the failure of neurotransmission probably contributes significantly to clinical symptomatology. In 1976, three groups of investigators in the United Kingdom reported that choline acetyltransferase (ChAT), the synthetic enzyme responsible for producing acetylcholine (ACh), was significantly decreased in the cerebral cortex and hippocampus of patients dying of AD. The level of ChAT was reduced below the level that could be accounted for by normal aging alone, and there was a linear correlation between the degree of enzyme loss and the severity of dementia. Moreover, Perry and colleagues showed that the reduction in ChAT and the degree of dementia correlated with the number of SPs present in the hippocampus of Alzheimer brain. ACh previously had been assigned an important role in the chemistry of cognition by Drachman, who found that the anticholinergic drug scopolamine, when given to young normal volunteers, produced a strik-

ing loss of the ability to form new memories. In 1982, Price and associates reported that in autopsied brains of AD patients there was a loss of large cells from the nucleus basalis of Meynert, a collection of neurons in the basal forebrain region of the brain that gives rise to the cholinergic input to the cerebral cortex and hippocampus (Figs. 1 and 7). Price and others hypothesized that the cholinergic deficiency in the hippocampus and cortex was fundamental to dementia of AD and that the primary site of pathology in AD is in the basal forebrain, with the cholinergic deficit occurring secondarily. SPs and NFTs could not be explained by this hypothesis and were assumed to be independent morphological concomitants of aging. Other investigators have since suggested that plaques and tangles might be morphological signposts of a "dying back" of cholinergic axons as they undergo retrograde degeneration, reflecting failure of the neuron's essential biological machinery.

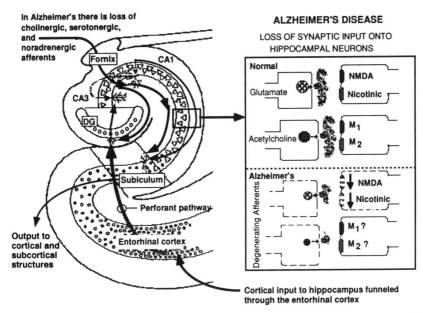

FIG. 7. Diagrammatic representation of the effects of Alzheimer's disease on acetylcholine and glutamate synapses in the hippocampus. All cortical input to the hippocampus must relay through the entorhinal cortex. The hippocampus receives input from the entorhinal cortex (perforant pathway), basal forebrain cholinergic neurons, and monoamine (serotonergic and noradrenergic) cell bodies of the brain stem. The intrinsic connections of the hippocampus provide a local hippocampal circuit: cortical input synapses on granule cells in the dentate gyrus, granule cells in dentate gyrus (DG) project to the CA3 pyramidal cells, CA3 neurons project to the pyramidal cells in the CA1 subfield, and CA1 neurons project to efferent relay nuclei of the hippocampus (the subiculum). Consequently, modifications of the input to the granule cells in the dentate gyrus (perforant pathway) or of the cholinergic (and monoaminergic) input to pyramidal neurons in CA1–CA3 subfields will affect this local circuit. The inset shows potential effects of Alzheimer's disease on the acetylcholine and glutamate synapses. Acetylcholine receptors (M_1, M_2, nicotinic) and the *N*-methyl-D-aspartate (NMDA) subtype of the glutamate receptor are depicted at these synapses. Alzheimer's disease, by causing degeneration of the glutamate pathway to the hippocampus, may either cause selective cell loss in the hippocampus or act directly at the NMDA and cholinergic nicotinic receptors to modify their densities. In contrast, there is no strong evidence that the degenerating cholinergic pathway innervating the hippocampus results in modifications in the density of the subtypes of the acetylcholine muscarinic receptors (M_1 and M_2).

A deficiency of ACh has been a consistent finding in AD and has led to numerous therapeutic efforts to reverse the symptoms of AD with cholinomimetic agents. Anticholinesterase drugs that block the catabolism of ACh and thus raise levels of ACh at the muscarinic receptor (see Chapter 6) have received the most attention in drug trials. ACh precursors (e.g., phosphatidylcholine) have also been used. Despite many well-designed clinical trials, none of these pharmaceuticals has proved to be more than transiently effective at improving memory or other cognitive functions.

The postsynaptically located cholinergic receptor recently became a logical target of experimental strategies. Cholinergic receptors have been broadly categorized into muscarinic and nicotinic types (see Chapter 6). Examination of the density of subtypes of the muscarinic receptor by radioligand binding in hippocampus and cortex of AD cases has revealed mixed results. Some groups have reported a reduction in the density of sites, whereas others have reported no change compared with age-matched controls. The original classification of the subtypes of the muscarinic receptor indicated the presence of two or three subtypes (M1, M2, and perhaps M3) based on pharmacological and biochemical data. It is now clear that there are distinct genes coding for five muscarinic receptors. Because it is not possible to distinguish pharmacologically among the five types, it is likely that radioligand binding studies cannot provide sufficient information about the status of these muscarinic receptor subtypes in AD. Molecular biological approaches that explore the expression, membrane insertion, and coupling of the muscarinic receptors to second messengers should provide important information about the status of these muscarinic receptor subtypes in AD. Results of radioligand binding studies to nicotinic receptors in AD have been more consistent. Significant reductions of the nicotinic receptor in both cortex and hippocampus have been reported (Fig. 7). The role this receptor might play in the clinical symptoms of AD is still unclear since the predominant receptor in brain is the muscarinic type.

Clinical studies of the last 40 years have provided strong evidence for the hypothesis that an intact hippocampus is essential for normal memory function in humans. In addition to the impairment of the cholinergic input to the hippocampus in AD, other afferent pathways are severely compromised. All neocortical input to the hippocampus is funneled through the entorhinal cortex and associated lateral occipitotemporal cortex (perirhinal region). Cells in layer II of the entorhinal cortex give rise to the perforant pathway that innervates the dentate gyrus of the hippocampus, establishing the first synapse of a multisynaptic pathway through the regions of the hippocampus. Hyman and associates showed that neurons in the entorhinal cortex degenerate in AD and are replaced by abundant plaques and tangles, which contribute to the isolation of the hippocampus from its cortical input (Figs. 5 and 7). The perforant pathway is rich in the excitatory amino acid glutamate. The glutamate theory of AD is receiving widespread attention at the present time, largely because of the suspicion

that glutamate plays a role in neuronal death in HD (see below) and in ischemia. Ischemia is known to cause relatively selective cell loss in the hippocampus and other regions receiving glutaminergic input. It has been established that glutamate, in high concentrations, is toxic to hippocampal neurons and is forced from intracytoplasmic storage vesicles of the terminals during the ischemic event. The proposal further assumes that glutamate is released in high amounts from perforant pathway, which causes cell loss within the hippocampus. By analogy, loss of hippocampal neurons in AD may result from pathological release of the transmitter or altered sensitivity of the hippocampal neurons to glutamate (Fig. 7). The first direct evidence to suggest loss of glutaminergic nerve terminals from the neocortex arose from the demonstration of reduced sodium-dependent binding of D-[^{3}H]aspartate to the glutamate/aspartate transporter located on glutamate nerve terminals in regions of the cortex. The uptake of D-[^{3}H]aspartate has been shown to be reduced in tissue from the temporal, frontal, parietal, and occipital cortex, as well as from hippocampus, but not from the striatal complex of AD patients. It is not clear whether this reduction is primary or related to the loss of pyramidal neurons in these regions (e.g., if they are glutaminergic) and therefore a consequence of the formation of NFTs. Moreover, current thinking would predict that in early AD an overproduction of glutamate leading to excitotoxicity of neurons will occur. Alternatively, increases in the density or biochemical coupling of the glutamate receptors might contribute to the neurotoxic effects of glutamate. Direct measurements of the densities of the three types of glutamate receptor (NMDA, kainate, quisqualate) have not indicated major alterations in the densities of these sites. However, measurement of the channel that is coupled to the NMDA receptor with [^{3}H]MK-801 has indicated a reduction in the density of this receptor–channel complex (Fig. 7). Whether this indicates a reduction in the number of receptor sites in response to an overproduction of glutamate or a loss of neurons expressing the receptor is still unclear.

HUNTINGTON'S DISEASE

Huntington's disease (HD) is an inherited (autosomal dominant) degenerative disease of the central nervous system that is named for the three generations of general practitioners who studied its prevalence among families in East Hampton, Long Island, New York, in the mid- to late nineteenth century. Subsequent work in other parts of the world has traced the origin of many cases to southern England, where a common progenitor lived in the mid-seventeenth century. Although there have been no clearly documented cases of new mutations since HD was first reported by George Huntington in 1872, the presence in isolated geographic regions of Huntington patients and families whose ancestry is not clearly traceable to southern England indicates that new mutations occur at a low but regular frequency.

Clinical Features

The clinical signs of Huntington's disease are diverse, but the most common are choreiform involuntary movements and dementia. Clinical expression of HD is usually insidious, beginning in the third or fourth decade of life, with an average duration before death of 17 to 20 years. Although the presumed single-gene defect of HD, recently localized to the short arm of chromosome 4 (see below), is completely expressed when present, wide-ranging clinical variability is the rule between and within affected families. In one survey of over 240 families, age of onset of symptoms among the affected members varied from the first to the eighth decade. Only a small minority were clinically affected in childhood, and most of these victims had paternal transmission of the gene. Rate of progression is more

rapid in these early onset cases, and the clinical profile of a typical case is dominated by a rigidity that resembles parkinsonism. Conversely, disease that starts after age 50 is relatively more benign and is associated with maternal transmission. The hastening effect of paternal transmission on clinical expression is currently unexplained.

The most recognizable and familiar signs of HD are the *choreiform involuntary movements* of the arms, legs, and trunk of the body as well as the muscles of the face. These manifest as widespread, quick, nonstereotyped, random, usually jerky movements of low amplitude that are subtle at onset but later interfere with coordination and function. The patient initially conveys a general impression of restlessness, but as the movements become more pronounced, focal twitching of various body parts becomes obvious. The result is facial grimacing, slurred speech, clumsy hands, unsteady walking, and abnormal posturing. The patient may attempt to hide an embarrassing involuntary movement by incorporating it into a concurrent or improvised purposeful action, such as combing the hair, clearing the throat, straightening a garment, and so forth. A mixture of choreiform movements, dystonic (twisted) postures, and ataxic or uncoordinated purposeful muscle activity is not uncommon in the middle phase of evolution of the clinical disease. The patient can no longer hide the movements; constant writhing and twitching are the rule. In the most advanced stage of the disease, movement is limited by increasing rigidity, and walking becomes all but impossible. Self-care is completely impossible.

Behavioral and psychological deficits may precede the onset of involuntary movements by years and therefore escape diagnostic recognition. An affected person may be described as impulsive, erratic, difficult, uninhibited, depressed, or clearly psychotic before the onset of involuntary movements clarifies the clinical picture. It is not uncommon for HD patients to be diagnosed initially as schizophrenic, with the diagnosis of HD becoming clear later with the expression of choreiform movements. Insightful patients are aware that something is seriously wrong, even when the total clinical picture is still vague. Huntington's patients tend to seek relief from depression and anxiety by drinking alcohol, sometimes heavily. Excessive drinking can aggravate any of the behavioral signs of the disease and can incorrectly suggest to observers and family members that alcoholism is the sole cause of the patient's aberrant behavior. A family history of HD raises suspicion that the altered behavior may be the first overt sign of the disease. However, the proper diagnosis may be delayed because many victims of HD and family members are unaware of the family's medical history, or may be misled by inadequate or erroneous information, e.g., the misinformation that only children are affected with HD. As the disease progresses, cognitive dysfunction gives way to gross dementia. In the final stages, the patient is usually mute and withdrawn because of disorientation, apathy, depression, severe rigidity, and total lack of coordination of the muscles of speech articulation.

Pathogenesis

Pathogenesis of HD involves the loss of neurons in the corpus striatum, a region involved in the control of movement. The pathology in HD is most concentrated in the region of the corpus striatum (caudate and putamen) (see Chapter 1), where medium-sized GABAergic spiny neurons, whose axons project outside the striatum, selectively degenerate and are replaced by a proliferation of glial cells. Loss of striatal neurons is neither regionally nor morphologically homogeneous. The dorsal striatum is the initial site of pathology, which spreads ventrally as the disease progresses. Even at the end, when the patient dies severely disabled, the dorsal striatum shows the greatest pathological change. Neurons in other parts of the brain are also affected (cerebral cortex, thalamus, brain stem, and spinal

cord), but much less so than in the striatum. Progressive loss of neurons causes generalized cerebral and focal caudate atrophy on computerized images of the brain (computed x-ray tomography and magnetic resonance imaging). This finding can be useful when the diagnosis of HD is suspected but not certain based on family history or clinical presentation.

The large striatal aspiny interneurons containing ACh, as well as the aspiny interneurons that contain somatostatin and neuropeptide Y, are largely spared in HD, whereas the medium-sized spiny neurons that contain GABA are lost. These spiny neurons also have peptide cotransmitters, either enkephalin (Enk; Fig. 8) or substance P (Sub P; Fig. 8). Enk-containing neurons projecting to the external globus pallidus and Sub P–containing neurons projecting to the pars reticulata of the substantia nigra degenerate early in the course of HD, whereas Sub P–containing neurons that project to the internal globus pallidus and the pars compacta of the substantia nigra are spared until late in the disease (Fig. 8). In contrast to PD, the nigrostriatal dopamine input to the striatum is generally unaffected.

Biochemistry and Molecular Pharmacology

The molecular pathology of HD is being clarified by focusing on the selective vulnerability of neurons of the corpus striatum. As with PD, the particular mechanism that leads to the premature death of certain neurons in the brain is unknown. The clear heritability of HD, however, reflects an ultimate genetic reason for the neuronal degeneration. One leading hypothesis holds that the medium-sized spiny neurons in HD are pathologically sensitive to the excitatory amino acid glutamate (as in AD; see above) that normally functions as a neurotransmitter in the corticostriatal pathway (Figs. 1 and 8). This hypothesis is supported by the following evidence: (1) cultured fibroblasts from patients with HD show a heightened sensitivity to ex-

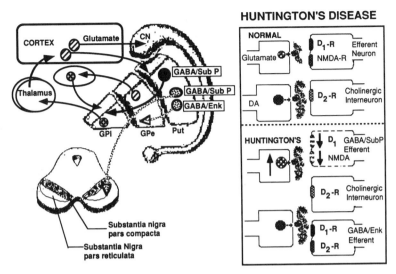

FIG. 8. Diagrammatic representation of the dopamine and glutamate synapses in Huntington's disease (HD). Some circuits of the basal ganglia are depicted. The axons projecting from the putamen to the globus pallidus external (GPe), globus pallidus internal (GPi), and substantia nigra pars reticulata all utilize GABA as well as different cotransmitters. These include (1) the pathway to the GPe containing GABA and enkephalin (GABA/Enk); (2) the pathway to the substantia nigra pars reticulata utilizing GABA and substance P (GABA/Sub P); and (3) the pathway to the GPi utilizing GABA and Sub P. As depicted in the inset, the dopamine nigrostriatal pathway is left intact in this disease, but the corticostriatal pathway may release more glutamate than in normal brain. Enhanced release may lead to the selective degeneration of certain types of neurons in the striatum. The selective loss of GABA/Enk pathway to the GPe and the GABA/Sub P pathway to the substantia nigra pars reticulata results in an imbalance in the output of the basal ganglia to the thalamus and of the thalamocortical pathways. The remaining striatal neurons continue to be sensitive to the effects of dopamine and contribute to the imbalance in the activity of the pathways. This may contribute to the motor symptoms (chorea) of this disease. The inset depicts the relative loss of certain neurons in HD and of those receptors normally expressed by the susceptible neurons (dopamine D_1 receptors and NMDA receptors).

posure to glutamate; (2) intrastriatal injection of kainic acid, an analog of glutamate, into animals causes morphological, physiological, and behavioral consequences that resemble the human phenotype of HD; and (3) blockade of, the corticostriatal glutamate pathway prevents kainate-induced neurotoxicity to striatal neurons. Conversely, abnormal release of toxic amounts of glutamate or the differential expression of subtypes of the glutamate receptor by the medium-sized spiny neurons might lead to a neurotoxic effect on these cells (Fig. 8). Recent studies have shown that the *N*-methyl-D-aspartate (NMDA) subtype of the glutamate receptor is depleted preferentially in HD and in a single case of a 32-year-old woman with presymp-

tomatic HD. In the latter, no morphological changes were identified on routine neuropathological analysis, but abnormalities of Enk-immunoreactive fibers projecting to the external globus pallidus and Sub P–immunoreactive fibers projecting to the substantia nigra were readily demonstrated.

Selective loss of the medium-sized striatal neurons and sparing of the interneurons may also have consequences for the expression of the two subtypes of dopamine receptor. The D_1 subtype is lost to a far greater extent in HD than the D_2 subtype, suggesting that dopamine causes choreiform involuntary movements, in part by activating the D_2 receptor (Fig. 9). Thus, drugs that block the D_2 receptor (phenothiazines and butyrophenones)

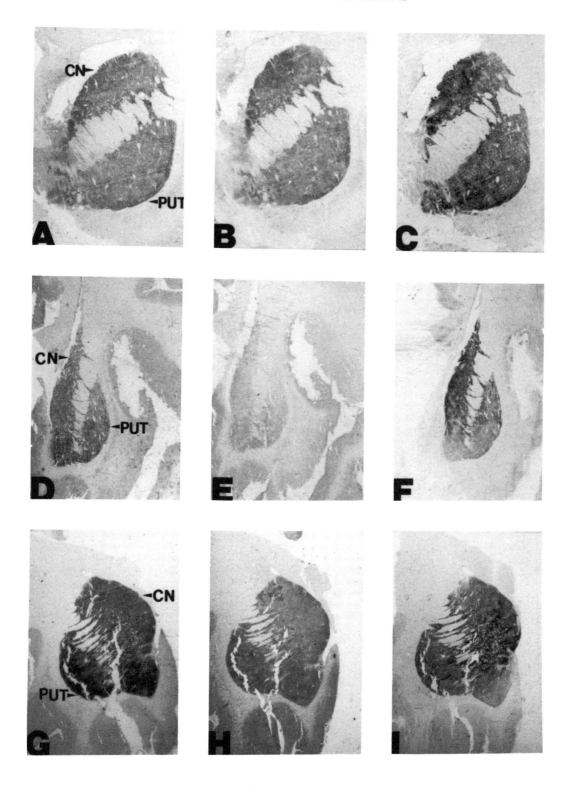

(see Chapter 18) can suppress the movements in some patients in the early and middle phases of the disease. Numerous drugs have been used to treat HD according to the prevailing knowledge of deficient or unbalanced neurotransmitters in the HD brain, but none has proved to have a sustained favorable effect on the symptoms or the rate of progression of the disease.

Genetic studies have established the specific location of the gene responsible for this disease on chromosome 4. Elucidation of the genetic basis of HD moved forward in the early 1980s, when James Gusella and his colleagues at Massachusetts General Hospital identified on the short arm of chromosome 4 a restriction fragment length polymorphism that was linked to the Huntington gene (see Chapter 16). Subsequent mapping efforts have determined the exact location of the gene on chromosome 4. They have recently identified the HD gene which involves an unstable DNA segment. The goal is to find and clone the gene so that the abnormal or missing gene product can be identified. This "positional cloning" approach might lead to effective therapy if the deficient gene product can be replaced or manipulated to ameliorate its destructive impact on striatal neurons.

SUMMARY

Neuronal degeneration occurs in selected regions of the brain and spinal cord to produce a variety of progressive neurological disorders. PD, AD, and HD have fundamentally different clinical patterns, divergent sites of neuropathology, and distinctive deficits in chemical neurotransmission. But these disorders are also tied together by their similarities: each is characterized by cognitive and motor impairments; each has prominent subcortical pathology and secondary distal pathway degeneration; each is associated with a variety of depleted neurotransmitters but with considerable overlap among them; each has a pathogenesis related in varying proportions to abnormal genes and the aging process.

PD is characterized by severe loss of dopamine-producing pigmented neurons in the midbrain (substantia nigra) and moderate loss of norepinephrine- and serotonin-containing neurons in the pons (locus coeruleus, raphe). Parkinsonian patients have the classic signs of rest tremor, rigidity, bradykinesia, cognitive dysfunction, and postural instability, usually starting after age 55. Treatments developed for this disorder (levodopa or direct dopamine agonists) were derived from animal models. Postsynaptic changes in receptor expression may contribute to the success of dopaminergic agents to reverse the symptoms of PD.

AD, the most age-related of the three disorders, affects neurons of basal nuclei in the diencephalon and of the hippocampus in the temporal lobe. ACh is the principal depleted neurotransmitter, but the monoamines and glutamate are also affected. The histopathological signature is the neurofibrillary degeneration (SPs and NFTs) of neurons throughout the brain, but mainly in the hippocampus. Alzheimer patients are primarily

FIG. 9. Photomicrographs of the expression of dopamine receptors and dopamine terminals in the striatum of a normal (**A, B, C**), Huntington's disease (**D, E, F**), and schizophrenic (**G, H, I**) case. Tissue sections have been labeled with radioligands that label D_2 receptors (A, D, G), D_1 receptors (B, E, H), or dopamine terminals (C, F, I) and exposed to film. The resulting images provide a detailed anatomic map of the distribution of these components of the dopamine synapse with higher numbers of sites showing up as dark gray. In Huntington's disease there is pronounced cell loss from the dorsal caudate nucleus (CN) and dorsal putamen (PUT), resulting in a "shrunken" appearance. The cell loss is selective so that neurons expressing D_1 receptors (compare E with B) are lost to a further extent than those expressing D_2 receptors (compare D with A). Dopamine input (compare F with C) is relatively normal. The schizophrenic case is shown for comparison. From Joyce JN, Lexow N, Bird E, Winokur A. Organization of dopamine D_1 and D_2 receptors in human striatum: receptor autoradiographic studies in Huntington's disease and schizophrenia. *Synapse* 1988;2:546–557.

demented; subtle parkinsonian and postural signs appear late in the course of the disease. Treatment of this disorder with agents that increase levels of ACh has not been successful. Consequently, research directed at elucidating the potential contribution of postsynaptically located receptors is proceeding.

HD is an inherited disease of striatal neurons that initially affects its victims at any time from youth to old age, producing dementia and choreiform involuntary movements. The abnormal gene causing HD has been localized to the short arm of chromosome 4. In contrast to either PD or AD, there is no significant reduction in the monoamine input to the striatum or cortex. The contribution of the selective loss of morphologically distinct neurons and NMDA receptors to the clinical manifestations of the disorder is being probed. The loss of neurons in the striatum leads to early selective reduction in one striatal efferent pathway that expresses the D_1 receptor. The imbalance in striatal output caused by the loss of one pathway and the preservation of other pathways, whose cell bodies may express the D_2 receptor, contributes to the choreiform movements.

BIBLIOGRAPHY

Original Articles

Ehringer H, Hornkiewicz O. Verteilung von Noradrenalin und Dopamin (3-hydroxytryptamie) in Gehirn des Menschen und ihr Verhalten bei Erkrankungen des extrapyramidalen Systems. *Klin Wochen* 1960; 38:1236–1239.

Gaspar P, Duyckaerts C, Alvarez C, Javoy-Agid F, Berger B. Alterations of dopaminergic and noradrenergic innervations in motor cortex in Parkinson's disease. *Ann Neurol* 1991;30:365–374.

Gerfen CR, Engber TM, Mahan LC, Susel Z, Chase TN, Monsma FJ Jr, et al. D_1 and D_2 dopamine receptor-regulated gene expression of striatonigral and striatopallidal neurons. *Science* 1990;250:1429–1432.

Gibb WR, Mountjoy CQ, Mann DM, Lees AJ. A pathological study of the association between Lewy body disease and Alzheimer's disease. *J Neurol Neurosurg Psychiatry* 1989;52:701–708.

Goldman JE, Yen S-H. Cytoskeletal protein abnormalities in neurodegenerative diseases. *Ann Neurol* 1986;19:209–223.

Hurtig H, Joyce JN, Sladek JR Jr, Trojanowski JQ. Postmortem analysis of adrenal-medulla-to-caudate autograft in a patient with Parkinson's disease. *Ann Neurol* 1989;25:607–614.

Joyce JN, Hurtig H. Differential regulation of striatal dopamine D1 and D2 receptor systems in Parkinson's disease and effects of adrenal medullary transplant. *Progr Brain Res* 1990;82:699–706.

Joyce JN, Lexow N, Bird E, Winokur A. Organization of dopamine D1 and D2 receptors in human striatum: receptor autoradiographic studies in Huntington's disease and schizophrenia. *Synapse* 1988;2:546–557.

Langston JW, Ballard P, Tetrud JW, Irwin I. Chronic parkinsonism in humans due to a product of meperidine-analog synthesis. *Science* 1983;219: 979–980.

Schmidt ML, Lee VM-Y, Trojanowski JQ. Relative abundance of tau and neurofilament epitopes in hippocampal neurofibrillary tangles. *Am J Pathol* 1990;136:1069–1075.

Tomlinson BE, Blessed G, Roth M. Observations on the brains of demented old people. *J Neurol Sci* 1970;11:205–242.

Van Hoesen GW, Hyman BT, Damasio AR. Entorhinal cortex pathology in Alzheimer's disease. *Hippocampus* 1991;1:1–8.

Vonsattel J-P, Myers RH, Stevens TJ, Ferrante RJ, Bird ED, Richardson EP Jr. Neuropathological classification of Huntington's disease. *J Neuropathol Exp Neurol* 1985;44:559–577.

Whitehouse PJ, Price DL, Struble RG, Clark AW, Coyle JT, DeLong MR. Alzheimer's disease and senile dementia: loss of neurons in the basal forebrain. *Science* 1982;215:1237–1239.

Young AB, Greenamyre JT, Hollingsworth Z, Albin R, D'Amato C, Shoulson I, et al. NMDA receptor losses in putamen from patients with Huntington's disease. *Science* 1988;241:981–983.

Books and Reviews

Agid Y, Javoy-Agid F, Ruberg M. Biochemistry of neurotransmitters in PD. In: Marsden CD, Fahn S, eds. *Movement disorders.* Vol. 2. London: Butterworth; 1981:166–230.

Chui HC. Dementia: a review emphasizing clinicopathologic correlation and brain–behavior relationships. *Arch Neurol* 1989;46:806–814.

Henderson VW, Finch CE. The neurobiology of Alzheimer's disease. *J Neurosurg* 1989;70:335–353.

Kopin IJ. Neurotransmitters and disorders of the basal ganglia. In: Siegel GJ, Agranoff BW, Albers RW, Molinoff PB, eds. *Basic neurochemistry,* 5th ed. New York: Raven Press; 1994 (in press).

Lee VM-Y. Unraveling the paired helical filaments of Alzheimer's disease. *J NIH Res* 1991;3:52–54.

Penney JB Jr, Young AB, Shoulson I, Starosta-Rubenstein S, Snodgrass SR, Sanchez-Ramos J, et al. Huntington's disease in Venezuela; 7 years of follow-up on symptomatic and asymptomatic individuals. *Mov Disord* 1990;5:93–99.

Selkoe DJ. Biochemistry of altered brain proteins in AD. *Annu Rev Neurosci* 1989;12:463–490.

Selkoe DJ. Biochemistry of Alzheimer's disease. In: Siegel GJ, Agranoff BW, Albers RW, Molinoff PB, eds. *Basic neurochemistry,* 5th ed. New York: Raven Press; 1994 (in press).

Subject Index

Note: Page numbers in *italics* refer to illustrations; page numbers followed by t refer to figures